BUILDING
SCHOOLS
MAKING
DOCTORS

UNIVERSITY *of* PITTSBURGH PRESS

BUILDING
SCHOOLS
MAKING
DOCTORS

KATHERINE L. CARROLL

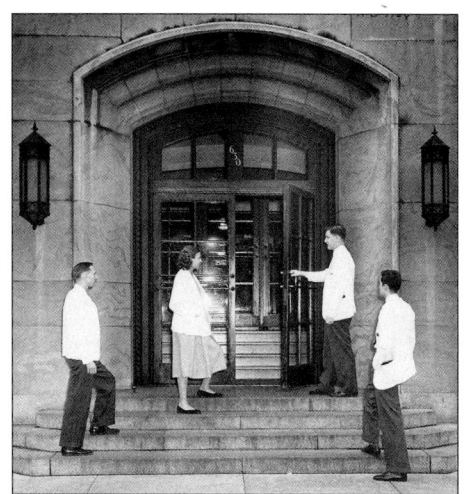

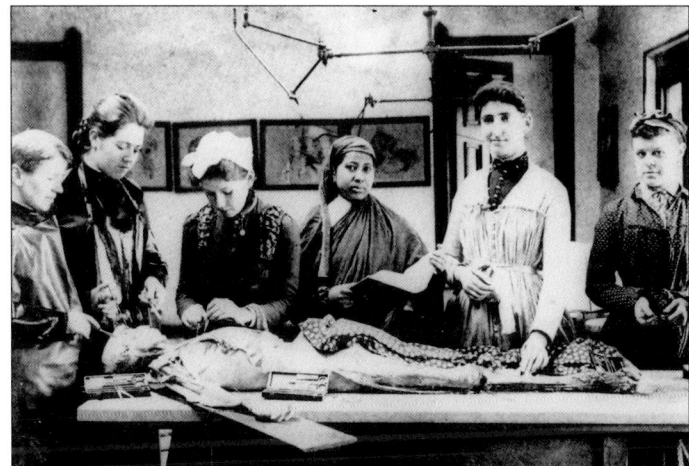

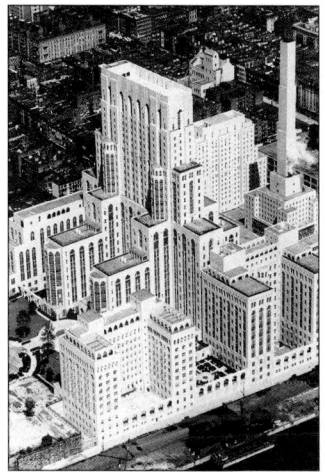

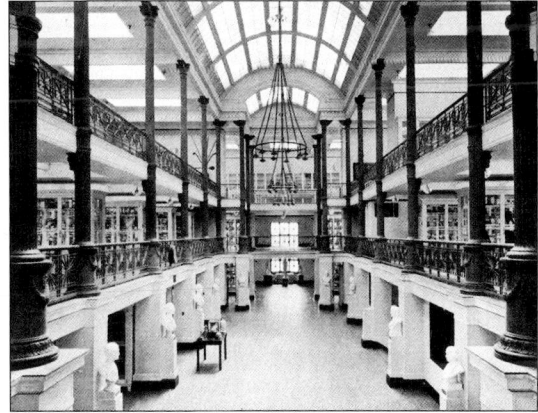

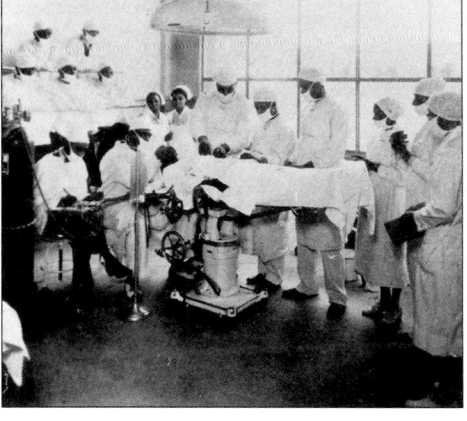

ARCHITECTURE *and the* MODERN AMERICAN PHYSICIAN

Graham Foundation

This publication has been supported by a grant from the
Graham Foundation for Advanced Studies in the Fine Arts

Published by the University of Pittsburgh Press, Pittsburgh, Pa., 15260
Copyright © 2022, University of Pittsburgh Press

Manufactured in the United States of America
Printed on acid-free paper
10 9 8 7 6 5 4 3 2 1

Cataloging-in-Publication data is available from the Library of Congress

ISBN 13: 978-0-8229-4705-9
ISBN 10: 0-8229-4705-6

Cover photographs (*from top left and then left to right*): Harvard Medical School, 1906,
Shepley, Rutan, and Coolidge, architects, plan, first floors, "Harvard University Medical
School, Original Medical School Buildings, Boston, MA, #0148, 1906" files, courtesy
of the Archives of Shepley Bulfinch Richardson and Abbott, Boston, Massachusetts;
College of Physicians and Surgeons, Columbia-Presbyterian Medical Center, 1928, James
Gamble Rogers, architect, entrance, photograph ca. 1949, Folder 2, Box 155, Historical
Photograph Collection, University Archives, Rare Book and Manuscript Library,
Columbia University Libraries; Woman's Medical College of Pennsylvania students at
dissecting table, ca. 1890, Photograph P-4870, WMCP Photograph Collection, Legacy
Center, Drexel University College of Medicine; New York Hospital–Cornell Medical
College, 1932, Coolidge, Shepley, Bulfinch, and Abbott, architects, Aerial Explorations,
Inc., photographer, courtesy of the Archives of Shepley Bulfinch Richardson and Abbott,
Boston, Massachusetts; Harvard Medical School, 1906, Shepley, Rutan, and Coolidge,
architects, Warren Anatomical Museum, Building A, William F. Whitney, *The Warren
Anatomical Museum of the Harvard Medical School and the Arrangement of Its Collection* (n.p.,
1911), frontispiece; senior medical and nursing students receive instruction in surgery,
Meharry Medical College, ca. 1931, [Marvin Willard?] Wiles, photographer, Photograph
12, Folder 2, Box 1, Historical Photographs 1800s Collection, Meharry Medical College
Library and Archives.

Cover design: Alex Wolfe

To Patrick, Luke, Beth, and Ian

CONTENTS

ACKNOWLEDGMENTS

IT IS A JOY TO ACKNOWLEDGE MANY OF THE PEOPLE WHOSE HARD work made possible researching and writing this book. Numerous archivists and librarians went far beyond reasonable expectations, especially in the final phases of this project, which occurred in the early months of the COVID-19 pandemic. I appreciated their professionalism and good cheer in such a difficult time. In particular, I recognize Abigail Cahill, Jack Eckert, Andy Harrison, Matt Herbison, Jessica Murphy, Steve Novak, Sandra Parham, Jesse Peters, Rob Roche, Tom Rosenbaum, John Schleicher, Mary Teloh, Jim Thweat, and Sonja Woods. Thanks to Walker Gilmore and George Kelly, I twice had the good fortune of receiving access to architectural plans just as I was giving up hope of locating them. Doris Bartuska, Robert Collins, Mary Coté, George Kelly, Bill Leslie, Steven Peitzman, and Cyril Stewart kindly met with me during my travels and shared their expertise. In the process of tracking down images and permissions, I benefited from the generosity of Annmarie Adams, Martha Holoubek Fitzgerald, and Maureen Meister. Several people have read part or all of the manuscript in various stages. I cannot adequately thank Keith Morgan, who participated in this project from the very beginning and whose training continues to shape my thinking on a daily basis. He, along with Jessica Sewell, read an early draft in its entirety and gave extensive feedback. William Moore and Patricia Hills also read an early draft, as did Carla Yanni, who has provided invaluable mentorship over many years. As the project neared completion, Jeanne Kisacky read the introduction and chapter 5. The reviewers for the University of Pittsburgh Press shared probing and useful comments. It was a pleasure working with Abby Collier and the rest of the talented team at the University of Pittsburgh Press.

I gratefully recognize the organizations that supported this project. The Graham Foundation for Advanced Studies in the Fine Arts provided a publication grant. Earlier assistance came from the Henry Luce Foundation/American Council of Learned Societies, the Francis

A. Countway Library of Medicine, the Rockefeller Archive Center, and the Pittsburgh Foundation.

I extend heartfelt thanks to my family and friends, particularly those who housed me on my many research trips, as well as Liz Chase, Kristin Hunter-Thomson, Kristen Kuhn, Melissa Leddy, Danielle Merzatta, Liz Mygatt, Kate Remillard, and Carla Steckman. Sam Stewart provided extraordinary child care. I have been buoyed by a caring circle of siblings—Megan Sabel, Thomas Zimmerman, and Frank Zimmerman, as well as their partners—along with Janet and the late Sey Zimmerman. My parents, Roberta Lynch Carroll and Jim Carroll, have done so much for me, not the least sharing with me their love of buildings. This project has spanned my children's earliest years. Luke, Beth, and Ian's enthusiasm for "mommy's book" and their excitement to see it (and their names!) in print has encouraged me more than they could know. I offer my deepest gratitude to Patrick Zimmerman, whose support has never wavered.

BUILDING
SCHOOLS
MAKING
DOCTORS

INTRODUCTION

IN THE LATE NINETEENTH CENTURY, AMERICAN MEDICAL EDUCATORS working to transform medicine into a scientific and prestigious profession recognized the role of architecture in achieving their goals. The schools they had occupied for most of the nineteenth century, some as simple as rented rooms over the local dry goods store, could not accommodate the education demanded by modern science. Reformed medical training necessitated numerous and varied laboratories, rooms for embalming and storing cadavers, housing for animals, libraries, and lecture halls, in addition to clinic and hospital access. G. Canby Robinson, dean of Vanderbilt University School of Medicine, explained in 1923 that architecture and pedagogy were so intimately intertwined that one could not necessarily ascertain which came first: "It is not always easy to determine whether the educational principles have dominated the types and arrangements of buildings, or whether the educational principles have been dominated by the facilities in which medical education is of necessity conducted." Robinson understood, however, that schools increasingly had the "opportunity . . . to construct new plants or thoroughly remodel old ones along lines which express the modern American conception of medical education."[1] In its investigation of medical colleges erected between 1893 and 1940, *Building Schools, Making Doctors* argues that the schools did more than promote innovative instruction; they also helped to codify medical science and alter physicians' professional identity.

Medical educators recognized that the public had little confidence in physicians in the late nineteenth century, and they did not believe that elevating educational standards was enough to change physicians' reputation. The faculty strove to teach their pupils the demeanor they

envisioned for elite physicians, and they made the educational environment an active participant in this agenda. Schools contributed to the formation of a shared professional consciousness among the new physician
class at the same time that they reinforced a hierarchy among doctors that
privileged white men over white women, Black women, and Black men.
Educators also used the buildings to inform the community about the
shifting status of physicians. Medical school leadership courted the public
throughout the construction effort and attempted to declare in brick and
stone the improved education and the rising social position of doctors.

Progressive pedagogical ideas and ambition for the profession compelled medical faculties and university presidents to orchestrate a wave of
construction in the late nineteenth and early twentieth centuries. Medical
colleges around the country rebuilt, substantially renovated, and expanded
their buildings. This massive effort required medical school and university
leaders to raise enormous sums of money. According to one estimate, medical colleges spent approximately $100 million on facilities and equipment
between 1900 and 1925.[2] By 1940, this figure had increased substantially.
Philanthropic foundations, state legislatures, and individual donors provided the bulk of the financial resources. Duke University's first president,
William P. Few, described the relationship between patron and institution
bluntly: "When you go out to get $40 million from a man, you will find
that he has some ideas of his own."[3] Indeed, patrons of medical education
developed a dialectical relationship with the medical school administrators
and university presidents working to secure funds to transform their colleges, and each group brought its own interests to the table.[4] Architecture
formed one part of the give and take. With a nod to that reality, this book
also demonstrates the impact of patronage—specifically that of John D.
Rockefeller's General Education Board—on medical school design.

Far from forgotten historical relics, the medical schools constructed in
the early twentieth century remain largely in use today. Often they form
only one section of a sprawling group of medical facilities and have endured
nearly continuous renovations (fig. I.1). The first dean of Duke University
School of Medicine and Hospital affirmed, "The only rooms in the Duke
Medical Center which now serve their original purposes are the toilets
which are too solid to move. I had nine different offices between 1927 and
1960."[5] For the last one hundred years, medical school administrators have
overseen one remodel after another and wrestled with the legacy of these
buildings—including the science, pedagogy, and professional character
they promote. In the end, the questions that frame today's construction
efforts mirror those that consumed faculties and architects in the early
twentieth century. Educators and architects then and now ask that the

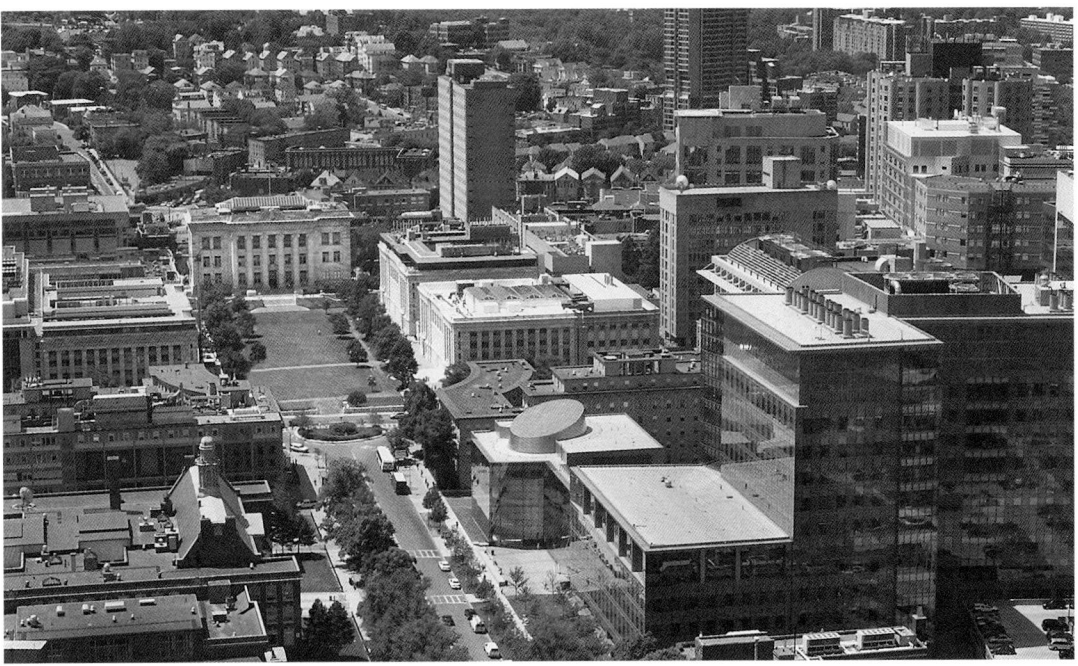

I.1.   Longwood Medical Area, 2007. Shepley, Rutan, and Coolidge's 1906 quadrangle for Harvard Medical
         School, at left, now anchors a neighborhood of medical institutions.

buildings encourage the latest medical science and pedagogy and help
shape the professional culture of the next generation of American physicians. Organized thematically, *Building Schools, Making Doctors* explains
how medical educators and architects first answered these questions.

    To date, medical historians who have examined the reform of Amer-
ican medical education and the changing status of physicians have not
given architecture sustained attention.[6] At the same time, architectural
historians, most recently Annmarie Adams, Jeanne Kisacky, and Carla
Yanni, have focused almost exclusively on medical spaces for patient
care rather than facilities for training.[7] By investigating the architecture
of medical schools, this book fills the gap and reinforces the ability of
architecture to highlight elements of medical history not easily plumbed
through the written record.[8] For example, an architectural reading of
medical schools reveals a previously unrecognized strategy—medical
college construction—by which physicians cultivated their cultural
authority in the late nineteenth and early twentieth centuries. It also
uncovers the professional hierarchies built into the educational structures
and expands our understanding of when and how professional identities
develop. Additionally, educators at the turn of the twentieth century
believed that medical schools supported specific forms of education and

science. An architectural analysis examines how such promotion took place and what ideas were being disseminated.

This last line of investigation also contributes to current discussions of how knowledge, and specifically science, is produced. In this and other ways, my work intersects with science and technology studies, particularly the diverse group of scholars, including Stuart W. Leslie, Thomas Gieryn, and Thomas Schlich, who explore the relationship between architecture and science through the lens of the laboratory. These scholars encourage my examination of professional culture, research agendas, architecture as a public face for science, the changing relationship between scientific practice and architecture, and the interactions between architects, scientists (medical educators), and donors.[9]

Furthermore, my research adds to the growing body of scholarship on the architecture of American schools. For a number of years, Helen Lefkowitz Horowitz's book on women's colleges and Paul Venable Turner's study of the collegiate campus, both first published in 1984, stood out for their focus on educational spaces and the college environment in particular.[10] Recently, however, architectural historians have begun to analyze educational buildings more frequently. These studies have considered educational structures ranging from elementary schools to universities. At the college level, Carla Yanni, Margaret M. Grubiak, and Clare Robinson have moved beyond purely educational buildings to explore dormitories, chapels, and student unions.[11] What architectural historians have not done is investigate facilities for graduate and professional training. This book offers the first comprehensive study of the architecture of an American professional school.

Whether writing about clinical spaces or school buildings, some architectural historians have embraced social history and material culture studies. These scholars, such as Annmarie Adams and Carla Yanni, position buildings within broad social and cultural dialogues at the same time that they examine both the design of the facilities and the objects within their walls.[12] I utilize this method as well. My research blends analyses of design with investigations of portraits, furniture, and uniforms as it positions early twentieth-century medical schools within conversations about pedagogy, science, professional identity, race, gender, and philanthropy.

In addition, this study rests heavily on the idea that the architecture of medical schools not only responded to changes in pedagogy, science, and professional character but also actively contributed to these shifts. When historians of medicine mention architecture, they typically assume that buildings passively follow pedagogical and scientific developments.[13] Although new pedagogical ideas often require a redesign of educational space, the historical record left by medical educators and architects in the early twentieth century complicates this interpretation. They believed that the schools themselves would alter students' conceptions of science, the types of practitioners they became, and their professional demeanor. Architectural historian Jeanne Kisacky has taken an analogous approach in her examination of American hospitals. Kisacky understands hospital design "as both a reflection of its sociocultural milieu and a shape-giving force on its inhabitants."[14] Similarly, I trace the intentions behind medical school design and the impact of the buildings on their occupants and the nonmedical community.

Transformations in Medical Education and Medical School Design, 1850–1900

In the 1860s, many American doctors received their medical education in a proprietary school. Initially developed as a supplement to the colonial era's apprenticeship system, the proprietary school had replaced the apprenticeship as the primary mode of American medical training by the middle of the nineteenth century. Unlike later medical schools, proprietary schools did not regularly maintain relationships with hospitals and universities, and when affiliations did occur, they resulted in limited clinical access and a nominal position within the university. Small groups, frequently numbering six to eight individuals, composed a faculty. The profits generated from student fees constituted the faculty's income. Without rigorous state licensing or other regulatory practices in place, the predominantly commercial enterprises encouraged lax admissions standards, big classes, and weak academic programs.[15]

Mid-nineteenth-century medical education centered on lectures delivered during a four-month term during the winter. The entire student body spent six to eight hours a day receiving instruction in a large amphitheater. Reprieve from this didactic method came from textbook readings and the occasional recitation. Schools usually provided seven courses: physiology and pathology; anatomy; materia medica, therapeutics, and pharmacy; chemistry along with medical jurisprudence; principles and practice of surgery; theory and practice of medicine; and diseases of women and children, along with obstetrics. Practical rather than scientific topics remained the focus. Students repeated the same course of lectures twice and earned their degree after passing perfunctory oral examinations. With the exception of dissection at some of the stronger schools, no hands-on laboratory work occurred. Similarly, students typically received no direct contact with patients. A handful of schools provided lectures

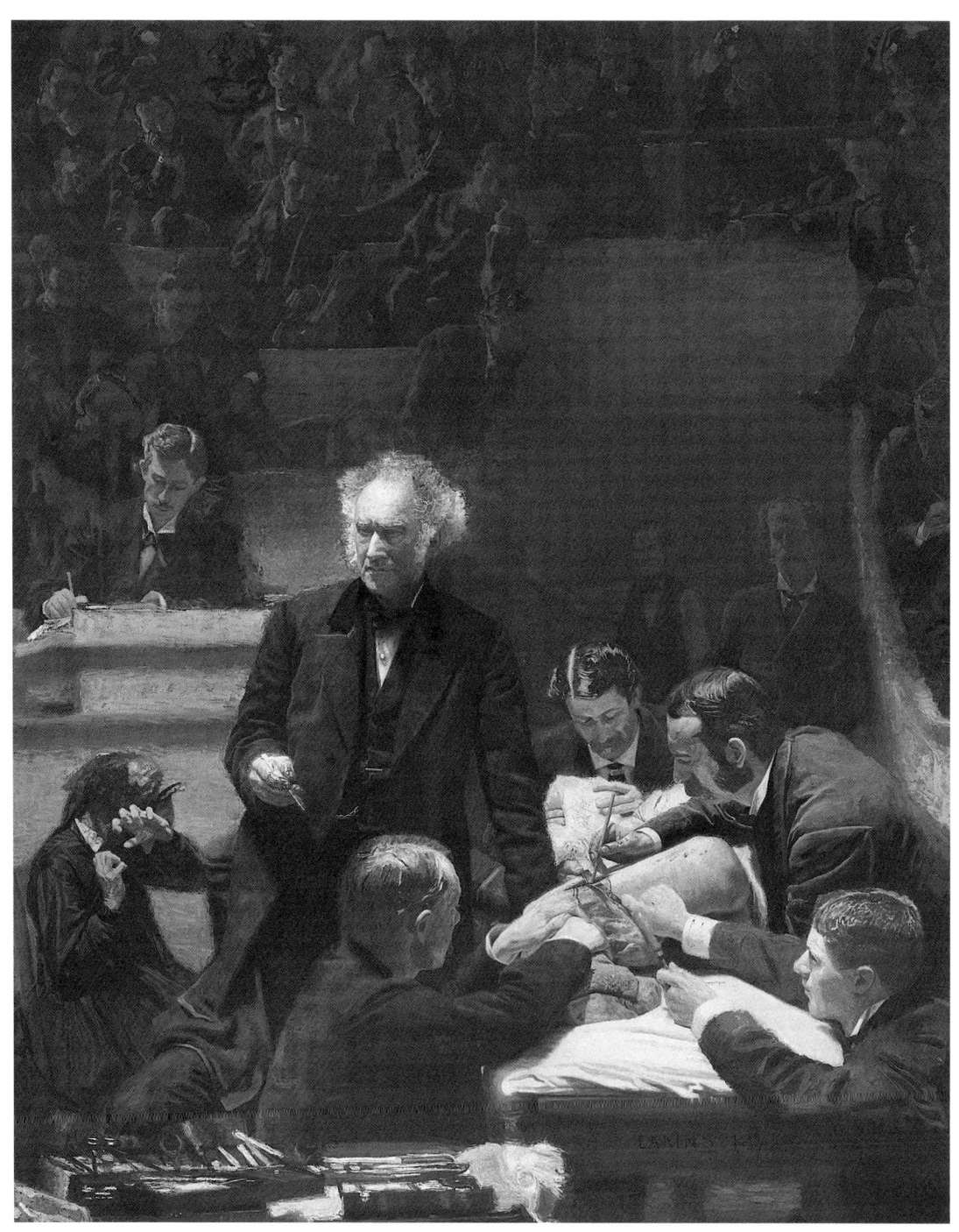

I.2.   Thomas Eakins, *Portrait of Dr. Samuel D. Gross* (*The Gross Clinic*), 1875. Oil on canvas, 96 by 78 inches.

in a hospital amphitheater or the occasional ward tour, but nowhere did hospital training compose a significant portion of the curriculum. The program did not even require that students demonstrate the ability to read and write. In fact, few had college experience, and those who did tended to represent the weaker college students, the superior students having chosen to pursue the more prominent professions of teaching, law, or the clergy.[16]

Realist painter Thomas Eakins's famous surgical scenes, *The Gross Clinic* (1875) and *The Agnew Clinic* (1889), depict the nineteenth-century surgical amphitheater. The surgical amphitheater, also called the operating theater, placed the patient and attending physician(s) at the center with observers in tiers of seats (fig. I.2). Kisacky explains that American hospitals often contained operating theaters, which enabled physicians to move surgeries out of the ward, by the early nineteenth century. The operating theater's popularity peaked in the United States from approximately 1860 to the middle of the 1880s.[17] Although the paintings are different in significant ways, not the least of which due to the absence (*The Gross Clinic*) and presence (*The Agnew Clinic*) of aseptic procedures, the two canvases present similar images of medical education. In both, celebrated Philadelphia surgeons step away from the patient to lecture students and other attendees, including the artist, who passively watch the surgery from the operating theater's steeply stacked seats. As Kisacky notes, medical students seated in a theater had to content themselves with an indistinct view of the patient.[18] One student later recalled the limited visibility for observers in the amphitheater: "It really made no difference what ailed the patient; the professor could use him as text for almost any disease and we would be none the wiser."[19]

More than portraying didactic clinical training, *The Gross Clinic* and *The Agnew Clinic* present physicians as exclusively white and male. White and Black women and Black men became physicians in this period, but white men dominated the profession. In *The Gross Clinic*, Eakins depicts Samuel D. Gross, professor of surgery at Jefferson Medical College, operating in Jefferson Hospital's six-hundred-seat amphitheater.[20] Jefferson Medical College did not graduate an African American male student until 1901. The first white woman graduated from the school in 1965 and the first Black woman in 1971. In *The Gross Clinic*, only the seated woman who covers her face in horror provides a female counterpoint to the men in the room. She is typically identified as the patient's family member, often the mother.[21] *The Agnew Clinic*, completed in 1889, shows an operation by D. Hayes Agnew, the John Rhea Barton Professor of Surgery at the University of Pennsylvania, and again no women appear as medical students or physicians. As art and architectural historian Margaret Supplee Smith

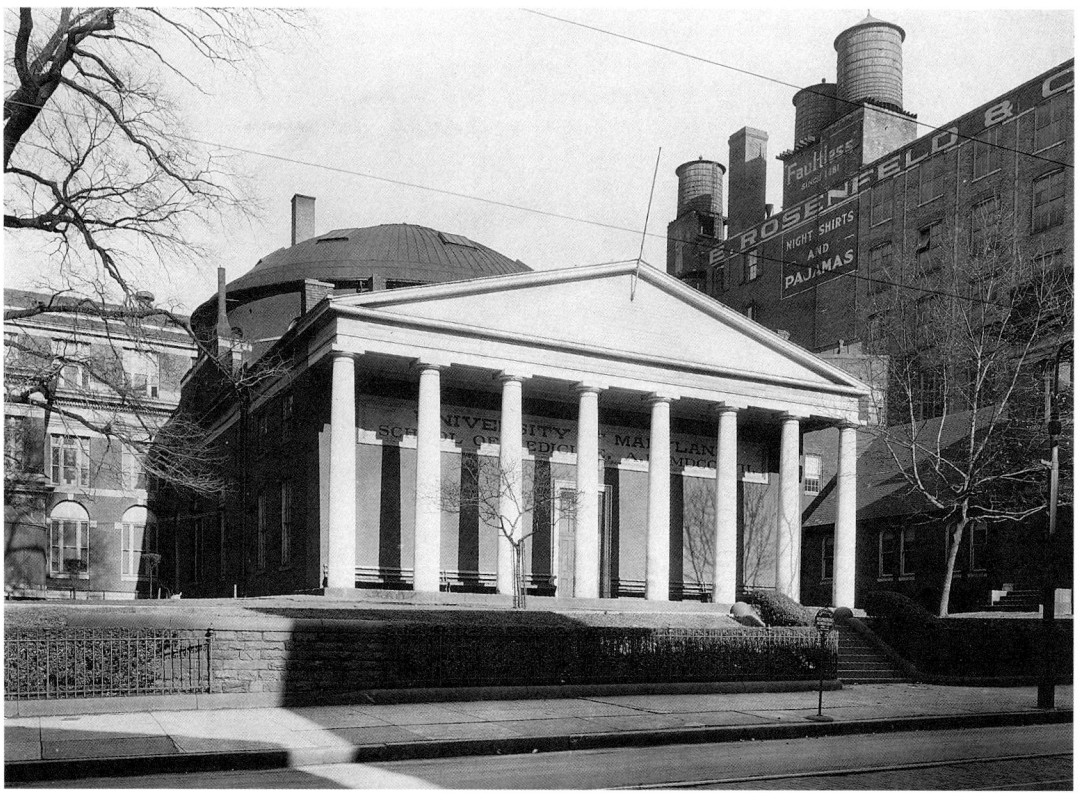

I.3.   College of Medicine of Maryland, 1812, Robert Cary Long Sr. [?], architect. Photograph ca. 1925.

describes, Agnew did not support the medical education of women. When Pennsylvania Hospital began formally admitting female students from Woman's Medical College of Pennsylvania in 1872, Agnew resigned his position. Agnew returned after six years, but in *The Agnew Clinic* Eakins paints the operating theater as Agnew preferred it; the only women are the patient and the nurse, a medical role Agnew did endorse for women.[22]

At midcentury, the primacy of the lecture shaped not only any hospital instruction that took place but also training in the medical school, where the architectural requirements were as limited as the educational program.[23] A school might provide its students with a library, museum, or laboratory, but all that a faculty had to have to run a school was a room in which to give lectures. Shortly after its founding, Syracuse University's College of Physicians and Surgeons rented rooms in the city's Clinton block from 1872 to 1875 and then spent the next twenty-one years in a renovated carriage factory.[24] When Howard University opened its medical program in 1868, it utilized makeshift arrangements as well. Howard's medical school occupied a former dance hall that it shared

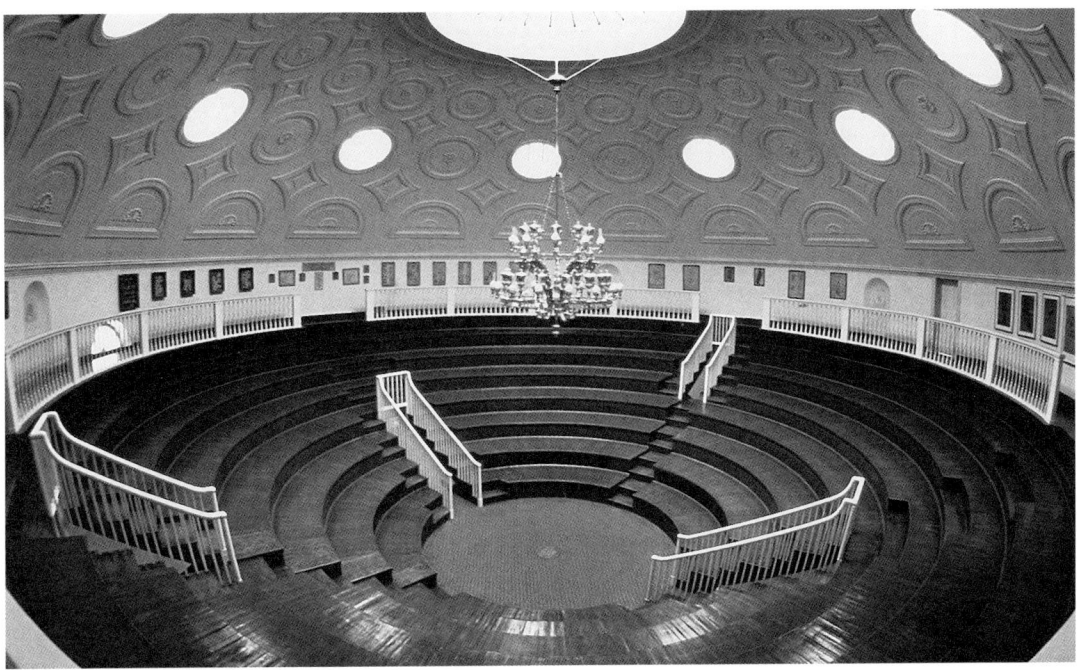

I.4.   College of Medicine of Maryland, 1812, Robert Cary Long Sr. [?], architect, anatomical theater.
         Photograph 1980s.

with other university departments, although it relocated the dissection course to a nearby shed when a professor living with his family in the repurposed dance hall complained.[25] At Howard, the medical school's accommodations improved quickly, however; the following year it moved into a purpose-built structure. Schools with the financial resources and the desire to create a discrete educational site—along with a unique physical identity—had long constructed purpose-built facilities.

These buildings confirm that didactic rather than experiential learning was the principal pedagogical mode. In 1812, the College of Medicine of Maryland moved into a purpose-built structure likely designed by architect Robert Cary Long Sr. (fig. I.3). Among the earliest purpose-built facilities for medical education in the nation, it primarily consisted of a pair of stacked auditoriums, including the country's fourth anatomical theater, following those at the Pennsylvania Hospital (1796), University of Pennsylvania (1806), and Dartmouth College (1811). In keeping with contemporary anatomical theaters in the United States and in Europe, where the building type dated back centuries, the College of Medicine of Maryland utilized an amphitheater design; tiers of benches encircled the room and provided students with the opportunity to observe dissections taking place in the center (fig. I.4). Medical historians generally agree that the anatomical theater served as the direct predecessor of the operating theater. Immense in size, Maryland's anatomical theater reportedly accommodated twelve hundred persons. Not all students sat, however. Some stood, leaning against the upper balustrade, where their carved graffiti left a silent testimony to the tedious lectures attended twice for the medical degree. In the building's lower auditorium, designated for chemistry, three sides of the hall offered tiers of seating for a slightly more modest one thousand pupils, with instruction taking place along the fourth wall. The remainder of the building contained a cramped area for anatomical work, a classroom, and a library.[26]

Beginning in the 1870s, the new system of American medical education began to develop, and existing medical school buildings quickly became obsolete. By 1891, John Shaw Billings, prominent physician and medical advisor for the design of Johns Hopkins Hospital, could write with confidence, "The days have long gone by when one or two amphitheaters or lecture-rooms and a small museum were all the outfit required for medical teaching."[27]

The reform of American medical education depended heavily on students' and physicians' experiences in Germany. As students and physicians sought ways to supplement their preparation for practice, one option had long been to study abroad, although the favored destination changed over time. In the eighteenth century, American physicians primarily traveled to Edinburgh. In the first part of the nineteenth century, their preference shifted to Paris, and in the second half of the nineteenth century, they set their course for Germany, the international leader in medicine at that time. Between 1870 and 1914, some fifteen thousand American physicians studied in Germany or at German-speaking universities in Switzerland or Austria. Standard advice encouraged prospective students to master the German language before leaving the United States, but in cities with many English-speaking faculty, such as Vienna, courses in the clinical subjects were frequently taught in English. The majority of American physicians pursued clinical instruction and returned home with training in one of the recently established clinical specialties, such as surgery, dermatology, and obstetrics. A smaller number undertook research in the German laboratories that focused on the basic biological sciences, in fields such as anatomy, physiology, pathology, and bacteriology. Members of this latter group joined the faculties of the American medical schools that would pioneer the transformation in medical education, including implementing German laboratory methods and founding active research programs.[28]

Fortunately for the reform-minded physicians, at the same time that they began promoting progressive methods of medical education, the

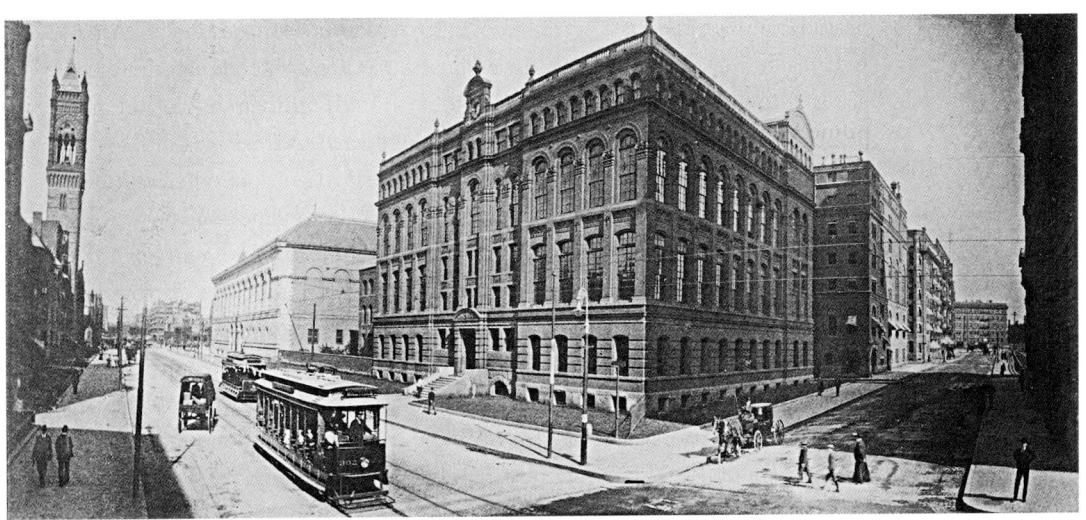

I.5.   Harvard Medical School, 1883, Ware and Van Brunt, architects.

modern American university was finding its footing. Medical educators discovered kindred spirits among the university leaders who advocated for their institutions of higher education as sites for investigation and the discovery of new knowledge. University medical schools, such as those of Harvard, Pennsylvania, and Michigan, started to teach the basic medical sciences, typically referred to in this period as the fundamental, laboratory, or preclinical sciences, and to adopt German laboratory methods in the classroom. As medical schools came under university control, they also improved their educational programs in other ways. They created graded schedules in which the curriculum became sequential rather than repetitive. Written examinations replaced oral assessments, admissions requirements became more stringent, and the program of study was lengthened. In 1893, Johns Hopkins Medical School inaugurated the program still largely in place today. It drew on both the German emphasis on laboratory experience and the British system of hands-on clinical instruction. The result was two years of laboratory work in the basic sciences followed by two years of bedside preparation, all within a university environment that encouraged original research.[29]

Medical training could not have been transformed, however, without the architecture that both responded to and promoted the innovative pedagogy. In 1871, Harvard Medical School began to reorganize its educational program, and in just over a decade the school had constructed a new facility. The school relocated in 1883 to Boylston Street in Boston, where it occupied a Romanesque revival building designed by Ware and

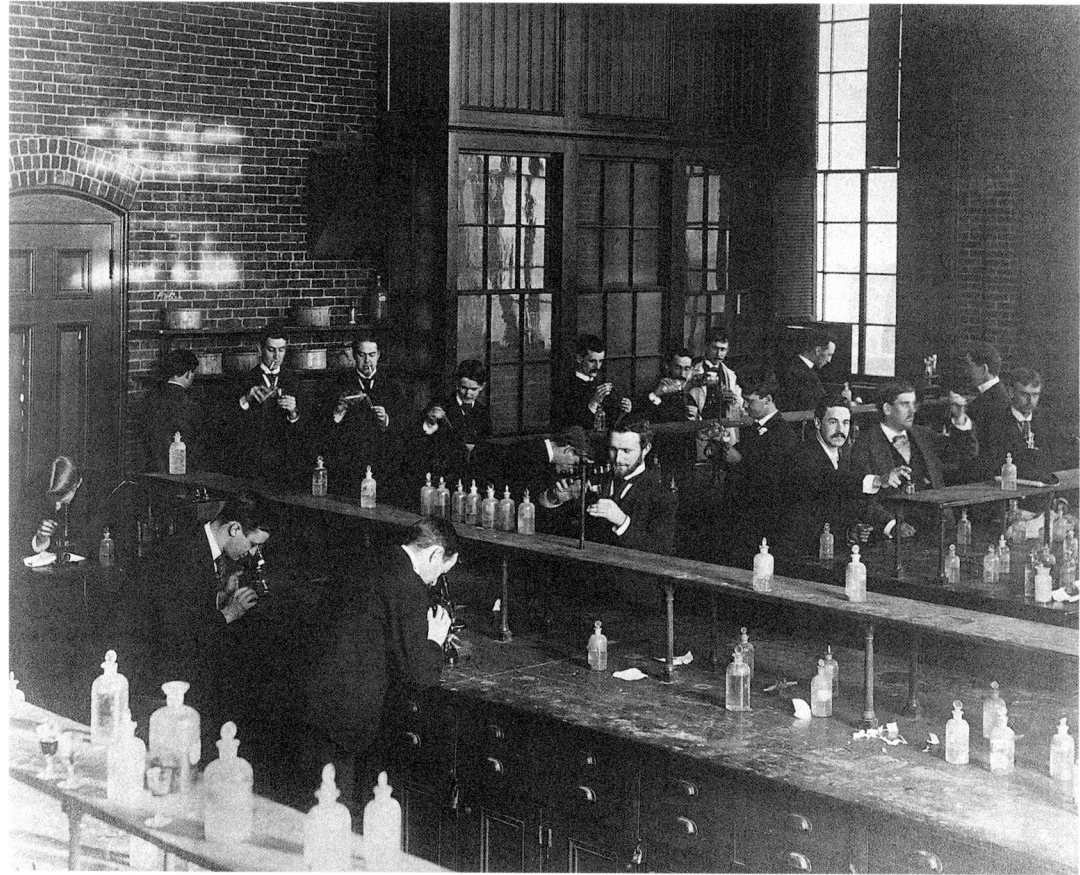

I.6.   Students in the chemistry laboratory of Harvard Medical School, ca. 1900.

Van Brunt and funded by gifts totaling nearly $300,000 (fig. I.5). With
resources for anatomy, physiology, chemistry, histology, and pathology,
the building offered more laboratory space than the school's previous
home (fig. I.6).[30] Contemporary reports described the building's essential role in the pedagogical shifts occurring at Harvard Medical School
and celebrated the carefully designed laboratories, lecture rooms, and
anatomical museum.[31] At the same time, the school's move from its location next to Massachusetts General Hospital among the tenements of
Boston's West End to the city's growing civic and educational center in
the exclusive Back Bay neighborhood gave the medical college greater
visibility within the city, particularly among its wealthiest residents. It
was a situation that the leadership hoped would inspire additional philanthropic support.[32] The building's prominent site and the coverage it
received in the popular and medical press also advertised the progressive
medical education pioneered at Harvard and elsewhere.[33]

Modern American medical education grew out of a conviction that experiential learning rather than didactic methods would create physicians fundamentally different from their medical forebears. In Europe, Germany reserved its famed laboratory training for advanced researchers and delayed major clinical instruction for the year after graduation, and Britain did not allow all students to assist with clinical work. By contrast, American educators insisted on significant laboratory and clinical experience for every medical student prior to graduation. When describing the redesigned system, Americans often focused on its educational rather than its research benefits.[34] A professor of anatomy at the University of Minnesota affirmed, "Never tell a student anything he can observe for himself; never draw a conclusion or solve a problem which he can be led to reason for himself; and never do anything for him that he can do for himself."[35] It may seem obvious that hands-on clinical preparation would benefit nascent practitioners, but it is perhaps more surprising that educators emphasized the importance of the laboratory both for aspiring clinicians and for future teachers and researchers. As Johns Hopkins anatomist Franklin P. Mall explained, "good habits in working, observing, and thinking" gained through laboratory opportunities benefited every student, irrespective of "whether his future career is in medicine, in laryngology, or in embryology."[36] In the end, reformers believed that not only a better physician but also an esteemed class of learned professionals, on par educationally with those in philosophy, law, and theology, would emerge from the improved program.[37]

As more medical colleges joined Harvard Medical School, the University of Michigan Medical School, and other pioneering institutions in constructing facilities on city streets and university campuses, the buildings proclaimed the remodeled pedagogy, the elevation of the profession, and the possibilities in American medicine. The architecture makes clear, however, that none of these ideas was straightforward. The structures themselves reveal debates about what conceptions of science would dominate, how much research would actually take place, and who would be included in this elite professional rank. These ideas shaped buildings' designs and, in turn, the daily lives of students and faculty for generations to come.

Scope and Content

Building Schools, Making Doctors focuses on the first fifty years of modern medical school construction. It starts in 1893, the year that Johns Hopkins Medical School opened and inaugurated the program of medical training still largely in place today. The terminus for this study is 1940. After World War II, a new period in the history of American medical education began when research programs rapidly expanded, an outgrowth of substantial federal funding not previously available.[38]

This book does not attempt to touch on every American medical school from the five decades addressed. It limits analysis to four-year regular (nonsectarian) programs located in a single city and leading to the degree of doctor of medicine (MD), rather than schools that offered only the first two years of medical instruction, that split their training between two cities, or that provided osteopathic, homeopathic, or eclectic medical education. *Building Schools, Making Doctors* does not examine the many medical schools that found themselves unable or unwilling to meet the increased standards and that subsequently closed. These schools did not typically construct facilities, and they had less of an impact on medical training in the years that followed. In addition, with the exception of Johns Hopkins Medical School, I focus on medical colleges that completely rebuilt their facilities in a single construction effort. New construction tends to articulate more clearly the pedagogical and architectural program and to generate more extensive written commentary than renovations or expansions of existing space. This decision also matches the historical record. By my estimate, approximately 75 percent of American medical schools engaged in a comprehensive building campaign between 1893 and 1940 rather than primarily renovating or augmenting existing facilities. Moreover, because countless histories have been written describing individual medical schools, I do not examine schools for which no secondary research exists. To put this framework in numerical perspective, close to forty-five schools fit these parameters, or more than half of the seventy-seven schools that offered the MD degree in 1933.

Building Schools, Making Doctors focuses on nine of these nearly forty-five medical colleges. Those chosen represent a mix of elite and nonelite schools; East Coast, midwestern, and southern locales; private and public institutions; historically Black and predominantly white colleges; robust and limited financial resources, and single-sex and coeducational student populations. They are Columbia University College of Physicians and Surgeons (New York City), Harvard Medical School (Boston), Howard University College of Medicine (Washington, DC), Johns Hopkins Medical School (Baltimore), Meharry Medical College (Nashville), Syracuse University College of Medicine (now SUNY Upstate University College of Medicine), University of Nebraska College of Medicine (Omaha), Vanderbilt University School of Medicine (Nashville), and Woman's Medical College of Pennsylvania (a predecessor institution to

Drexel University College of Medicine in Philadelphia). Together these schools demonstrate the major developments in medical school design while allowing for a diverse investigation of pedagogy, conceptions of science, philanthropy, gender, race, and professional identity.

Some physician readers will wish that their alma mater received greater attention, and other historians of medicine or architecture might focus on a different cross section of schools. I believe, however, that this group generates a broad-based analysis that speaks comprehensively to the issues at stake in medical school design between 1893 and 1940. This collection of schools also acknowledges that the elite colleges may often produce the most innovative buildings, but they are not necessarily indicative of the experience of many medical students. Average and weak schools, no less than their more prestigious counterparts, shaped both how students learned and the types of physicians they became.

Two ahistorical restrictions exist within the investigation itself. First, *Building Schools, Making Doctors* does not generally examine the architectural changes made to medical schools after they opened. This decision denies the reality of medical colleges. Medical colleges undergo nearly continuous modifications of use and renovations of space. To future scholars is left the task of tracing these adaptations and alterations. Moreover, this book analyzes the medical school to the relative exclusion of the hospital. Because architectural historians first studied hospitals as discrete institutions, I largely continue this practice. In actuality, though, modern medical training requires instruction in the laboratory and at the bedside, and as such it demands both medical school and hospital facilities. In an attempt to mitigate this historically false bifurcation within the field of architectural history, I discuss the ways in which medical schools integrated clinical space into their campuses and facilities even if I do not retrace the shifts in hospital design so thoroughly explored by others.[39]

In the end, this book illuminates the major developments in medical college design in the late nineteenth and early twentieth centuries and investigates the role the school buildings played in creating the modern physician. The chapters progress thematically. Chapters 1 and 2 examine the types of medical schools constructed in the United States between 1893 and 1940 and the pedagogical and scientific ideas they encouraged. Chapter 1 analyzes the relatively small but often prestigious group of schools with vocal faculties that embraced the institute plan, a multistructure alternative to the single building for preclinical training that emphasized the physical and conceptual separation of the various areas of scientific study. By 1920, however, the institute plan had lost its supporters, and the single building went largely unchallenged. Chapter

2 explores the well-established single building for preclinical departments and the novel "medical school–hospital" (my phrase), which in the mid-1920s began placing preclinical and clinical facilities under one roof. In contrast to the institute plan, both unified designs endorsed the integration of the branches of medical science. Chapter 3 turns our attention to two critical but heretofore largely unrecognized forces in the physical development of early twentieth-century medical schools: the work of Boston-based architectural firm Shepley, Rutan, and Coolidge and its successors and the patronage of John D. Rockefeller's General Education Board. Shepley, Rutan, and Coolidge designed an unmatched eight medical schools between 1906 and 1932. The General Education Board's gifts not only contributed to the dominance of the unified plans but also privileged the elite research schools attended primarily by white men, a policy that hampered the building programs at the nation's two coeducational Black medical colleges and one predominantly white medical school for women. Chapter 4 argues that educators utilized the school buildings as they strove to promote reformed medical education, scientific medicine, and the notion of the elite physician to the public. Simultaneously, faculty leaders both responded to and shaped local communities when they oversaw the construction of new facilities. Chapter 5 reveals that medical schools fostered an elevated professional identity among students and faculty at the same time that they favored white men and privileged physicians over other medical personnel. The epilogue discusses the ongoing use of the medical colleges from this transformative period and sets in historical context the present surge in medical school construction through a case study of the recently founded Dell Medical School at the University of Texas at Austin.

By creating a thematic study of American medical colleges, I raise questions with wide applicability. If medical school design codifies conceptions of knowledge and pedagogical ideas, then how can we apply this type of analysis to other educational spaces? If the General Education Board shaped the architecture of medical schools without formalizing an architectural agenda, what other philanthropic foundations implemented similarly unstated initiatives for the facilities they funded? If professional identities begin to form in the educational setting, then where else should we look outside of the workplace for the inculcation of professional consciousness? Finally, I hope that investigating the historical roots of the dialogues taking place in medical colleges today will give current educators, architects, and donors additional insight when crafting the next generation of medical school buildings.

1

AN ALTERNATIVE
TO UNIFICATION

The Institute Plan and the Division of the Medical School

AT THE TURN OF THE TWENTIETH CENTURY, THE FACULTIES AT Johns Hopkins Medical School and Harvard Medical School rejected the use of a single building for preclinical studies—an arrangement long utilized by American medical colleges. Inspired by the institutes they had experienced in Germany, the leaders at Johns Hopkins and Harvard decided to divide their schools into multiple structures that each housed a department or two. The institute design never became as popular in the United States as the unified plans—the single building for preclinical training and later the medical school–hospital that combined laboratory and clinical facilities into one structure. However, the institute plan's prominent display at Johns Hopkins and Harvard captured the interest of medical faculties nationwide. Administrators debated the institute plan's cost, efficiency, and conception of science, particularly its emphasis on separating the subjects that composed medical education and research.

The institute plan differed from its unified counterparts in significant ways, but several characteristics existed across progressive medical schools regardless of type. The original medical school campus at Johns Hopkins highlights the construction of extensive laboratories with provisions for emerging disciplines, along with the placement of the medical school in proximity to the hospital and with the pathology laboratory as a conceptual and physical bridge between the two. It also demonstrates attention to light, ventilation, and furnishings in the laboratory—all of which were tied to expected student behavior—and investment in pioneering technology for storing cadavers. The 1906 Harvard Medical School quadrangle underscores additional elements of medical school design found in both institute and unified plans, beginning with the shift in the footprints of medical school buildings and the adoption of double-loaded corridors as the twentieth century opened. Moreover, the Harvard quadrangle reveals the prevalence of the museum and the unit system of laboratory organization. Certain components of medical school design became relatively standard even as medical educators celebrated the distinctiveness of their respective construction efforts and of the building type they chose.

Educational Philosophy in Practice and Student Life in the Modern Medical School

Proprietary schools did not immediately disappear with the advent of modern medical training. Physicians continued to establish proprietary schools, and the number of medical colleges did not peak until 1906. For several decades, proprietary and reformed medical schools existed simultaneously.

Students in progressive medical colleges received a dramatically different education from the one offered by proprietary schools. Students at proprietary schools spent six to eight hours a day for four months of the year in a large amphitheater listening to lectures, a monotonous experience generally relieved only by textbook readings, recitations from time to time, and, at some schools, dissection. After repeating this course twice and successfully answering a short series of oral questions, students earned their degrees.[1] Conversely, reformed medical education included four distinct years of training, with each year designed to build on the previous year. The initial two years centered on laboratory instruction in the preclinical sciences—anatomy, biochemistry, physiology, pathology, bacteriology, pharmacology, and pathophysiology—along with an introduction to taking patient histories and to physical examination (fig. 1.1). Students then spent the second two years of medical school learning clinical subjects. They focused on surgery, internal medicine, obstetrics and gynecology, pediatrics, and psychiatry. More specialized clinical fields, such as anesthesia and orthopedics, received less time.[2]

Although the transition to experiential learning took place more slowly in the clinical departments than in the preclinical subjects, clinical training also became a hands-on endeavor. During the second half of the nineteenth century, medical schools had initially remained reliant on didactic clinical instruction, and amphitheaters grew in size. In 1871, the new amphitheater at Bellevue Hospital in New York City reportedly offered seating for eight hundred, and in 1873 the amphitheater at the University of Pennsylvania Hospital could accommodate seven hundred.

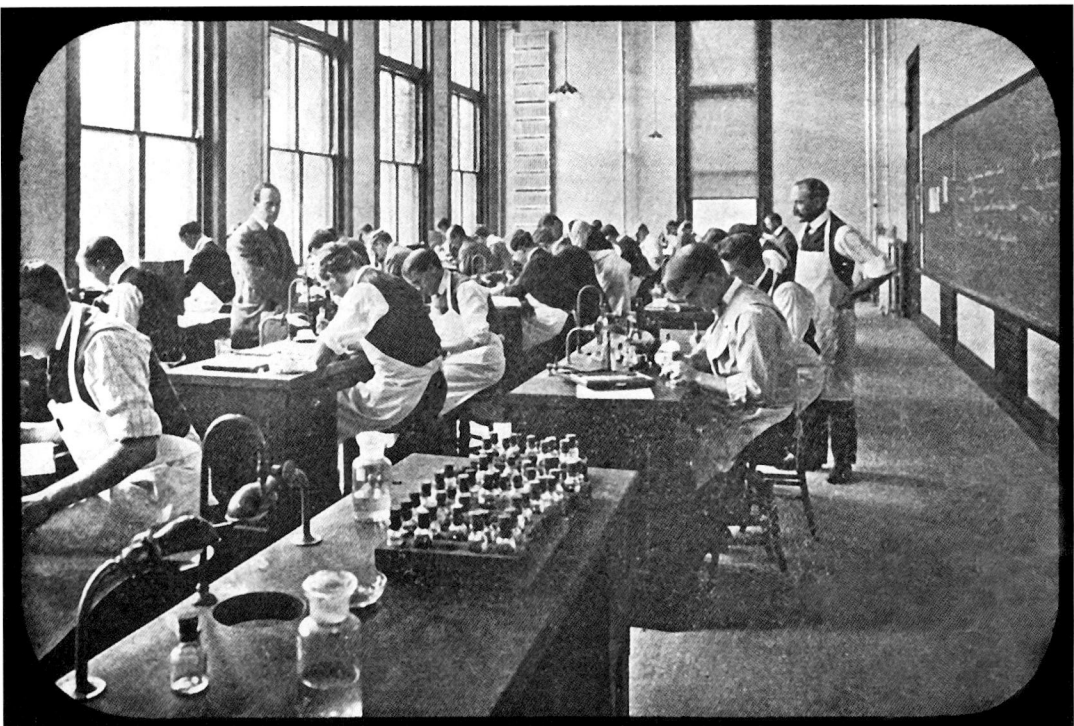

I.I.   Students in a laboratory in Building D, Harvard Medical School, ca. 1906.

The amphitheater at Jefferson Hospital seated six hundred in 1876 (see fig. I.2). When Johns Hopkins Medical School opened in 1893, however, founding faculty member William Osler inaugurated the clerkship, a system that involved medical students in patient care. The clerkship spread slowly, but in time it enabled medical students at reformed colleges to participate in treating patients in the clinic and on the wards. In surgery, the shift away from didactic instruction eventually merged with the desire to reduce the number of observers and the challenge they posed to an aseptic operating area. Simultaneously, the overall increase in the number of surgeries performed encouraged hospitals to include more operating rooms. To accommodate these demands, the operating theater gave way to surgical suites composed of multiple operating rooms along with preoperative facilities, sterilizing rooms, and other related spaces.[3] In the operating room, medical students and nurses learned in small groups by standing at the elbow of the attending physician or watching from a nearby viewing stand (fig. 1.2).

   With its emphasis on hands-on laboratory and clinical training beginning in the late nineteenth century, modern medical education embraced active learning and what would later be designated "progressive

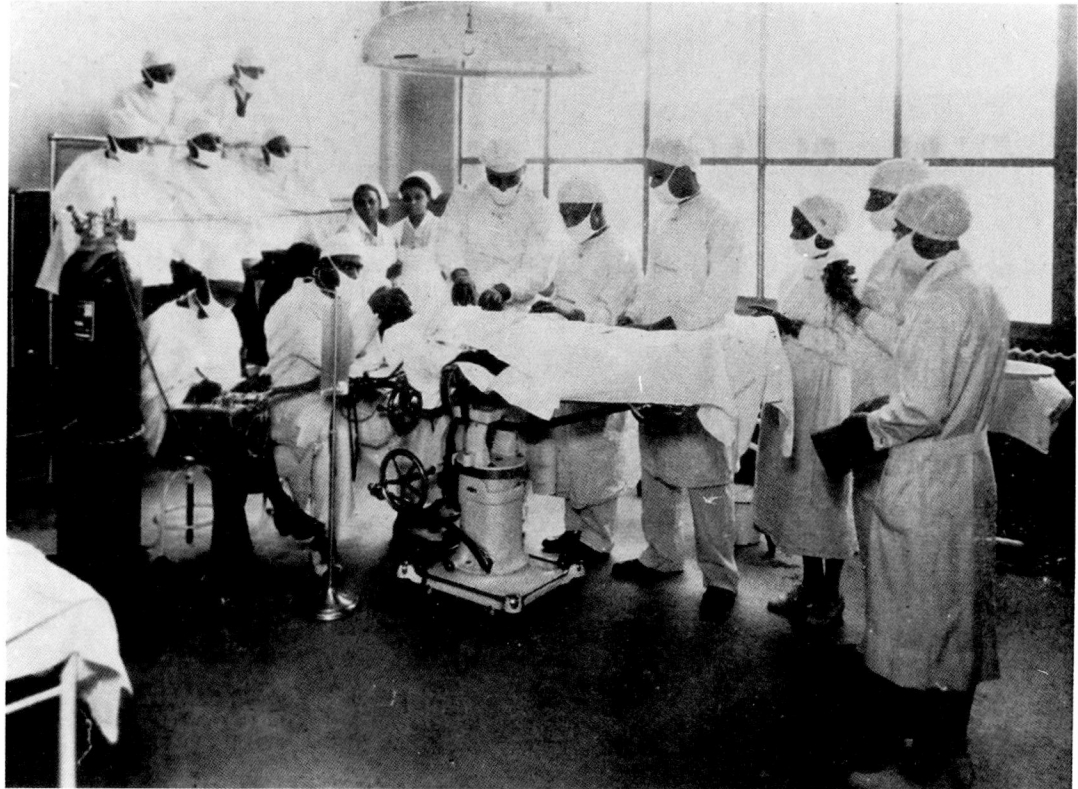

1.2.   Senior medical and nursing students receive instruction in surgery, Meharry Medical College, ca. 1931.

education." John Dewey, progressive education's leading proponent in the early twentieth century, called for many changes, including experiential rather than passive learning, group work rather than recitation by individuals, and discussion. These ideas influenced the entire education system, from the elementary through the college years, in the first part of the twentieth century.[4]

As medical training developed, it involved all subjects, even those that predated reform. At the University of Michigan starting in 1889, medical students in the anatomy course undertook dissection and preparation of materials themselves, a far more time- and resource-intensive practice than learning through lectures and demonstrations.[5] Not coincidentally, this shift in the teaching of anatomy took place the same year Michigan opened a new building for anatomy.

Faculty hoped that experiential training—participation in laboratory work, contact with patients, instruction and discussion in small groups— would benefit students throughout their professional lives. Prominent medical educators spoke passionately of the need to create practitioners who, no different from their classmates who would embark on research careers, knew how to solve problems in an organized, scientific fashion. For practitioners, this training would help them to navigate the inherent uncertainty of medical practice, in which events and disease in the human body do not consistently mirror the descriptions found in textbooks. As medical historian Kenneth Ludmerer reminds us, however, "it is not easy to teach students how to think critically, particularly in a discipline so laden with important facts as medicine. The history of twentieth-century medical education is one of striving to attain these ideals rather than one of actual realization."[6]

Although the basic four-year structure of medical education established in the late nineteenth century remained in place, the curriculum was not static across time or identical at all schools. The curriculum's content evolved as medical science developed and the prevalence of certain diseases shifted. In addition, despite the guidelines set by state licensing boards, variation existed from one school to the next. For example, depending on where the student enrolled, in 1940 they would spend between 90 and 326 hours studying bacteriology. The details of medical education, including what to teach in each lecture, the ratio of students to laboratory bench or cadaver, and how to transition the students from preclinical to clinical training, also received constant attention from medical educators. As educators debated what core knowledge all physicians should know and how to balance the teaching of scientific principles with more practical training, their concerns paralleled broader conversations in higher education as university faculties considered what general education should be given to all liberal arts students and weighed instruction in the liberal arts against more utilitarian pursuits.[7]

Regardless of the medical college attended and the specific modes of instruction, however, all students would likely have agreed that medical education required long hours and nearly complete dedication of time and energy. In the preclinical years, students typically arrived at school at 8:00 a.m. on weekdays and remained in laboratories and lectures until the late afternoon. Saturdays brought a half-day schedule. Faculty frequently discouraged romance and marriage.[8] Francis D. Moore, Harvard Medical School class of 1939, recalled, "Married students were rare in those days. There was still a bias against marriage by medical students. In a class of 120 only two of us were married at the beginning . . . ; a third . . . was married the next summer."[9] Compared to colleges, medical schools offered little by way of extracurricular activities beyond the occasional yearbook or student newsletter. Medical faculties worked to provide some relief from the stress of medical training through the parties, teas,

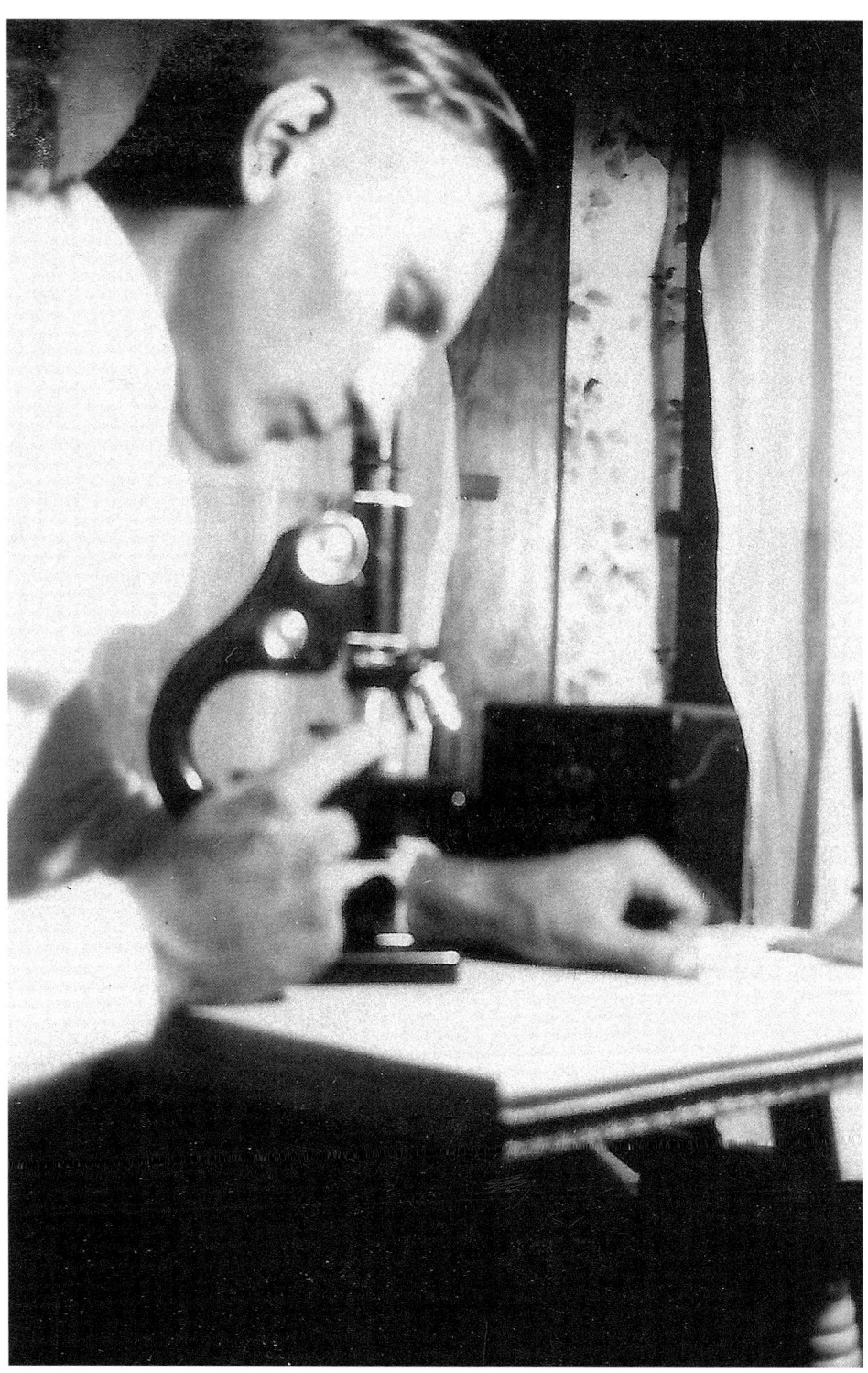

1.3.   Joe Holoubek at his microscope, ca. 1936.

and luncheons they organized for students, and medical fraternities and sororities supplied additional support and diversion—at least for those invited to join and with the means to participate.[10]

During their academic day, most medical students experienced some version of the block or concentrated system, which became more prevalent than the concurrent schedule for the preclinical years.[11] With the block system, students studied fewer courses at a time by spending more hours each day on a given subject. For example, before Harvard Medical School adopted the block system just prior to 1900, its students began their education balancing anatomy, histology, physiology, and physiological chemistry. After the introduction of the block system, students studied anatomy and histology during the first half of their first year and physiology and physiological chemistry during the second half of the year.[12] Not only did the block system focus students' efforts, but it also gave the faculty extended chunks of time when they could focus on research.[13] Not every school's arrangement of courses was identical, but all strove to create an ordered and systematic program of study.

The student's experience of the curriculum, particularly the extensive laboratory instruction reinforced by lectures and an emphasis on swift mastery of the material, becomes clear in the writing of Joe Holoubek, who began his medical training at the University of Nebraska College of Medicine in the fall of 1934 (fig. 1.3). Late in his life, Holoubek used his medical school class notes as the basis for a memoir. His description of the first six weeks of medical school, when Nebraska students took embryology and bacteriology, is representative of his preclinical training. Embryology took place during the morning and began with a lecture from 8:00 to 9:00 a.m., when Holoubek "would take from three to ten pages of handwritten notes." After lecture, the students moved to the laboratory for three hours, during which time they turned their attention to "drawing everything we saw in microscope." He elaborated: "Each day we were assigned slides of the subject that had been discussed during the lecture. We each made a notebook that contained a total of forty-eight drawings or plates in color of the various stages of development of the chick, pig and a few human embryos. Each plate was followed by a two page written description of what we had seen and drawn. These were handed in and graded." Holoubek identified embryology as the school's "elimination course" and explained that "comprehensive examinations were held every Friday. . . . It didn't take long for those who could not or did not want to study to drop out." Students turned their attention to bacteriology during the second part of the day and had a combination of lecture and laboratory instruction along with "several meetings in the medical amphitheater in the hospital where we were presented with clinical cases that were due to infections of the bacteria that we were studying. This was the fun part."[14]

From Holoubek's memoir a picture emerges of an intensive, largely experiential education with a focus on practical applications. In his second year, he returned to the same laboratory and the same teachers with whom he had studied bacteriology a year earlier and began an introduction to immunology. Holoubek recounted the laboratory exercises related to typhoid fever and concluded, "We studied typhoid fever thoroughly because it was prevalent in the state and patients were available from which material could be obtained." In addition, he described extensive clinical laboratory work, including when "we prepared and standardized the reagents of the Wassermann test [for syphilis] and did it. Patients with the disease were plentiful in the clinics and material was available."[15]

For students, time in the laboratory served two purposes. It was a means to understanding many of the preclinical sciences, and it was training in the techniques necessary to carry out the laboratory work, such as white and red blood cell counts, urinalyses, and cultures, that increasingly formed the basis of clinical care and for which students would be responsible beginning in their third and fourth years of training. They spent long hours learning to think about the body according to the current tenets of science, which demanded medical practice based on methodical investigations in the clinic coupled with the recognition that the laboratory was an educational and diagnostic tool in itself.

At some schools, students also gained firsthand experience of the laboratory as a site of investigation, either through the design of their courses or exposure to their professors' work. Johns Hopkins Medical School anatomist Franklin P. Mall described the mind-set of faculty who conceived of their courses as expressions of the research process: "The aim is to make the course one continuous problem for each student to investigate, aiding each one with good material, and teaching him how to study, wherever necessary."[16] Certain students, inspired by the research of the faculty, developed projects of their own. For Moore at Harvard, "research was a key component of our medical education because our teachers were deeply involved in the biomedical sciences." He explained that "participation in research is now a requirement at many medical schools. While this was not so in the 1930s, doors were opened and research was made possible. In our second and third years Bill Carleton and I carried out a research study that occupied Sundays and holidays for many months."[17]

Much was at stake in these buildings for the young men—and a few women. (Harvard admitted no women at this time; Nebraska did, but Holoubek remembered none in his class.[18]) Medical educators put a tremendous amount of energy into the design of medical schools. They believed that the buildings helped to facilitate how students learned and shaped students' understanding of medical science.

"High Thinking and Low Living" at Johns Hopkins Medical School

In the summer of 1893, as Americans flocked to Chicago for the World's Columbian Exposition, a group of physicians in Baltimore had a different focus: the upcoming opening of the long-anticipated Johns Hopkins Medical School. This school often enjoys prime billing in histories of American medicine for the influence of its graduates and the impact of its program, which included rigorous admission standards (for the first time incoming students had to have a bachelor's degree), experiential learning over two years of preclinical and two years of clinical instruction, university affiliation, and commitment to generating original research.[19] Although rich in ideas, the school was strapped for cash and constructed its campus piecemeal over several years.

In 1873, Johns Hopkins, a Baltimore businessman and the largest shareholder in the Baltimore and Ohio Railroad, died and left funds for the creation of an eponymous university and hospital. Hopkins requested that the university contain a medical school and that this medical school work closely with the hospital.[20] The university and the hospital, however, struggled to follow his mandates. In both cases, only the income from Hopkins's gifts could be used for construction, which constituted a financial challenge compounded by a reduction in income from the university's and the hospital's respective endowments during their early years. Significant proportions of both institutions' resources came in the form of Baltimore and Ohio Railroad stock, which produced diminishing dividends between 1886 and 1891. After having to delay its intended opening for four years, the hospital welcomed its first patients in 1889, but the university was unable to begin offering medical training at that time.[21] In the end, four more years passed before students arrived at the Johns Hopkins Medical School in 1893, a development famously made possible by a group of women, led by Mary Elizabeth Garrett, who raised the $500,000 necessary to open the school (see chapter 3). Because the terms of Garrett's gift stipulated that not more than $50,000 of the original benefaction could be spent on buildings, the medical school

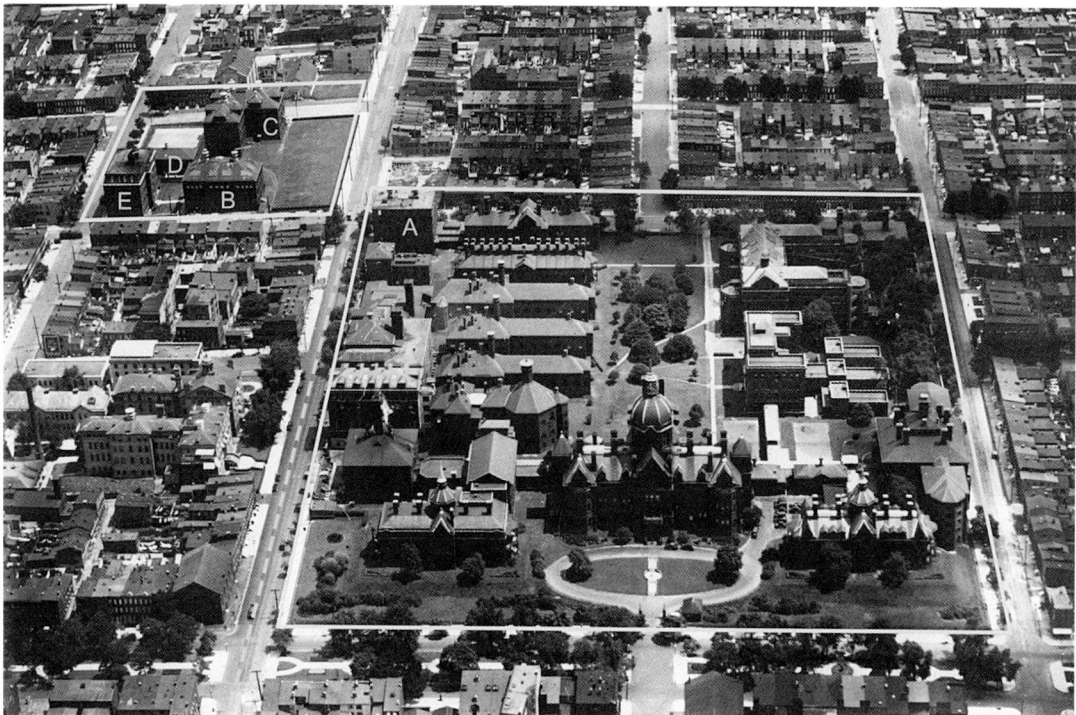

1.4. Campus of Johns Hopkins Hospital and Johns Hopkins Medical School, ca. 1921, modified by author to show hospital block (large box), medical school campus (small box), Monument Street (dashed line), expanded pathology laboratory with 1910 addition of a fifth floor (A), Women's Fund Memorial Building (B), Physiological Building (C), first Hunterian Laboratory (D), and second Hunterian Laboratory (E).

had to adopt a slow construction schedule.[22] The gradual expansion of space was acceptable since the school added a class a year and did not immediately need to support four classes of students.[23]

The university completed the medical school campus over the next six years. In the fall of 1893, the construction of two floors on top of the existing two-story pathology building located on the back corner of the Johns Hopkins Hospital property supported the instruction of first-year students. Pharmacology and physiological chemistry occupied the third floor and anatomy, the fourth (fig. 1.4).[24] The following year, the school dramatically increased its facilities with the completion of the Women's Fund Memorial Building, so named to satisfy another mandate of Garrett's gift to open the medical college.[25] The faculty placed the Women's Fund Memorial Building on the medical school lot, which sat diagonally across the intersection from the pathology laboratory. Although designed for the anatomy department, the Women's Fund Memorial Building's construction also made it possible for pharmacology to move into its first

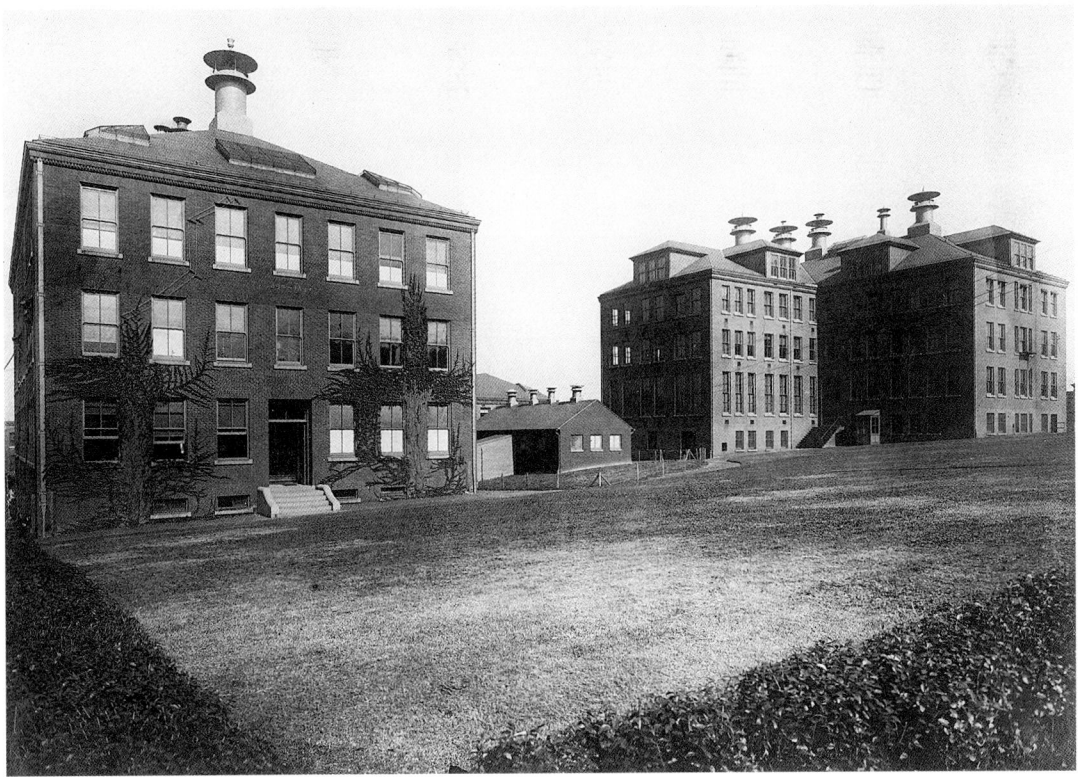

1.5.   Left: Women's Fund Memorial Building, Johns Hopkins Medical School, 1894, George Archer, architect. Right: Physiological Building, Johns Hopkins Medical School, 1898 or 1899, George Archer, architect. Photograph ca. 1912.

floor temporarily and vacate the enlarged pathology laboratory where it had been residing.[26] In 1896, the Johns Hopkins Hospital superintendent reported the addition of four classrooms to the outpatient clinic to accommodate students.[27] The following year he described the expansion of one hospital building by two stories in order to provide the hospital and medical school with a "clinical laboratory" composed of classrooms, student laboratory, small library, darkroom, and rooms for research.[28] During the course of the 1898–1899 academic year, the so-called Physiological Building was finished to the east of the Women's Fund Memorial Building (fig. 1.5). Despite its moniker, the structure actually housed pharmacology, as well as physiology and physiological chemistry. This building enabled physiology to relocate from the university to the medical campus, and for the first time the medical school was united on a single site.[29]

Relatively little information exists about the three major spaces erected for the young medical school: the addition to the pathology laboratory, the Women's Fund Memorial Building, and the Physiological Building. Further frustrating research efforts is that, unlike most of the buildings discussed in this study, none of the three facilities remains. The pathology laboratory burned in 1920, and the Women's Fund Memorial Building and the Physiological Building were razed in 1979 and 1959, respectively. Of these structures, the Women's Fund Memorial Building is the best documented, through the coverage it received in the local and medical press. Despite these research challenges, the early Johns Hopkins Medical School buildings are revealing. They indicate that the leaders of the medical school returned from their studies in Germany with an appreciation not only for that country's system of scientific inquiry but also for its separation of universities into discrete institutes.

With physiology still taught at the university when the Women's Fund Memorial Building opened in 1894, the medical school's leadership recognized that the structure did not fully satisfy needs. The medical educators and architect conceived of the Women's Fund Memorial Building as the first step in the construction of a complete medical school campus. School cofounder William Osler later described the ideal campus plan he had sketched during the organization of Johns Hopkins Medical School. Had money not been an object, he would have preferred four principal buildings, one centered on each side of a square outlined by cloisters that contained busts and statues of medical luminaries. The building on the Monument Street side of the square across from the hospital would be "a beautiful structure in stone devoted to the library and museum."[30] At the time of the construction of the Women's Fund Memorial Building, the medical school had publicly adopted Osler's vision. Two accounts of the projected campus, one of which was published in the local newspaper, generally followed Osler's ideas.[31] Together these descriptions express a desire to create a square composed of a prominent building at the front of the lot, for the administration and/or the museum and library, flanked by a series of ancillary buildings, each devoted to a specific laboratory subject or two.

Although the placement of the Women's Fund Memorial Building and the Physiological Building far back from Monument Street left room for an administration building to be erected in front of them, later construction did not follow the original plan for a quadrangle. In 1905, the first Hunterian Laboratory was built between and behind the earlier two buildings, and in 1916 the second Hunterian Laboratory was completed on the corner of the site behind the Women's Fund Memorial Building. Despite this trajectory, Osler still had hope for at least part of his

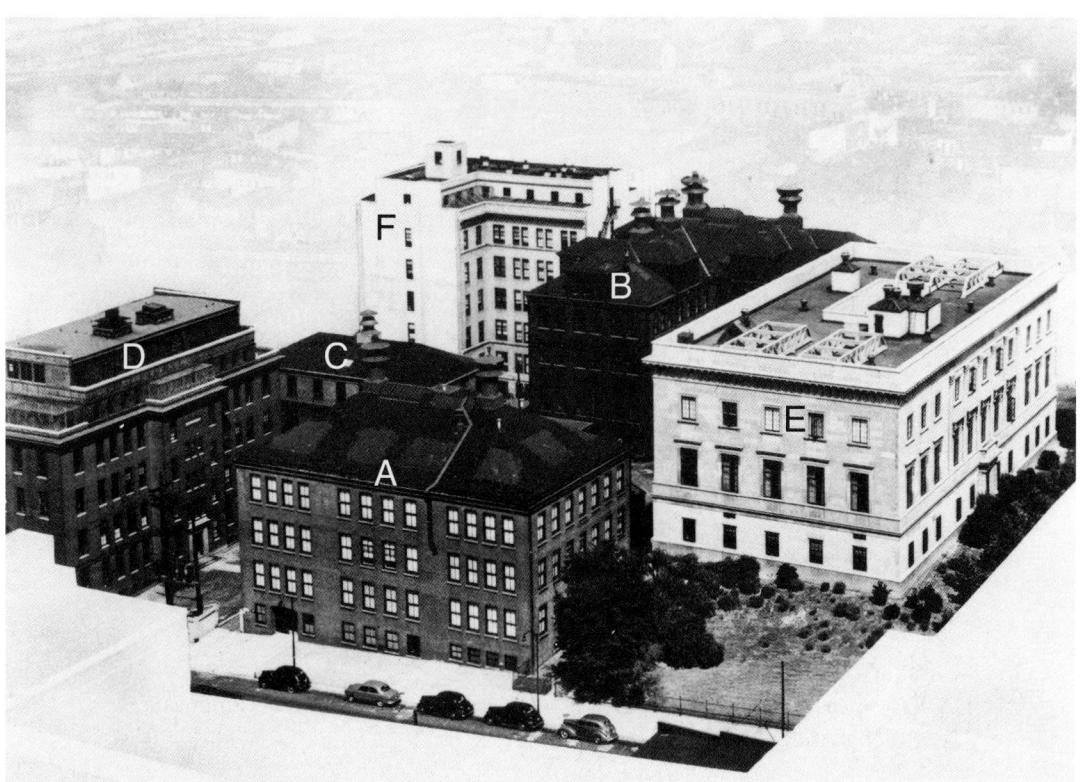

1.6.   Johns Hopkins Medical School campus, ca. 1940, modified by author. The William H. Welch Medical
        Library (E) and the new Physiology Building (F) were completed in 1929. Earlier buildings are the
        1894 Women's Fund Memorial Building (A), the 1898 or 1899 Physiological Building (B), the 1905
        Hunterian Laboratory (C), and the 1916 Hunterian Laboratory (D).

original vision. In 1911, he observed that the main building, a library and
museum along Monument Street, "could yet be realized. As the museum
collections grow, and as year by year the books increase in number such a
building will become a necessity, and in it these special libraries will find
their appropriate home."[32] Osler's optimism was not misplaced. In 1929,
some forty years after he formulated his plan for Johns Hopkins Medical School, the William H. Welch Medical Library filled the reserved
space at the front the medical school campus. The same year, the new
Physiology Building opened, the first step in a planned "reconstruction
of the Medical School laboratories into a U-shaped building" that would
outline the back three sides of the plot and create "ultimately a proper
setting" for the library (fig. 1.6).[33] In some sense, time has achieved what
the early faculty could not. A coordinated reconstruction of the laboratory buildings never occurred, but Johns Hopkins's original medical school
campus now contains the William H. Welch Medical Library along

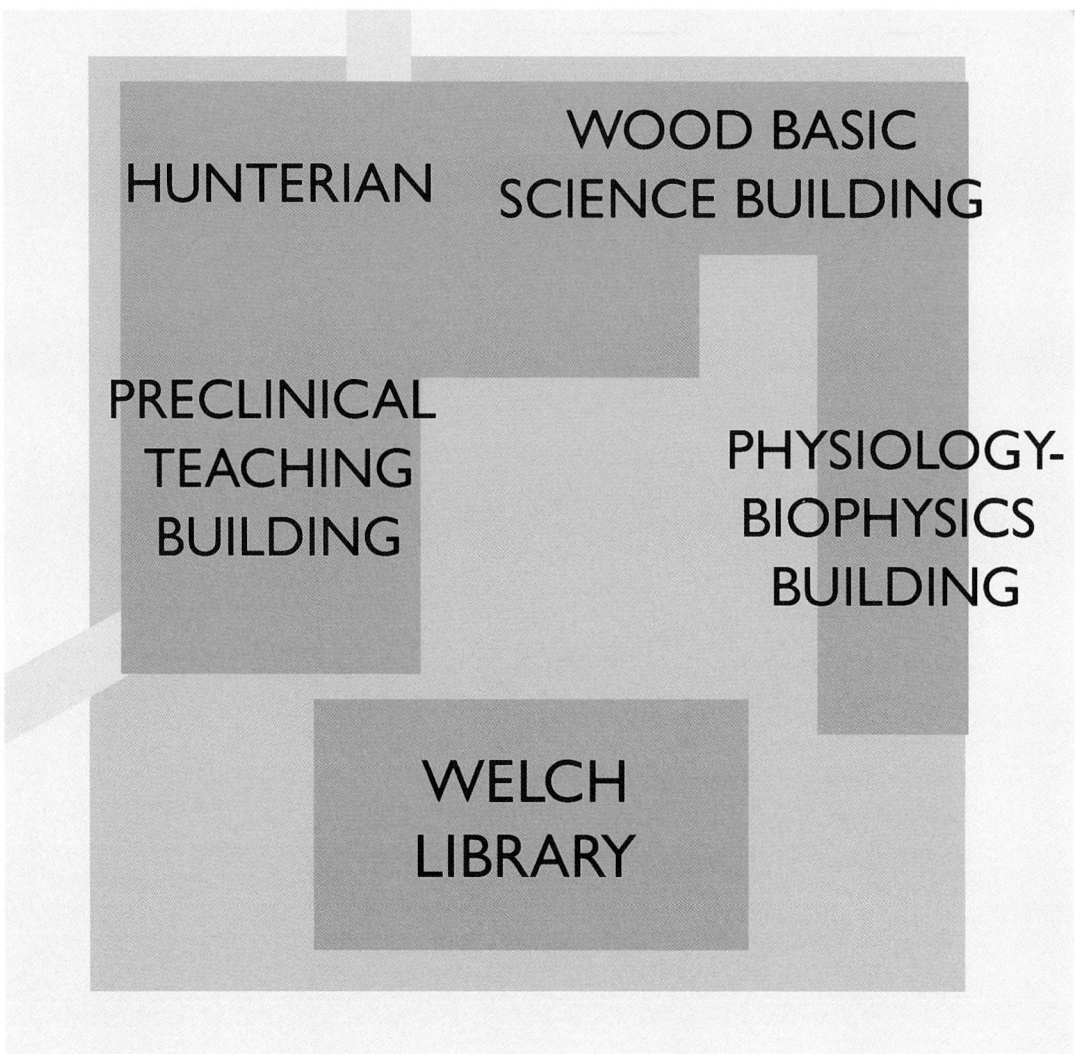

1.7.   Original Johns Hopkins Medical School campus lot, ca. 2019.

Monument Street and a roughly U-shaped conglomerate of buildings
behind it (fig. 1.7).

   As construction of the initial medical school campus between 1893
and 1899 ended, the faculty persisted in seeking separate structures
for different departments. But William Welch, another of Hopkins's
founding physicians, had made clear that another option existed. In 1891,
Welch outlined what buildings the medical school needed. The first part
of his proposal, ultimately enacted, called for expanding the pathology
laboratory, erecting a building for anatomy (the eventual Women's Fund
Memorial Building), and making do with existing facilities. He then

suggested constructing "a building or buildings for pharmacology and experimental therapeutics, for hygiene, for lectures and recitations and the general purposes of medical instruction not provided for in existing buildings." He concluded, however, with an alternative: "the anatomical building might be planned with reference to additions for these purposes."[34] In the end, the faculty chose to erect more structures rather than enlarge the Women's Fund Memorial Building, a choice John Shaw Billings, medical advisor for the design of Johns Hopkins Hospital, would have approved. In 1891, Billings described the facilities for an ideal medical school. Outside of clinical resources, the school would need a minimum of four laboratory buildings and "a building for general lectures, library, etc." Billings continued, "It is, of course, possible to consolidate all these into a single three- or four-story building, and thus save money, especially in cost of ground, but the results are not so good."[35]

Osler and Welch made the decision to construct distinct buildings for the various departments, a choice that drew on the German institute design familiar to those, such as Osler, Welch, and Billings, who had studied or traveled in Germany. In Germany, American medical men became familiar with universities made up of many institutes, each of which focused on a particular discipline. A separate physical and administrative unit within the university, an institute typically enjoyed its own facilities; housed expensive equipment, including scientific devices and extensive libraries; contained a large staff; and benefited from a generous budget.[36] A site plan of the University of Kiel published in 1890 depicts the German university's physical division into institutes (fig. 1.8).

In the nineteenth century, German universities developed into centers for original research, and, with this change, institutes increased in number in both philosophical and medical faculties.[37] Between 1860 and 1914, at least 173 institutes were founded among the medical faculties of German universities. Frequently, these institutes supported new fields of study, such as hygiene or otolaryngology. At the same time, huge sums of money went to established institutes, such as those devoted to anatomy or surgery, to erect buildings and improve working conditions.[38] German universities were the primary creators of the institute model, but it migrated to universities that drew on the German system, particularly in Scandinavia, Russia, eastern Europe, Switzerland, and the Netherlands, and inspired significant change in university research and teaching in the United States.[39] Many scholars have recognized that the German commitment to laboratory investigation had a lasting impact on American medical education. A closer look at the architecture, however, reveals that American physicians also brought home from Germany an

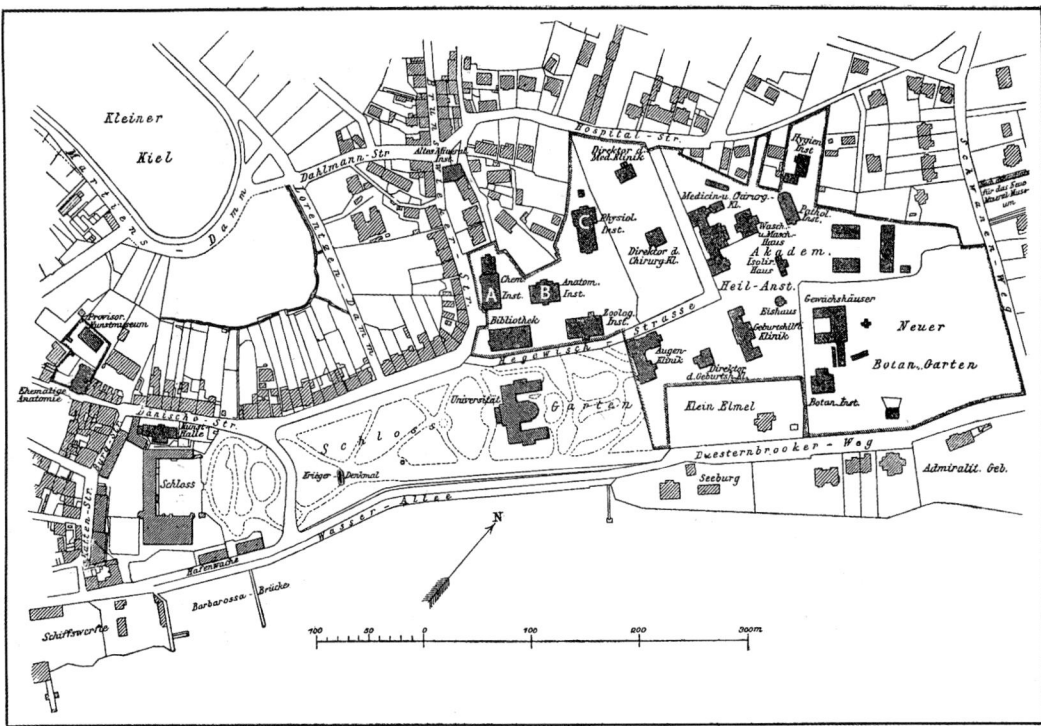

1.8.   Site plan of the University of Kiel, Germany, ca. 1890, modified by author to show the Chemistry
Institute (A), the Anatomical Institute (B), and the Physiological Institute (C).

appreciation of that country's division of the campus into separate structures for different academic disciplines.

In this sense, the medical schools that embraced the German institute plan deviated from broader American campus-planning trends. As
architectural historian Paul V. Turner writes, "In the mid-nineteenth
century, the German university system began to influence American
education in significant ways, but architecture and planning were not
commensurately affected. To a remarkable degree, college planning in
America has an independent history . . . less subject to European fashion
than other fields of architecture and design."[40] The institute form adopted by the medical schools at Johns Hopkins, Harvard, and elsewhere
defied American independence in college planning, but medical school
planning overall in the late nineteenth and early twentieth centuries
does not fundamentally alter Turner's analysis. The German institute
plan failed to become the dominant medical school type in this period.
American medical educators relied primarily on the single building for
preclinical studies and, in the mid-1920s, developed a medical school

type—the medical school–hospital—that expanded on the theme of unification.

Between 1893 and 1899, the Johns Hopkins medical faculty oversaw the construction of the school's first campus, eventually composed of discrete buildings for pathology, anatomy, and physiology and pharmacology. Although not the grand, formally organized campus that Osler had imagined, the buildings served the school well. The structures were pioneering at the time of their completion, but as other schools rebuilt, the Johns Hopkins buildings came to typify many of the features of medical school design between 1893 and 1940 regardless of whether the school utilized an institute plan or one of the two unified types: the single building for preclinical studies and the medical school–hospital.

A critical element of progressive medical education was training in the laboratory and at the bedside. As noted earlier, it was at Johns Hopkins that Osler famously inaugurated the clinical clerkship, whereby third- and fourth-year medical students participated in the treatment of patients. The physical proximity of medical school and hospital and the students' extensive access to the wards—a privilege most hospitals refused to give in this period—facilitated the novel form of clinical training at Johns Hopkins. Many years earlier, Johns Hopkins himself had called for the coordination of the hospital and the medical school in his directive to the hospital trustees: "In all your arrangements in relation to this hospital, you will bear constantly in mind that it is my wish and purpose that the institution should ultimately form a part of the medical school of that university for which I have made ample provision by my will." With this statement, he linked the separate corporations of the Johns Hopkins University and the Johns Hopkins Hospital and guaranteed that medical students would be welcome on the wards.[41]

The hospital trustees did not forget the benefactor's vision, and they ensured that the hospital would be designed with medical education in mind. When the trustees reviewed the plans for the hospital generated by five American hospital experts, Billings's report stood out for its commitment to integrating the hospital and medical school. Billings called for constructing and equipping the hospital for education and research in addition to patient care.[42] Billings, in collaboration with well-known Baltimore architect John R. Niernsee, designed the hospital to accommodate medical students. One contemporary description affirmed, "The hospital not only provides rooms for the sick, but gives means for higher medical education. There is a large amphitheatre . . . and provision is made for thirty students to reside in the hospital and devote themselves, under proper guidance, to the study of disease and the practical care of the sick."[43] In the end, however, demand for resident housing meant that medical students never lived in the administration building.[44]

The construction of the pathology laboratory on the back corner of the hospital lot near the medical school further aligned the two entities. In March 1876, the Johns Hopkins University trustees sanctioned the purchase of the site on the far side of Monument Street for the medical school. The hospital trustees approved the final block plan for the hospital the following February. Although the block plan was never fully realized, the pathology laboratory was constructed in accordance with this plan on the corner of the hospital site closest to the medical school.[45] The purchase of the medical school land likely influenced the placement of the pathology laboratory in proximity to the projected medical school campus. Johns Hopkins historian Alan M. Chesney explains that before Welch became professor of pathology in 1884, the plan for educating medical students centered their pathology instruction on the medical school property.[46] In this context, locating the pathology laboratory between the hospital and medical school made sense for the pathologist who needed to work on both sites. The appointment of Welch ultimately changed where medical students would receive their training in pathology but reinforced the placement of the pathology laboratory. Welch insisted that the pathology department's educational efforts take place as close as possible to the hospital. The 1893 alterations to the pathology laboratory created instructional space for medical students in the building on the hospital site.[47] Adjacent to the medical school campus, the pathology laboratory formed a link between the preclinical and clinical studies.

In modern medical schools, the pathology department often sat between the preclinical and clinical facilities, regardless of whether the school utilized an institute design or one of the two unified plans. On the one hand, this location for pathology was efficient. Pathology departments conducted autopsies, and the bodies for the postmortem came from the hospital. But the department's intermediary location had conceptual roots, too. Helen Ingleby, professor of pathology at Woman's Medical College of Pennsylvania, described in 1932 the significance of pathology to a student's education: "no one can be a competent physician without thinking pathologically as well as clinically, and visualizing the changes in the organs of the patient she is examining."[48] Ingleby described a dialectical relationship between the pathology laboratory and clinical practice: "the work of the Department of Pathology . . . is based on two fundamental principles: first, the enormous importance of pathology to clinical medicine; second, that medicine and surgery

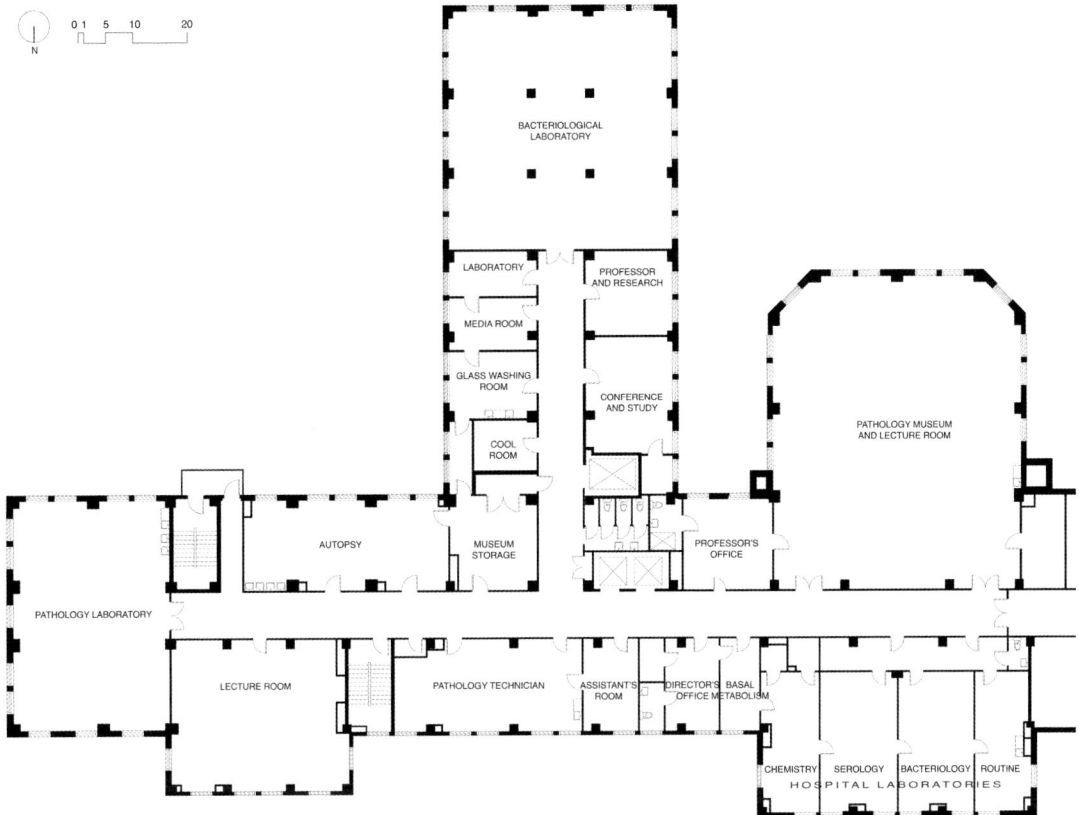

1.9.   Woman's Medical College of Pennsylvania, 1930, Ritter and Shay, architects, plan, second floor,
departments of pathology (along east-west corridor) and bacteriology (along north-south corridor),
redrawn. Note also the hospital laboratories on the opposite side of the corridor from the pathology
museum and lecture room. Hospital laboratories were often located at the intersection of the preclinical
and clinical zones in the medical school–hospital.

are to it as the breath of life." Ingleby connected her observations to the
building's design: "since this is so, and since the pathologist's opportunity
for increasing his knowledge can ordinarily only come from contact with
clinicians, the first essential in building a pathology department is that
it shall be accessible to the clinical staff—easily accessible."[49] Ingleby
assumed that the pathology department would sit within the preclinical
section of the building, but she argued that it be located near the wards.

Two years earlier, Woman's Medical College of Pennsylvania had
moved to a purpose-built facility that satisfied Ingleby's vision. The
structure combined a medical school and hospital into one building
that was bifurcated vertically, with the medical school on one side and
the hospital on the other. The principal corridor on each floor ran the

breadth of the building and connected the preclinical laboratory and hospital facilities. Ingleby believed the pathology department had a "pleasing and convenient lay-out of workshops and offices."[50] Arranged along the main corridor of the second floor, the department had immediate access to the clinical area through double doors just beyond one of the entrances to the large pathology museum and lecture room (fig. 1.9).

If the placement of the pathology laboratory represented a bridge between the medical school and the hospital at Johns Hopkins as well as other medical institutions, then the joint appointment of staff further knit together the two organizations. In his 1910 review of American and Canadian medical schools, Abraham Flexner lauded the arrangement in Baltimore: "The medical staff of the hospital and the clinical faculty of the medical school are identical; the scientific laboratories ranged around the hospital are in close touch with clinical problems, immediate and investigative. The medical school plant is thus an organic whole, in which laboratories and clinics are inextricably interwoven."[51] The coordination of the laboratory and the hospital represented a cornerstone of the program at Johns Hopkins. Architectural historians have overlooked the Johns Hopkins Medical School campus in favor of the far more famous hospital, but the medical educators who founded the school understood the two to be indivisible, united by a pedagogical program that emphasized experiential training in the laboratory and on the wards. The school demonstrates medical educators' interest throughout the period 1893–1940 in intertwining preclinical and clinical training, an agenda at once conceptual, pedagogical, and architectural.

Modern medical educators were also committed to carefully designed laboratories for teaching and research. At Johns Hopkins Medical School, the faculty devoted their limited budget for the 1894 Women's Fund Memorial Building to progressive facilities for education and research rather than architectural ornament. The Women's Fund Memorial Building housed the anatomy department and resulted from a collaboration between anatomist Franklin P. Mall and architect George Archer, who had a long relationship with both the Johns Hopkins Hospital and the medical school and whose work also included the 1893 addition to the pathology laboratory and the Physiological Building constructed at the end of the decade.[52] The local newspaper only somewhat overstated the austerity of the Women's Fund Memorial Building when it reported that the edifice "will be without architectural decoration on the exterior."[53] As Welch put it, "the building is not likely to attract anyone's attention from its architectural beauty."[54] In 1929, when the William H. Welch Medical Library and the Physiology Building opened amid hopes for reconstructing the entire

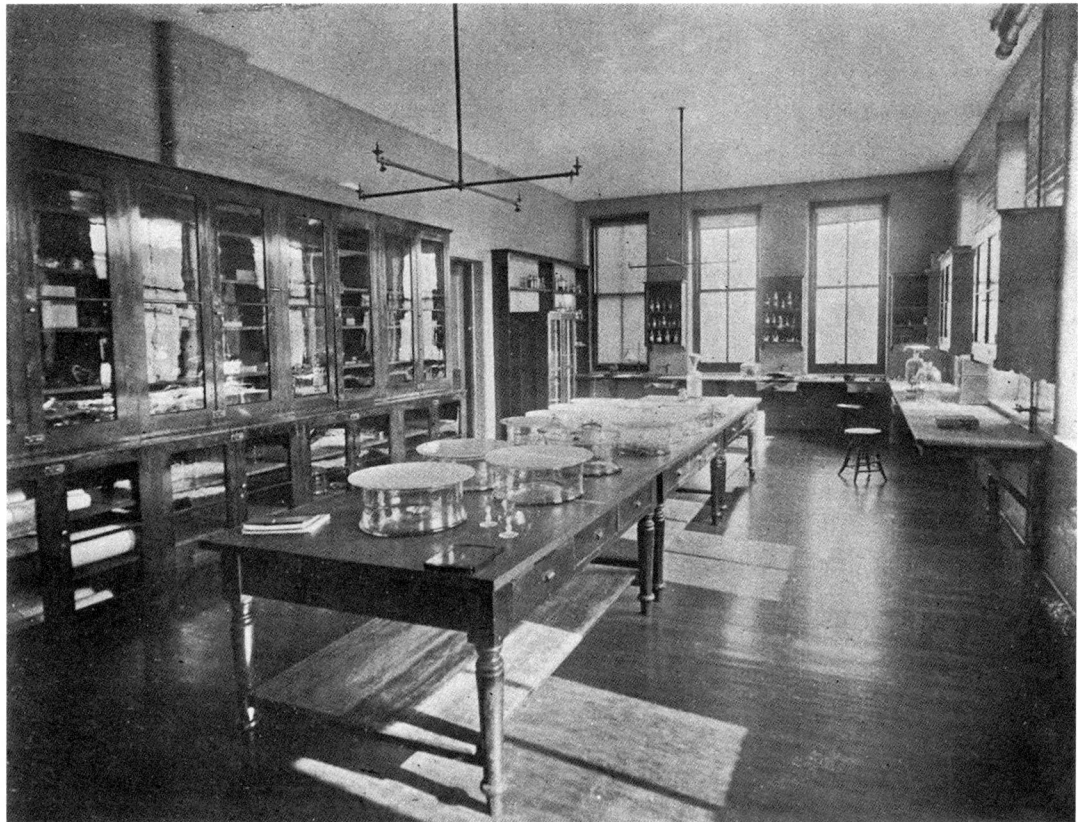

I.10.   Women's Fund Memorial Building, Johns Hopkins Medical School, 1894, George Archer, architect,
         second floor, private laboratory.

medical school campus and at a time when the school was enjoying significant philanthropic support, the faculty indicated their desire to rebuild
along grander lines (see fig. 1.6). For the Welch Medical Library, architect
Edward L. Tilton decided to forgo the plain, predominantly brick exterior
of the Women's Fund Memorial Building. Instead, he faced the campus's
new focal point in Indiana limestone, and, taking his inspiration from the
Italian Renaissance, he included on the frieze "ornaments similar to those
of the Farnese Palace."[55] What the Women's Fund Memorial Building
may have lacked in aesthetics, however, it made up in innovative design.

    So great was his pride in the Women's Fund Memorial Building that
Mall wrote at length about it in the *Johns Hopkins Hospital Bulletin*. As Mall
explained, "the object of the laboratory [building] is to teach students, to
train investigators, and to investigate."[56] To accommodate research, the
structure contained four private or experimental laboratories separate from
the teaching laboratories (fig. 1.10). For medical students, the teaching

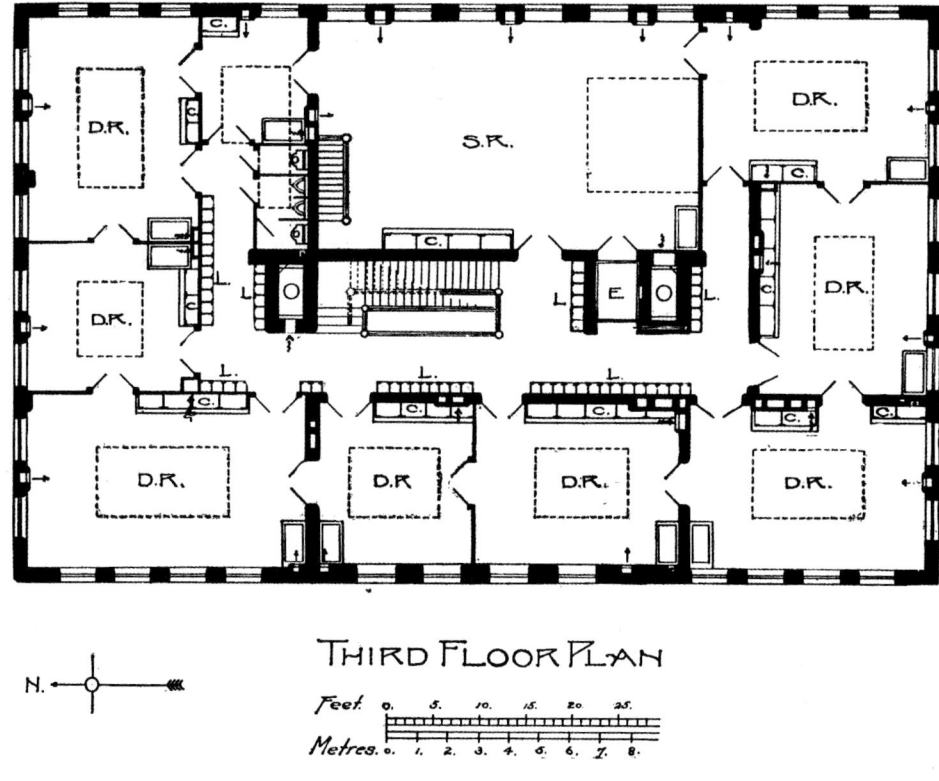

THIRD FLOOR PLAN

N.

Feet 0. 5. 10. 15. 20. 25.

Metres. 0. 1. 2. 3. 4. 5. 6. 7. 8.

FIG. 10.

DR, Dissecting room. SR, Study room. C, Cases. L, Lockers. E, Elevators.
The dotted rectangles around DR indicate the extent of the light wells. The lighter partitions indicate that the walls are thin and can be removed easily.

1.11.   Women's Fund Memorial Building, Johns Hopkins Medical School, 1894, George Archer, architect, plan, third floor.

laboratories provided the opportunity for hands-on learning. To Mall, and others, students retained far more from experiential learning than from lectures, even when the latter included demonstrations: "Lectures with demonstrations are certainly valuable—more valuable than the lectures with text-books alone. Yet analyzing the object itself is infinitely more valuable than to watch the results exposed by another. Wrestling with the part which is being studied, handling it and viewing it from all sides, and tabulating and classifying the parts worked out, give us the greatest reward. All this may be accomplished by practical laboratory work. If we can make the student work thoughtfully and carefully, a great result is achieved. . . . He is upon the stage, not in the audience."[57] Medical educators may have increasingly emphasized laboratory training, but the lecture did not disappear. As Mall pointed out, the pharmacology department housed temporarily in the building's first floor held lectures in a spacious room planned ultimately to accommodate histology.[58] Outside of this laboratory-turned-lecture hall, the building contained no dedicated lecture space. In the anatomy department, lectures were given in the laboratory.[59]

Not surprisingly, considering Mall's commitment to laboratory work, the Women's Fund Memorial Building contained pioneering laboratory accommodations. Writing in 1896, Mall lamented that, unlike in Europe, "in America we cannot boast of the multitude of buildings erected especially for the teaching of anatomy and investigation in this subject." Although he recognized a few significant exceptions, Mall decried the lack of resources for anatomy in the United States and declared, "The dissecting room is as a rule poor."[60] In its very construction, then, the Women's Fund Memorial Building, with its ample space for dissection, was progressive. But the exceptional characteristics of the building went further. Mall explained that, although dissection traditionally took place in a large room, he had adopted a different approach. Likely frustrated by the noise, general commotion, and lack of personal attention associated with large laboratories, he divided the upper floor of the building into nine relatively small dissecting rooms, with eight or ten tables in the largest room and one table in the smallest (fig. 1.11). Mall reported that students preferred the smaller rooms and that professors' fears about student behavior while they rotated between rooms were unsubstantiated.[61]

Mall not only changed the size of the anatomy room; he also created a different laboratory environment. Most anatomists in the late nineteenth century presided over highly unpleasant laboratories. Through the example he set, Mall helped to rectify this situation, but it lingered at some medical schools into the first decade of the twentieth century. Abraham Flexner, in his 1910 report on American and Canadian medical colleges, assessed the dissecting rooms found at a number of the lowest-tier schools: "The conditions in them defy description. The smell is intolerable; the cadavers now putrid." At one college he discovered that the anatomy room "did duty incidentally as a chicken yard: corn was scattered over the floor—along with other things—and poultry fed placidly in the long intervals before instruction in anatomy began."[62] In contrast to the odor and filth Flexner encountered in these spaces, Mall insisted on meticulously clean and well-organized anatomy laboratories (fig. 1.12). Movable wooden bookstands reduced clutter on the dissecting tables and placed reference materials and students' notes within easy reach. The pine floors were saturated weekly with paraffin, and if they became unclean in the interval, then they were scoured immediately with lye and the paraffin reapplied.[63] Most likely the janitors, who were William Hartley and his wife, undertook these tasks. Alan M. Chesney, Mall's student at Johns Hopkins and later dean

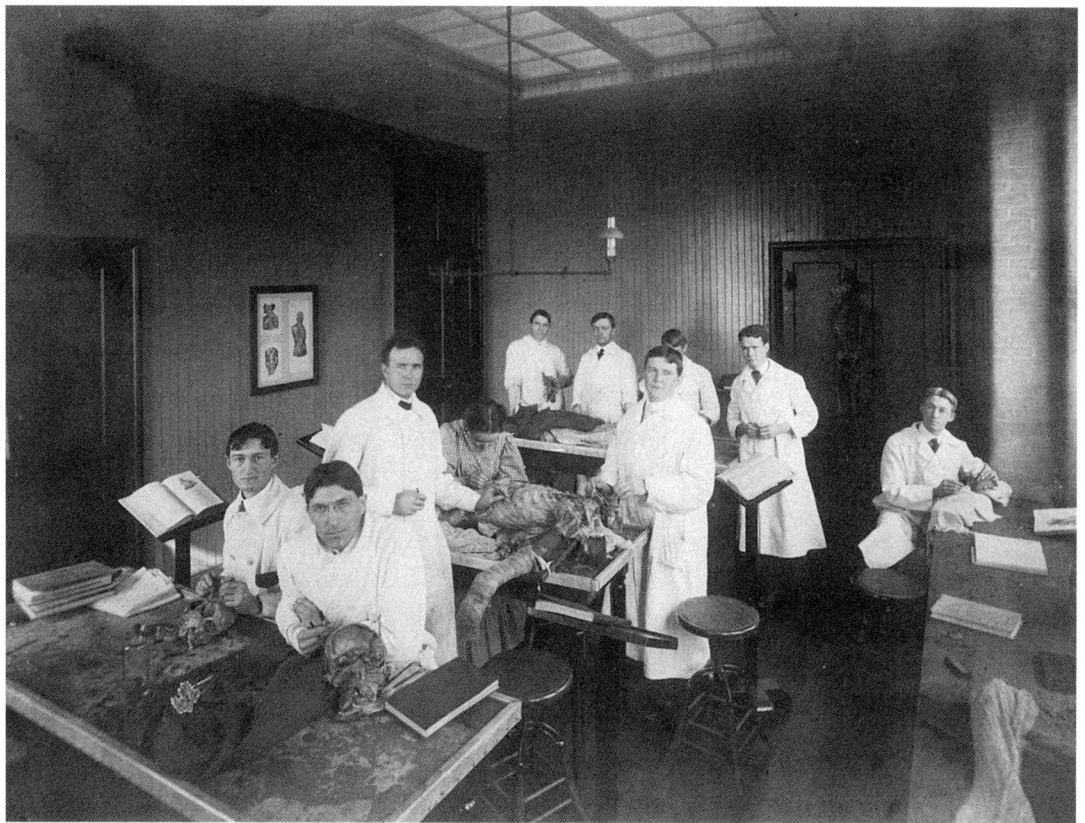

1.12.   Students in anatomy laboratory, Johns Hopkins Medical School, ca. 1900.

and historian of the school, reported that the couple "followed [Mall's] instructions to the letter. Woe betide any student who did not leave the building promptly at 5 P.M. when they took over!"[64]

Mall recognized that clean and carefully furnished rooms facilitated student learning, something observers at Howard University acknowledged in 1924 during the renovation of that school's anatomy laboratory: "The [dissecting] tables have also been painted and shelves for books, hooks for hats, coats, etc., have been constructed. Side tables for notes, directions, etc., will be close at hand for the convenience of the students. Drop lights will be provided, and a system of sanitation put into effect which will make working conditions conducive to greater efficiency."[65] Mall, however, made clear that successfully reconceptualizing the anatomy laboratory involved more than design, maintenance, and furnishings. It also encompassed student behavior.

G. Canby Robinson took Mall's anatomy course when he entered Johns Hopkins Medical School in 1899, and he explained the behavior required by Mall in the novel environment: "The dissecting rooms in Mall's department set a new style. The light, airy, adjoining rooms on the top floor of the anatomical laboratory in which eight to twelve students worked together in well-ordered and clean surroundings were in striking contrast to the usual dissecting halls of that time, where indignities were often played on the social outcasts who ended their terrestrial sojourn in dissecting rooms. Only once was the academic tone of our dissecting room disturbed." Robinson recounted the memorable event. When the sounds of a street organ made their way through one of the room's open windows, a classmate took the spleen from Robinson's table and threw it out the window at the musician. A police officer witnessed the event and returned the spleen to Mall. Robinson continued, "Mall came immediately to the dissecting room with more than usual to say, and ordered those involved in the episode . . . to report immediately to his office. The thrower and his partner, my partner, and I, who had abetted the act, went together to his office to diffuse the blame, and received a scholarly discourse on proper behavior in a dissecting room, on public decency, and on the responsibility of scientists."[66] As Robinson makes clear, Mall sought to create a decorous, academic atmosphere by maintaining a clean and smoothly functioning laboratory and raising standards of behavior.

To this end, Mall even prohibited smoking, an expected activity in anatomy laboratories in this period (see fig. 4.15). Arthur Hertzler, a medical student at Northwestern in the early 1890s, described the convention: "Many a properly raised young man blew his first tobacco smoke across the dissecting tables. Tradition had established that it was impossible to endure the odors of the dissecting room unless one smoked. I chose the lesser odor and did not smoke."[67] The flammability of materials in the room, particularly the paraffin applied to the floor and possibly the embalming fluid, which contained carbolic acid (phenol) and alcohol, may have further encouraged Mall's ban.

Achieving Mall's intended environment also required close attention to light, ventilation, and heat. Mall reported that he continued the practice of many American medical schools and placed anatomy on the building's top floor to take advantage of the illumination provided by skylights. Additionally, the numerous and wide windows of the Women's Fund Memorial Building "reach[ed] nearly to the ceiling, thus giving ample side light for each room."[68] Mall took great care in designing the ventilating and heating systems, the latter created in collaboration with Baltimore's Bartlett, Hayward, and Company, best known for its ironwork but also active in other fields, including engineering. The heating system for the Women's Fund Memorial Building began with cold air

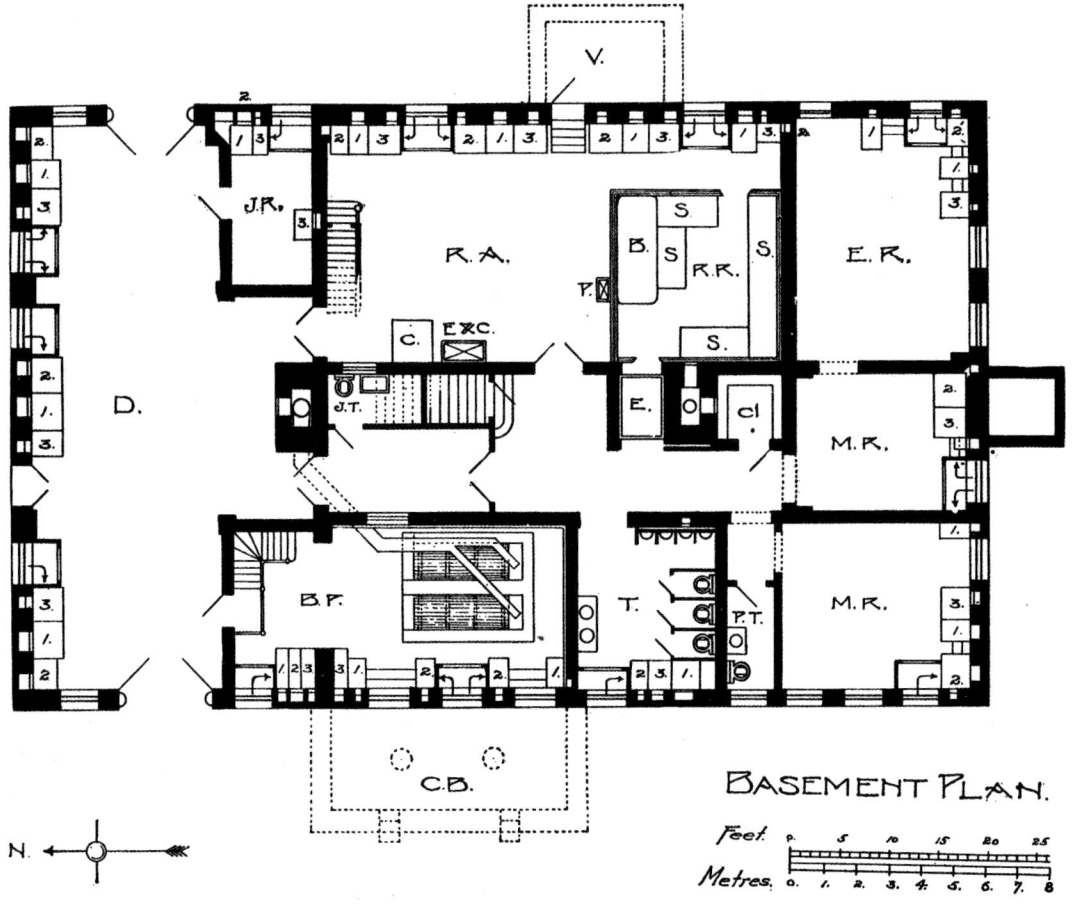

FIG. 1.

D, Driveway.   *RA*, Refrigerating apparatus.   *C*, Condenser.   *E & C*, Engine and compressor.   *P*, Pump.   *B*, Brine tank. *RR*, Refrigerating room.   *S*, Shelves.   *ER*, Embalming room.   *MR*, Machine room.   *BP*, Boiler pit.   *T*, Toilet.   *PT*, Private toilet.   *E*, Elevator.   *Cl*, Closet.   *JT*, Janitor's toilet.   *JR*, Storage room.   *V*, Chemical vault.   *CB*, Coal bins.

    The figures 1, 2 and 3 in the boxes communicating with the hot-air shafts indicate that the shafts communicate with the first, second and third floors respectively.

1.13.   Women's Fund Memorial Building, Johns Hopkins Medical School, 1894, George Archer, architect, plan, basement.

entering the building through the basement windows. The chilly air was warmed by steam coils, and it then moved through a unique shaft to each room. With regard to ventilation, on the opposite side of the room from the site where the heated air arrived was the "ventilating register," which communicated either directly or via a duct with one of two airshafts. A steam coil heated the air in each central shaft and generated a continuous upward current, thereby ventilating the structure.[69] Across the street, the Johns Hopkins Hospital enjoyed its own carefully designed heating and ventilating systems, developed with the assistance of an earlier iteration of Bartlett, Hayward, and Company. As one report affirmed, the hospital "is a good laboratory for teaching the practical applications of the laws of hygiene to heating, ventilation, house-drainage, and other sanitary matters."[70] Mall may well have studied the hospital systems when he planned the Women's Fund Memorial Building. Writing after two years in the anatomy building, Mall reported that its systems had performed well. He called the heating and ventilating "very perfect" and boasted that no gases or smells had passed between floors through one of the central shafts.[71]

Regardless of how much effort went into planning the dissecting rooms, however, they had little educational value without cadavers. As Mall explained it, the Johns Hopkins Medical School suffered from a lack of anatomical material much of the year, with a relative abundance during the hot summers, which meant a need for careful preservation of bodies at all times.[72] An enclosed driveway in the basement of the Women's Fund Memorial Building allowed for the discreet transfer of anatomical material into the basement, designed specifically for embalming and storing cadavers (fig. 1.13). Mall advocated preserving each body by injecting it with carbolic acid diluted with glycerin and alcohol, covering it in "vaselin," wrapping it in paper, adding more "vaselin," wrapping it in muslin, and then freezing it. Freezing the body required a specially designed room and cooling apparatus, both built by the Remington Machine Company of Wilmington, Delaware (fig. 1.14). Cold brine pumped through a series of pipes affixed to the ceiling cooled the storage room. A tank of brine within the cold room further absorbed heat when the brine was not running through the ceiling coils. To help maintain the low temperature, the designers carefully insulated the vault and the door, which measured more than a foot thick. The shelves could hold approximately two hundred bodies. During the planning of the cold storage, Mall learned much from the similar setup at Columbia University's College of Physicians and Surgeons, but this type of storage was still in its infancy, and Mall admitted that his apparatus could be improved. Nevertheless, he was pleased: "after we are accustomed to a cold-storage plant for the preservation of anatomical material it is difficult to understand how we ever got along without it."[73]

In fact, good preservation techniques went hand in hand with the clean, well-organized educational space Mall desired. Hertzler's description of dissecting in the early 1890s at Northwestern proves the point. There, as was typical, the janitor had responsibility for the cadavers: "The dissecting room in our day was a mess. The preservation of material was then not understood, certainly not by our custodian."[74] In the absence of sound preservation, cadavers could either rot, resulting in a dirty and disagreeable anatomy experience, or dry out, making dissection difficult.

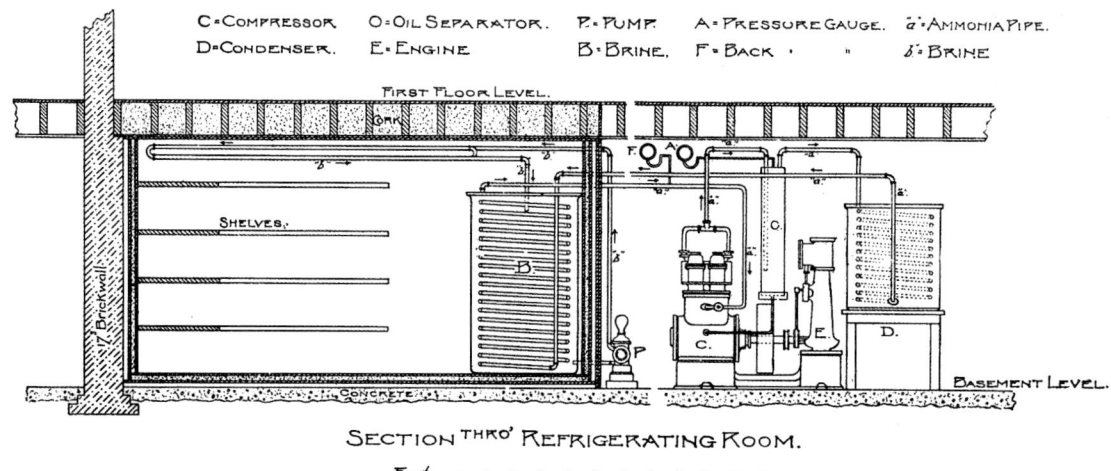

ANATOMICAL LABORATORY

JOHNS HOPKINS UNIVERSITY.

C = COMPRESSOR.   O = OIL SEPARATOR.   P = PUMP.   A = PRESSURE GAUGE.   *a* = AMMONIA PIPE.
D = CONDENSER.   E = ENGINE   B = BRINE.   F = BACK   "   *b* = BRINE

FIRST FLOOR LEVEL.

SHELVES.

BASEMENT LEVEL.

SECTION THRO' REFRIGERATING ROOM.

Feet.
Metres.

FIG. 4.   PLAN OF COLD-STORAGE APPARATUS AND VAULT.
In addition to the insulation, as shown in the diagram, there is another two-inch air space covering all six sides of the vault.

1.14.   Women's Fund Memorial Building, Johns Hopkins Medical School, 1894, section through refrigerating room.

The Women's Fund Memorial Building demonstrates the effort educators made to design effective laboratories, but progressive medical education in this period also meant providing space for emerging disciplines. Between the 1860s and the opening of Johns Hopkins Medical School, medical colleges began teaching numerous new subjects. In the clinical years, gynecology, pediatrics, psychiatry, hygiene, and other areas joined medicine, surgery, and obstetrics. In the preclinical years, the scope expanded from a focus on anatomy, the only laboratory science examined in depth in the 1860s, to include physiology, physiological chemistry, pathology, pharmacology, and bacteriology.[75] More specifically, by 1870, nearly ninety years after Harvard Medical School opened, it had grown from two to nine departments. Between 1870 and 1900, the school expanded by thirteen departments, and Harvard's faculty struggled to accommodate the additional areas of teaching and research in the Boylston Street facility built in 1883.[76]

At Johns Hopkins Medical School, Mall emphasized the anatomy department's commitment to histology (microscopic anatomy), an area of study not offered at many schools. As Mall explained, "anatomy, taught for many centuries, has recently been made a new science through the

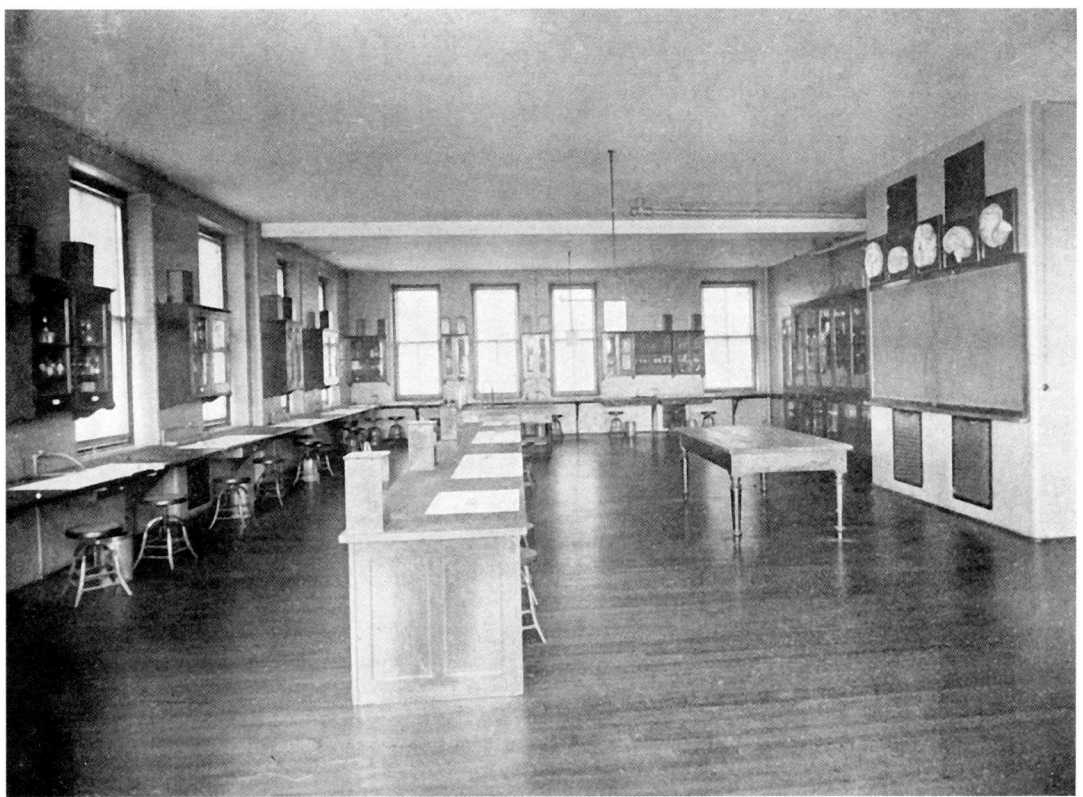

1.15. Women's Fund Memorial Building, Johns Hopkins Medical School, 1894, George Archer, architect, second floor, histology laboratory.

studies in embryology and histology. . . . The great influence of histology is not yet fully felt[,] . . . but its importance has been shown over and over again in the branches fundamental to medicine."[77] This commitment to histology resulted in a laboratory in the Women's Fund Memorial Building with room for enough benches to seat up to fifty to sixty students. Here students in the first-year histology course listened to lectures with demonstrations and engaged in laboratory work (fig. 1.15). Another optional but highly popular course provided the opportunity to examine one type of tissue and to prepare specimens. As with gross anatomy, Mall conceived of histology as an exercise in investigation: "We find that with the research method of teaching we can lead the student much further into the subject than without it. Students do better work when you expect much of them than when you expect little."[78]

As medical education and medical school design changed in the United States in the late nineteenth century, shifts in medical training and the architecture of medical schools also occurred in other places. In his examination of Owens College Medical School's 1874 building and its 1894 expansion in Manchester, England, historian James Hopkins reveals that the faculty who had studied in Germany brought home from that country ideas about laboratory design. Moreover, he highlights the alterations in design undertaken at Owens College Medical School when the faculty began to conduct research, embrace hands-on laboratory instruction, and add fields of study to the curriculum.[79] If American medical educators knew about the changes under way in locations such as Manchester, however, they did not mention them.

Among American medical colleges, Johns Hopkins Medical School offered an exceptional education by the standards of the 1890s, with experiential preclinical and clinical training provided over a period of four years. As Mall and others recognized, the buildings played an essential role in progressive medical training. When creating the campus plan, the Johns Hopkins medical faculty put tremendous effort into the design of the buildings and drew on the institute model they had encountered in Germany. The Johns Hopkins facilities, however, were far from ornate. As Howard A. Kelly, one of the founding faculty, observed in 1913, medical schools required sufficient facilities and equipment, but they did not need extravagance. He declared, "Some of the best work ever done there [at Johns Hopkins Medical School] was in the early days of 'high thinking and low living' by a few choice spirits."[80] The innovations of the Women's Fund Memorial Building did not diminish the fact that the Johns Hopkins faculty struggled to construct the medical school with limited funds and never developed the quadrangle they originally envisioned.

The leadership at Harvard Medical School was happy to fill this architectural gap. Unlike Johns Hopkins Medical School when its campus was built in the 1890s, Harvard Medical School suffered no lack of finances when it relocated in the early 1900s. A pioneer in the medical education reforms of the late nineteenth century and determined to maintain its place in the top tier of American medical colleges, Harvard Medical School in 1906 occupied an unparalleled facility: the grand, formally organized quadrangle based on the German institute design that had eluded the medical educators at Johns Hopkins.

Harvard Medical School and the Full American Expression of the German Institute Design

By 1901, the Harvard Medical School leadership had launched a campaign for a new home. Although they had believed that the 1883 building on Boylston Street would serve the school for quite some time, in under

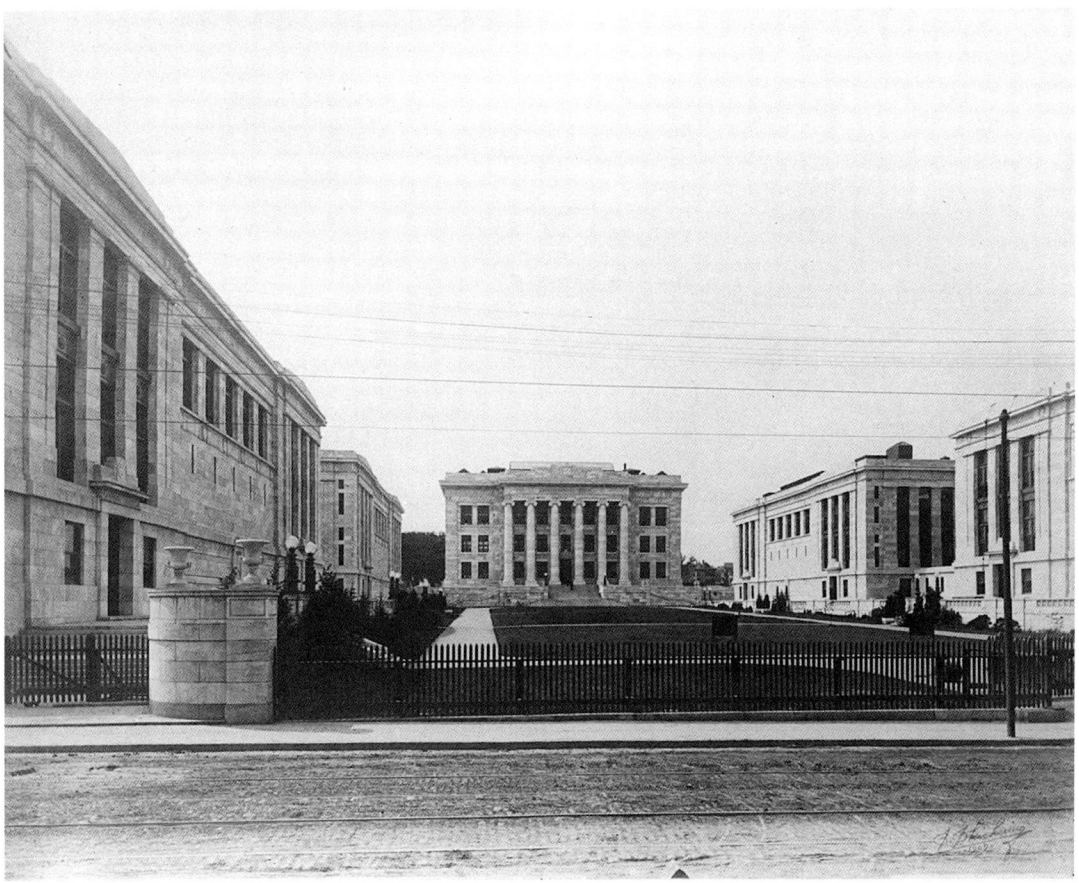

1.16.   Harvard Medical School, 1906, Shepley, Rutan, and Coolidge, architects.

two decades the growth in the student body and the rapid changes in medical education had rendered the facility obsolete.[81] In 1906, Harvard Medical School moved to an entirely new campus in the Longwood section of Boston.

Funded primarily by substantial donations from a handful of individuals, the medical campus contained five buildings constructed for a staggering sum in excess of $2.6 million or nearly twenty times the combined cost of the Women's Fund Memorial Building and the Physiological Building at Johns Hopkins Medical School (fig. 1.16).[82] The classical revival–style marble ensemble designed by Shepley, Rutan, and Coolidge invoked one of the most famous American collegiate quadrangles: Thomas Jefferson's Academical Village at the University of Virginia. The size of the buildings heightened the quadrangle's imposing feel. Each structure provided as much space as the medical school's entire previous home.[83] At five times the size of the school's 1883 structure on

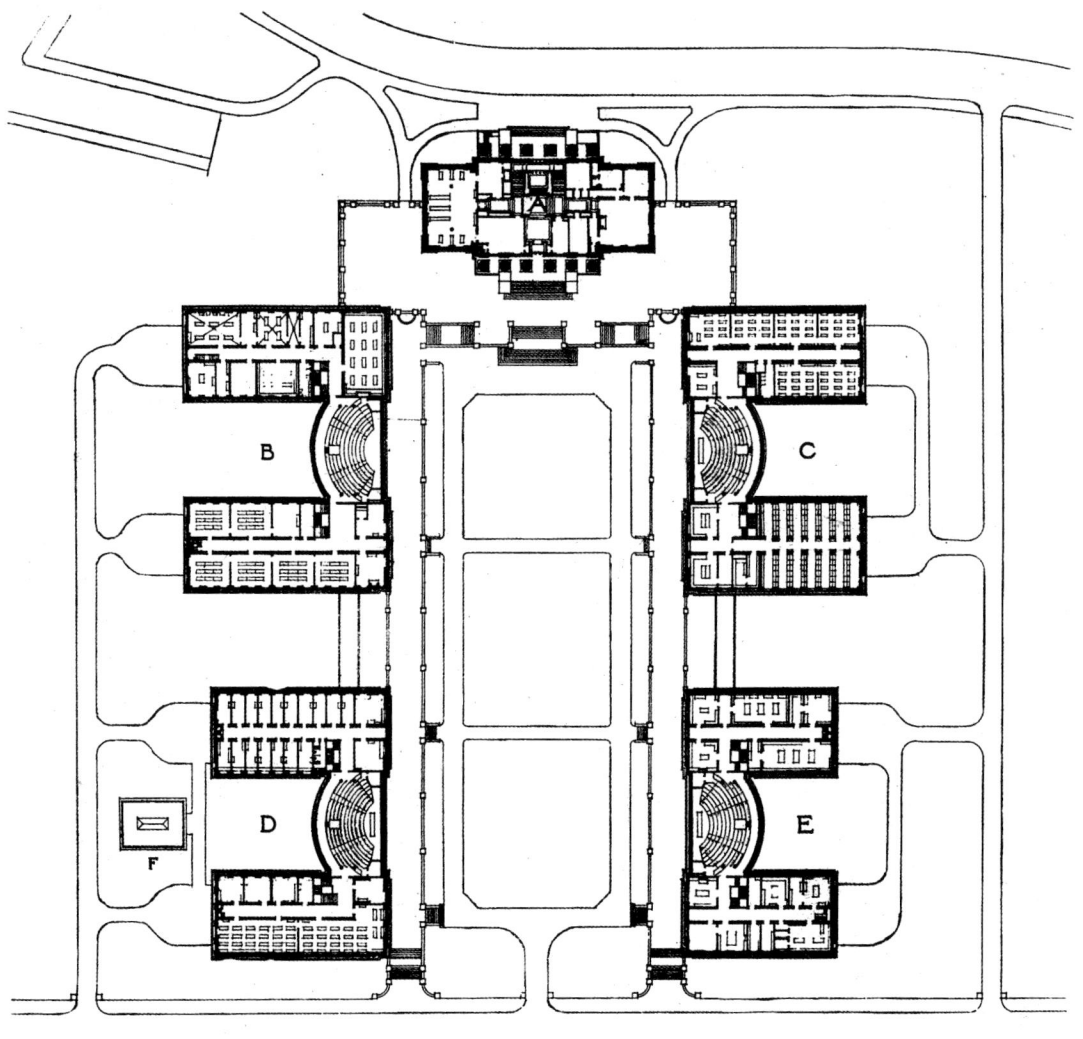

A - ADMINISTRATION BUILDING
B - ANATOMY AND HISTOLOGY BUILDING
C - PHYSIOLOGY AND PHYSIOLOGICAL
     CHEMISTRY BUILDING
D - BACTERIOLOGY AND PATHOLOGY BUILDING
E - HYGIENE AND PHARMACOLOGY BUILDING
F - ANIMAL HOUSE

PLAN OF FIRST FLOORS

1.17.   Harvard Medical School, 1906, Shepley, Rutan, and Coolidge, architects, plan, first floors.

Boylston Street, the 1906 Longwood facility was aspirational, a reflection not of what the school was at the time of its move but of what it wanted to become. As Daniel Bluestone has noted, the 1906 building allocated far more space for laboratories relative to lecture halls than the 1883 building, which by 1900 had no room to accommodate the growing emphasis on laboratory instruction, the increasing number of academic departments, and the expanding commitment to faculty research.[84] Although some schools did enlarge their facilities incrementally on their original site, many medical colleges shared Harvard's sudden transformation when they relocated and rebuilt, trading antiquated facilities for often far bigger and more complete modern educational buildings.

The extraordinary size of the school notwithstanding, Harvard's medical faculty, after rapidly running out of space in their previous building, had wanted to ensure that the new campus would serve the school for generations. The projecting wings on the back of four of the structures could be made longer and then connected without disrupting the center of the quadrangle (fig. 1.17).[85] This time, the faculty achieved their goal: Harvard Medical School still remained on this site after nearly 120 years, and additions to the buildings have proceeded without compromising the quadrangle's interior, as the medical school leaders and architects had hoped (see fig. I.1).

In line with the German institute design, separate structures divided the campus by academic discipline. The building at the head of the quadrangle held primarily the administration and the museum. Each of the other structures provided space for two fields of study. The wings of these U-shaped buildings housed the laboratories, with library and lecture hall in the connecting section.[86] Only one laboratory building varied from this overall layout. In contrast to the disciplines grouped in Buildings B, C, and D, respectively, those in Building E had "so little in common that the libraries remain[ed] distinct."[87] The designers placed the separate libraries in the wings of Building E and reserved for a future hygiene laboratory the area above the lecture hall that usually contained the joint library.

Unlike the Johns Hopkins Medical School leadership, who never explicitly mentioned the school's indebtedness to the German institute model, at Harvard Medical School the faculty acknowledged the roots of the school's design. American physicians in this period applied the word *institute* to a range of characteristics of a medical school, but one use of the term denoted a distinct physical structure housing a specific discipline. A Harvard Medical School publication explained: "To Professor H. P. Bowditch belongs the credit . . . in association with Professor J. C. Warren, of devising a scheme along the broad lines on which the plans of the new School have been worked out. He proposed a group of buildings arranged somewhat on the plan of the modern German medical school—that the various departments should be housed in separate 'Institutes'—such as the Institute of Anatomy, the Institute of Physiology."[88] Both Bowditch and Warren had studied in Europe, but Bowditch's correspondence in particular suggests that the footprint and

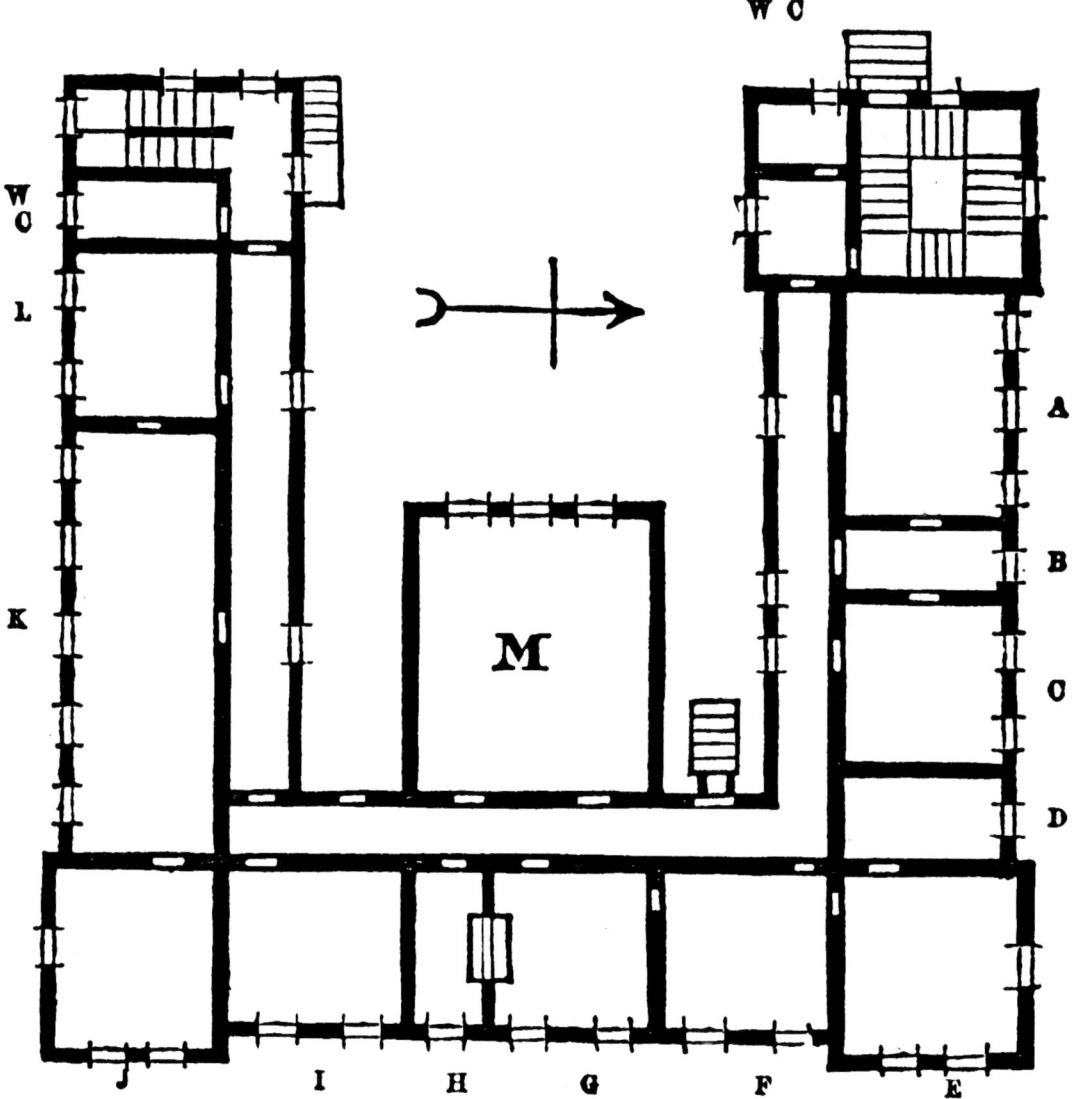

1.18.   Physiological Institute, University of Leipzig, Germany, 1869, plan, first floor.

interior arrangement of the Harvard Medical School buildings were also drawn on the German prototype.

In 1870, when Bowditch was working in the recently opened Physiological Institute at the University of Leipzig under the direction of renowned physiologist Carl Ludwig, he wrote to the *Boston Medical and Surgical Journal* to describe his experience. He explained that few Americans traveled to Leipzig, as they preferred instead the larger cities, such as Berlin and Vienna, with better clinical opportunities. For fledgling chemists and physiologists, however, Bowditch promised that Leipzig offered the best resources in all of Germany.[89] Indeed, when Ludwig joined the medical faculty at the University of Leipzig in 1865, he created a physiology institute that influenced many young doctors and universities besides Bowditch and Harvard. Ludwig's institute not only made a number of major discoveries, but it also became the preeminent location for investigation and training in physiology.[90] In 1869, Ludwig's institute moved into a new building. In the two decades after 1870, eleven similar institutes erected at different German-speaking universities followed the model of Ludwig's institute.[91] In his letter to the *Boston Medical and Surgical Journal*'s editor, Bowditch took care to describe the structure in detail and asserted that "it is universally acknowledged to be the most complete establishment of the kind in Europe."[92]

The 1906 laboratories at Harvard that Bowditch would later help to plan included several basic components found at Ludwig's institute. The Physiological Institute in Leipzig had a U-shaped plan, with a lecture hall projecting from the rear of the central portion of the first floor (fig. 1.18). As in the Boston buildings, the wings and connecting corridor of the German institute's first floor contained various types of laboratory space in addition to storage and a small library.[93]

Ludwig's Physiological Institute was not the only German institute with a central lecture hall. For example, the first floor of the University of Berlin's Anatomical Institute, built in 1865, contained a central auditorium with laboratory and collection spaces in the wings.[94] Ludwig's institute, however, appears to have been the direct point of contact between this basic plan and the Harvard medical faculty.

The U-shaped design served Harvard Medical School well. On the one hand, it divided each of the laboratory buildings into zones. With the U footprint, the central portion of the structure provided an excellent location for large communal spaces, namely the library and lecture hall. The central area was easily accessible to all faculty and students, while the wings offered more privacy when professors and pupils retreated to their respective laboratories, segregated by discipline, research project, or course.

Laboratory work also required plenty of light. During the design of Harvard Medical School's 1906 campus, Shepley, Rutan, and Coolidge conducted on-site experiments in an attempt to ensure that the buildings were separated enough for sunlight to enter the basement windows even in the winter.[95] The U-shaped plan with its narrow wings punctuated by large windows permitted light, as well as fresh air, to enter all of the laboratory space in the building.

As laboratory teaching and research grew in the United States, the medical school leadership and architects responsible for the designs

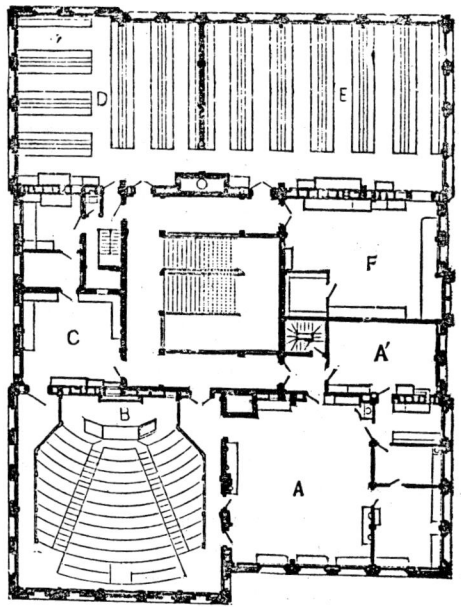

SECOND FLOOR.

A. Laboratory, Physiology.
A'. Mechanic's Room.
B. Lecture Room.
C. Anteroom, Chemistry.
D. Laboratory, Medical Chemistry.
E. Laboratory, General Chemistry.
F. Laboratory, Special Chemical Analysis.

1.19.　　Harvard Medical School, 1883, Ware and
Van Brunt, architects, plan, second floor.

moved away from the rectangular footprints of buildings such as the 1894 Women's Fund Memorial Building at Johns Hopkins Medical School and Harvard Medical School's 1883 Boylston Street facility (fig. 1.19). Although a skylight might provide some extra light to the center of a building with a rectangular footprint, as was the case on Boylston Street, the core of the building lacked sufficient light to house laboratories. Medical educators and architects began to favor structures with narrow wings that typically contained double-loaded corridors. With a double-loaded corridor, a hall runs down the center of the wing with doors opening onto rooms on both sides. When fitted with large windows, the rooms on either side of the hallway receive generous amounts of light (see fig. 1.1). This light-filled design became typical of modern medical schools, where the hallway also sometimes terminated at a large teaching laboratory where light entered from three sides (see figs. 1.9, 2.12, 2.13, 2.14, and 3.5). Medical school designers could, and did, arrange narrow wings in many shapes besides a U, including the I footprint (e.g., Howard University's 1927 medical school) and the grid footprint (e.g., Vanderbilt University's 1925 medical school). These shapes allowed not only access to light but also relatively easy expansion of the wings in the future.

Like medical schools, mental hospitals constructed according to the linear plan utilized a series of narrow wings containing rows of windows. Also called the Kirkbride plan after physician Thomas S. Kirkbride (1809–1883), whose influential book promoted the design, the linear plan became standard for American asylums in the mid-nineteenth century. The asylums remained in use at the beginning of the twentieth century and would have been familiar to architects and physicians in the early 1900s. With this plan, the building contained a series of wings composed mostly of double-loaded corridors, with each successive wing set slightly back to form a wide V (fig. 1.20). Treatment required patients to have ample access to the natural environment for its restorative vistas and healthy breezes. This principle dictated not only the placement of mental hospitals in rural locations but also the V shape, which ensured that all

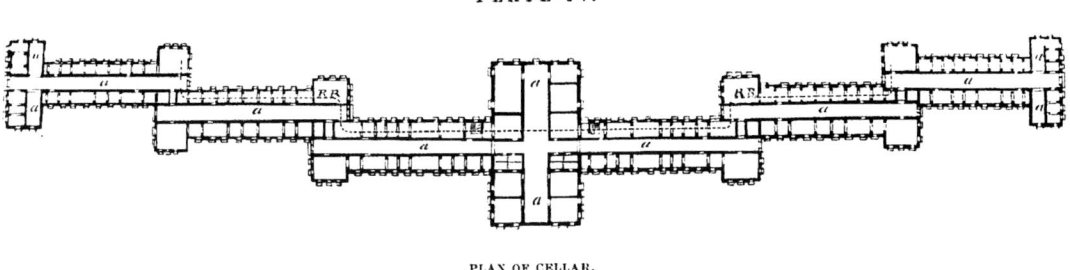

1.20.   Hospital on the linear plan, Samuel Sloan, architect, plan, cellar (*top*) and basement or first floor (*bottom*), published in Thomas Kirkbride's impactful book, *On the Construction, Organization, and General Arrangements of Hospitals for the Insane.*

rooms had unobstructed views of the landscape around the asylum.[96] For mental hospitals, the V footprint's intensive use of land mattered little on their expansive sites. In contrast, medical schools typically sat on closely bounded city lots, on college campuses surrounded by other structures, or on open plots with considerable space reserved for hospital construction. The linear plan demanded far too much land for its adoption by medical school designers considering ways to connect the laboratory wings. Instead, they turned to more compact footprints.

More than thirty years would pass between the publication of Bowditch's letter describing Ludwig's institute and the completion of the Longwood buildings, but the Harvard Medical School facilities were still considered very much of their time, with the link to Germany recognized. Faculty member J. Collins Warren, like Bowditch, was instrumental in the construction of the 1906 facilities. Warren wrote that "a plant of . . . a series of buildings for the School [was] similar in general plan to those which Dr. Bowditch pointed out existed in some of the *most recently* organized of the German medical schools."[97]

Although the Harvard Medical School faculty celebrated the quadrangle's indebtedness to German medical schools, architect Charles

Coolidge disagreed, stating that German laboratories "were not adaptable to our needs." He contrasted the Harvard buildings with the German ones. As he saw it, "their system is different from ours, the professor living in the school, with his private laboratory joining the main laboratory, and the whole plant being finished without reference to future extension, which renders their problem easier to solve."[98] It is hard to imagine that the German faculty did not plan for additions to their structures, and in fact, professors did not always live in German medical institutes.[99] In comparing the Harvard Medical School facilities with those of Germany, the faculty and Coolidge likely responded to different agendas, one striving to highlight similarities and the other, dissimilarities. Coolidge wanted to ensure that his firm's design did not appear derivative. The Harvard Medical School faculty, however, had chosen this campus plan—with its separate buildings and U-shaped laboratory structures—not only because it was familiar to them from their time abroad but also because it represented a design that had proven successful for physicians in the world's leading medical nation. They eagerly underscored the architectural connection.

The faculty's decision to construct a medical school in keeping with the German institute plan had a tremendous impact on students' daily academic lives. The institute plan reinforced and promoted the curriculum. Students at Harvard Medical School had a block schedule during their preclinical years, and in keeping with reformed medical education, they spent significant time in the laboratory, along with time spent in demonstrations, conferences, and lectures.[100] The laboratory buildings at Harvard Medical School paired the same subjects that were grouped in the block schedule. During students' first semester of medical school, they studied anatomy and histology, and Building B housed both (see fig. 1.17). Inside the building, the two departments shared the central lecture hall and library. The use of the latter would in particular have brought faculty from both disciplines in contact with each other and encouraged the transfer of ideas between departments. Pedagogy and architecture together signified to students and faculty that these disciplines were closely related within modern medicine.

The buildings carried the relationship between pedagogy and architecture a step further. As students advanced through their training, they moved through the buildings progressively. Journalist Ralph Bergengren hinted at this situation shortly after the medical school opened: "Each department building thus bring[s] together the subjects most closely allied in the school curriculum and [is], to all intents and purposes, the home of the individual student while he is mastering them."[101] For the first term of their first year, students learned anatomy and histology in Building B, where they spent their entire academic day, with the exception of excursions to Building A, the administration building. They studied physiology and physiological chemistry in the second half of the year, when they moved to Building C. Their second year began with courses in bacteriology and pathology in Building D. In the second half of the second year, students did not follow a block schedule and instead balanced the remainder of the preclinical work with the beginning of their clinical training. A portion of their time, however, was spent in Building E, where they learned pharmacology and hygiene and completed their trek around the medical school's quadrangle.[102]

Each medical school's faculty organized the progression of courses carefully. Medical educators generally assumed that courses taught concurrently would explicitly or implicitly establish connections with each other. In fact, some criticized the block system because it limited the number of courses a student took each semester and reduced the students' ability to understand relationships between many fields of study.[103] Harvard Medical School, like most medical schools, however, used the block schedule, and faculty member W. T. Councilman described in 1907 the conceptual bases for the course sequence:

> Form and structure come first in the study of objects, so in the first term in the School the time is spent on the study of anatomy. The second term is devoted to physiology or the study of function. In the first term of the second year the student takes up pathology, in which the disorders of form and function are considered. In the second term of the second year he learns and practises the methods which are used in clinical work. This is a natural transition of subjects, and the student goes to clinical work feeling that there is no violent break of connection, but that it is merely a continuation of the kind of work he has been doing.[104]

Despite Councilman's assertion, the correlations between subjects were not "natural" or fixed, and not all schools organized the preclinical subjects the same way. For example, when Syracuse University opened its new medical school facility in 1937, its second-year students learned physiology and bacteriology during the first half of the year and pathology, clinical pathology, and pharmacology during the second half. By aligning physiology with bacteriology, the medical faculty at Syracuse paired the normal functioning of the body (physiology) with an examination of the bacteria that disrupt it (bacteriology). In contrast, the faculty at Harvard

Medical School coupled bacteriology with pathology, which is the study of the impact of disease on the body.[105] Harvard Medical School's quadrangle codified and encouraged the school's particular curriculum and the scientific relationships that underpinned it.

Medical educators debated the curriculum constantly, and each medical school formulated its own version of the reformed system of training. Because medical faculty believed that medical school buildings participated in the pedagogical effort, they worked hard on the buildings' designs. Compared with other factors, such as endowment, faculty, access to laboratories and hospitals, and equipment, however, these curricular and architectural differences likely did not create significant variation among graduates. In other words, in the training of modern physicians, the ability to construct, equip, staff, and maintain a facility not too far from a teaching hospital mattered more than the exact form of the medical school. Nevertheless, the tremendous planning—and expense—that went into medical school buildings highlights medical faculties' commitment to architecture as a pedagogical tool.

The physical relationships between departments established by medical educators also encouraged efficient movement of students and faculty. If the most closely aligned disciplines—at least as defined by Harvard Medical School—shared the same building within the 1906 quadrangle, then collaborating faculty had only short distances to travel to interact with one another. In addition, concentrating students' classes within a single building reduced their movement around the quadrangle over the course of the day. Moreover, as Harvard Medical School faculty member and dean Henry A. Christian explained, the block schedule itself improved efficiency. It "increase[d] the amount of time actually available for study" by minimizing students' daily travel: rather than moving between several rooms during the day, students spent the morning in one laboratory and the afternoon in another.[106]

Efficiency, a Progressive Era obsession that permeated American society, remained a concern for medical educators and architects throughout this period. The consolidation of the Johns Hopkins Medical School on one campus and its location near the hospital served to reduce the movement of students and faculty and to increase their efficiency. Once medical educators affirmed the need for hands-on clinical training, they strove to consistently locate medical schools near hospitals and sometimes connected them with corridors or tunnels. The Harvard Medical School leadership worked to ensure that a hospital soon joined its new medical school, and in 1913 the Peter Bent Brigham Hospital opened directly behind the medical school quadrangle.

As at Johns Hopkins Medical School, the faculty at Harvard Medical School celebrated the school's laboratories for teaching and research, proximity to clinical resources, space for expanding areas of study, room for teaching in small sections, and technology designed specifically for medical education. The last generated an enthusiastic response from art and architecture critic Frederick W. Coburn. Inspired by the "light heart throb of the power plant" constructed for Harvard Medical School and current and future hospitals, Coburn used the human body as a metaphor for the mechanical system designed by engineers Densmore and LeClear. Within this metaphor, the ventilation system allowed the facility to breathe. It transmitted clean air to lecture and study spaces and purged foul air from dissecting rooms, animal cages, and laboratories containing noxious chemicals. Coburn's attention also settled on cadaver preservation, that mechanically challenging and relatively unique component of medical education. Coburn outlined the system at Harvard Medical School for cooling brine in the powerhouse and pumping it to refrigeration rooms in the medical school buildings. For Coburn, the medical school, which he believed "probably exceeds any other institution in its special requirements of a sanitary nature," provided a glimpse into the future when homes would be cooled as well as heated. Impressed by the plant, Coburn affirmed, "All the physical conditions seem to have been made as favorable to teaching as is humanly possible at this time."[107]

Despite the tremendous variations in size, grandeur, construction time line, and comprehensive planning, much united the facilities designed for Johns Hopkins Medical School and Harvard Medical School, including a shared commitment to the institute plan. In the end, the choice to house the academic departments in a series of separate buildings promoted an understanding of the medical sciences as relatively discrete areas of study. The American campuses shared this architectural and conceptual division with their German prototypes. Historian Charles E. McClelland has written of German universities that "the walls of the institute . . . buildings . . . were mute representatives of the walls between disciplines, even within the same faculty."[108] If the educators planning the medical schools at Johns Hopkins and Harvard accepted this idea, others took issue with it and relied instead on the unified medical school types—the single building for preclinical studies and the medical school–hospital, both of which encouraged a different notion of medical training and science. Nevertheless, although medical schools diverged in their campus plans and the conceptions of science they supported, they uniformly championed the laboratory and hands-on learning, two undertakings that involved the museum.

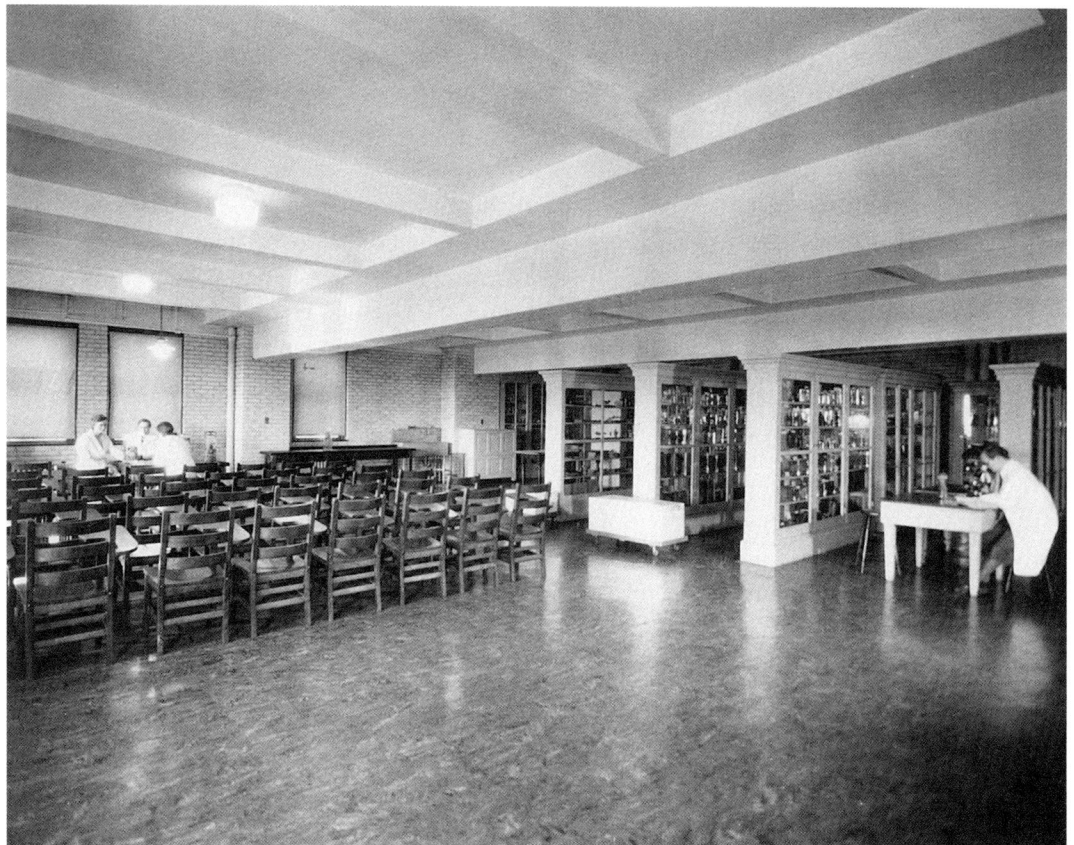

1.21.   Woman's Medical College of Pennsylvania, 1930, Ritter and Shay, architects, pathology museum and
         lecture room. Photograph ca. 1932. At far right a student or faculty member uses the microscope, while
         in the back a group examines specimens in jars on the table.

The Museum as an Extension of the Laboratory

While other organizations, such as physician groups, may have maintained a medical museum, most were part of medical colleges. The museums contained anatomical material, pathological material, or both.
Generally much of the collection was made up of wet specimens—human body parts obtained from autopsies and preserved in jars filled with
transparent fluid. A short text accompanied each specimen to provide
background on the condition and patient. Museums often also included skeletons, models, and medical instruments. The museums allowed
students and faculty to study typical, atypical, and diseased parts of the
body in three dimensions to facilitate both teaching and research (fig.
1.21).[109] Some medical schools allowed public admission to the museum.

Museums predated medical education reform, but historian of science Erin Hunter McLeary has argued that even when American medical education began to embrace the German emphasis on laboratory research, museums remained relevant. Museum proponents did not see a contradiction between the museum and the laboratory because they did not conceive of the clear division between observation and experimentation delineated by many medical historians. Techniques of observation and the skills associated with microscopy were fundamental to both museum and laboratory work. Even more, educators intended the museum to function as a site of active learning, where students drew, described, prepared, and handled specimens, all in keeping with the tenets of progressive medical education. Especially when cadavers were hard to obtain and dissection opportunities slim, the museum provided a critical alternative mode of hands-on instruction. Additionally, as the twentieth century began, medical faculties understood the taxonomic efforts of museum curators as scientific work and a form of original investigation.[110]

In his study of the medical museums at the University of Michigan, Peter M. McIsaac affirms that museums played a critical role in the development of modern medicine at Michigan and elsewhere, and he argues that today's narrow definition of the laboratory makes it difficult to reconstruct a time when the laboratory encompassed the museum and its specimens.[111] When Harvard Medical School's 1906 quadrangle opened, the pathology department's sole criticism of the campus revealed the connection the faculty made between the museum and the laboratory: "It is unfortunate that it has seemed advisable to place the pathological collection in the Warren Anatomical Museum [in Building A], which is so far distant from the Pathological building [Building D]. To obviate this difficulty to some extent, provision has been made in the laboratory for housing a teaching collection of pathological specimens."[112] Likely also a response to the Warren Anatomical Museum's location in Building A, the anatomy and histology departments maintained space for teaching collections near their laboratories in Building B.

Typically, neither design nor size set the museum apart from the rest of the medical school. The majority of American medical colleges constructed between 1893 and 1940 contained single-story museums, without the mezzanines that distinguished the most famous of these spaces, and they were usually rectangular in footprint. Furthermore, museums required ample illumination for examining specimens. With its rectangular footprint and many windows, the museum matched in basic form any number of other rooms in the building. Only the furniture—rows of cases for organizing and viewing specimens—set these rooms

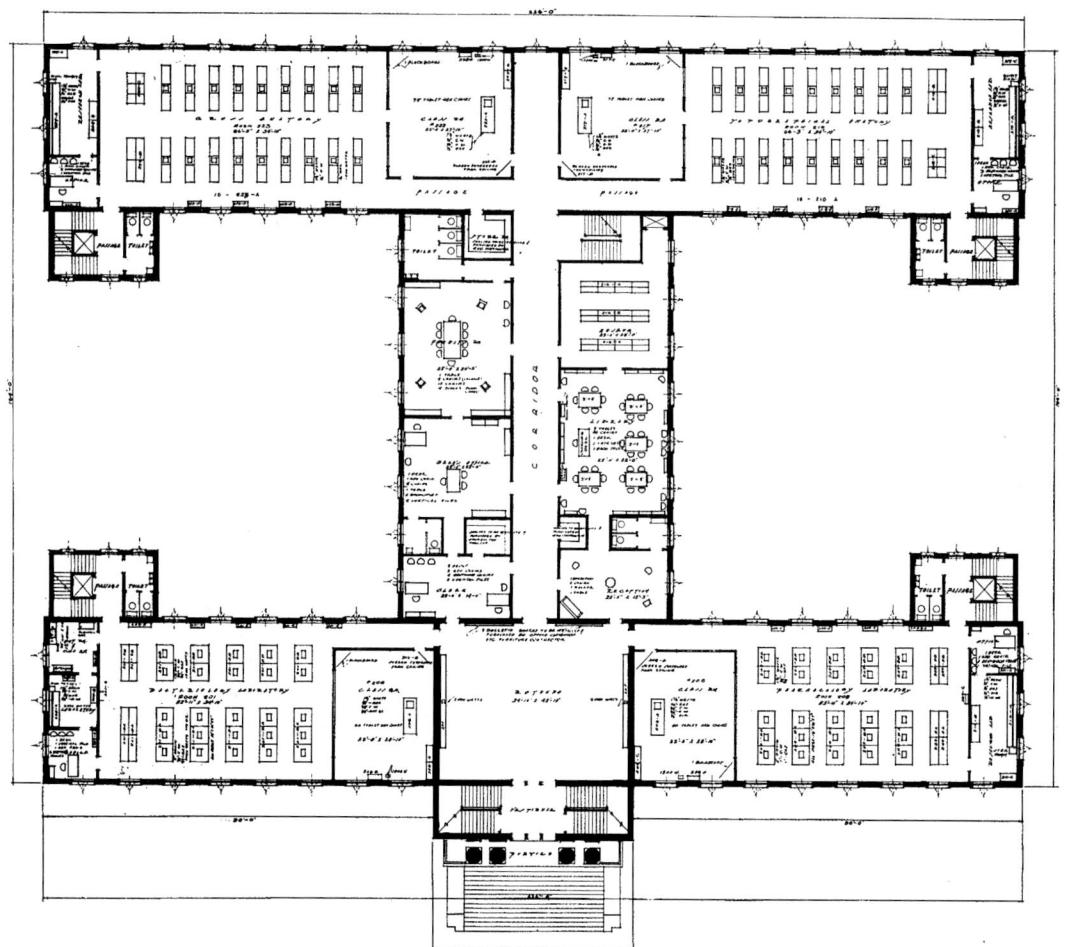

PLAN OF FIRST FLOOR, SHOWING EQUIPMENT

1.22.   Howard University College of Medicine, 1927, Albert I. Cassell, architect, plan, first floor. Note museum just below stairwell in central wing with rows of cases in the middle of the room.

apart (fig. 1.22). Sometimes the museum also enjoyed a separate space for receiving or preparing specimens. At Howard University's medical school, an elevator connected the museum on the first floor directly to the preparation room in the basement. The museum, however, generally commanded only a small percentage of the school's overall square footage. The modest museum facilities likely struggled to house growing collections and may account in part for McLeary's observation that "medical museums were often smelly and cramped, unpleasant."[113] The architecture suggests that in most schools the museum was a necessary but not dominant component of education and research.

On occasion museums occupied more lavish facilities. Extensive

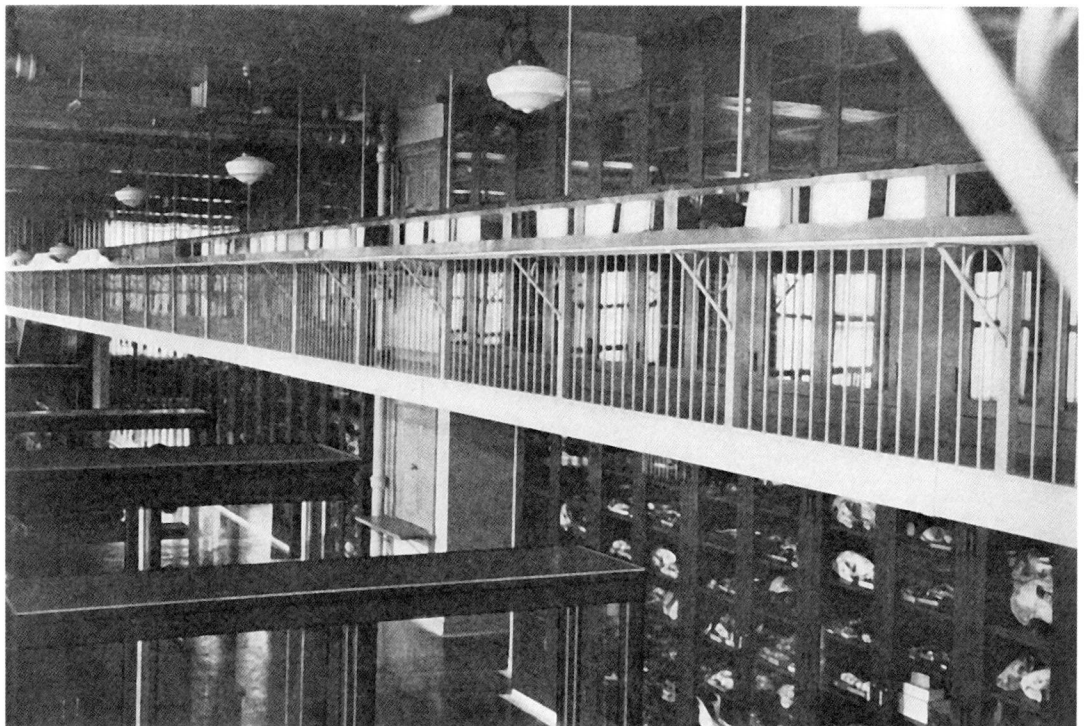

1.23.   Western Reserve University School of Medicine, 1924, Coolidge and Shattuck, architects, Hamann
Museum of Comparative Anthropology and Anatomy.

collections, significant financial resources, and enthusiastic faculty or
curators characterized the schools that constructed larger and sometimes more ornate museums. These museums might follow the design
identified by Adams as typical of medical museums: a rectangular space
augmented by a narrow mezzanine that she calls the doughnut in the
box. Not new, this design had, for example, been employed for numerous
well-known museums of natural history.[114] In 1924, Western Reserve
University School of Medicine's Hamann Museum of Comparative
Anthropology and Anatomy, as well as the school's smaller pathology
museum, adopted this form (fig. 1.23).

Few, if any, American medical schools enjoyed a museum that
matched in size or magnificence the Warren Anatomical Museum, constructed in 1906 by Harvard Medical School. In 1888, John Shaw Billings
had proclaimed the Warren Anatomical Museum "the best museum
connected with a medical school in this country."[115] Nearly twenty years
later, Harvard Medical School's facility provided the museum with an
impressive home, one fit for the famous collection. In Building A, the administration building at the head of the quadrangle, the central staircase

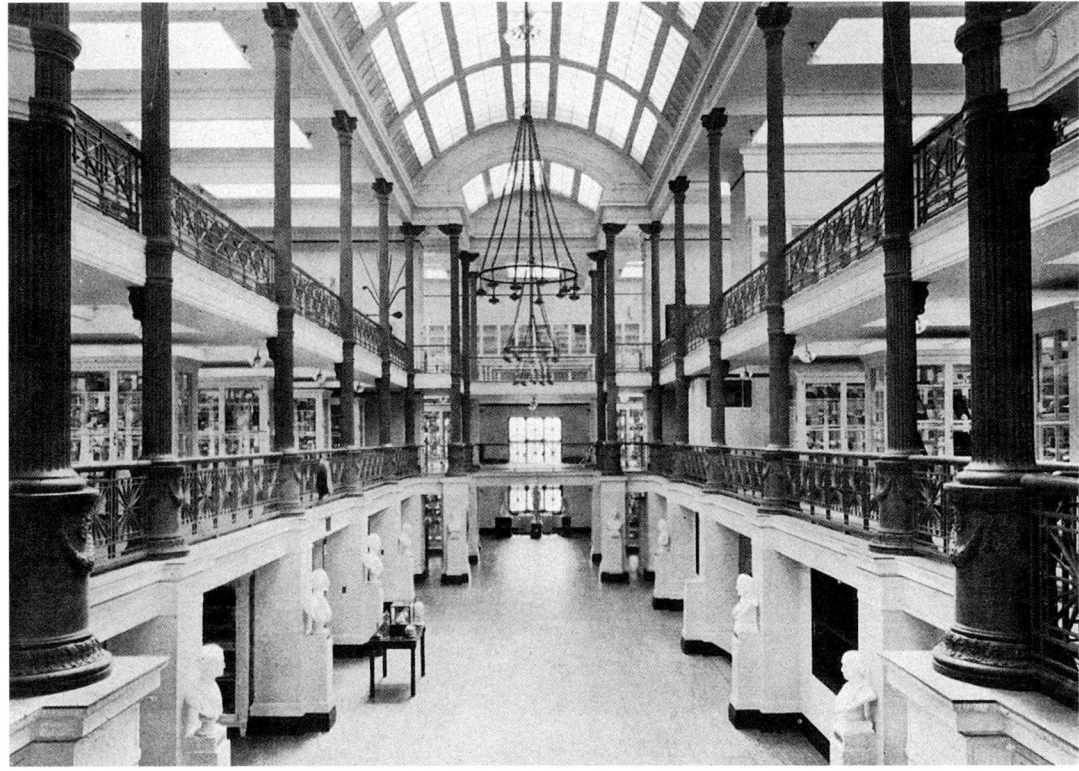

1.24.   Harvard Medical School, 1906, Shepley, Rutan, and Coolidge, architects, Warren Anatomical
         Museum, Building A.

terminated at the Grand Hall on the third floor (fig. 1.24). Here the
Warren Anatomical Museum extended from the base of the hall through
two galleries for an extraordinary twenty-two thousand square feet of
floor space.[116] From the Grand Hall's marble floor, ornamented cast iron
columns and railings drew the eye upward to immense skylights. Light
flooded the museum from the glass vault in the center of the ceiling, the
glazing over the upper galleries, and the windows in the alcoves on the
first gallery and the main floor. Floor lights—large sections of glass in the
floor—punctuated much of the second gallery and allowed light to pass to
the first gallery. As the museum's curator noted in 2015, "the grandeur of
the space . . . and its placement as the focal point of the Harvard Medical
School quad was a clear statement in 1906 as to its importance as an anatomy and pathology classroom and laboratory."[117] At the 1906 dedication
of the quadrangle, Thomas Dwight, a professor of anatomy, called the
museum "the crown of a medical school, the chronicle of its progress."[118]

     Some departments dispersed the museum collections throughout
the laboratories and other spaces rather than construct a dedicated

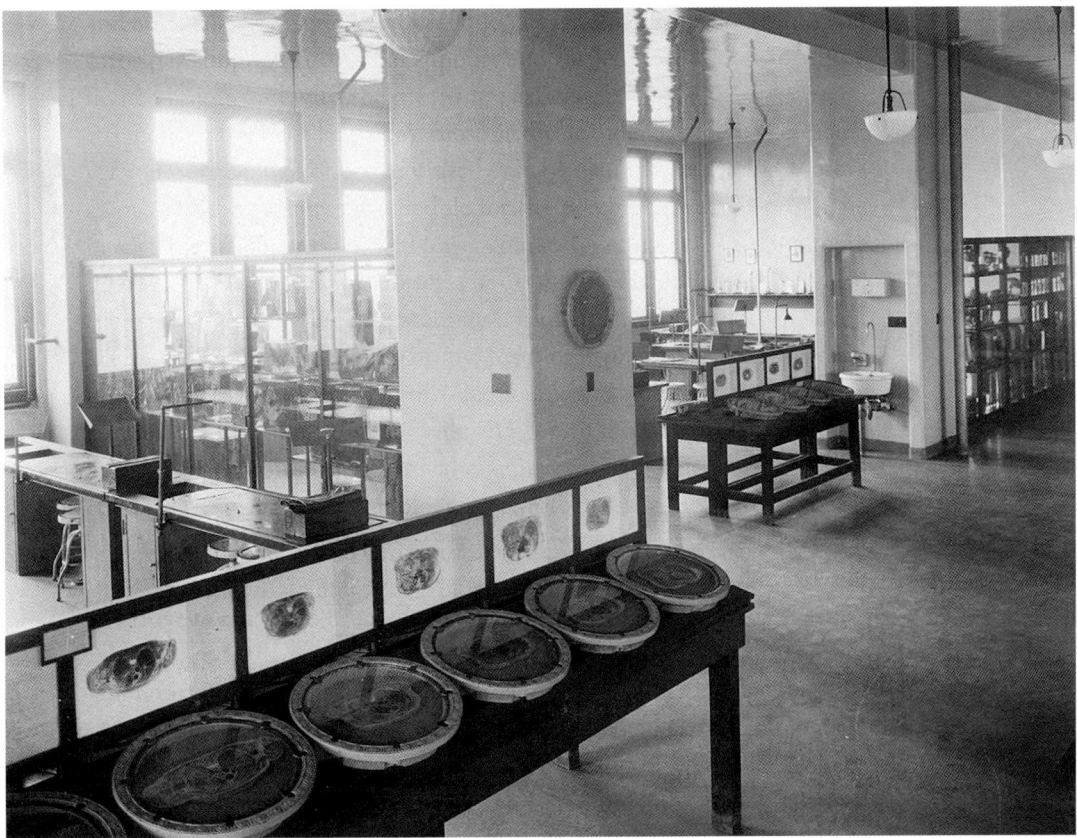

1.25.   Washington University School of Medicine, 1914, Theodore C. Link, architect, gross anatomy laboratory
          with cases and displays for museum collection. Photograph ca. 1920.

room for the museum. At the medical schools of both Washington
University in St. Louis and Johns Hopkins University, the pathology
departments maintained separate museum facilities, but the anatomy
departments did not. This choice may have devalued the museum
architecturally, but it integrated the collection more seamlessly into
the teaching and research of the department. In 1926, the professor of
anatomy at Washington University in St. Louis described the anatomy,
neuroanatomy, and histology facilities, which had been only slightly
modified since the buildings opened in 1914. The teaching and research collections still occupied what appear to have been their initial
locations: cases throughout the departments' various rooms, including
the histology and gross anatomy laboratories; the secretary's office,
which housed the histology and embryology research collection; and
a small study room next to the dissecting laboratory, where specimens from the demonstration collection could be left for students to

examine (fig. 1.25). The Washington University professor of anatomy underscored the ready accessibility of the collection: "museum
specimens illustrating the gross structure of the body are placed in
the cases in the [dissecting] laboratory where they may be consulted
at any time."[119]

Similarly, in the Women's Fund Memorial Building at Johns Hopkins Medical School, Mall spread the collection throughout the cases
that lined the dissecting room walls (see fig. 1.11). Although Mall reserved
one room on the third floor as a study room where part of the anatomical
collection could be exhibited and analyzed, Mall pointed out that this
room "loses much of its force, because all the dissecting rooms are study
rooms," with each containing cases of models and specimens.[120] Moreover, in practice the study room hosted special, short-term dissections
and differed little in function from the regular dissecting rooms. For
Mall, the emphasis remained on so-called "fresh" material, or recently
obtained specimens and cadavers, rather than long-preserved material
and models from the museum: "there is no special demand for it [the
study room] as long as the students can make their own dissections."[121] As
McLeary has documented, others shared Mall's opinion. The museum's
utility depended in part on the lack of better opportunities in the clinic,
the autopsy room, or the dissecting laboratory.[122]

In time, museums disappeared from medical colleges. By the 1920s
and 1930s, even as many schools continued to expand their collections,
educators increasingly understood museums as static repositories rather
than active sites of knowledge production. Many museums remained
open until the 1960s, but their relevance to education and research had
begun to diminish decades earlier. In their teaching, faculty increasingly
used fresh material, now more readily available, rather than preserved
specimens, and shifts in pathology research along with the growth of
clinical pathology also rendered the museum less significant. Museums'
tendency to become cramped and malodorous and expensive to maintain
discouraged their continuation as well.[123] Moreover, in his study of the
extensive medical collections at the University of Michigan, McIsaac
places the museum in the context of individual careers and research
agendas. Simply put, the museum struggled in the absence of faculty
willing to commit time and resources to the collections.[124] Additionally,
advances in photography improved the illustrations in medical textbooks
and may have further reinforced the movement away from teaching in
medical museums.[125] As the museum's teaching and research functions
declined, administrators reallocated museum space to more pressing
educational demands.[126]

The Unit System and the Arrangement of Laboratory Space

If Harvard Medical School was atypical in its grand and expansive Warren Anatomical Museum, it was typical in its reliance on the unit system to organize laboratory space. The unit system was a modular approach to medical school design developed during the planning for Harvard's 1906 quadrangle. The many proponents of the unit system celebrated its rationalization of the laboratory; they believed that the unit system created economical, efficient, and flexible facilities. The unit system became the dominant tool for laboratory design in American medical schools of all building types in the early twentieth century.

Harvard Medical School faculty member William Townsend Porter conceived of the unit system, but his colleague Charles S. Minot publicized it with articles in 1900 and 1901.[127] In his first article on the subject, Minot identified museums as the inspiration for the unit system, although later an architect equated the unit system to the arrangement of office buildings.[128] Minot, however, did not focus on architectural precedents or parallels. Instead, he positioned the unit system as an excellent solution to familiar problems of medical school design. As Minot knew firsthand from planning the histology laboratory on the top floor of Harvard Medical School's 1883 facility, medical schools at the time consisted of an assemblage of unique rooms suited to specific purposes (see fig. 1.19). These buildings, however, quickly became obsolete, Minot explained, as medical education evolved, especially with the rapid addition of more fields of study, each with its own laboratory requirements. Modern medical education's emphasis on hands-on laboratory training, along with growth in the number of students, further increased the need for new laboratory buildings. Minot reported that many laboratory buildings were under construction, with more expected in the near future. He hoped that the unit system would allow educators and architects to design schools that would function better in the immediate and the long term than current structures.[129]

In Minot's ideal plan, the laboratory became factorylike in its rationalization of space. A foundational component of the unit system was the expectation that students would receive their instruction in small groups, what he called "sections," in rooms of moderate size rather than in one big group in a large laboratory or in small groups within a large laboratory. Minot set the section size at twenty-four students and proposed that each student have seventeen and a half square feet in which to work. He also reserved space for passing through the room and for sinks and for cabinets in which to store apparatus. Ideally, each

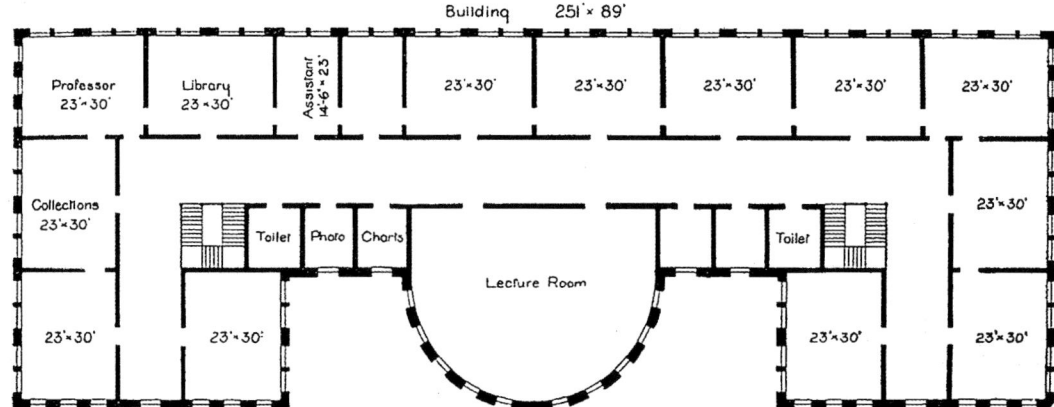

1.26.   Medical school designed according to the unit system, ca. 1901, published in article by Charles S. Minot.

laboratory would function independently, without the need for students to obtain equipment from other rooms. (Minot understood laboratories as complete environments, and he also designed laboratory furniture.) After a little rounding of numbers, Minot set thirty feet by twenty-three feet as the ideal unit. Minot optimistically assured the reader that a unit room of this size would meet nearly every physical demand of medical education: "It will be of convenient dimensions for a class of elementary study, a smaller class of advanced students, or a still smaller number of research men, or of assistants. It can be subdivided into two smaller rooms by temporary partitions. It will be convenient for collections, for a library or reading room, or for a small lecture room."[130]

The unit system went hand-in-hand with the transition to medical schools composed of double-loaded corridors within narrow, light-filled wings arranged in footprints that allowed for easy expansion, such as a U or a grid. As Minot explained, "the best plan will probably be found to be that of long corridors with rooms on each side, after the manner so common in large hotels."[131] With the exception of the lecture hall, the medical school would consist of a series of unit rooms along both sides of a corridor (fig. 1.26). Extension of the building could occur through the construction of additional unit rooms. By installing large windows along the room's thirty-foot side, every desk in the relatively shallow room would have ample light.[132]

For Minot, the unit system had architectural, pedagogical, and administrative advantages over medical schools planned without the module. Architecturally speaking, Minot believed that the unit system simplified the architect's project by reducing the program to a series of identical, well-lighted, and easily accessible rooms. The architect could adopt any number of footprints and, Minot asserted, enjoy "great freedom as to the exterior of the building, which generally seems as important to the architect as the interior arrangements are important to the owners and users of a building." Construction costs would also decrease due to the uniformity of materials in a structure mainly composed of units rather than variously sized rooms. Pedagogically, the unit system reinforced teaching students in modestly sized sections, which Minot strongly advocated. From an administrative perspective, Minot championed the unit system's complete flexibility. Changing the function of a room simply required replacing the furniture, even if the room was reassigned to a different department, a point Minot underscored with six diagrams of possible room arrangements "somewhat arbitrarily" attached to particular disciplines (fig. 1.27). Ease of expansion augmented the flexibility of the unit system.[133]

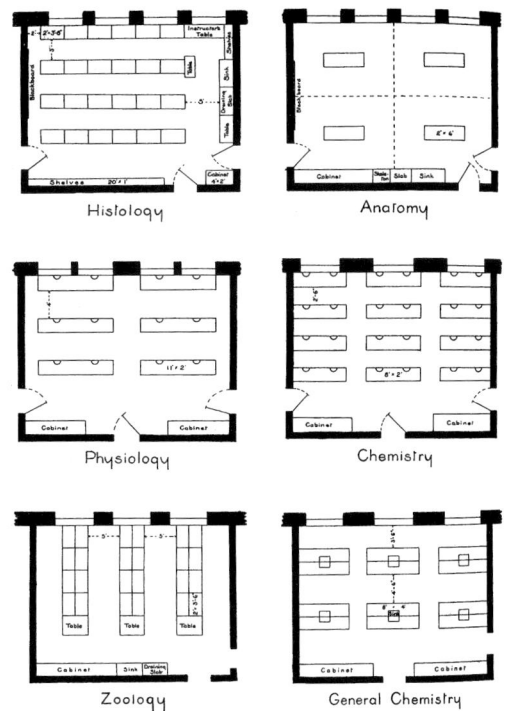

1.27.   Unit rooms with various arrangements of furniture, windows, and doors, ca. 1901, published in article by Charles S. Minot.

Harvard Medical School's use of the unit system, however, did not precisely mirror Minot's vision. Architects for Harvard Medical School and elsewhere adopted a far smaller unit than Minot's thirty by twenty-three feet. Harvard Medical School architect Charles Coolidge recalled, "I talked with Dr. Warren, Dr. Bowditch, and Dr. Minot. Dr. Minot had the idea we could build a unit." He then stated, "I took a small unit of 12 feet, and built those buildings with the piers outside 12 feet apart in the centres."[134] A contemporary description reported that the architects set the unit size for the rooms in the Harvard buildings at ten feet wide and twenty-three feet deep, with a single window within each ten-foot section.[135] The difference in unit widths may be attributed to the variation between interior and exterior measurements or the possible passage of time between the construction project and Coolidge's statement. In the end, the architects replaced Minot's single larger unit, which could be subdivided if desired, with a smaller unit, which could be multiplied as needed. The architects also extended the flexibility of the building by creating non-load-bearing walls between

the units, as the same contemporary description explained: "The partitions of terra-cotta separating each unit were intended to be so arranged
as to enclose any given number of units, and to be removed or replaced
from time to time as necessity required, thus giving accommodation for
small sections, laboratories, professors' rooms, and research work of all
kinds."[136] According to a 1905 assessment of the unfinished quadrangle,
the placement of the heating and ventilating ductwork in the walls along
the corridors—in addition to the building's steel frame—made possible
the construction of the non-load-bearing terra-cotta walls between the
unit rooms. Single-unit rooms functioned well for use by one professor
or instructor, while three-unit rooms, measuring twenty-three by thirty
feet, in keeping with Minot's ideal, were typically the most economical
size for laboratory and small group instruction.[137] In the end, however,
Harvard's buildings contained many unit variations, including a six-unit
room in Building D, a five-unit room in Building E, and even a massive
chemistry laboratory in Building C that encompassed an entire wing
with no subdivisions at all (see fig. 1.17).

Minot's passionate argument in favor of the unit system found a
receptive audience. Beyond its flexibility and potential for expansion,
the unit system may have been embraced by medical educators because
it created a way of allocating space according to the needs of a certain
number of occupants and then clearly communicating this information.
In a letter to Harvard University's president, Minot asserted that, with
the unit system, "difficulties about assigning space to the different
departments and providing accommodations for the new departments
immediately vanish."[138] The unit system also facilitated the transfer of information between architects and medical educators.[139] Architects could
ask educators how they wanted a specified number of units subdivided,
and medical educators could explain that they needed a certain number
of rooms built according to a particular multiple of units.

Other medical schools quickly adopted the unit system.[140] In 1903,
Minot wrote to Harvard University's president to let him know that the
University of Toronto had constructed its medical school buildings with
the unit system. Presumably in recognition of his work on the unit system,
Minot had received an invitation to participate in the dedication events.[141]

A 1907 trip west by Minot likely increased interest in the unit
system. He lectured to medical students and sometimes faculty at six
universities, using as visual aids lantern slides of the recently completed
Harvard Medical School. He offered "a general address on the new ideals
in medical education and practice for which our buildings stand." Minot
reported that the "audiences seemed very much interested in the account

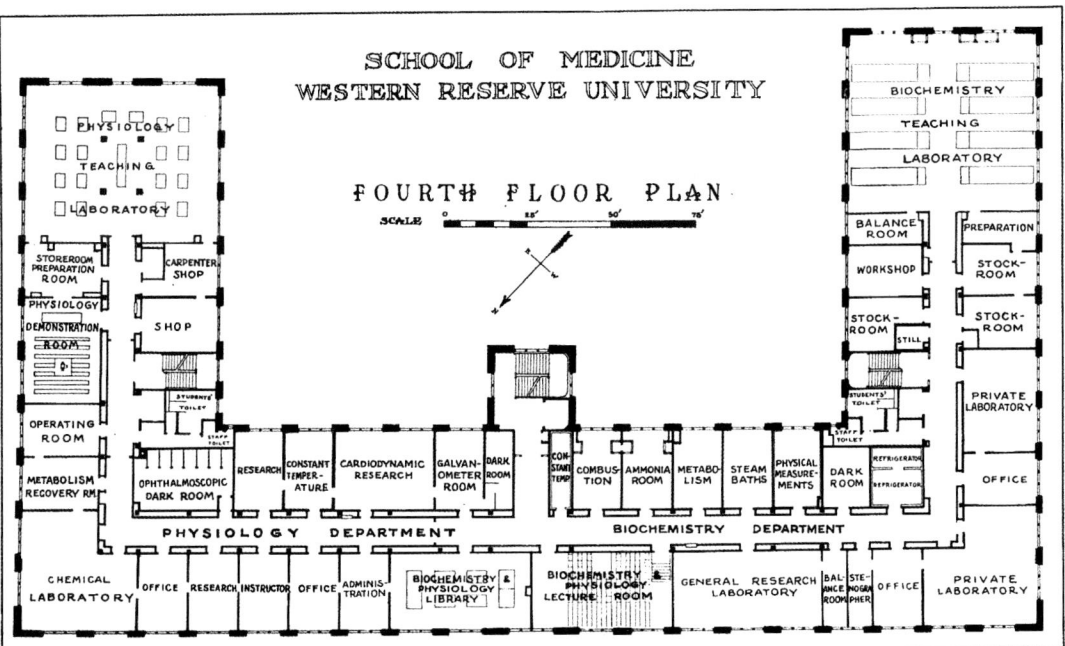

1.28.   Western Reserve University School of Medicine, 1924, Coolidge and Shattuck, architects, plan, fourth floor.

of the Medical School, and as, apparently, the nature of our plant was very imperfectly known in the West, I hope that some good results may follow from what I call my 'advertising trip.'"[142] Minot's lectures almost surely included a description of the unit system.

The unit system's popularity held. Two decades after the dedication of Harvard Medical School's 1906 quadrangle, the University of Rochester opened a medical school designed with the unit system. George W. Corner joined the Rochester medical faculty two years before classes commenced and later described the development of the school. He emphasized the unit system's cost savings and its usefulness for the administration: "To save time and money as well, [medical school dean George Hoyt] Whipple had the architects . . . lay out a plan of crisscrossing axes in a simple modular form, so that the concrete forms for pillars and girders could be moved along section by section. . . . The very efficient plumbing was as uniform as possible throughout. Window spacing was consistent throughout the building. Each department head had only to fit the needs of his laboratory or clinic into the modular space allotted him."[143] In 1929, Alan E. Munby, long-term member of the Science Standing Committee of the Royal Institute of British Architects, gave an address to the institute entitled "The Design of Science Buildings."

Nearly thirty years after Minot had published his first article on the unit system, Munby championed it: "In large buildings the adoption of a unit will often simplify construction and assist in the allocation of space. . . . With such a unit it is possible to obtain a rapid mental picture of space allocation to different subjects in the early stages of planning. As changes are inevitable[,] as much elasticity as possible should be obtained by the use of partitions which are not constructional."[144] To illustrate his point, Munby included in the publication of his talk the fourth-floor plan of Western Reserve University School of Medicine (fig. 1.28). Coolidge and Shattuck, a successor firm to Shepley, Rutan, and Coolidge, the architects of Harvard Medical School's quadrangle, designed Western Reserve University's 1924 single-building medical school. Shepley, Rutan, and Coolidge—and its later iterations—was the premier architectural firm for American medical schools in the early twentieth century. The firm's continued reliance on the unit system also encouraged educators and other architects to embrace this planning tool.

The Impact of Medical School Design on Medical Practice

Tremendous changes in how physicians practiced medicine took place in the nineteenth and early twentieth centuries. Although science has encapsulated a variety of meanings throughout medical history, in the course of the nineteenth century it came to represent the experimental sciences undertaken in the laboratory. With this shift, sound medical practice came to rest primarily on the fundamental laws that regulated a biological organism rather than a practitioner's personal judgment and experience.[145] Many of the innovations that altered medical practice in this period stemmed from advances in basic science achieved through research in the laboratory. Although physicians had relatively few therapeutic or curative agents at their disposal, their understanding of disease increased. Louis Pasteur's and Robert Koch's pioneering work in bacteriology eventually led to more effective public health measures and antiseptic surgery, which expanded the safety—and scope—of operations. A number of diagnostic technologies also developed in the nineteenth century, including the stethoscope, ophthalmoscope, and laryngoscope, along with the microscope and x-ray. By the first decade of the twentieth century, laboratory tests could detect tuberculosis, cholera, typhoid, diphtheria, and syphilis. Physicians came to rely less on patients' descriptions of symptoms and their own unaided observation and more on the information they collected through various instruments and tests.[146]

Medical historian Joel Howell has studied medical technology between 1900 and 1925, the period in which medical technology became a
component of routine patient care in the hospital. Howell demonstrates
that the clinical adoption of the latest technology was not automatic, immediate, or uniform. One factor in this overall change in medical practice,
however, was the advent of modern medical education. By the end of the
nineteenth century, Howell explains, "physicians had been educated in
a new medical world, one in which the laboratory had become familiar
territory. . . . Medical schools . . . were coming to emphasize science
as a means of knowing and of teaching." Medical faculties oversaw the
construction of teaching laboratories, and aspiring physicians increasingly received training in clinical laboratory techniques. Medical schools
taught students to conceptualize the body through the lens of science
and to utilize the most recent technology, a particularly important skill
at a time when physicians were responsible for medical testing, including
doing blood counts and operating the x-ray machine.[147] When Harvard
Medical School opened its 1906 quadrangle, students could learn to run
the x-ray machine, a technology enthusiastically described in medical
literature but not yet in wide clinical use, in a specially designed suite in
the basement of Building A.[148] Moreover, Joe Holoubek, University of
Nebraska College of Medicine class of 1938, described his training in clinical laboratory techniques, including the Mantoux and Schick tests related
to tuberculosis and diphtheria, respectively, and the Wassermann test for
syphilis. He concluded, "We obtained a very thorough foundation of this
type of clinical laboratory testing, have prepared the reagents and did the
tests ourselves."[149] With their emphasis on laboratory science, medical
schools—like many hospitals in this period—promoted an understanding
of the patient less as a person and more as an illness requiring diagnosis.[150]

Scholars have carefully investigated the relationship between shifts
in medical practice and developments in hospital design in this period.[151]
Until this point, however, they have largely ignored medical schools, presumably because they understood them as mute boxes with little impact
on either students' education or their future practice of medicine.[152] In
contrast, faculty put tremendous effort into these expensive structures
and conceived of them as pedagogical tools. As one observer of Yale
University's medical buildings wrote, "although the success of a School
of Medicine . . . is measured by the quality of its product and not by its
buildings, Yale has acted on the theory that well-planned physical facilities constitute an important asset in medical teaching and research."[153]
In his analysis of Harvard Medical School's 1906 quadrangle, journalist
Ralph Bergengren laid bare the relationship between architecture and

pedagogy: "Behind the marble walls of these department buildings . . . one might readily trace, in the object lessons of individual equipment, storage rooms, special laboratories and special arrangements for the illustration of lectures, the whole plan of modern medical instruction, its remarkable combination of minute research with broad general knowledge leading together to the actual hospital work that completes the medical student's education."[154] Faculties' and their contemporaries' appreciation of the educational significance of the medical schools notwithstanding, in broad strokes it is not very surprising that laboratory facilities encouraged students to practice scientific medicine. What is perhaps of greater interest, although difficult to document, are more specific ways that the architecture of medical schools may have impacted medical practice.

Jonathan Reinarz has asked a similar question of medical museums. Building on the argument that a medical gaze developed within the hospital in the late eighteenth and early nineteenth centuries and increasingly depersonalized the interaction between physician and patient, Reinarz proposes that this relationship may have begun before students stepped onto the wards, when they learned to privilege observation during their training in the museum. Reinarz posits further that students' early engagement with passive subjects in the form of cadavers and museum specimens may have promoted an understanding of the patient as an object for investigation.[155] Museum architecture may well have reinforced the experience Reinarz references by facilitating display and taxonomy, a process that places the specimen completely within the physician-curator's construction of knowledge.[156]

Much of this chapter investigated the institute plan for American medical schools. Enthusiasm for this type, however, never became widespread. One deterrent was medical educators' growing belief that a unified design, rather than a series of distinct buildings, would present students with a different conception of science, one that would ultimately improve how they practiced medicine. Although the outcome of such a claim is challenging and perhaps impossible to document, we need to take it seriously. Faculties believed that the form of a medical college had an impact on the type of physicians students became, and as new educational and scientific ideas became dominant, the design of medical schools shifted.

———————

In 1893, the faculty at Johns Hopkins Medical School decided not to construct a single building for preclinical studies, the prevailing design for American medical schools at the time, and instead to erect a campus composed of a series of discrete buildings following the German institute plan. A handful of medical schools, including those at Harvard University in 1906, Washington University in St. Louis in 1914, and Emory University in 1917, made the same choice. The champions of the institute plan were vocal and came largely from elite schools, but by 1920 the celebration of the institute plan had ended. So complete was the movement away from the institute plan that in 1949 prominent medical educator Herman G. Weiskotten reported, "An official of a long established medical school which had developed its various laboratories and clinical departments in separate buildings recently stated that the faculty of this school had even considered the advisability of abandoning their entire plant and starting over again in the development of a well integrated physical plant."[157]

The institute plan had always had critics. At Harvard Medical School, the decision to construct five separate structures in 1906 was not without discussion, and the faculty considered several other plans.[158] In 1902, Minot wrote to Harvard's president and lamented that the quadrangle would include four rather than two laboratory buildings. Four laboratory buildings would result in wasted space, Minot argued, whereas two would prove more convenient for the occupants and save $200,000.[159] Undoubtedly other medical educators shared Minot's concerns about the institute plan's extraneous square footage and cost.

Additional factors also discouraged long-term enthusiasm for the institute plan. After 1900, young American doctors no longer needed to travel abroad in search of strong medical training, and the number of physicians studying in Germany decreased. The outbreak of World War I in 1914 all but ended this transatlantic migration.[160] Although American physicians had generally stopped training internationally in the period after World War I, faculty engaged in planning facilities did sometimes visit Europe, including Germany, as they refined their designs.[161] Still, the institute plan failed to inspire another generation of adherents, perhaps in part because German institutes were autonomous administrative and financial units, unlike most American departments.[162] In the end, however, the dismissal of the institute plan by American medical leaders likely stemmed primarily from their continual efforts to improve medical training, to innovate, and to stimulate donors, and they made coordination in medical education and architecture the overriding refrain.

Even during the decades of support for the institute plan, the single building for preclinical studies never disappeared. Some faculties continued to erect single buildings, although in footprint and interior spaces these structures had little in common with the single-building schools constructed before education reform. The new single-building medical colleges, like the schools built according to the institute plan, embraced the unit system and other elements of modern medical school design and encouraged students to recognize the laboratory as the root of education, research, and practice. Because all medical school facilities shared a commitment to the laboratory and experiential learning, the significance of the difference between the institute plan and the single building may seem small. But for educators, the design variations had meaning. They believed that the form of the schools would impact how their students conceptualized science and later practiced medicine. For roughly twenty-five years, the institute design represented a celebrated alternative to the single-building medical school.

2

UNIFICATION TRIUMPHS

*The Single Building for Preclinical Studies
and the Medical School–Hospital*

MEDICAL EDUCATORS HAD NEVER STOPPED CONSTRUCTING SINGLE buildings for preclinical studies, but support for this building type began to grow around 1920. The burgeoning enthusiasm for the single-building medical college contributed to the decline in popularity of the institute plan, but the prominence of the institute type in Germany and at a handful of elite medical schools in the United States made it a frequent topic in discussions of medical school design for decades to come. As educators championed the single building for preclinical studies and later endorsed the medical school–hospital, they did so in part by contrasting these designs with the institute plan and its division of the campus. Ultimately, the majority of medical colleges that comprehensively rebuilt their facilities between 1893 and 1940 constructed one of the two unified designs: the single building for preclinical studies or the medical school–hospital. This choice promoted efficiency, lower construction costs, and flexibility along with a conception of education and science that emphasized the interconnectedness of the branches of medicine.

Medical Education Reform after 1900

In the first decade of the twentieth century, the number of medical colleges began to decline. After peaking in 1906 at 162, only 131 schools remained in 1910. Many more stood on the precipice of closure, with 37 registering a total enrollment of fewer than 50 students.[1] Put simply, the economics of medical education had shifted. Reformed medical education required more laboratories, equipment, and clinical resources, plus the recruitment of new faculty with different training, and these costs undermined the profit-making function of the proprietary schools. Proprietary medical colleges generally merged, closed, or affiliated with a university in an attempt to acquire more funds.[2] This trajectory received a boost in 1910 with the publication of the Flexner Report. State licensing laws had been on the books since the 1870s, but the report's caustic review of American and Canadian medical colleges served as an impetus for stronger licensing laws. One requirement for licensure specified that physicians have a degree from an "approved" medical college, a stipulation that helped to reduce the number of medical colleges still further.[3]

When planning new structures, medical school leaders made a critical calculation in order to ensure financial solvency. They examined anticipated expenses (maintenance of preclinical and, possibly, clinical facilities and equipment, faculty salaries, and in some places also research budgets) and the expected revenue (tuition fees along with endowment income or state appropriations) in order to determine two interrelated numbers: how many students to enroll and how large a medical school, and sometimes a teaching hospital, to construct.[4] Changing entrance requirements in the opening decades of the twentieth century made these calculations more difficult, however. In 1900, only 15 or 20 percent of medical colleges demanded a high school diploma to enroll, and only Johns Hopkins Medical School insisted on a college degree. The following year, Harvard Medical School required a college degree and Western Reserve University School of Medicine, three years of college work. No other medical school stipulated any college training. Before 1900, there simply were not enough qualified applicants for a widespread increase in admissions standards. By the early 1900s, the American education system had improved significantly thanks to the growth in the number and quality of high schools and colleges. Medical schools began to raise their entrance requirements, and by 1915 more than 42 percent of all medical schools required at least two years of college training. Nevertheless, through the end of World War I medical schools adopted more stringent admissions standards ahead of available applicants, and many schools saw substantial decreases in enrollment. By 1918, the number of students with the necessary college background had risen, and medical classes were at capacity once again.[5]

Perhaps in part due to an awareness of this trajectory, medical school leadership sometimes anticipated an expansion of class size when they oversaw the design of medical colleges, a view likely also based on the recognition that it was more cost effective to construct larger-than-necessary spaces initially than to add square footage later. Harvard Medical School had made this choice when it built its 1906 quadrangle. In 1915, an article in the *Harvard Alumni Bulletin* reported that the "school can accommodate still more students than are at present enrolled. But already signs of substantial increase appear, and this year's catalogue contains the statement that the right is reserved to 'refuse applicants, if the number admitted is as large as can be effectively taught.'"[6] The University of Rochester inaugurated its medical college in 1925 in a building planned for classes of 75 students.[7] But the initial class contained only 22 students, a low enrollment no doubt shaped in part by the fact that the school, not just the building, was new. Edward F. Adolph was a member of the original Rochester medical faculty and taught physiology until 1960. He recalled the experience of the medical school's steady growth: "From the first class of 22 medical students, the number admitted each year progressively increased, to 45 in 1935. Ten years later the number had risen to 65, partly in deference to the demand for physicians in wartime. Actually, the ratio of teachers to students also continuously increased; nevertheless, the intimacy between faculty members and students seriously diminished."[8] Even medical colleges with far smaller construction budgets than Harvard or Rochester built schools that would allow for an expansion of the student body. In 1930, Woman's Medical College of Pennsylvania relocated to a facility designed for classes of up to 50 students and a total enrollment of 200, but in the 1930–1931 school year it registered just 120 students.[9] Particularly for schools like Woman's Medical College that were struggling to keep the doors open, planning for larger class sizes may also have reflected the desire for an increase in revenue from tuition fees. Nationwide, however, by the 1930s medical colleges were turning away almost half of those who applied.[10]

Overcrowding within certain medical institutions, including mental hospitals and some general hospitals, is well documented in the early twentieth century, but overcrowding in medical education did not become a widespread issue until shortly before 1940. The number of medical students across the country dropped between 1904 and 1920. In the same period, the average number of students per medical school fell from 175.9 to 162.3. Between 1920 and 1930, the number of medical schools continued to decrease, but enrollment increased. Sociologist William G. Rothstein explains that in the early twentieth century revenue from tuition was less critical for medical schools than in the preceding century, but it still represented the schools' greatest single income source. As a result, schools enlarged enrollment in the two decades after 1920 to expand revenue, which led to the criticism in a late-1930s American Medical Association (AMA) report of "abnormal growth in the size of the student bodies in institutions without sufficient clinical, laboratory or financial resources for their proper instruction."[11] Schools' efforts to build their revenue during the Great Depression no doubt accounted in part for this trend. The average number of students per school between 1880 and 1940 peaked in 1935 at 297.2 before declining to 276.2 in 1940. In terms of medical school graduates, the country produced roughly the same number of doctors in 1940 (5,097) as it had in 1906 (5,364), but the ratio of graduates to population decreased.[12]

In the early decades of the twentieth century, the Flexner Report stands out for its impact on medical education. The AMA reorganized in 1901 and three years later created the Council on Medical Education. In 1906, the council's representatives reviewed all of the country's medical colleges and generated a report that it shared with the schools but did not publish. Not wanting to criticize the nation's medical colleges directly, the council asked the Carnegie Foundation for the Advancement of Teaching to undertake its own investigation of medical colleges. The Carnegie Foundation agreed and hired Abraham Flexner to execute the project. Together with a member of the AMA Council on Medical Education, Flexner visited every medical school in the United States and Canada, and in 1910 the Carnegie Foundation published his report, known colloquially as the Flexner Report.[13]

How Henry Pritchett, president of the Carnegie Foundation for the Advancement of Teaching, found Flexner remains unclear. Born in Louisville, Kentucky, in 1866, Flexner earned his undergraduate degree from Johns Hopkins University in 1886. After graduation, he returned to his hometown and spent nineteen years running a private high school. In 1905, Flexner shut down his school and enrolled at Harvard. He focused his graduate studies on philosophy and psychology and their connection to educational issues. In 1907, he went to Europe to examine educational systems. Flexner published his first book, *The American College*, in 1908, the same year Pritchett hired him to survey medical schools. Flexner remained a member of the Carnegie Foundation staff for the next four years.[14]

The Flexner Report codified the reform movement already in progress and accelerated the transformation of medical education across the country. The report functioned in two ways. First, it described and celebrated the system of medical education recently created at elite, university-affiliated American medical schools. Second, it enumerated unflinchingly the deficits and assets of each American and Canadian medical college. A quintessential piece of muckraking journalism, the Flexner Report generated significant public attention. The public now joined with medical educators, Flexner, the AMA, and others in demanding that state boards create stringent licensing laws.[15]

The AMA Council on Medical Education used its system for rating medical schools to step into a powerful gatekeeping role. It designated medical schools as Class A (acceptable), Class B (in need of improvement), and Class C (requiring total reorganization). After 1914, for-profit schools automatically received a Class C rating. State licensing boards determined which medical schools qualified as satisfactory based on the AMA rankings. Beginning in 1914, thirty-one states refused to recognize Class C schools. Moreover, from its formation in 1915, the National Board of Medical Examiners tested only physicians with a degree from a Class A institution. A strong AMA rating became essential for a school's success.[16]

The AMA's system of rating medical colleges encouraged the renovation of existing structures and the construction of new facilities even if it did not prioritize buildings among its various criteria. In his investigation of the AMA Council on Medical Education, medical historian Kenneth Ludmerer has shown that limitations with regard to the physical plant in and of themselves were unlikely to shift a school's ranking. Although the Council on Medical Education examined all elements of a medical college and might criticize it for any deficit, a school's Class A ranking would be jeopardized only by failing to meet the council's expectations in three areas: a sufficient endowment, an adequate teaching hospital, and a minimum of six full-time basic science faculty undertaking research.[17] For schools struggling to obtain or maintain a Class A ranking, however, the facilities often represented one component in a constellation of shortcomings. On 29 November 1921, N. P. Colwell, the secretary of the Council on Medical Education, reviewed Meharry Medical College, an acutely underfunded medical school for African Americans in Nashville, Tennessee. He saw many recent improvements, including alterations to the anatomy and auditorium facilities: "Anderson Hall for anatomy and the Auditorium building show similar evidences of effective readjustment. At previous inspections it was difficult to know whether these were dormitories or laboratory buildings. At present, the dormitory function has been entirely abolished; the laboratories are more complete; they are clean and show evidences of careful oversight. The apparatus is in orderly arrangement and has been placed in charge of responsible persons. A limited amount of new equipment has been provided."[18] In their efforts to raise Meharry Medical College from Class B to Class A, the president and faculty had made significant changes, some to the facilities. Nevertheless, they were not enough. Following his November 1921 review, Colwell upheld the school's Class B ranking. He cited the need for more funds so the school's hospital could stay open through the summer, and he called for upgrading the library, an increase in clinical training, and more full-time instructors.[19]

A school's physical plant alone would not be the determining factor in its rating from the AMA, but faculty either did not know this or did not want to test it. No doubt faculty also realized that meeting some of the other AMA criteria, such as research by basic science faculty, was difficult without acceptable facilities. The specifications set by the Council on Medical Education spurred schools to renovate, as at Meharry, or rebuild, as at Howard University College of Medicine, which after 1923 was the nation's only other medical school for Black students. In his 1922–1923 annual report, Howard University's president wrote, "Our School of Medicine continues to maintain the same high standards which caused it to be rated as a Class A school. . . . Owing to lack of laboratory facilities and teaching force, the School has been obliged to limit its classes to fifty. . . . This works a great hardship upon many deserving students which can be remedied only by a modern building. The present buildings date from 1869 and are obsolete so far as the requirements of modern medical teaching are concerned."[20] In Howard's case, the university president used the educational guidelines set by the Council on Medical Education to explain why the medical school curbed class size based on laboratory space and teaching staff and why it needed a larger and better-equipped facility in order to raise enrollment. It worked. By 1927, Howard University had funded and constructed a new medical college building. Similarly, the leadership of Woman's Medical College of Pennsylvania proudly described its 1930 facility in the context of the AMA council's criteria: "This new building invites inspection as an example of economical construction. . . . This has been accomplished . . . without curtailing the enormous laboratory, hospital, and library requirements of a Class 'A' Medical College."[21]

Within the AMA's criteria the architectural guidelines were very general. In 1910, the AMA Council on Medical Education published a pamphlet, *An Outline of the Essentials of a Satisfactory Medical College*, that called for "cleanliness, good care and proper ventilation of all college buildings," "thoroughly equipped laboratories," a library room with "suitable tables and chairs," "a working medical museum," and "evidences that all facilities are being intelligently used in the training of medical students."[22] Because any structure that provided for modern training would meet these prescriptions, educators and architects did not mention these requirements when developing building designs. The AMA standards encouraged faculties to update their schools, but they did not dictate the details of the structures.

In his 1910 report, Abraham Flexner offered more specific ideas about medical school design than did the AMA Council on Medical

Education. As we will see in chapter 3, Flexner's report became the template for the distribution of huge sums of money for medical education, particularly by John D. Rockefeller's General Education Board. As this philanthropic effort got under way, Flexner's ideas about architecture shaped the redesign of American medical colleges. One major pedagogical and architectural concept embraced by Flexner was coordination of departments.

The Single Building for Preclinical Studies

In the early twentieth century, the majority of American medical colleges employed single buildings for the preclinical studies covered during the first two years of medical training. Despite the prestige of the schools that adopted the institute design and the later enthusiasm for the medical school–hospital, faculties chose the single building for preclinical sciences approximately twice as often as they selected either of these other types. Schools with purpose-built facilities had utilized a single building design even before the reform of medical education. For example, Harvard Medical School's 1816 and 1847 buildings followed this type, as did the school's first reform-era facility in 1883. During the reform movement, prominent medical colleges such as Western Reserve University School of Medicine, in 1924, as well as struggling medical schools, including Howard University College of Medicine, in 1927, erected single buildings for preclinical studies. Like schools with institute plans, colleges with single buildings for preclinical studies frequently located near hospitals, sometimes with corridors or tunnels connecting the facilities. Syracuse University College of Medicine represents a typical medical school; it provides an example of this most common medical school design and illustrates the challenge many schools faced in terms of meeting the financial demands brought about by the changes in medical education.

In 1896, the Syracuse medical faculty oversaw the construction of the school's first purpose-built home (fig. 2.1). The progressive structure included significant space for hands-on learning, with five large teaching laboratories and three rooms dedicated to museum collections. The placement of the teaching laboratories on the ends of the floors allowed ample light to enter from three sides (fig. 2.2). The rectangular building also contained three lecture halls, dedicated laboratory-office space for the faculty, and separate study rooms for male and female students. The basement housed modern facilities for storing cadavers, and the building was said to have heating and ventilation systems similar to those promoted by John Shaw Billings.[23]

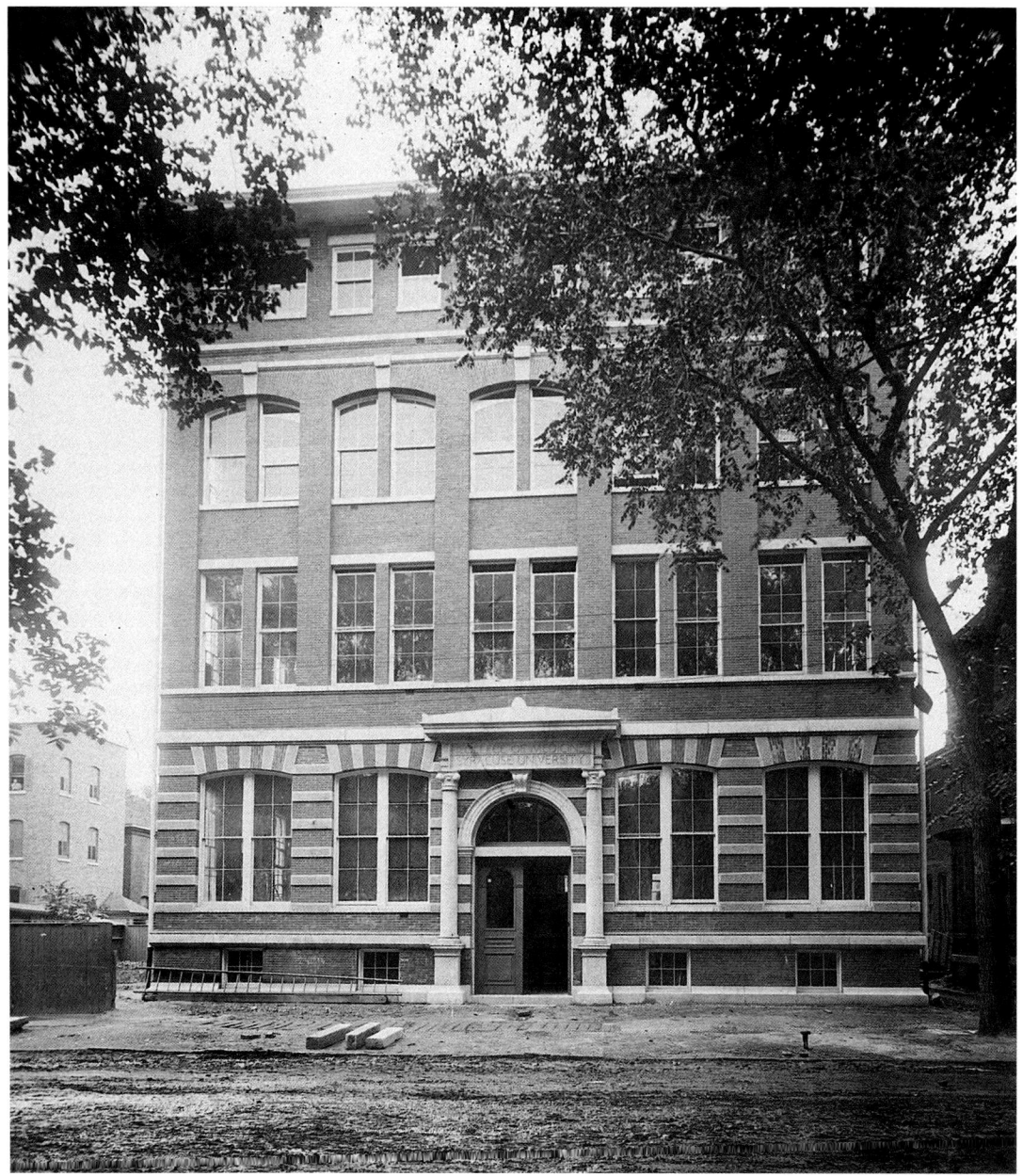

2.1.   Syracuse University College of Medicine, 1896, Albert Brockway and John Benson, architects.

Unlike many schools, Syracuse University College of Medicine fared
relatively well in its assessment for the 1910 Flexner Report. Flexner gave
the school's laboratory offerings a positive review, reserving criticism
for the clinical portion of its medical training. When comparing New
York State medical schools, Flexner lauded Syracuse for its university

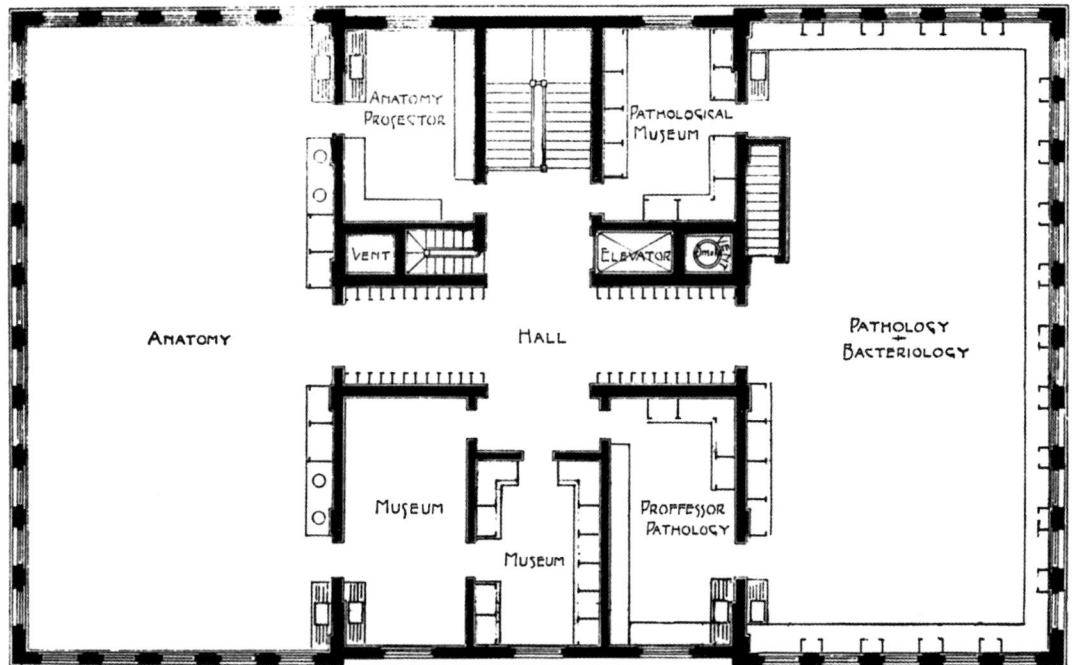

PLAN OF FOURTH FLOOR

2.2.   Syracuse University College of Medicine, 1896, Albert Brockway and John Benson, architects, plan, fourth floor.

affiliation and its financial practices. Not only did the medical college use all of the profits generated from student fees for improving the school rather than padding the professors' pockets, but it also attracted outside gifts. For these reasons, Flexner asserted that, of the New York State medical schools not located in New York City, only Syracuse University College of Medicine might survive the period of education reform.[24] But Flexner did not anticipate the trouble Syracuse University would subsequently have raising money for its medical college.

    In time the Syracuse medical faculty found the 1896 building, constructed in the early decades of educational change, lacking. They desired to relocate the medical college to a larger and more modern structure close to multiple hospitals. Although the faculty, alumni, and university had raised $40,000 to erect the 1896 building, in later decades outside support on the scale necessary to rebuild the medical school did not materialize.[25] Adjacent to Syracuse University a constellation of clinical facilities offered convenient first steps toward a medical center with the ideal geographic alignment of hospital(s) and medical school, but the medical college remained across town in its increasingly outdated and overcrowded building.[26] Ward L. Mould graduated from Syracuse University College of Medicine in 1936, the year before it finally moved. He later recalled the limitations of the college's antiquated home, albeit with fondness:

> The College was still (to my way of thinking) the step-daughter of the University. It was not housed in an elegant structure of the "Hill" [site of the main Syracuse University campus]. It was far removed, in a plain red brick building. . . . There was no inspiring inscription over a stately portal nor even a brass plaque attesting the generosity of some patron Unit.
>
> Instead it sat smack dab on the sidewalk with the street number on the door. The interior was as lacking in inspiration as the drab exterior. Classrooms and laboratories were furnished with the basic necessities (mostly old) and little else. In spite of its Spartan character, I think of that place with kindness in my heart and doubt if a more elegant facility could mean more to me![27]

The administration, however, could not take such a positive view of the situation. As Herman G. Weiskotten, dean of Syracuse University College of Medicine, affirmed in September 1936, "the present requirements for an approved medical college are such that our College could not have hoped to maintain its present rating . . . without a more satisfactory physical plant. The new building now under construction will fill this need."[28] By 1928, American medical colleges had improved to the point that the AMA Council on Medical Education stopped ranking schools as Class A, B, or C.[29] The council still endorsed schools, however, and the deficient facilities referenced by Mould and Weiskotten were likely just one inadequacy jeopardizing Syracuse's recommendation by the AMA.

Fortunately for the medical college, the New Deal offered Syracuse University the financial means to build its long-anticipated structure. The university obtained an $825,000 loan through the Public Works Administration to construct the medical school. Designed by Dwight James Baum and John Russell Pope, an architectural partnership that already had an established relationship with Syracuse University, the relatively modest building for preclinical studies finally allowed the medical college to relocate to the site of the university and the growing medical center in 1937 (figs. 2.3 and 2.4). The structure remains in use by the medical school today.

The building housed all of the facilities for the first two years of medical education under one roof, a significant improvement for the school. According to Weiskotten, lack of space in the college's previous home had forced the faculty to move the bacteriology and clinical pathology departments to the outpatient facility near the 1896 medical

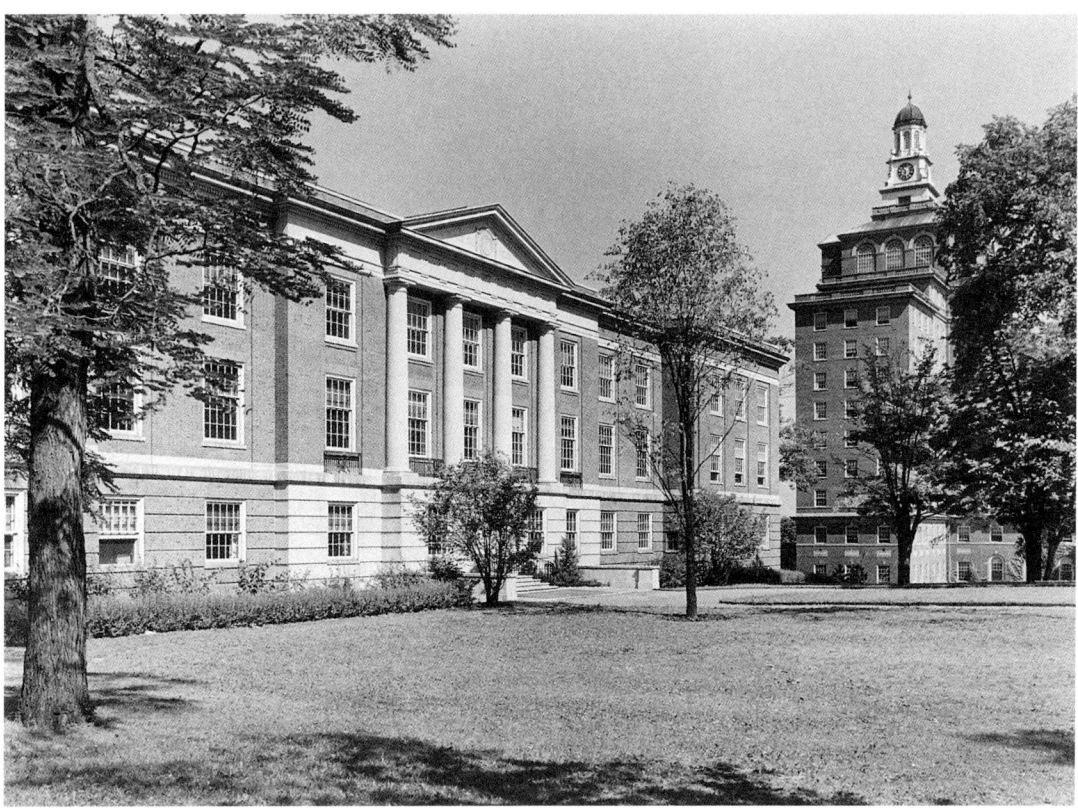

2.3.   Syracuse University College of Medicine, 1937, Dwight James Baum and John Russell Pope, architects, with Syracuse Memorial Hospital at right.

school and to place the physiological chemistry department more than a mile away, on the main university campus. Weiskotten lamented, "This separation of departments has been a great handicap in the development and conduct of the school."[30]

Beyond reuniting the medical school, the 1937 building improved on the 1896 structure. It provided more teaching laboratories, additional rooms for research, and expanded library facilities, as well as museum, administration, and extracurricular spaces. Moreover, it incorporated many of the ideas utilized in Harvard Medical School's 1906 buildings. Most simply, Syracuse's new structure formed a U shape, with a first-floor auditorium along the back of the central section and with the narrow edifice containing mainly double-loaded corridors.

The Syracuse University College of Medicine facility also followed the Harvard Medical School quadrangle in its physical coordination of the courses grouped in the curriculum. Both medical schools had block schedules that, although not identical, paired preclinical courses. As a

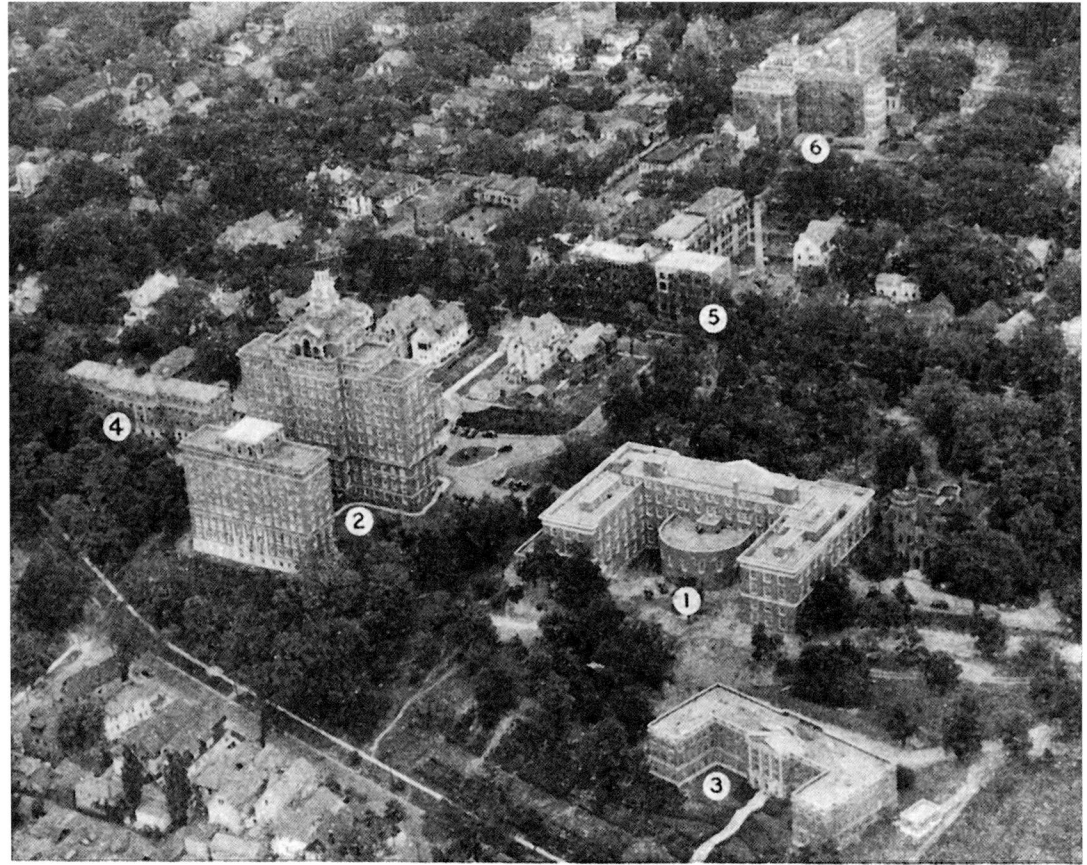

¹SYRACUSE UNIVERSITY COLLEGE OF
MEDICINE
²SYRACUSE MEMORIAL HOSPITAL
³CITY COMMUNICABLE DISEASE HOSPITAL

⁴STATE PSYCHOPATHIC HOSPITAL
⁵CROUSE-IRVING HOSPITAL
⁶UNIVERSITY HOSPITAL OF THE GOOD
SHEPHERD

2.4.   Syracuse University College of Medicine (1) and neighboring hospitals (2–6), ca. 1937.

Syracuse University publication noted, "in these [preclinical] courses the various subjects are correlated, so that the relation of each subject to the others and of all to the purpose of grounding the student in the sciences essential to the practice of medicine, is ever kept in view."[31] Like the Harvard Medical School quadrangle, Syracuse University College of Medicine's building reinforced the curriculum. The north corridor of its U-shaped structure accommodated anatomy in the basement, histology (and presumably embryology) on the first floor, and physiological chemistry on the third floor. During the first semester of their first year, students learned anatomy concurrently with histology and embryology; during the second semester of the first year, they studied anatomy, neuroanatomy, and physiological chemistry. As a result, they spent their entire first year in the north wing. Bacteriology utilized the south and central corridors on the second floor, with physiology in the south corridor one floor above. These subjects occupied students during the first semester of the second year, during which time they also began their clinical training. In addition to more clinical instruction, the next semester emphasized pathology, housed along the central corridor and north wing of the second floor; clinical pathology, located throughout the second floor; and pharmacology, placed one story above, along the central corridor.[32] As at Harvard Medical School, courses that the faculty understood as representing conceptually related disciplines were located adjacent to one another in the curriculum and in the architecture, reducing the intellectual and physical distance between the subjects. At the same time, Harvard Medical School and Syracuse University College of Medicine did not pair the subjects the same way in the curriculum or in the building, a reality that highlights the impact of local differences, perhaps based on relationships between faculty or understandings of science, on pedagogy and architecture. The facility at Syracuse makes clear, however, that single-building medical schools, while well established in a basic sense, differed dramatically in the early twentieth century from their nineteenth-century, prereform, and even early reform-era predecessors.

Several factors from the practical to the conceptual encouraged medical schools to construct single buildings that conformed to the modern standards of medical education rather than the institute plan. The faculty at Western Reserve University School of Medicine made this choice, as Frederick Clayton Waite, a professor of histology and embryology, later described in his history of the medical college: "The proposal for a new building in 1912 brought discussion as to whether the plan should be for a single building housing all the laboratory departments, or for a series of buildings or 'institutes.' Architects stated that a series of buildings would increase the cost of construction and also the cost of subsequent maintenance. Also it was the opinion that separate buildings would diminish the solidarity of the institution. Therefore a definite agreement was made that all laboratory departments should be located within one building."[33] In addition to highlighting concerns about cost, Waite emphasized the faculty's interest in expanding cooperation among the various departments. As preclinical departments multiplied in the early twentieth century, the decision to construct a single-building medical school supported unification in the face of specialization. Medical colleges, including Syracuse University College of Medicine and Western Reserve University School of Medicine, that chose single buildings promoted greater levels of coordination among all departments than did

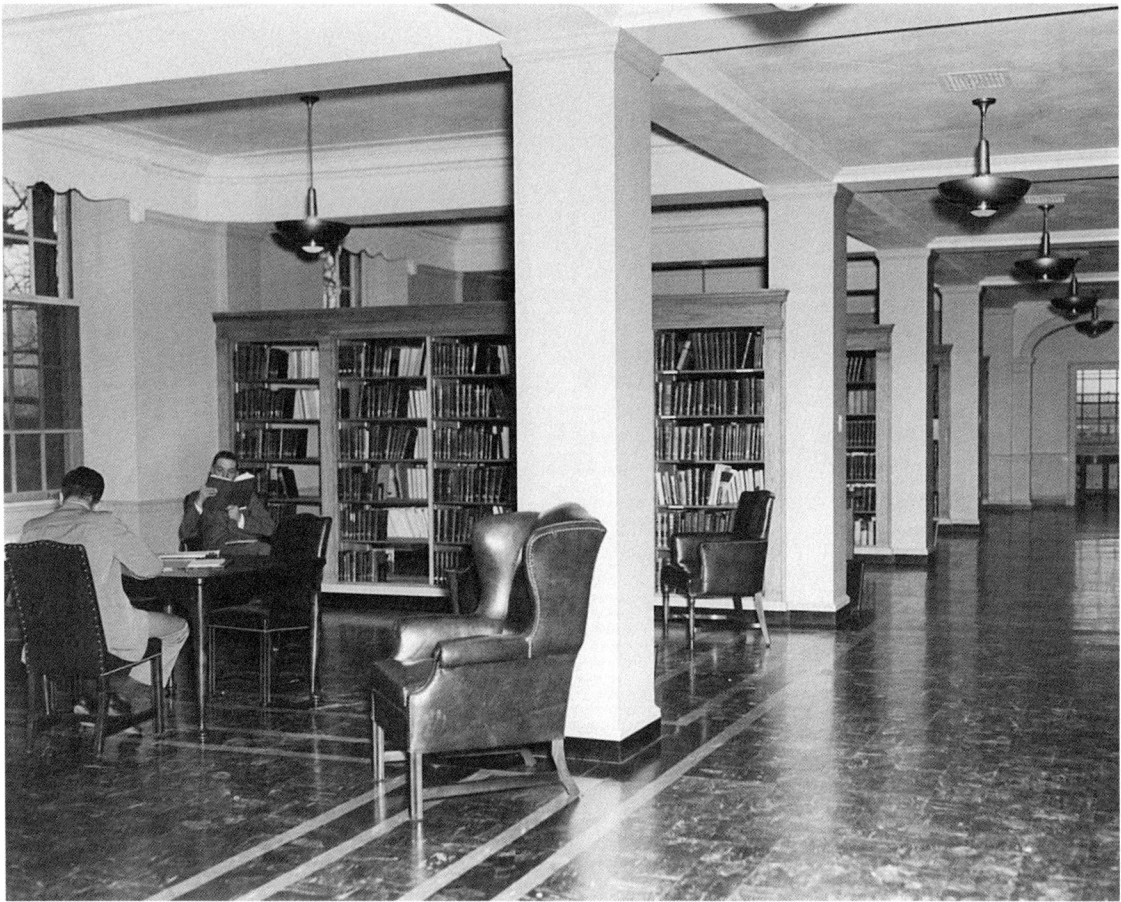

2.5.   Syracuse University College of Medicine, 1937, Dwight James Baum and John Russell Pope, architects, library. Photograph ca. 1937.

those with institute designs. Even if the anatomists dissecting in the north corridor of the basement rarely ventured to the bacteriology department in the south and central corridors of the second floor, all Syracuse professors entered the medical school facility through the same doorways and moved through the same hallways. Moreover, although not every single-building medical school contained a central library, most eventually did, as was the case in Syracuse's 1937 building, which meant that faculty from across disciplines also read books and journals together (fig. 2.5).[34] Unlike the institute design, the single building for preclinical studies reduced unnecessary duplications of space and encouraged the integration of departments increasingly celebrated by American medical educators.

Single buildings offered greater convenience for students as well. In Harvard Medical School's institute plan, students had to leave the

laboratory structures and walk to Building A when they needed to access
the administration, the museum, or the students' smoking room, locker
room, or reading room. In single-building medical schools, one structure
housed all laboratory, administrative, study, and social spaces. Additionally, the single-building design allowed for more seamless changes
to the students' schedule. The year after Syracuse University College
of Medicine moved into its 1937 edifice, it altered the schedule for the
preclinical courses. Although classes no longer aligned as closely with
the architecture, students had far less distance to travel in their revised
schedule than if the departments had resided in separate structures.[35]

The single building also offered educators the opportunity to promote a different conception of medical science. Wilburt C. Davison,
dean of Duke University School of Medicine during its construction
in the late 1920s, explained the philosophical difference between an
institute design and a plan that consolidated the medical school under
one roof. He asserted that those who supported a unified design wanted
their students to understand the branches of medicine as parts of a
whole rather than as discrete disciplines.[36]

The vagaries of local history further affected the choice of building type. At Syracuse University, hospitals arrived first in the designated area of the medical center. When it came time for the medical
school to move, there was no need to construct a hospital simultaneously. Other localities, however, built medical schools and hospitals
at the same time. In the early 1920s, the opportunity to construct a
medical school and hospital concurrently at Vanderbilt University
resulted in a pioneering design that over the next decade became
recognized as the most innovative medical school type in the United
States. The novel building coordinated medical school and hospital
into one structure, taking the idea of unified medicine and consolidated
buildings in a direction at once both very familiar and fundamentally
different.

The Creation of the Medical School–Hospital

In the 1920s and into the early 1930s, before the Great Depression fully
gripped the nation, medical school construction, like hospital construction, boomed thanks to the support of individual donors, appropriations
from state legislatures, and grants from major foundations—particularly
John D. Rockefeller's General Education Board.[37] In the midst of this
uptick in construction, Vanderbilt University's medical school dean,
G. Canby Robinson, conceived of the first medical school–hospital.

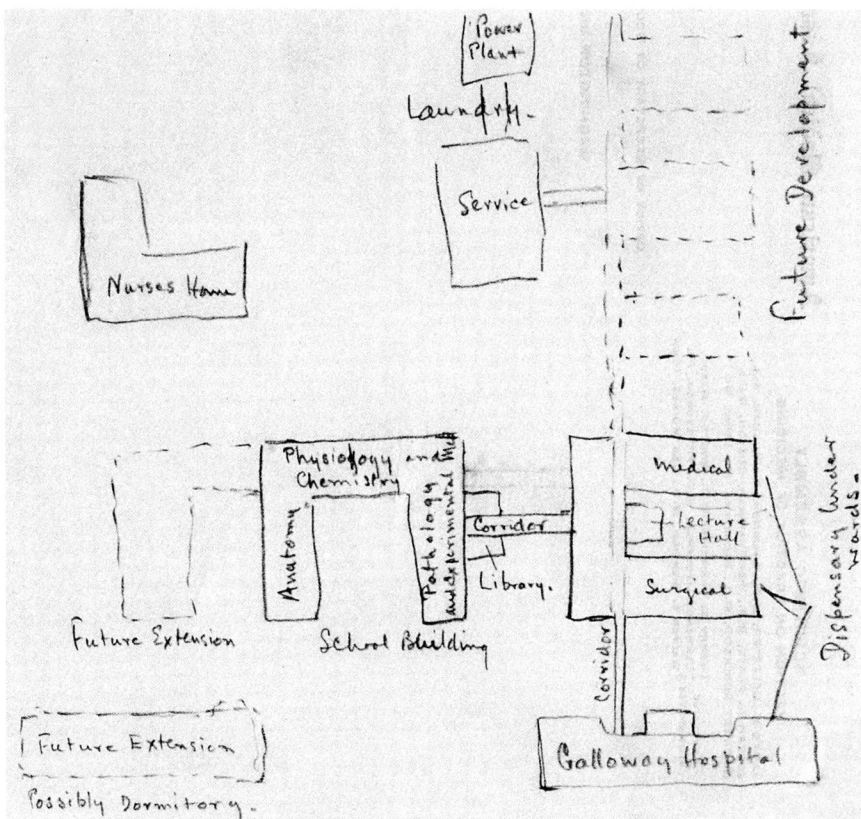

2.6.   Sketch for proposed Vanderbilt University medical facilities, spring 1920.

Before Vanderbilt's medical school was reorganized, three buildings housed medical instruction on the South Campus, two and a half miles by automobile from the main university. Two buildings contained pre-clinical departments, and one accommodated laboratories for anatomy, histology, and pathology, along with the outpatient clinic (also known as the dispensary in this period) and a forty-bed hospital. Only one of the buildings had been constructed for Vanderbilt's medical college.[38] Schools struggling to adopt the requirements for progressive medical education while having minimal funding at their disposal often located laboratory and clinical facilities, sometimes rather incongruously juxtaposed, in repurposed buildings.

Early plans for Vanderbilt University's reformed medical school de-pict a conventional facility. Two unsigned sketches made in fall 1919 and spring 1920 reveal the intention to keep the college on the South Campus and to construct a relatively typical single building for preclinical studies near the existing Galloway Memorial Hospital. In the later sketch, a

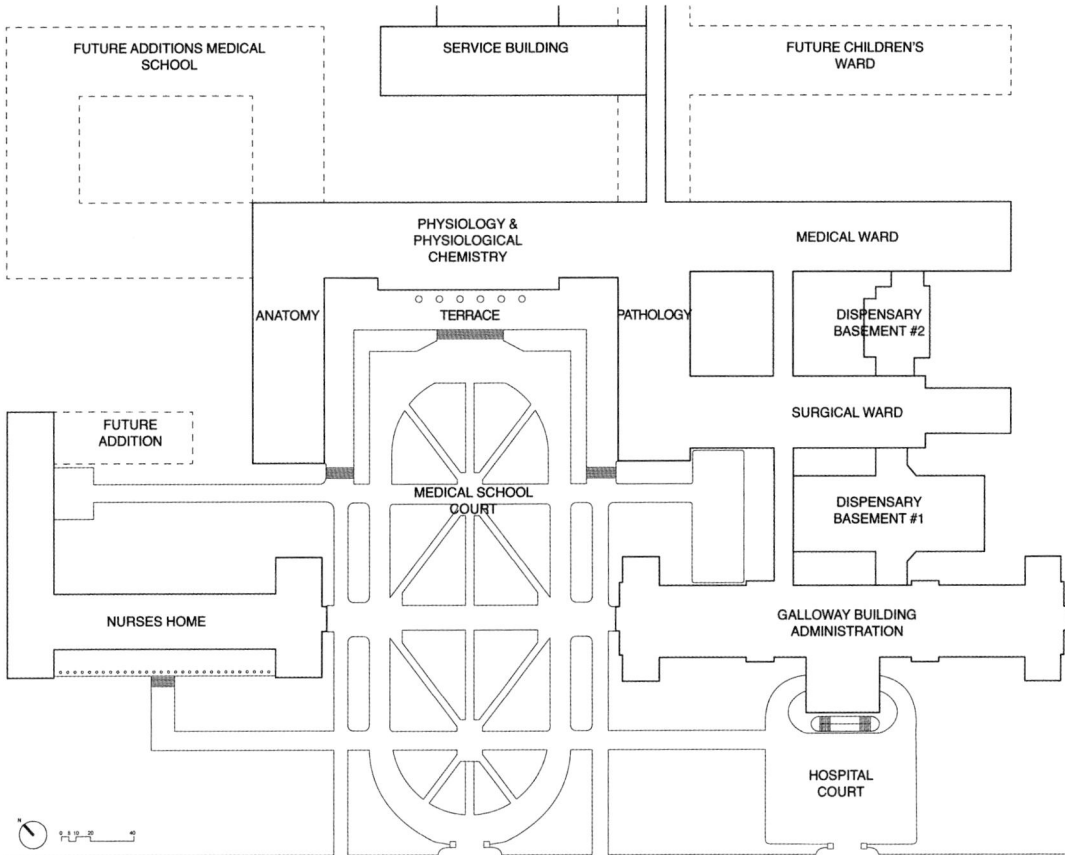

2.7.   Southwest section of plot plan for proposed Vanderbilt University medical facilities, summer 1920,
        Coolidge and Shattuck, architects, redrawn. The northeast section (not shown) included the laundry,
        kitchen, power house, additional service buildings, and animal house, along with the future school of
        public health and tropical medicine and future wards.

corridor connected the school with a proposed hospital extension (fig.
2.6).[39] Since Robinson's initial meeting with hospital consultant Winford
Smith and members of the architectural firm Coolidge and Shattuck in
the first part of 1920, they had explored, according to Robinson, "the
desirability . . . of coordinating closely the laboratory and clinical departments."[40] By the summer of 1920, Coolidge and Shattuck had plotted a
plan for a medical campus that, although reminiscent of Harvard Medical
School's quadrangle with its dramatic courtyard, terrace, and columned
Building A, presented a pioneering design: it eliminated the corridor
between the hospital and the medical school. Instead, the hospital wards
attached directly to one side of the U-shaped medical school (fig. 2.7). In
its fledgling form, the unified medical school–hospital was born.

To enact this vision for a combined medical school–hospital, however, Robinson needed funding. In September 1920, he sent a proposal
to Vanderbilt University chancellor James H. Kirkland and the General
Education Board, where Abraham Flexner now ran the medical education program. Robinson called for a complete redesign of the Vanderbilt
University School of Medicine—conceptually, pedagogically, and architecturally. Early in his report, he made a bold statement:

> A guiding principle which I believe is to be an important factor in advancing
> medicine and medical education is coordination of departments, and this con-
> ception has been kept in mind in the planning of buildings and in the organi-
> zation of departments. Although much has been accomplished by the German
> "Institute" method, in which each department is a defined entity, often physical-
> ly removed from the other departments, much more may be accomplished by a
> medical school which forms one "Institute," grouped about and participating in
> the study of disease, especially the study of disease in living human beings. No
> medical school has yet been developed with this as a fundamental conception,
> and the time is now at hand for the establishment of such a school.[41]

Robinson imagined a medical school that would function as a single
institute, offering not only the various preclinical disciplines but also
clinical training, which Robinson referred to as "the study of disease
in living human beings."[42] To make his idea a reality, Robinson suggested the physical coordination of the preclinical laboratories with the
clinical work, as well as continuity of staff. In his scheme, the head of
a preclinical department would oversee all of the research undertaken
in that department's area, no matter whether that work developed in
the preclinical or clinical section of the school. This novel physical and
administrative organization would make possible a change in the curriculum much anticipated by reformers. In Robinson's view, the teaching
system would "allow the integration of laboratory and clinical studies
which will be mutually beneficial, and which will tend to mold a new
type of medical practitioner."[43]

If the single building for preclinical studies, as at Syracuse University
College of Medicine, promoted the coordination of the various laboratory subjects, then the medical school–hospital focused on the unification
of preclinical and clinical teaching and research. Certainly this was not
an original idea. The desire to align the two components of medical
education had for decades encouraged progressive educators to place
medical schools and hospitals in proximity to each other. The innovation
of Vanderbilt's medical school–hospital came from its emphasis on this

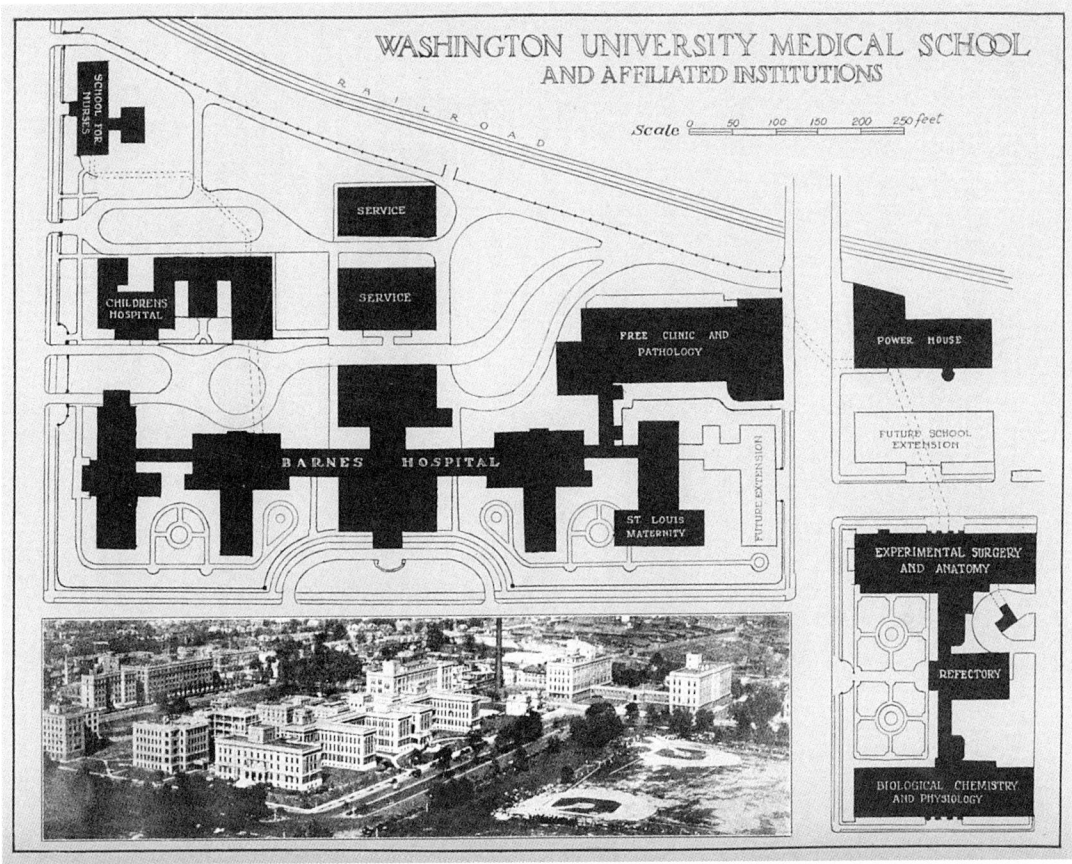

2.8.   Washington University Medical School (*bottom right*) and affiliated institutions (*upper left*), ca. 1926.

aspect of medical education, a shift that Robinson believed would create
a better physician.

Robinson visited a number of medical colleges and hospitals as the
Vanderbilt plans developed, but his time as a faculty member and dean
at Washington University Medical School in St. Louis before coming
to Nashville likely fueled his determination to create a fully coordinated
medical school and hospital.[44] Robinson affirmed that his administrative
experience at Washington University Medical School had shaped his
September 1920 proposal.[45] His time in St. Louis may also have influenced his ideas about the physical plant. After Washington University
Medical School moved to its new facility in 1914, it—like Johns Hopkins
Medical School—occupied a school with an institute design located close
to its teaching hospital (fig. 2.8). At Washington University Medical
School, however, greater physical coordination existed between the various school and hospital structures than at Johns Hopkins. A corridor

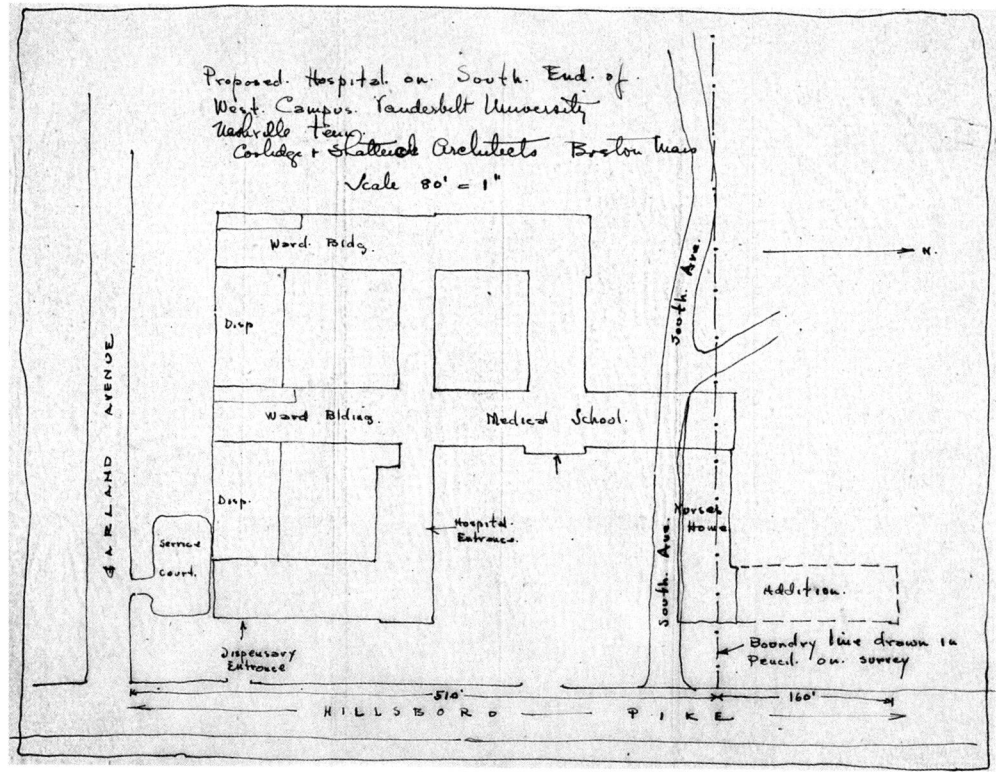

2.9.   Sketch for proposed Vanderbilt University medical facilities, winter 1921, Coolidge and Shattuck, architects.

linked the two laboratory buildings and refectory of Washington University Medical School. In addition, tunnels joined the medical school structures to the power plant and then to the pathology building, which communicated with the hospital. A description of the facilities published by the medical school declared, "A system of corridors and tunnels connects the buildings of the group so that they are practically *under one roof*."[46] Corridors joined the five structures of Harvard Medical School as well, but no publications emphasized this design element. Although in its basic form an institute design with multiple laboratory buildings, Washington University Medical School may have been understood by educators somewhat differently than the institute plans at Johns Hopkins and Harvard, and educators' ideas about architecture may have been changing more quickly than the school buildings themselves.

Robinson's idea for a combined medical school–hospital resonated with major funding organizations. In spring 1921, the General Education Board augmented a previous gift to Vanderbilt University School of Medicine, bringing the board's total support to $5.5 million, and

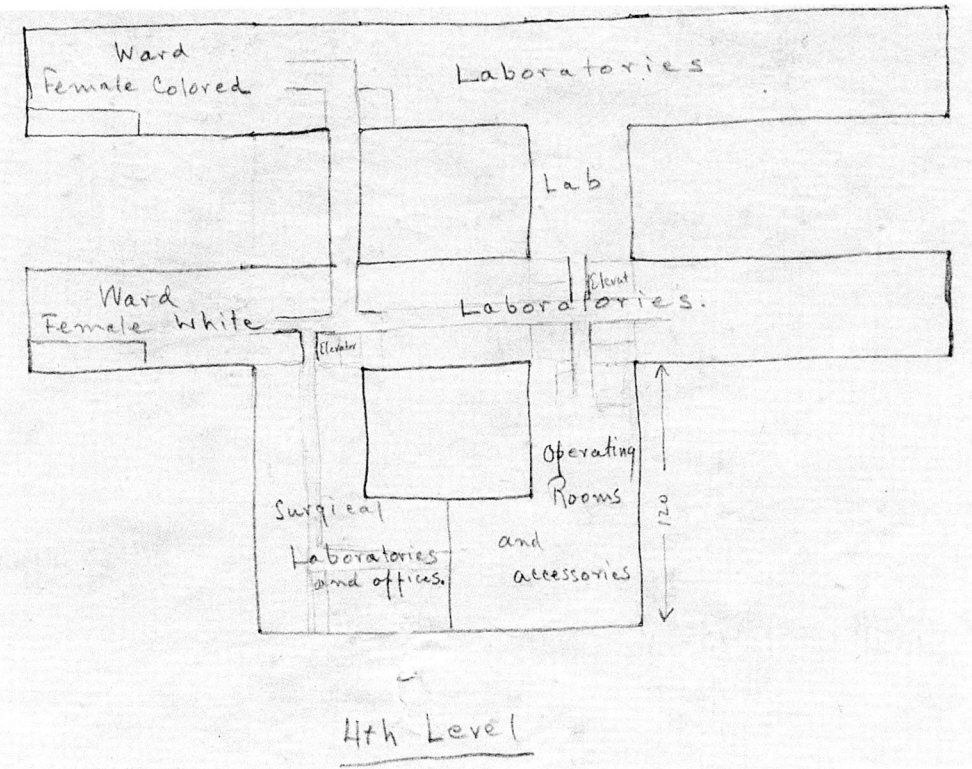

2.10.   Sketch for medical school–hospital at Vanderbilt University, June 1921, by G. Canby Robinson, fourth floor.

the Carnegie Corporation gave $1.5 million. Together with an earlier $1 million donation from Andrew Carnegie, these funds provided the money needed to erect on Vanderbilt University's main campus a plant that enacted Robinson's vision. In the end, construction of the entire complex—comprising medical school–hospital, adjacent nurses' home, and nearby combination power plant and laundry—cost approximately $3.35 million, with the remainder of the gifts reserved for endowment.[47]

Between making his proposal in fall 1920 and receiving the funds in spring 1921, Robinson collaborated on additional architectural plans with Coolidge and Shattuck, Chancellor Kirkland, and consultant Smith. In the winter of 1920–1921, Coolidge and Shattuck sketched a design for the West Campus, home to the main university, that continued to feature the medical school–hospital concept (fig. 2.9). Two north-south corridors connect the medical school concentrated to the north with the hospital facilities to the south. In June 1921, Robinson expanded on this idea when he created a number of sketches to establish the final form for the structure (fig. 2.10).[48] In this plan, medical school and hospital became a fully

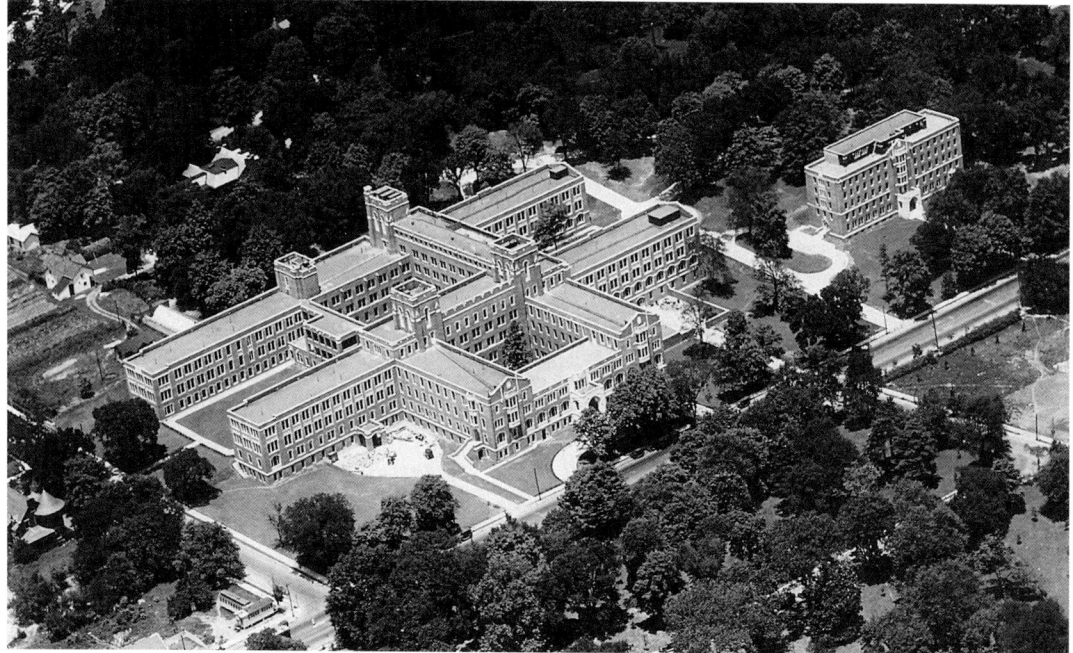

2.11.   Vanderbilt University School of Medicine and Hospital and Nurses' Home, 1925, Coolidge and
Shattuck, architects, with medical school–hospital at center left and nurses' home at far right.

coordinated facility organized around two main north-south corridors
that aligned the laboratories directly with the wards. Robinson found a
way to execute physically his conception of medical education, and the
facility opened on the main university campus in 1925 (fig. 2.11).

Although growing out of established trends in medical training
and medical school architecture, the 1925 Vanderbilt building provided a novel educational environment. Robinson explained his ideas in a
number of publications, including an article in the prestigious *Journal of
the American Medical Association* that contained architectural plans of the
first and third floors of the new facility. Robinson used this prominent
platform both to generalize about the direct relationship between the
design of a medical school and the type of pedagogy it facilitated and to
detail the structure at Vanderbilt and the innovations it made possible
in medical education.[49]

Vanderbilt University's medical school–hospital aligned the preclinical and clinical departments more closely than they had been coordinated
at any previous medical college. Laboratories for the preclinical sciences
composed three sides of a court oriented toward the north, while the
hospital was grouped at the southern end of the building. The clinical
laboratories—spaces in which to undertake routine labs and investigative

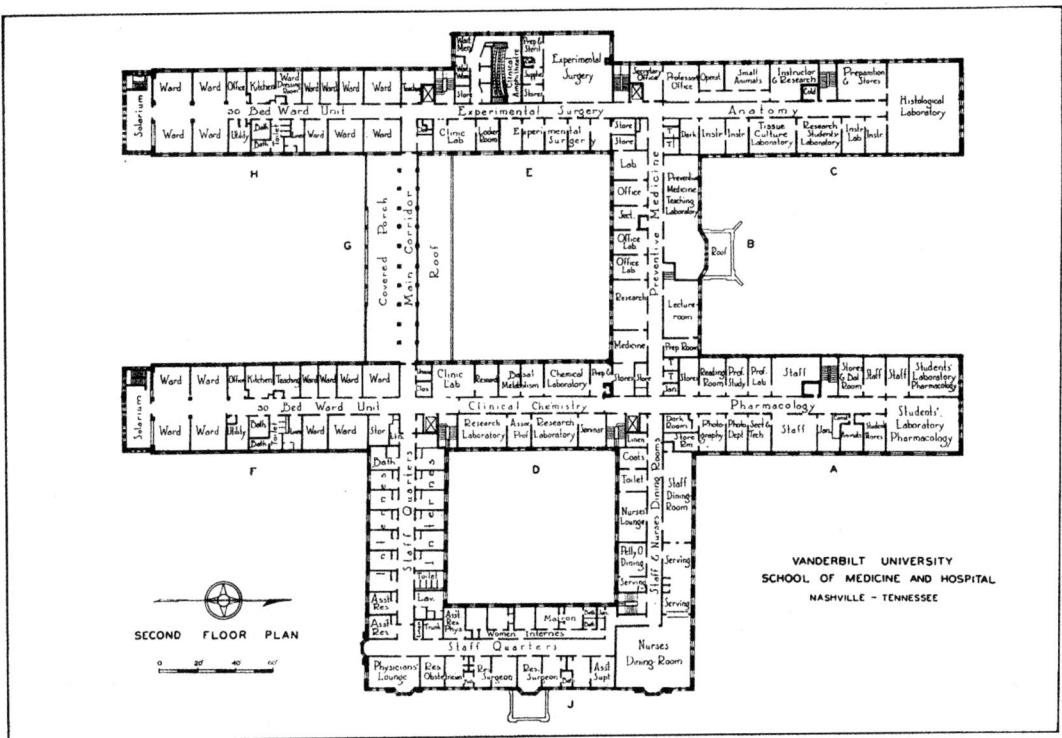

2.12.   Vanderbilt University School of Medicine and Hospital, 1925, Coolidge and Shattuck, architects, plan, second floor.

work related to patients—stood between the two sections, with each clinical laboratory adjacent to the preclinical subject with which it was most strongly connected conceptually. On the main north–south corridors of the second floor, the suites of rooms dedicated to the preclinical disciplines of pharmacology and anatomy (specifically histology, or microscopic anatomy) led to the affiliated disciplines of clinical chemistry and experimental surgery, respectively, and then to the wards (fig. 2.12). On the third floor one could move directly from the wings that housed preclinical physiology and bacteriology, along with pathology, to clinical physiology and bacteriology, respectively, and then to the wards (fig. 2.13). Robinson hoped that this design would encourage the tightest possible coordination among the preclinical departments, the clinical laboratories, and the hospital and result in the continuous transfer of ideas between the preclinical laboratory and the bedside.[50]

If merging separate institutes into a single building for the preclinical departments, as at Syracuse University College of Medicine, allied the medical sciences in the face of specialization, then the combined medical school–hospital at Vanderbilt extended this objective. The constant

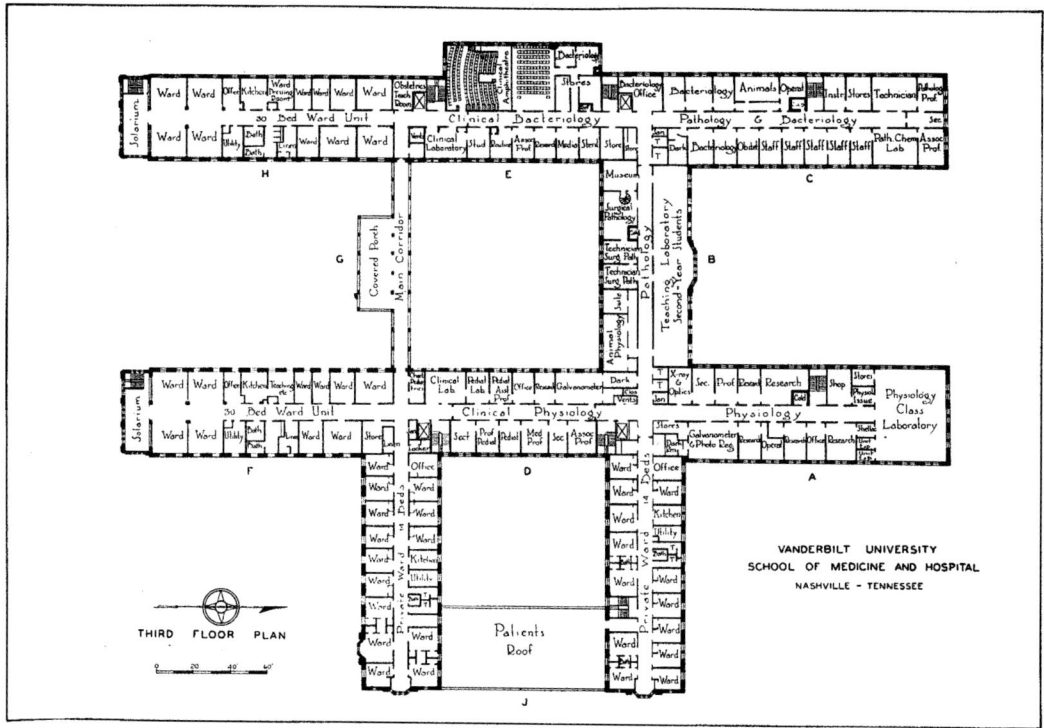

2.13.   Vanderbilt University School of Medicine and Hospital, 1925, Coolidge and Shattuck, architects, plan, third floor.

contact between the various preclinical and clinical departments, so the argument went, would make it impossible for faculty and students to ignore the interconnectedness of the disciplines. Four years after the plant opened, Robinson published his perspective on the facility: "[The plans of the building] have been developed with the idea of stimulating a coordination of the various departments of the laboratories and hospital in such a way that an intellectual interrelation may be readily developed and cooperation of departments be effected. The physical continuity of departments which has been established goes far to eliminate barriers between the preclinical and clinical studies, and allows all departments to exert a constant influence on the training of future physicians."[51] As noted earlier, Wilburt C. Davison, dean of Duke University School of Medicine, wrote of the conceptual significance of a unified design in presenting medicine as one integrated enterprise rather than as a series of discrete parts. This idea applies to the single building for preclinical subjects, such as at Syracuse, but Davison directly referenced the medical school–hospital in comparison to the institute type. He asserted that the medical school–hospital was designed to "enable them [students] from their first day to observe medicine as a whole."[52] By aligning the preclinical and clinical departments, rather than highlighting their distinctiveness, the medical school–hospital presented the various modes for studying the human body, and returning it to health, as an indivisible network.

This idea of correlation, of engaging "medicine as a whole," was not the same as understanding the "patient as a whole," the concept that Robinson would advocate in the late 1930s. In his work on this concept, Robinson encouraged students and physicians to investigate a patient's social and psychological history alongside the biological factors typically explored.[53] Both architectural correlation and the patient as a whole, however, challenged the reductionist tendency in scientific medicine, features of which, according to medical historian John Harley Warner, included commitment to the laboratory, dependence on instruments for diagnosis, and the division of the profession into specialties. As Warner explains, beginning at the turn of the twentieth century educators at elite medical schools firmly entrenched in scientific medicine strove not to refute scientific medicine but to temper its growing reductionism.[54] Educators' rejection of the institute design and enthusiasm for the unified plans, especially the medical school–hospital, represented an antireductionist perspective and resulted in buildings that encouraged a form of scientific medicine that celebrated not specialization but coordination.

Davison, dean of Duke University School of Medicine during the construction of its medical school–hospital, also lauded the efficiency of that plan.[55] The single building for preclinical studies increased efficiency compared with the institute design, but the combined medical school–hospital economized movement even more. Meharry Medical College opened a medical school–hospital in 1931, and five years later its president wrote that "considerable time is saved when the facilities for teaching students are concentrated under one roof, over the system of having certain laboratories in separate buildings and where students must go varying distances for their hospital services."[56] Although students typically completed some amount of clinical training in area hospitals, particularly those dedicated to specialized subjects, such as obstetrics and psychiatry, or particular diseases, such as tuberculosis, clinical work was usually concentrated in the primary teaching hospital and, in the case of the medical school–hospital, within the same building.

The relatively small size of the Vanderbilt medical school–hospital further reinforced the ease with which faculty and students could travel from one area to another. As Rudolph Kampmeier, who joined the

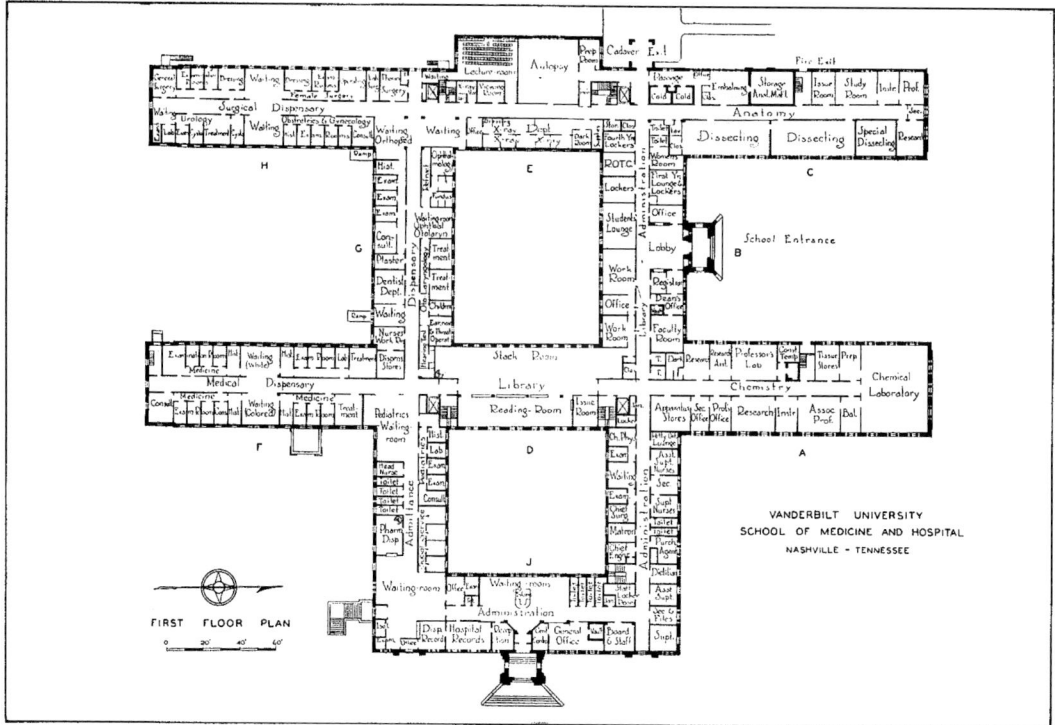

2.14.   Vanderbilt University School of Medicine and Hospital, 1925, Coolidge and Shattuck, architects, plan, first floor.

Vanderbilt medical faculty in 1936, recalled, "The institution physically was compact; it took only moments to visit a colleague's laboratory."[57] Additionally, the plant reduced duplications of space and equipment inherent to facilities with multiple buildings.[58] Although Vanderbilt University School of Medicine adopted the block schedule before it occupied the new plant, the faculty chose not to arrange the preclinical departments according to the alignment and sequence of the courses in the curriculum.[59] Students did not progress through the facility in conjunction with the evolution of their preclinical classes as did students at Harvard Medical School and Syracuse University College of Medicine. Perhaps the Vanderbilt medical faculty felt it unnecessary to cluster preclinical subjects in this way due to the compact nature of the plant, or the goal of efficient movement from preclinical department to related clinical discipline may have eclipsed the desire to coordinate the preclinical fields.

The commitment to efficiency also meant that educators and architects designing medical school–hospitals generally placed the most communal facilities where medical school and hospital converged. A

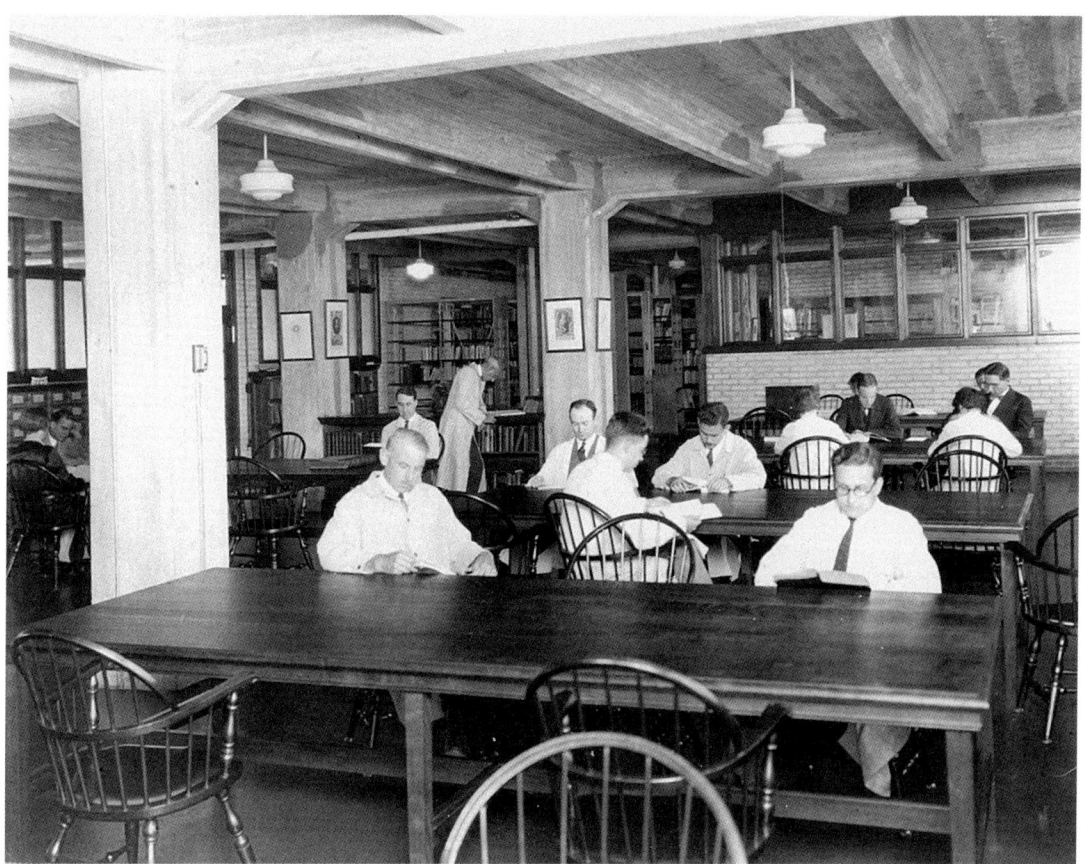

2.15.   University of Rochester School of Medicine and Dentistry and Strong Memorial Hospital, 1925,
         Gordon and Kaelber, architects, library reading room.

favorite choice for this location was the library. Davison and Robinson,
the deans responsible for the construction of medical school–hospitals
at Duke and Vanderbilt, respectively, emphasized the significance of a
single, centrally placed library to the integration promoted by this building type. Describing the Vanderbilt building, Robinson explained, "The
library occupies a central position on the first floor, almost analogous
to the hub of a wheel, and no provision for departmental libraries has
been made" (fig. 2.14).[60] Similarly, the founding dean at the University of
Rochester School of Medicine and Dentistry discouraged budgeting for
departmental libraries and sited the facility's lone library in the middle
of that medical school–hospital (fig. 2.15). Faculty and students at Rochester so appreciated the library's location that when expansion became
necessary in the late 1950s, the school's leadership decided to enlarge the
library without moving it.[61]

The Rise of the Central Library

The decision to construct a central library for the medical school–hospitals at Vanderbilt, Duke, Rochester, and elsewhere rather than to rely primarily on departmental libraries represented a relatively recent trend in medical school design. This shift served the needs of the medical school–hospital well and was particularly celebrated by the designers of this building type, but it occurred across all three medical school types: institute plans, single buildings for preclinical studies (see fig. 2.5), and medical school–hospitals. For medical educators, increased contact among faculty was just one of several benefits of the central library.

Before education reform, not all medical schools had libraries. When describing some of the remaining proprietary medical colleges in 1910, Abraham Flexner reported that "in general no funds are set aside for the purchase of books." At the College of Physicians and Surgeons, Los Angeles, he found "the word 'Library' is prominently painted on a door which, on being opened, reveals a class-room innocent of a single volume."[62] The absence of a library was no longer acceptable, however—a reality acknowledged by the AMA, which included in its criteria for ranking medical schools a provision for library facilities. A library had become critical to modern medical training due to the rapid expansion of medical knowledge. As medical historian Joel Howell explains, a faculty member in the mid-nineteenth century might have requested that a student read Hippocrates (the famed Greek physician who lived ca. 460–375 BCE) to gain insight into clinical medicine, but by the arrival of the twentieth century, progressive educators would more often send their students to review a recently published textbook or examine the swiftly growing body of scientific journals.[63]

As medical knowledge swelled and some schools started to undertake original research, reformed medical colleges began to depend on departmental libraries. By the mid-nineteenth century, Harvard Medical School had developed a general collection primarily for student use, and when the school moved to its building on Boylston Street in 1883, one room served the needs of the library. Over the next two decades, however, the Harvard medical faculty also established departmental libraries.[64] The departmental libraries resided in the offices of the department heads or in multifunction rooms adjoining their offices. One faculty member later reported, "On account of their situation in semi-private rooms they [the libraries] were far from being available to the many instructors, assistants, research workers and students who daily required them. The books were to a considerable extent uncatalogued, and indices to the periodical literature were seldom complete." When the school relocated in 1906, each of the quadrangle's four laboratory structures contained one or more departmental libraries. Within a year, librarian services were expanded and "modern library methods" introduced. Nevertheless, the libraries remained closely connected to individual faculty, as most of the anatomy library belonged to Professor Charles Minot rather than the school.[65] Separate from the departmental libraries, a student reading room, perhaps now home to the general collection, was located in Building A.

A similar trajectory took place at Columbia University's College of Physicians and Surgeons. In 1887, the medical school relocated to a single building for preclinical studies, and the purpose-built facility provided no dedicated library space, only a study room where students could review personal materials. By 1912, however, the school was maintaining several libraries. According to medical school librarian Alfred L. Robert, the college now housed "a students' reference library and . . . five department libraries, located on different floors of the building." The student reference collection had formed in 1901 when Columbia University's librarian transferred 260 volumes to the medical school. As for the five departmental libraries, Robert explained, "the department libraries have developed largely from the private collections of the professors, who in many cases have generously place [sic] the books at the disposal of students and colleagues." In fact, in 1912 two of the departmental libraries still resided in professors' offices. Additionally, Robert recognized the close connection between libraries and research and wrote confidently that "well equipped special libraries . . . are necessary supplements to the laboratories."[66] Regardless of whether the school occupied one building or several, departmental libraries seem to have been the norm at reformed schools when the twentieth century began.

In the early 1910s, however, American medical schools started to place increasing emphasis on the central library. In 1912 at Columbia University's College of Physicians and Surgeons, Robert opened a centralized periodical room containing journals and dissertations. Robert also reported that he had commenced work on a "union catalogue of everything in the college," the intent being that it would reside in the student reference library. By clarifying the contents of the various collections, the catalog would reduce unnecessary trips to another medical library in the city. Moreover, through his efforts, Robert already had determined that of the school's 328 journal subscriptions, 114 were duplicates.[67] Around 1913, Harvard Medical School began to centralize its libraries as well.[68]

By the 1920s, the central library, sometimes called the general library, had come to dominate medical schools in both practice and design. Some schools gave up departmental libraries altogether. In 1926, architect Henry R. Shepley, who was part of Coolidge, Shepley, Bulfinch, and Abbott, the premier architectural firm for medical schools in this period, wrote an article with the assistance of Robinson in which he argued strongly for the central library. He asserted, "The practice of maintaining departmental libraries is now generally considered unsound. It [the library] should be centrally placed with respect to the students and staff, adjacent to the administration, and in sufficiently close relation to the museum that the cataloguing, arranging and issuing of books and specimens may be done by the same staff."[69] Of the sixty-six four-year medical schools examined in the late 1930s for the Weiskotten Report, an AMA-sponsored review of American medical education, all had centralized collections to some extent, and twenty-nine reported no departmental libraries.[70]

Many faculties, however, wanted both a general collection and specialized collections, and the Weiskotten Report documented thirty-seven schools that had departmental libraries in addition to a central library.[71] In 1924, Western Reserve University School of Medicine in Cleveland moved into a single building for preclinical studies, with departmental libraries. As Torald Sollmann, who was both professor of pharmacology and material medica and school librarian, explained, "the decision was not against the establishment of a central library, but against the absorption of the departmental libraries." In fact, Western Reserve University School of Medicine had on its campus a separate general library in the form of the Allen Memorial Medical Library, completed in 1926 for the Cleveland Medical Library Association. In his effort to encourage the maintenance of departmental libraries, Sollmann systematically rebuffed each of the arguments typically made against them, specifically "inconvenience for extra-departmental use; expense of duplication of volumes; expense and efficiency of librarian service; and space requirement." In support of departmental libraries, Sollmann focused on their usefulness for research. Sollmann noted that the department could organize and manage the library in the way that worked best for that group of faculty. Close at hand, never closed, and under department control, these libraries were readily accessible and could respond more quickly than a central library not only to shifts in instructional demands but also to changing directions of research.[72]

Others disagreed with Sollmann's assessment of research needs. After Anna C. Holt's appointment as librarian at Harvard Medical School in the early 1930s, she spent twenty-five years in that role. In describing the move toward library centralization that began at Harvard Medical School around 1913, Holt articulated a different conception of the requirements of medical research: "Very decided changes were taking place in the trend of modern medicine and men teaching and doing research in the laboratories had become investigators in many fields. Their demands were universal and they required information in various branches of science for the solution of a single one of their problems. Thus the need became imperative for the Medical School to have a larger centralized library to serve all the departments equally, instead of one small general library and many scattered collections, all showing a tendency toward greater and greater duplication of material."[73] Robinson, Davison, and other proponents of coordination would have endorsed Holt's assessment.

Consistent with national trends, most departments at Harvard Medical School added their collections to a central library. The central library opened in 1914 in Building A, which was substantially renovated for this purpose in 1928 by Coolidge, Shepley, Bulfinch, and Abbott, an iteration of the firm that had designed the quadrangle. By the late 1940s, Harvard Medical School's central library had incorporated several collections, including those of the dental school and the Peter Bent Brigham Hospital, and had begun providing library services to the School of Public Health, established in 1922. Five branch libraries remained—two within the original quadrangle and three located elsewhere—but all were under the umbrella of the central library rather than their respective department or other organization.[74] In 1947, Western Reserve University remodeled part of its medical school building to create a central library.[75]

Perhaps nowhere did the rise of the central library leave a greater architectural legacy than at Johns Hopkins Medical School, where the William H. Welch Medical Library opened in 1929. The large and imposing structure combined the libraries of the Johns Hopkins Hospital, the School of Hygiene and Public Health, and the Medical School, which included a department of the history of medicine created simultaneously with and housed within the new library (fig. 2.16).[76] As a discrete building, however, the Welch Medical Library was unusual. In keeping with medical educators' and architects' resistance to the division of the campus according to the institute plan, medical school designers generally located libraries within medical school buildings. In 1940, the Weiskotten Report recorded that fifty-one of sixty-six four-year medical schools had a central library physically located in the medical school. Of the remaining fifteen schools, only six had a separate structure reserved entirely for the medical library.[77]

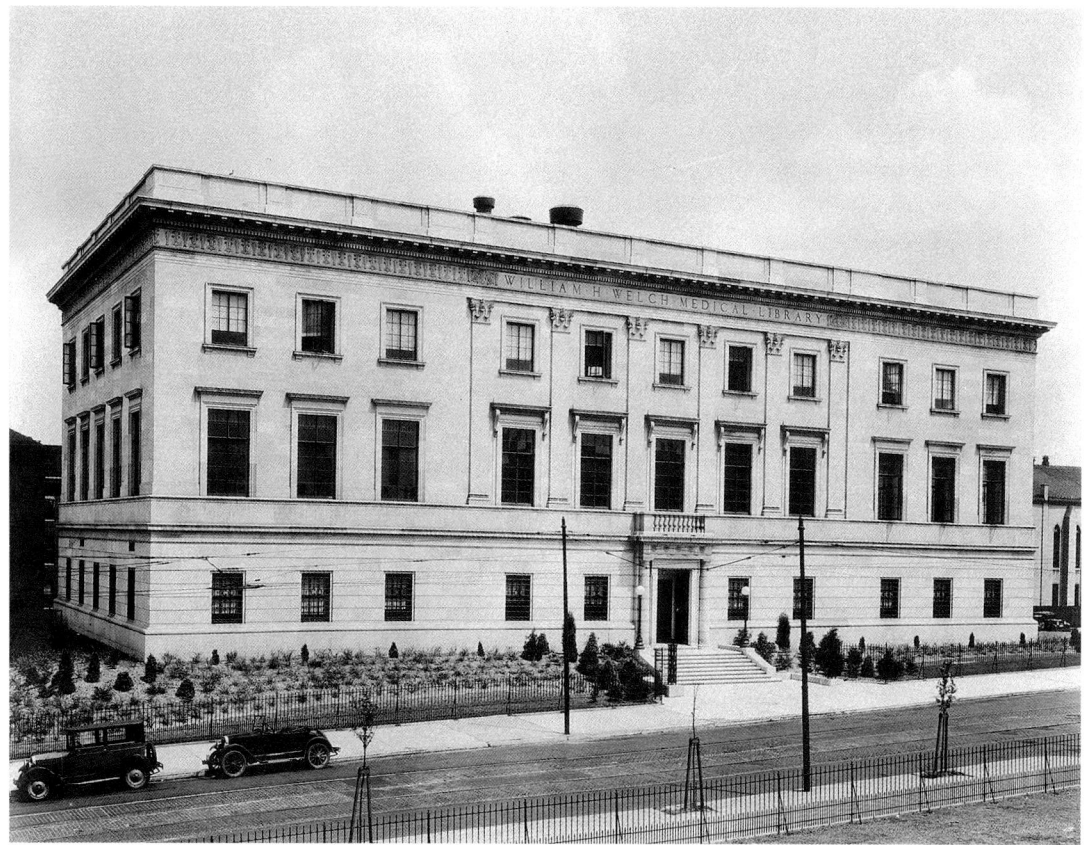

2.16.   William H. Welch Medical Library, Johns Hopkins Medical School, 1929, Edward L. Tilton, architect.

The shift toward centralization in medical libraries mirrored the
trend toward centralization in university library systems. Unlike in
medical colleges, however, centralization in university libraries frequently resulted in separate, large, and often prominently sited libraries.
Construction at American universities of the "great centralized research
libraries," in the words of sociologist Andrew Abbott, took place just
before and during the interwar years. These included libraries at the
University of Chicago (Harper, 1910), Harvard University (Widener,
1915), Johns Hopkins University (Gilman, 1916), the University of Michigan (unnamed, 1920), the University of Minnesota (Walter, 1924), Yale
University (Sterling, 1931), and Columbia University (Butler, 1934).[78]

Another significant distinction existed in the centralization of
university versus medical school collections. In the medical school, the
creation of a central medical library provided a general collection at
a distance from faculty members' laboratory and teaching space, but
when medical schools retained departmental libraries, discipline-specific

collections remained close at hand for researchers in the department. In the university, however, departmental libraries might be located some distance from the department. Abbott explains that "if most of these newly centralized libraries followed Widener's lead in containing departmental or seminar facilities, they nonetheless removed those facilities from the faculty's home space. Faculty now had to leave their main classroom buildings to do graduate training and library research."[79] In medical colleges, the maintenance of departmental libraries allowed faculty to spend more time in their departments rather than seek out materials in the centralized collections, a scenario read as either positive or negative depending on the particular faculty member or librarian.

Medical librarians may have pushed harder for centralization than faculty. Although the sample size here is very small, librarians Robert and Holt advocated for centralization, while a faculty member, Sollmann, argued for departmental libraries, a position he reportedly shared with the other department heads at Western Reserve University School of Medicine.[80] In the early twentieth century, medical librarianship rose alongside the medical profession, fueled by the increase in research, expansion in the amount of medical literature, and growth in the number of medical libraries.[81] A desire to reinforce their role as the primary administrators of the medical school's library collections and to shore up their professional position likely fueled librarians' commitment to centralization. In turn, some medical faculty may have resisted centralization to maintain greater control of the departmental collection. In the end, departmental libraries remained at many medical colleges, and discussion about the relationship between departmental and central libraries in medical schools continued through at least the end of the twentieth century.[82]

The dialogue about the centralization of the medical school library represented in microcosm the larger conversation in the 1910s and 1920s about coordination of medical school departments in response to specialization. Pioneering neurosurgeon Harvey Cushing made this point clear in his address at the dedication of the William H. Welch Medical Library in 1929. He lamented the "progressively increasing decentralization" of the last quarter century, what he described as "a successive splitting off from both preclinical and clinical departments of new groups, many of which slowly have attained sufficient strength and dignity to be recognized as independent units."[83] Cushing also echoed Robinson's assessment of the need for unification in the face of growing division between the preclinical and clinical sciences, and he summarized the contemporary situation bluntly: "More and more the preclinical chairs in most of our schools have come to be occupied by men whose scientific interests may be quite unrelated to anything that obviously has to do with Medicine, some of whom, indeed, confess to a feeling that by engaging in problems that have an evident bearing on the healing art they lose caste among their fellows. They have come to have their own societies, separate journals of publication, a scientific lingo foreign to other ears, and are rarely seen in meetings of medical practitioners with whom they have wholly lost contact."[84] Coordination in the form of a library offered a solution, particularly in the case of the Welch Medical Library, which housed a new department of the history of medicine, an area of study that was itself a unifying and humanizing force to Cushing. He envisioned a library "that will serve as a common meeting ground, where the different streams of knowledge may coalesce."[85]

The Medical School–Hospital and the Trifecta of Modern Medical Education

At the end of the nineteenth century, university-based medical schools began to celebrate their dedication to teaching, research, and patient care. In the opening decades of the twentieth century, medical schools' collective commitment to this constellation of activities deepened as more medical colleges affiliated with hospitals and cultivated research programs. Educators experimented with different ways of expressing this tripartite endeavor architecturally in the decades leading up to World War II. With the medical school–hospital at Vanderbilt University, these functions came fully under a single roof, an architectural development quickly emulated in several locations. In New York City, Columbia University's College of Physicians and Surgeons and Presbyterian Hospital opened the unified Columbia-Presbyterian Medical Center in 1928. In their fundraising efforts for the project, Presbyterian Hospital's boosters explained to the public the benefits of the facility: "The Medical Center will be made up of a group of coordinated institutions whose concern will be the welfare of the patient, as well as service to the cause of medical education and research."[86] Not surprisingly, these three undertakings were far more complicated—and contested—than fundraising materials suggested.

Teaching

If a medical school in immediate proximity to or connected by corridor with the hospital aligned laboratories and wards, then the medical school–hospital took this association a step further. The physical integration, according to proponents of the building type, would boost students' educational experience. The year after the Vanderbilt medical school–hospital opened, Robinson made his annual report to the university's chancellor and explained, "The students are thrown in close contact with the faculty as a whole; they obtain a grasp early in their course of the ultimate aims of medical education; they see the coordination of the laboratories and the hospital wards, and soon learn to appreciate their mutual dependence."[87] The design of the building would help to ensure that students' training in the basic sciences did not become divorced from clinical applications, a concern about laboratory instruction in this period. In 1927, prominent medical educator W. C. Rappleye outlined the results of a survey of more than five hundred general practitioners who had completed medical school between 1915 and 1922. He reported that the physicians criticized the "redundant laboratory work" of the preclinical courses, which failed to provide an "understanding of the sciences themselves."[88] In 1940, the Weiskotten Report described the situation more bluntly: "In too many instances the preclinical courses were merely a mimicry of nonmedical university courses practically devoid of any medical and clinical implications. Without wishing to in any way minimize the importance of pure science, it is important to point out that the primary objectives involve the laying of a foundation for the future practice of medicine and that such a program calls for preparation of the student for his introduction to clinical medicine in the third year."[89] The report separated out the stronger schools from this assessment, however, and noted that "many of the teachers in higher ranking departments found that the fundamental principles of the basic medical sciences frequently could be as well, if not better, taught in connection with human phenomena."[90] If and how to correlate basic science training with clinical applications remained an active topic of dialogue in the early twentieth century. Medical educators in any building type could have created more clinically relevant basic science courses, but to some medical educators the medical school–hospital itself encouraged this practice.

Other medical educators remained unconvinced by the purported advantages of the medical school–hospital, however. In 1929, the architect and medical consultant responsible for the new medical facilities at the University of Iowa described the "considerable difference of opinion [that] seemed to exist regarding the relative desirability of including the school building and the hospital in a single unit such as had been advocated by prominent teachers and carried out in the planning and building of a number of recent medical schools and teaching hospital units."[91] The Iowa medical faculty did not adopt the medical school–hospital plan and instead chose to erect one building for preclinical studies and connect it by tunnel with a nearby hospital. The architect and medical consultant explained:

> The arguments of those who advocate the single unit plan often seem logical enough but on critical analysis they are shown to be largely theoretical. . . . It is assumed that continuity between the clinical and preclinical departments will effect a closer relationship between them, but if this were so, which after all is doubtful, the department of physiology for instance could not be joined to general medicine without effecting a separation of medicine from surgery. In turning out practitioners of medicine, it is after all just as important to retain a close association between medicine and surgery as it is to retain a close association between medicine and physiology or surgery and anatomy.[92]

Even Robinson, perhaps the medical school–hospital's biggest promoter, had reservations about integrating laboratory and clinical training. In an article published two years before the completion of the medical school–hospital at Vanderbilt University, Robinson lauded the coordination of laboratories and hospital "in bringing about successfully the much desired correlation between departments," but he offered a cautionary note as well:

> It is possible . . . that this close linking of the laboratories and the clinics will . . . tend to have the undesirable influence of distracting both students and staff from engaging in the less spectacular and less practical activities of the laboratories, and to place too near them the allurements of clinical medicine. . . . The desire to impress on the student the practical application of his early medical studies may result in leading him astray, diverting his attention and giving him clinical notions before he is ready or capable of receiving them. There is much more to be said for carrying forward the laboratories into the clinics than there is for carrying the clinics into the laboratories, and it is hoped that a plan which will effect the former may not unduly produce the latter condition.[93]

Robinson appears not to have addressed this concern again in his writings, and once the Vanderbilt facility opened, he wrote only positively of the relationship between laboratories and hospitals.

Not only did medical educators express uncertainty about the instructional benefits of the medical school–hospital, but students' experience of the preclinical and clinical alignment also remains difficult to distill. On the one hand, the proximity of school and hospital to each other constantly reminded students of the preclinical and clinical components of their study. One 1951 Vanderbilt University School of Medicine graduate later explained that when students left the lecture hall in the center of the west corridor of the third floor (see fig. 2.13), they had only to look to one side to see the preclinical department of pathology and to the other to see the surgical ward. Students had the opportunity to learn in a place where doctors were working; they could easily see what was going on in the other sections of the building.[94] With doors enclosing some of the wings, however, this looking may have been more metaphorical than actual, but correlation did occur in other ways. At least one preclinical department at Vanderbilt reported, "The compactness of the building . . . makes it easy" for cooperation with the clinical faculty, who "at appropriate places in the course . . . present clinical material or lectures showing the relation between the subject being studied and the clinic."[95]

On the other hand, the presence of preclinical and clinical facilities does not necessarily mean that students went back and forth between these sections of the building on a regular basis. Woman's Medical College of Pennsylvania relocated to a medical school–hospital in 1930. The architects and medical educators responsible for the design bifurcated the plant vertically, with the college on one side and the hospital on the other. On each floor, a single hallway connected the two sides, but a set of doors demarcated the boundary between school and hospital (see fig. 1.9). Students did not routinely move between the two sections. One class of 1954 graduate recalled that the swinging doors on each floor effectively separated the college and hospital, as well as the students' preclinical and clinical training. She underscored this point when she noted that students spent their preclinical years in casual clothing and their clinical years in a white coat.[96] Earlier students likely had a similar experience, judging from the guidelines printed in the 1945–1946 *Freshman Handbook*. For the first year, it advised "almost any type of general school clothes" but cautioned that "during the upperclass [*sic*] years students are reminded of their professional status and should dress accordingly."[97] The locations of the stairs and the elevators within Woman's Medical College enabled occupants to travel vertically to all floors of the college or hospital, respectively, without entering the opposite side of the building, and apparently many students rarely crossed from one side to the other.

Medical educators championed the innovative pedagogical environment of the medical school–hospital, but simply placing the medical school and hospital under one roof did not automatically change either the way that faculty taught their courses or the students' daily experiences. Although the medical school–hospital design undoubtedly encouraged correlation of preclinical and clinical training, it could not inherently achieve this shift any more than could the medical school adjacent to and possibly linked by corridor with the hospital. Even Robinson, who saw physical integration of clinical and preclinical departments as the "first requisite" of a coordinated curriculum, admitted that "the question of physical contact will not accomplish the solution of the problem."[98] Success depended on adjusting the curriculum as well. Sociologist Thomas F. Gieryn, in his work on science facilities, asserts that "tethers," which are connectors between buildings such as corridors and tunnels, are "not just physical and functional linkages . . . ; they may also become symbolic."[99] In the case of medical schools attached by corridor with or in the same structure as a hospital, the symbolism of an educational enterprise that combined laboratory and clinic was clear. Equally clear, however, was the fact that novel design does not necessarily result in new teaching methods.

Research

In the late nineteenth and early twentieth centuries, designers of medical schools believed that an environment privileging investigation, irrespective of building type, would have a positive impact on medical students. According to Robinson, "The students are . . . exposed to the spirit of research, and seem to catch this spirit, which it is hoped they will carry into their future work as practitioners of medicine."[100] Thomas Ordway, dean of Albany Medical College in upstate New York, explained further: "[Medical education] should mean the acquiring by the student as early as possible of the research point of view so that as a practitioner he may realize that each patient or even each change in the condition of a patient is a new problem to be solved. Such an attitude should prevent to a considerable extent routine orders in the management of patients and allow practitioners to make real contributions to the development of medicine."[101] Quoting Johns Hopkins Medical School cofounder William Osler, Robinson made an additional claim: through "the atmosphere of research," the student "should come face to face with the cold logic of science which 'Keeps the mind independent and free from the toils of self-deception and half-knowledge'" and provides an antidote to the "many other deceptions of well-advertised half-science or half-truths whose toils we must constantly avoid."[102] For the designers of medical school–hospitals, the building type offered an opportunity not only to introduce students to research but also to facilitate a more specific research goal. Although architectural change does not inherently shape research any more than it does teaching, the faculty planning the medical school–hospitals asserted that the design would mitigate the increasing specialization in medicine by encouraging interdepartmental collaboration on a level not possible in other medical school building types.

From today's perspective, we can hardly imagine how research took place in early twentieth-century medical schools, when federal funding was not a possibility. In the 1970s, the colleagues of Edward F. Adolph, a University of Rochester School of Medicine and Dentistry physiologist, repeatedly asked him about research funding in the first part of the century. A member of the faculty at Rochester since its beginning in 1925, Adolph explained that "every faculty member tacitly understood that research activities were part of his work, on a par with teaching and patient care, and that the School would do what it could to provide facilities for those activities." All department heads, and particularly the dean, "set an example in research initiation." Adolph went on to describe some of the specific features of the school that encouraged research: "Every faculty member, I believe, was free of teaching some months of the year. The result was that all worked at and talked about research projects. Where equipment was required, teaching instruments could be employed. Supplies could often be drawn from stocks of chemicals and glassware in the department storeroom. Animals could be used in moderate numbers. . . . Many a person experimented on himself and friends; borrowing of materials sometimes led to collaboration."[103] Rochester's pathology department established a relationship in 1926 with Eli Lilly and Company that came to include stipends to expand research on anemia.[104] Individual departments also obtained modest research grants, and around 1929 the dean procured a foundation gift for a fluid research fund. A faculty committee distributed small amounts annually, with particular emphasis on interdepartmental work.[105]

The interest in interdepartmental collaboration was not new or unique to Rochester. In the early twentieth century, specialization continued, and the preclinical and clinical fields also grew further apart.[106] In 1912, Henry H. Donaldson, neurologist at the Wistar Institute of Anatomy and Biology, an independent research institute in Philadelphia, explained how coordination, in this case a medical school and hospital near a university, could mitigate the effects of specialization: "Specialization requires to be supplemented by cooperation. The passing comment or appreciation, the incidental conversation, are most potent. They prevent useless labor and reveal unsuspected relations. This form of intellectual stimulus, always difficult to cultivate even under favorable conditions, becomes well nigh impossible in the face of geographical

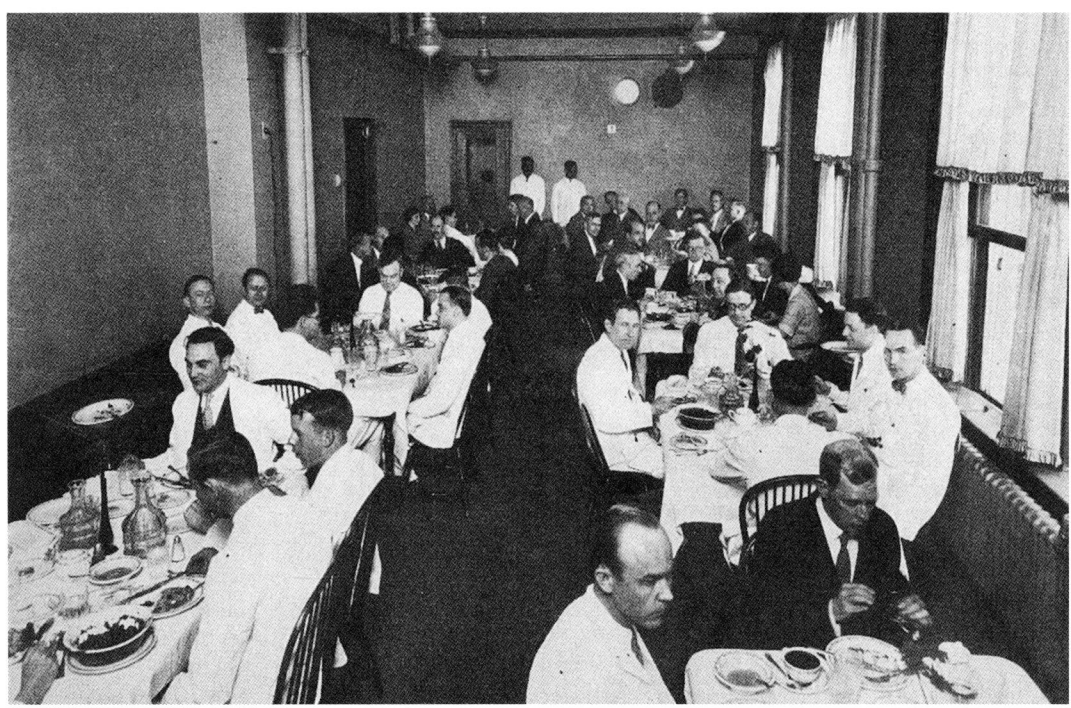

2.17.   Vanderbilt University School of Medicine and Hospital, 1925, Coolidge and Shattuck, architects,
           physician dining room. Photograph ca. 1929.

separation. The farther the sciences divide, the more imperative is the
concentration of all workshops at one spot."[107] Educators who supported
unified medical school designs, and particularly the medical school–
hospital, would have agreed with Donaldson's assessment of the impact of physical proximity, in contrast to the mind-set of the faculty at
Harvard Medical School, where a 1906 publication affirmed that the
quadrangle, with its institute design, enabled "each Department . . . to
arrange its courses of study and to perform research work without that
friction which is inevitable when all are crowded into one building."[108]
The institute design emphasized separation, even isolation, of faculty
as they engaged in teaching and research, but the unified designs, and
especially the medical school–hospital, promoted interaction. After three
years in the Vanderbilt medical school–hospital, Robinson reported, "the
faculty has developed a unity of understanding and of cooperation to an
unusual degree." He went on to say that "the facilities and the special
knowledge of the staff of each department have been utilized freely by
members of other departments. A group consciousness has developed
which has been distinctly beneficial in cultivating a spirit of stimulation
in research and in teaching." Robinson highlighted the daily luncheon

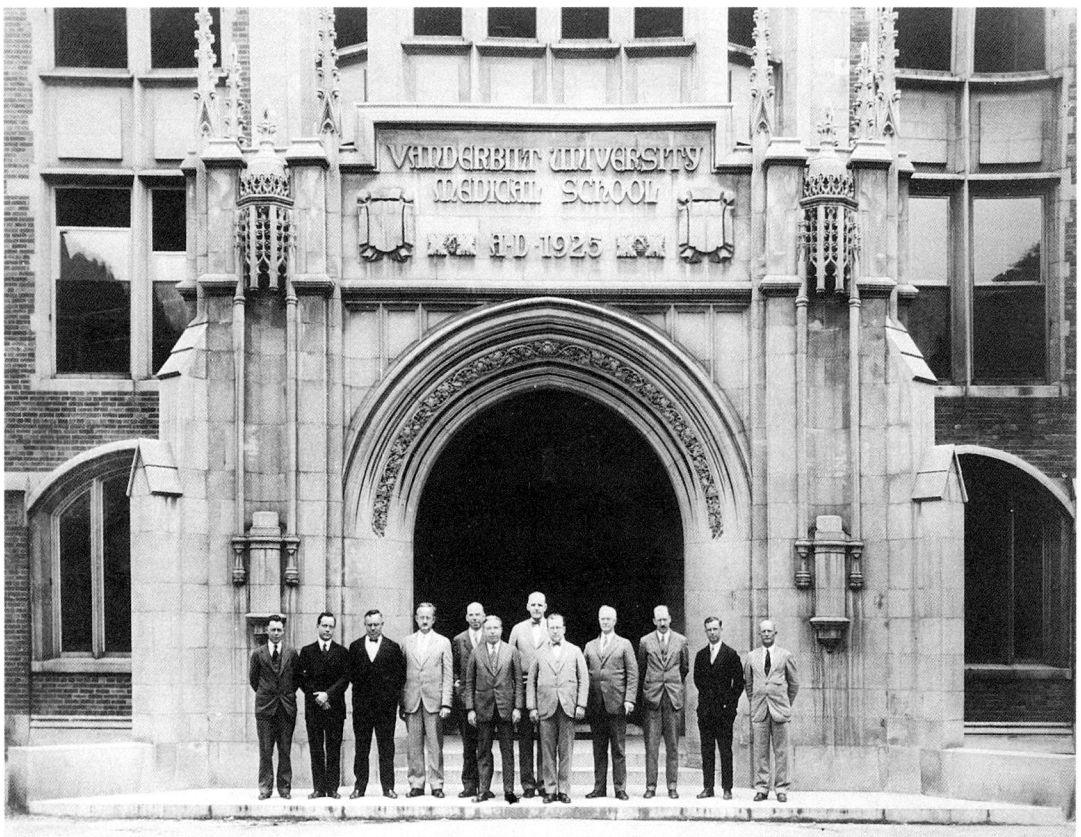

2.18.   First group photograph of the senior faculty at the reorganized Vanderbilt University School of Medicine,
         ca. 1925, in front of the medical school entrance of the recently completed medical school–hospital.

attended by faculty from all departments as a central component of the
cooperative environment.[109]

Many familiar with the Vanderbilt University School of Medicine's
first decades in the facility joined Robinson in underscoring the significance of the communal lunch in the physician dining room (fig. 2.17).
As affirmed by the hospital's first chief resident in medicine, Tinsley
Harrison, who went on to spend the next sixteen years at Vanderbilt,
"interns, residents, and faculty members all ate in the single hospital
dining room. There were no fixed places. One day I might have lunch
at the same table with the Chairman of a preclinical department, or a
junior full-time teacher and one or more interns and assistant residents.
The next day there would be a different group."[110] With some frequency,
the university chancellor also joined the assembled faculty, which in
1925 included just nineteen professors, associate professors, and assistant
professors (fig. 2.18).[111] Rudolph Kampmeier, appointed to the Vanderbilt

medical faculty in 1936, later stated, "As all have agreed, the dining room was the most important spot in the whole school. Here a small band of scholars could meet to discuss, debate, and criticize concepts in research or clinical practice in an atmosphere of friendship." To Kampmeier, the interactions in the dining room, the school's small size, the slower pace of the school's early years, and the accessibility of the department chairmen facilitated the free exchange of ideas that accounted for the productivity that quickly translated into Vanderbilt University School of Medicine's prestigious reputation.[112]

Adolph had a similar experience at the University of Rochester, where, as at Vanderbilt, the school of medicine occupied a relatively small medical school–hospital. He recalled, "In 1925 there were about twenty members in the faculty of the School. They filled two or three tables of the lunchroom. That was where they learned from one another and aired their varied opinions, and where the dean sampled prevalent views before each problem came to the Advisory Board for decision."[113] Also, both Rochester and Vanderbilt had a monthly meeting of their respective university medical society, which provided the opportunity to learn about research from around the medical school. At Rochester, the regular interdepartmental seminar brought preclinical and clinical faculty together until faculty growth led to its eventual replacement by departmental seminars.[114]

The compact medical school–hospital facilities at places such as Vanderbilt University and the University of Rochester were designed to bring people together in the dining room, long hallways, and central library. In 2002, Robert D. Collins reviewed the existing literature on Vanderbilt's medical school and noted a shared conclusion: "the building design, coupled with facilitation of communication between preclinical and clinical faculty, was key to creating the harmonious and collegial atmosphere for which Vanderbilt was (and is) known."[115] Within this atmosphere, significant research took place between 1925 and 1935, including what Collins considered "five major discoveries" that established the school's national reputation. Among these discoveries was William DeMonbreun's path-breaking work on the fungal infection histoplasmosis. In describing his research on histoplasmosis, DeMonbreun emphasized the impact of interdepartmental collaboration at two junctures in his various investigations.[116] Collins's analyses reinforce the assessment of the 1925 medical school–hospital offered by the dean of Vanderbilt University School of Medicine forty years after the facility opened: "All in all, the plan was a success. It did provide for close relationship of functions and personnel and contributed greatly in my opinion to the closely knit, integrated and coordinated mechanism or organization in medical teaching, as well as medical care and research, for which it was designed and for which it represented a new concept."[117]

In the early twentieth century, major discoveries occurred at medical schools housed in all building types, but in the 1920s many educators celebrated the medical school–hospital for its encouragement of collaboration in research. The unified medical school designs, and the medical school–hospital in particular, reveal the effort made by educators to mitigate the impact of specialization on teaching and research. In the case of the medical school–hospital, the emphasis on cooperation brought the clinics into unprecedented proximity to the laboratory, a point that concerned some. In 1929, the architect and the medical consultant for the University of Iowa's medical school and hospital, two separate structures connected by a tunnel, described the faculty's criticisms of the medical school–hospital building type and concluded, "Is it not conceivable that the tendency has been too much to bring the patient and the guinea pig into juxtaposition?"[118] For proponents of the medical school–hospital, the answer to this question was no.

Patient Care

In the nineteenth century, medical schools often located close to hospitals, a convenience for the physicians—and any students—active in both institutions, but almost invariably the hospitals tolerated only the most cursory teaching and research in their buildings. Medical school leaders intent on education reform and hands-on clinical training for students waged vigorous campaigns to persuade hospital trustees or voters and legislative bodies to alter hospitals' missions. They achieved their goal. By 1921, every medical college in the nation could boast a teaching hospital either controlled or owned by the school. Educators' success in acquiring teaching hospitals depended on several factors. Critically, hospitals had shifted from being locations for indigent care to serving as sites for the latest technology and procedures. This change meant that hospitals wanted what progressive medical schools could offer, such as access to top physicians, including those in the basic sciences, and laboratory facilities. In the end, hospitals agreed to become sites of significant medical education and research out of the conviction that teaching hospitals provided superior clinical care, thanks to a large staff of academic physicians who were constantly available and to inquisitive students observing their instructors' work. Big, ambitious, and already invested in new technology, the hospitals that affiliated with medical schools hoped their roles in medical education and research would also propel them to international prominence. On the most pragmatic level, technology and clinical laboratories were costly, and mergers enabled hospitals and universities to share the expense. Additionally, a number of substantial philanthropic gifts to hospitals stipulated that they align with modern, scientific medical schools. In time, a Class A ranking by the AMA required control of a satisfactory teaching hospital, and many medical schools that could not meet this condition ultimately closed.[119]

The dramatically expanded relationship between medical schools and hospitals reinforced the existing tendency for medical schools to settle in the vicinity of hospitals, and medical schools in the process of reorganizing almost always built on sites near hospitals. At first the medical colleges constructed either single buildings or institute plans adjacent to hospitals. Then, in the 1920s, complete physical unification of medical school and hospital began to occur. This trajectory did contain a few exceptions, however. Architectural historian Jeanne Kisacky has reviewed the relationship between medical schools and hospitals in the 1870s and 1880s and affirmed that medical schools usually enjoyed their own facilities close to the hospital, but she points out the unusual case of the 1876 Jefferson Medical College and Hospital, designed by architects Frank Furness and George E. Hewitt, which was, "in essence, a three-story pavilion hospital stacked on top of a two-story medical school."[120]

Coincidentally, another Philadelphia school, Woman's Medical College of Pennsylvania, also aligned physically with a hospital at an early date. In 1862, after a short closure due to the Civil War, Woman's Medical College reopened in rented rooms within the Woman's Hospital of Philadelphia. Often excluded from observing in hospital amphitheaters and wards and from house staff positions, women faced greater challenges than their male counterparts in obtaining clinical access. The Woman's Hospital, founded in 1861 in large part to supply the students of Woman's Medical College with clinical instruction, provided the medical college with a hospital affiliation, which was rare for medical schools at the time. When the college needed a new home, the hospital offered it a favorable rental arrangement. In the early 1870s, however, the hospital recognized little benefit from students on the wards and moved to push out its tenant when space became tight. Woman's Medical College wanted to maintain its unusual arrangement for clinical teaching, so in 1875 it occupied a purpose-built structure located very near the hospital. Demonstrating that physical proximity alone cannot dictate relationships, the affiliation between Woman's Medical College and the Woman's Hospital dissolved completely in the early twentieth century. Woman's Medical College constructed its own hospital one floor at a time between 1907 and 1913

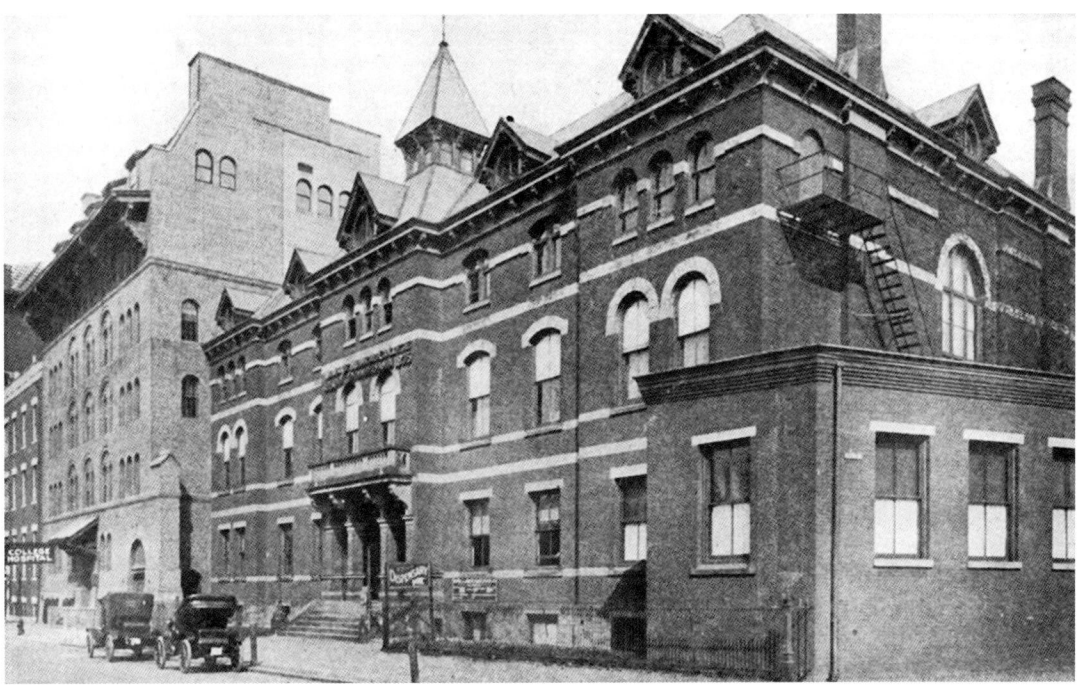

2.19.   Woman's Medical College of Pennsylvania, 1875, Addison Hutton, architect, with adjoining "college hospital" (*left*) completed 1913.

on a lot between Woman's Medical College and Woman's Hospital (fig. 2.19).[121] The college and hospital may have connected directly with one another, as outside physicians who reviewed the school in 1919 described the "college and hospital *building*."[122] Regardless, in neither the Jefferson Medical College and Hospital example, which stacked the medical school and hospital, nor the Woman's Medical College scenario, where a hospital erected piecemeal came to occupy the adjacent lot, did physical integration occur between the preclinical and clinical departments on the level celebrated at Vanderbilt University in the mid-1920s. Medical educators recognized that the medical school–hospitals constructed at Vanderbilt, Rochester, and elsewhere represented a novel architectural form for medical schools.

The fully coordinated medical school–hospital became popular in part because it supported ideas prevalent in both medical school and hospital design. At the same time that medical schools moved away from facilities composed of multiple buildings, so did hospitals. In the early twentieth century, separate pavilion wards, such as those at Johns Hopkins Hospital (see fig. 1.4) and Peter Bent Brigham Hospital, gave way to a variety of consolidated designs. Jeanne Kisacky has investigated this shift and writes, "While not every new American hospital in the 1920s was a high-rise, the era of the detached pavilion hospital was near its end. Even new low-rise American hospital facilities typically housed all spaces under one roof." Beginning in the mid-1920s, medical schools merged with hospitals in relatively low buildings, as at Woman's Medical College, Vanderbilt, Rochester, Duke, Meharry, and Colorado, and in tall structures, as at Columbia-Presbyterian Medical Center and New York Hospital–Cornell Medical Center.[123] The 1920s witnessed a wave of construction for hospitals as well as medical schools, and designers of these institutions celebrated unified plans for similar reasons. For the leaders of hospitals and medical schools, consolidation offered efficiency, economy, centralization, and collaboration in the face of scientific medicine's increasing specialization and burgeoning spatial demands. Hospital structures, Kisacky explains, responded just as medical schools had to the "growing medical awareness of the systemic, holistic nature of many ailments." Modern hospitals, like medical schools, were also carefully designed to create efficient relationships between many departments. In addition, despite advances in lighting and ventilation, hospitals and medical schools typically utilized buildings with narrow wings in order to provide ample access to sunlight and air, a similarity in design that made it relatively straightforward to align hospital and medical school facilities.[124] Conveniently, according to at least one medical educator, hospitals benefited most from "a southern exposure insuring an excess of sunlight and fresh air for its wards," while "a school of medicine should demand . . . a northern exposure to secure clear steady light for its laboratories and scientific workrooms"—a conviction that meant the hospital's and school's light requirements complemented one another.[125] The medical school–hospitals constructed at Vanderbilt, Meharry, and Columbia-Presbyterian followed this north-south orientation for the laboratories and wards.

Among medical school–hospitals, not all coordinated the constituent institutions to the same extent. Although some facilities, such as those at Vanderbilt University and Woman's Medical College, contained long hallways that directly linked school to hospital, other designs reduced the connection between the medical college and the wards, as prominent hospital architect Edward F. Stevens noted in his descriptions of the University of Colorado School of Medicine and Hospital and Columbia-Presbyterian Medical Center. Of the former, located in Denver, he explained that "the hospital . . . is well cut off from although physically connected on each floor by corridors to the administration building, and thus to the school" (fig. 2.20). Nevertheless, Stevens contended, "from

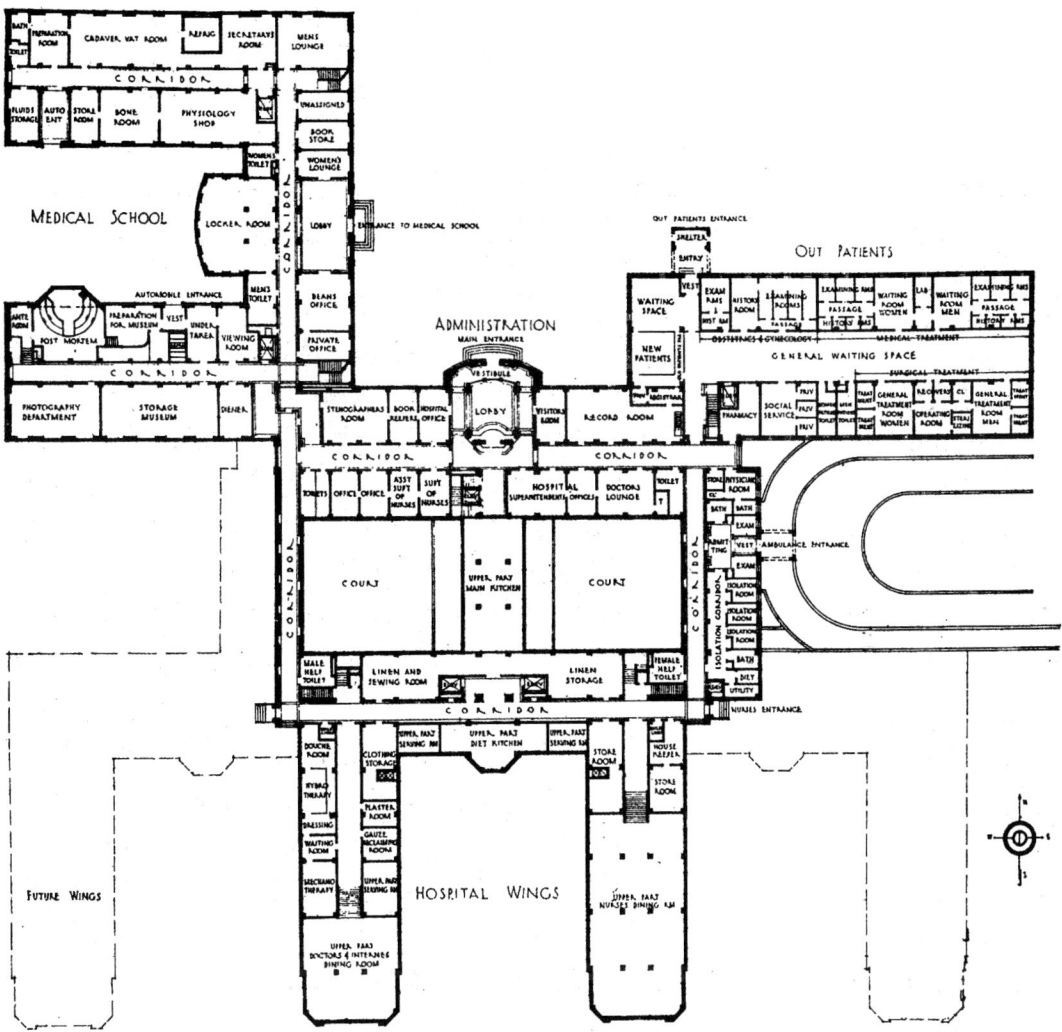

Ground floor plan.

2.20.   University of Colorado School of Medicine and Hospital, 1924, Maurice B. Biscoe, William E. Fisher, and Arthur A. Fisher, architects, plan, ground floor.

a careful study of the plans one will note the intimate relation of one department to the other, which are so planned that each department may function independently or in co-relation to the other."[126] As for the New York structure, which he called "one of the greatest developments of the medical school and hospital combination in this country," Stevens explained that "while there is a physical connection between the medical school, the clinic unit and the hospital, to go from one department to another one must pass through the administrative unit of the hospital

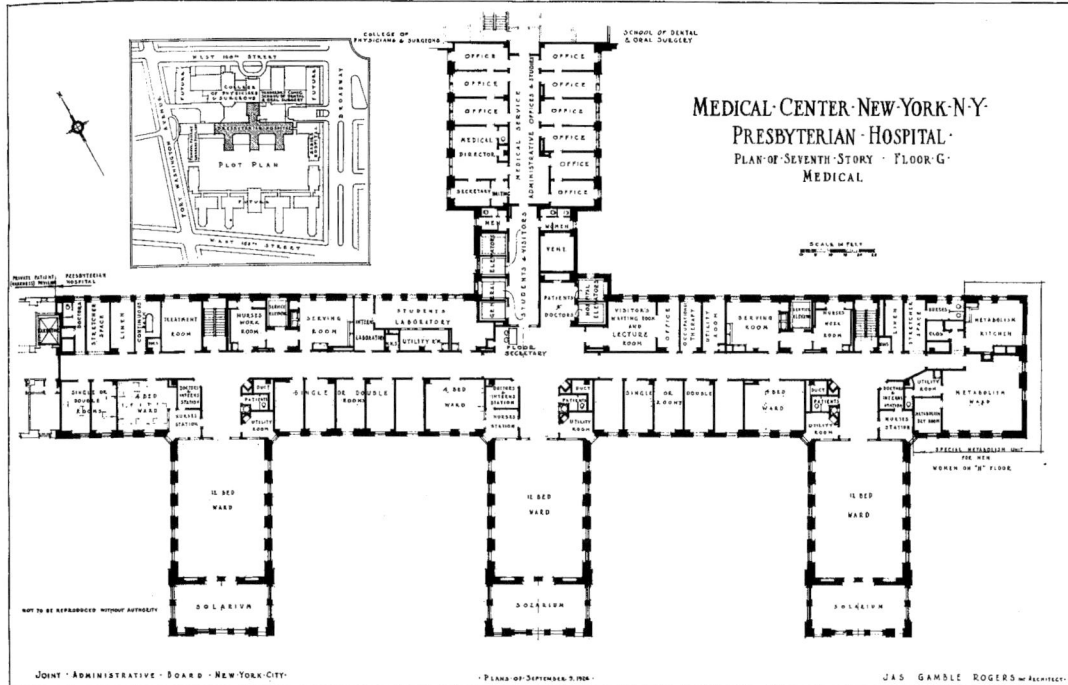

2.21.   Presbyterian Hospital, Columbia-Presbyterian Medical Center, 1928, James Gamble Rogers, architect, plan,
          seventh floor. The multistory wing to the northeast, referred to as the "stem," connected the medical school
          and hospital. On this floor the stem contained offices for the medical service administration.

floor, thus guarding very largely the privacy of the hospital" (fig. 2.21).
Stevens pointed out that the lecture rooms and clinical amphitheaters
were centrally located with regard to the school, outpatient clinic, and
hospital, but "to enter the hospital from the medical school or clinic,
the student must pass from his classroom or laboratory, through the
corridor upon which the staff offices are located, into the central lobby
of the hospital. This connection is made only in one location on each
floor." Stevens reversed his emphasis on separation, however, when he
concluded, "The medical school, with its laboratories and lecture rooms
on the many stories and with its vital connections to both clinic and
hospital, affords every opportunity for the closest co-operation of all
departments."[127]

     Stevens's convoluted readings of the designs reflected the contra-
dictions in the Denver and New York medical school–hospitals. At
Columbia-Presbyterian, the multistory wing, referred to as the "stem,"
that provided the critical link between school and hospital vacillated
between bifurcating and uniting the two institutions. On some floors
it housed facilities—such as the telephone exchange and instructional

space for the nursing school—that failed to align medical school to hospital in any pedagogically meaningful way. On other floors—such as those containing the McCosh Memorial Amphitheater for surgical demonstrations and rooms where students could sleep and study while on call for maternity cases—the stem served as a conceptual bond between school and hospital.

The stem at Columbia-Presbyterian represented in microcosm the ambivalence that surrounded merging the medical school and hospital into a single facility in the 1920s. As the medical school and hospital moved physically closer together than ever before, two elements in particular mitigated total integration. Kisacky does not differentiate between medical schools located on the same campus as hospitals and medical school–hospitals, but she argues that, when medical schools and hospitals rebuilt together, the level of physical distinction between the two institutions typically mirrored their administrative relationship. Affiliations between two strongly independent institutions, such as Columbia University's medical school and Presbyterian Hospital, usually resulted in greater physical autonomy than affiliations where one organization controlled both medical school and hospital, as at Vanderbilt and Colorado.[128] Reinforcing Kisacky's analysis, Stevens emphasized that at Columbia-Presbyterian Medical Center, "the institutions of the group . . . will not lose their individual identities."[129] These distinctions were not absolute, however. The University of Colorado created a less integrated plant than Vanderbilt University, despite the fact that both universities oversaw their respective hospitals and medical schools. No doubt local politics, departmental and personal relationships, and pedagogical and scientific agendas shaped these designs. The University of Colorado's architects also may not have known about Vanderbilt University's highly unified design when they drew the plans for the Denver facility.

Ongoing concerns about students on the wards further encouraged educators and architects to resist full physical integration in some medical school–hospitals. In a 1927 article for *Architecture* on the nearly completed Columbia-Presbyterian Medical Center, Robert Leroy wrote that the stem linking the medical school and hospital "gives ready access, while 'controls' prevent students from entering the hospital excepting in the ordered course of their work." Leroy noted that medical students would not be welcome in the private patients' wing, and he explained that "there will be galleries in certain operating-rooms from which students may observe the work, under favorable conditions, and in such a way that their presence cannot be detrimental in any way."[130] Leroy was not writing for a medical audience, and he may have intended his words to ease the fears of prospective patients. Educators and architects designing medical school–hospitals may have limited students' access to patients out of a recognition that some members of the public felt anxious about having students in the hospital.

Additionally, some physicians may have had apprehensions of their own about medical students on the wards. Medical historian Kenneth Ludmerer has explained that every American medical school had begun offering clinical clerkships by 1926, but most did not give students significant responsibility. Rarely did students have permission to enter the wards at night, and a 1924 fundraising booklet for Columbia-Presbyterian Medical Center explained that students on Presbyterian Hospital wards were primarily observers. Although Ludmerer contends that by the mid-1920s "fears engendered by the presence of medical students in the wards, so common a generation earlier, had virtually disappeared," he also mentions the existence of "periodic second thoughts about whether medical students really did belong on the wards," a situation that challenged relationships between medical schools and hospitals. Even as clinical education became firmly established, physician leaders worked to balance the demands of medical training with the needs of patients. Exchanges between the Peter Bent Brigham Hospital superintendent and physician-in-chief reveal the impositions placed on patients by student clinical clerks, whose examinations interrupted patients' meals and sleep. Numerous complaints from the wards described noise and commotion caused by clerks.[131] An architectural analysis underscores the lingering doubts of some members of the public and physicians about students having unrestricted ward access.

Despite these concerns, however, medical schools and hospitals had become intertwined, and research and training now took place on the wards. When coordinated on one campus and—in the case of the medical school–hospital—under one roof, the school and hospital became known as a "medical center." Although the term had been used at least once in the 1890s to describe a neighborhood with medical school, outpatient, and hospital facilities, decades would pass before the phrase took on its modern usage or became widespread. When Columbia-Presbyterian Medical Center opened in 1928, it was the first institution to put the phrase in its name (fig. 2.22). Modern medical centers usually contained a medical school, a general teaching hospital, and specialty hospitals united by the foundational concept of coordinated teaching,

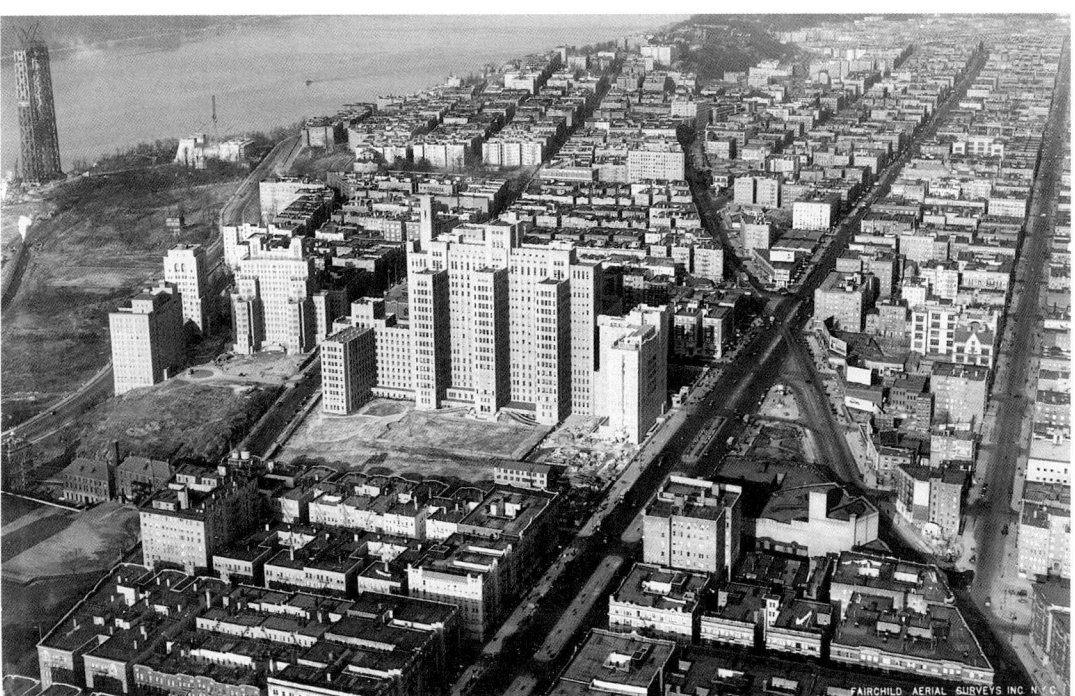

2.22.   Columbia-Presbyterian Medical Center, 1928.

research, and patient care. In the case of Columbia-Presbyterian
Medical Center, it initially included the medical school, Presbyterian
Hospital, the Sloane Hospital for Women, the Vanderbilt Clinic (the
outpatient department), the Neurological Institute, and Babies Hospital.
Following World War II, "academic medical center" replaced the earlier
"medical center."[132]

The Joint Administrative Board, the body responsible for oversee-
ing the affiliation between Columbia University's medical school and
Presbyterian Hospital, thought carefully about Columbia-Presbyterian
Medical Center's pioneering name. When the board decided to finalize
the name for the complex in 1926, its executive officer listed the various
unofficial titles applied to the project, and all contained the phrase "medical center," a term that the board subsequently noted carried positive
associations.[133] Columbia's leadership was at least partially responsible
for the phrase's early application to the project; more than a decade earlier, in 1915, it had published *A Medical Center for New York*, a pamphlet
describing the affiliation and the intended complex.[134] Presbyterian
Hospital also adopted the phrase before the official decision to use the
name.[135] When the Joint Administrative Board moved to finalize the
name, the executive officer pointed out that "within the past few months

the term 'Medical Center' has been advertised by Pittsburgh, Syracuse and Chicago, where similar movements are actively under way."[136] After the board decided to use the phrase, it considered formal action against the one "medical center" in the telephone book in New York City, to protect the name.[137]

The fundraising material created by Presbyterian Hospital, which raised nearly $4.5 million from the public toward the new facility, sought to educate potential donors about the triumvirate of activities undertaken in a medical center. One pamphlet, titled *Build New York a Medical Center*, explained that "a group of medical institutions including a general hospital, a medical school, special hospitals and research laboratories built around a common center and co-operating in care of the sick, medical education and research, is an accepted definition of a medical center." It declared that this initiative "means organized war on disease," and "it is the modern method of fighting disease." The pamphlet went on to detail the particular advantages of the medical center to the patient, to the student, and for research, respectively.[138]

The medical center of the 1920s celebrated the idea of coordinated teaching, research, and patient care, an idea with its roots at Johns Hopkins Medical School, Harvard Medical School, and elsewhere. Although the phrase "medical center" first appeared as a formal title with Columbia-Presbyterian Medical Center, a medical school–hospital, the term in time was applied to any campus that combined facilities for teaching, research, and patient care, regardless of building types. In 1937, Syracuse University opened a single-building medical school near affiliated hospitals, and physician Edward S. Van Duyn confidently declared, "With the opening of the new Medical College . . . the central unit of our developing Syracuse Medical Center becomes a completed fact."[139]

The idea of a unified facility for teaching, research, and patient care became a foundational component of academic medical design, and it remained prevalent until at least the end of the century. In 1999, Allan M. Brandt and David C. Sloane wrote, "It is a remarkable phenomenon, and one that can be explained only by the nature of certain historical contingencies, that the same institution in which the urban poor seek care at the door of the emergency room has, at the same moment, researchers conducting studies of the new molecular biology." According to Brandt and Sloane, this seeming paradox stems from the idea of the modern hospital as a place where science and medicine are interwoven. In this framework, basic research—research without direct clinical application—would seamlessly translate into clinical research, which in time would create cutting-edge patient care. Brandt and Sloane continue, "In some ways, situating these laboratories in hospitals reflects an anachronism, a time in which it was assumed that the scientist would also be a physician, easily moving from bench to bedside; within academic medicine such careers have become increasingly unlikely. Nonetheless, just as vestiges of the nineteenth-century hospital are found today, so this ideal of the physician-investigator is no small part of the academic hospital's structure and design. Academic medical centers promised to combine effectively teaching, research, and patient care, each goal benefitting the other."[140] Future generations would debate whether the medical center had met this promise.[141] But as the medical centers took shape in the 1920s and 1930s, enthusiasm and optimism soared.

The Medical School–Hospital as a New American Building Type

Medical schools in the opening decades of the twentieth century sought to coordinate physically with hospitals on the same campus or within the same building.[142] Like medical educators, architects actively discussed the design of these buildings. In 1928, prominent hospital architect Edward F. Stevens published the second revised edition of his book *The American Hospital of the Twentieth Century* with a chapter, "The Medical School Hospital," that had not appeared in earlier editions. In this chapter, Stevens described the designs of hospitals planned with special attention to laboratory and research space; hospitals and medical schools adjacent to one another; hospitals and medical schools connected by corridor; and fully integrated medical school–hospitals. Stevens devoted the greatest space to the facility at Vanderbilt University, with an extensive reprint of an article about it.[143] Stevens's emphasis on the Vanderbilt arrangement—in addition to his discussions of the medical school–hospitals at the University of Colorado and Columbia-Presbyterian Medical Center—suggests the novelty of this design.

The medical educators and architects responsible for the medical school–hospitals understood that they had created a new building type, a point made clear by several men who claimed to have invented the form. In October 1922, Charles Coolidge, a principal with the architecture firm responsible for Vanderbilt's facility, wrote to that university's chancellor. Hospital consultant Winford Smith had shared with Coolidge the blueprints of the medical school–hospital for the University of Colorado along with an article to be published in *Modern*

Hospital on the Denver facility. Coolidge asserted, "In some way or other it seems as if the architect must have seen one of our reports on the Vanderbilt buildings as it is based on the same lines and is stealing our thunder." Smith encouraged the publication of the Vanderbilt plans in *Modern Hospital*.[144] In February, the article on the Nashville school appeared in *Modern Hospital*, two months before the article on the Colorado school.[145] Whether the Colorado facility's chief architect, Maurice Biscoe, had seen the Vanderbilt plans is not known, but priority of design lies with the dean of Vanderbilt University School of Medicine. Robinson completed the June 1921 sketches that formulated the relationships within and footprint of the Vanderbilt complex before Biscoe began drawing the plans for the Colorado structure that fall.[146] Publicly Robinson would explain, "A plant embodying many of the same features was simultaneously projected for the medical school of the University of Colorado at Denver."[147]

Similarly, planning for the medical school–hospital at the University of Rochester did not get under way until fall 1921, when the founding dean, George Whipple, arrived and after Robinson had executed his Vanderbilt sketches.[148] Accounts vary as to whether the Rochester architects had access to the Nashville design. In 1927, Whipple wrote, "This plan [for the University of Rochester facility] was adopted practically simultaneously by the School of Medicine of Vanderbilt University . . . and the School of Medicine of the University of Colorado," a claim he would repeat again in his autobiography three decades later: "Vanderbilt and Rochester evolved the same general plan for these buildings, working independently."[149] In 1929, Robinson put on record that "after the plans of the new Vanderbilt school were drawn, they were adopted for the new medical school of the University of Rochester, changes being made only to meet their local conditions and to afford a somewhat larger plant. The architects of the Vanderbilt plant cooperated freely with those of the Rochester plant."[150] Considering the almost identical, and at the time unusual, footprint of the medical facilities at Vanderbilt and Rochester, it is difficult to have much confidence in Whipple's assertion. The efforts to claim the first medical school–hospital also reflected the competitiveness among American medical schools as they introduced reforms designed to strengthen their programs and outstrip their rivals.[151]

In the end, Colorado, Rochester, and Vanderbilt opened medical school–hospitals between 1924 and 1925, and the enthusiasm for the design spread quickly. Duke University School of Medicine dean Wilburt Davison later wrote, "Like all medical schools built since 1919, e.g., Colorado, Vanderbilt, Rochester, Columbia, and Cornell, the [Duke] Medical Center

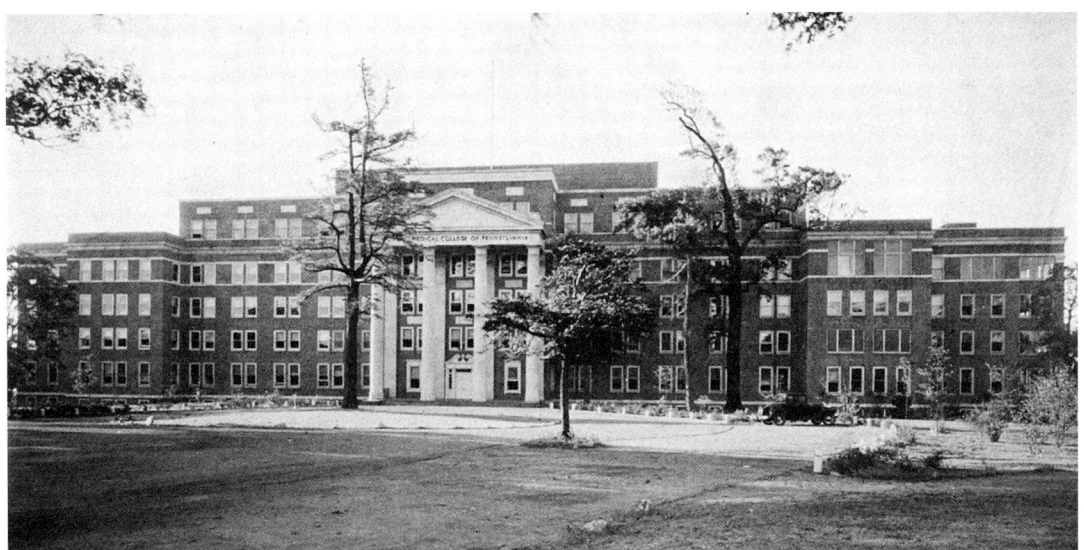

2.23.   Woman's Medical College of Pennsylvania, 1930, Ritter and Shay, architects. Photograph ca. 1932.

was arranged compactly with all departments, especially the library, under one roof."[152] Davison exaggerated. Not every medical college between 1919 and the opening of New York Hospital–Cornell Medical Center in 1932 constructed a medical school–hospital, but the fact that Davison framed it this way is significant. Educators and architects experimented continuously with medical school design between 1893 and 1940, and in the 1920s the medical school–hospital became the new gold standard.

In addition to the six facilities mentioned by Davison, I have identified two other medical school–hospitals constructed in a single campaign before 1940: Meharry Medical College and Woman's Medical College of Pennsylvania. Meharry's architects, Gordon and Kaelber, knew the medical school–hospital intimately, having completed such a design for the University of Rochester before undertaking the project for Meharry. At Woman's Medical College, the initial sketches for the college's proposed home contained a medical school separate from the hospital but joined by a corridor or perhaps a multistory wing. The school's leadership planned to build the medical college and at least part of the hospital in the first wave of construction.[153] A shortfall in the school's fundraising likely prompted the faculty to reconsider these plans.[154] Architect Howell Lewis Shay also encouraged the school's leadership to place medical school and hospital in one structure; he felt "great difficulties would arise having [clinical] cases in one and desk work in another building."[155] In 1930, Woman's Medical College moved into a modest medical school–hospital (fig. 2.23). As the dean reported the week of the groundbreaking, "the economical methods of construction, developed in the erection of several new medical school buildings in a number of cities, have been carefully studied, and where possible followed or improved upon, and it is our belief that the new Woman's Medical College and Hospital will be a demonstration of what can be done without the vast expenditure that has marked some of the large university plants."[156]

The rapid adoption of the medical school–hospital type stemmed in part from its flexibility. Woman's Medical College of Pennsylvania built a relatively compact and inexpensive facility. The entire structure cost just under $900,000 to construct and included a hospital with 143 beds. Conversely, architect Edward F. Stevens projected that the Columbia-Presbyterian Medical Center had "every prospect of being the most complete medical unit under one large comprehensive scheme in this country, and perhaps in the world."[157] Columbia University raised $4 million to build and endow the medical school within the medical center, which in total cost $25 million to construct and included 1,674 beds. Not surprisingly, the enormous facility offered little of the close contact remembered in more modest institutions such as Vanderbilt, of which Tinsley Harrison wrote with all seriousness, "The great virtue of the place was its smallness."[158] Famed pediatrician Benjamin Spock graduated from Columbia University's College of Physicians and Surgeons in 1929, a year after the Columbia-Presbyterian Medical Center opened, and he then spent two years at Presbyterian Hospital as a medical intern. He recalled, "Nobody on the staff liked the new Presbyterian Hospital at first. It had lost its intimacy in the move and seemed too large, too modern, too impersonal." In particular, he noted, "in the old Presbyterian, . . . interns and residents had dined with the attending physicians; now they were relegated to a huge general cafeteria quite audibly close to the dishwashing facility."[159]

Reinforcing its flexibility, the medical school–hospital appeared around the country, in northern, southern, coastal, and mountain locations. The distinctive grid footprint employed at Vanderbilt, Rochester, Meharry, and Duke proved popular in design if not entirely in function. Architects and faculty created the inner courtyards to provide access to light and air, but the dean of Duke University School of Medicine, Wilburt Davison, declared, "Our worst error was in having three interior courtyards patterned after those of Rochester, New York, which has a cooler climate. But in the Durham summers, before air-conditioning was installed, they were a foretaste of Hades."[160]

Medical educators also saw the emphasis on unified designs, and the medical school–hospital in particular, as uniquely American. Jeanne Kisacky has described the construction of tall, centralized American hospitals in the 1920s and argues, "At a time of great nationalism, high-rises were seen as distinctly American and high-rise hospitals provided a visible and tangible differentiation of American from European development." She continues, "Experiences in World War I and its aftermath had eroded the long-lived American infatuation with European hospital institutions and their traditional low-rise, decentralized pavilion facilities."[161] Similarly, in the 1920s American medical school design moved self-consciously away from the German institute plan. Educators positioned the unified designs as American and not German, an indicator of American physicians' decreased reliance on Germany as a leader in laboratory and clinical medicine and perhaps, too, of anti-German sentiment in the wake of World War I. In February 1923, the same month the plans for Vanderbilt's new facility appeared in *Modern Hospital*, Abraham Flexner quoted a report he was preparing:

> While, generally speaking, this movement [modern medical science?] owes most to Germany, the United States has, in education, made an original contribution. The Germans first made independent sciences of anatomy, biochemistry, pathology, pharmacology, medicine, pediatrics; but though each has rounded itself out, chemically and biologically, each has also jealously preserved its own autonomy, as though coöperation would clip the wings. The best schools in the United States have adopted the German scheme of differentiation; but they have been less fearful of harm through contacts. On the contrary, they seek, more and more, to establish, whether for education or research, coöperative relationships.
>
> The separate institutes, which compose the medical faculty in Germany, tend thus in America to merge in an organic plant, in which laboratories and clinics interact without loss of scientific integrity.[162]

In addition, Davison and Robinson differentiated the medical school–hospital from the German institute plan. When Davison wrote his *Reminiscences* in 1966, he described the unified medical school–hospitals constructed at Duke University and elsewhere in the United States and asserted, "All this was in contrast to the German medical schools which are a scattered series of isolated institutes for each subject and are separated from each other by departmental ambitions and jealousies."[163]

As they looked away from Germany, American medical leaders could have found similarities with facilities for medical education in other countries. In his chapter on the "medical school hospital" for the 1928 edition of *The American Hospital of the Twentieth Century*, Stevens explored the relationship between medical school and hospital with examples in Montreal, London, and Kingston (Ontario), alongside four examples in the United States and one example in China by an American architectural firm.[164] But educators did not make these comparisons. The medical school–hospital represented a new American building type in that it fully integrated medical school and hospital for the first time in the United States. In the minds of medical educators, most architects, and donors, they had forged a distinctly American architectural, pedagogical, and conceptual understanding of modern medical education.

Physicians were justifiably proud in 1940 when they looked back on the "almost complete revamping of medical education in the United States," as Ray Lyman Wilbur, physician and president of Stanford University, expressed it in his foreword to the Weiskotten Report. Although concerned about the deleterious effects of the Great Depression on progress in medical education, Wilbur affirmed, "American medicine is assuming more and more a position of leadership and distinction in the world. A decline in the quality of medical education in many European countries has increased the responsibility of our medical schools to keep medical education abreast of the rapid advances in the knowledge applicable to medicine."[165] Critical to the revolution in medical education—and the US medical community's effort to become an international leader—were the medical schools and hospitals where physicians trained. In 1949, Herman Weiskotten asserted, "Nothing will cement the relationships of the various units of a medical school's development quite like cement. Furthermore, nothing will prevent barriers between departments quite like eliminating them in construction plans."[166] Medical faculties understood school buildings as frameworks for research and pedagogical tools.

The medical schools erected between 1893 and 1940 promoted multiple visions of medical education and science. The institute plan codified and encouraged a pedagogical and scientific ideal based on classifying and separating the branches of knowledge on which medical practice was founded. In contrast, those faculties that constructed unified buildings—either single buildings for the preclinical departments or medical school–hospitals—endorsed an approach to medicine that saw the study of medicine, and, by extension, the human body, primarily as an indivisible whole. Although they debated exactly how unification should occur, by the 1920s educators and architects had embraced physical coordination over separation, and the majority of American medical schools built before 1940 were unified facilities. In the end, the schools' designers attempted to do more than provide efficient space for instruction and investigation in scientific medicine; they sought to shape the education and research formulated in their halls and nurture a particular understanding of medicine among students and faculty. The line between educators' and architects' aspirations and occupants' realities is challenging to distill and no doubt varied from school to school and even from person to person, but faculty and students in progressive medical schools worked and learned in vastly different spaces than their proprietary predecessors had. The development of modern American medicine could not have taken place without the simultaneous and intertwined transformations in medical education and medical school design.

Between 1893 and 1940, medical colleges across the United States rebuilt their facilities. Many of the schools became founding members of the new medical centers that combined teaching, research, and patient care on one campus, and sometimes within a single building, in cities around the country. With most of the structures built during the reform movement still used for medical education today, the impact of these original facilities continues to be felt. Far from historical relics, the medical schools of the early twentieth century play an active role in creating the American physicians of today and the foreseeable future.

3

DONORS, ARCHITECTS, AND
MEDICAL SCHOOL DESIGN

IN THE EARLY DECADES OF THE TWENTIETH CENTURY, MEDICAL school leaders continuously set their sights on bigger and more complex facilities as they worked to meet, if not exceed, current educational standards and competed for students, funding, and prestige. Constructing expensive schools required both new sources of money and architects. Within these groups, John D. Rockefeller's General Education Board (GEB), a philanthropic foundation, and the Boston-based architectural firm Shepley, Rutan, and Coolidge stand out for their impact on medical education.

In a period when the federal government offered very little aid to medical colleges, the General Education Board provided the only national program to fund medical schools. Abraham Flexner, famous for his 1910 report on medical training in the United States and Canada, ran the GEB's medical education program. Under Flexner, the General Education Board strategically supported schools around the country in an attempt to create educational—and architectural—models of medical instruction. To this end, Flexner worked to put in place the vision for American medical training that he first outlined in the Flexner Report. The architectural result was an emphasis on coordination of departments and unified designs. Moreover, Flexner's program at the GEB privileged elite research schools, which primarily enrolled white men. The GEB's policies left the nation's two coeducational Black medical colleges and one predominantly white medical college for women without the financial resources to construct buildings that matched the standard set by the research schools.

Similar to the GEB's dominance in medical philanthropy, Shepley, Rutan, and Coolidge distinguished itself among architectural firms as the nation's premier designer of medical schools. The successor firm of the office of H. H. Richardson, Shepley, Rutan, and Coolidge (1886–1915), along with its next two iterations (Coolidge and Shattuck [1915–1924] and Coolidge, Shepley, Bulfinch, and Abbott [1924–1952]) completed a record eight medical schools, seven in the United States and one in China, between 1906 and 1932. Among these eight schools, the firm created all three medical school types: the institute plan, the single building for preclinical studies, and the medical school–hospital, including the prototypical medical school–hospital at Vanderbilt University. Thoroughly versed in the features of the modern medical school, the firm offered medical colleges depth of knowledge augmented by prestige. The firm's reputation benefited from close relationships with Rockefeller organizations and with leading American medical schools, particularly Harvard Medical School.

Financing the Burgeoning Costs of Medical Education

With the reform of medical education, medical colleges attempted to teach, provide patient care, and generate original research. This tripartite focus—and the emphasis on individual, hands-on instruction rather than large lectures—meant that medical school budgets far outstripped the income earned through student fees. Training now required laboratories, equipment, teaching hospitals, expanded faculty, and research funds. These initiatives necessitated huge sums of money.[1]

Medical colleges had not generally received philanthropic support in the United States before the redesign of medical education, and the schools that inaugurated the nation's new pedagogical program also had to develop medical philanthropy. In 1874 Harvard Medical School began a fundraising campaign that would result in its 1883 edifice on Boylston Street (see fig. I.5). The campaign benefited from strong leadership and the school's improved reputation after its recent transition to a true university department. Harvard Medical School's faculty focused their efforts on Boston's professionals and business leaders, and the community responded. A number of relatively modest contributions resulted in the construction of the 1883 building, which ultimately cost nearly $300,000.[2]

Occasionally, less progressive schools obtained funds as well. Beginning in 1884, the College of Physicians and Surgeons of New York, at the time affiliated in name only with Columbia University, received a series of gifts from the family of Cornelius Vanderbilt that amounted to more than $2 million.[3] Prominent physician William A. Pusey recalled the donations in 1927: "At that time it was a unique experience for medical education and, indeed, a very unusual one for medicine at all. . . . Our first comic paper, *Puck*, had a front page cartoon in which it represented Mr. Vanderbilt going up the steps of the medical school with his bags of money and a college president pulling at his coat tails and telling him: 'You are going into the wrong place; nobody ever gives money there.'"[4] If the early fundraising successes at Harvard University and the College of Physicians and Surgeons of New York were atypical, they had become commonplace by the time Pusey wrote his remarks.

In the opening decades of the twentieth century, medical education came to enjoy previously unimaginable financial support. As medical colleges left their commercial roots behind, moved into the university, and strengthened their educational programs, deans and faculty members worked to generate enthusiasm for their new endeavor and lobbied aggressively for more funds. University presidents eager to expand the influence of the university through distinguished professional schools joined them in their campaigns. The leadership communicated effectively the ambitions of their changing institutions, but they also benefited from growing concerns about public health, recognition of the research undertaken at elite medical schools, and optimism about future discoveries. The Flexner Report, however, provided the primary stimulus for greater contributions to medical colleges. In the Progressive Era tradition of sensational surveys, the Flexner Report shocked the country. The report described the inadequacies of many of the nation's medical colleges in frank terms and focused on the shortcomings of American medical education rather than the improvements that had already been achieved. In its wake, strong and struggling medical colleges alike initiated fundraising campaigns with unprecedented goals, and state legislatures, individuals, and philanthropic foundations took action. By 1930, medical schools overall were no longer finding themselves hampered by a lack of funds.[5]

Medical colleges in the West, unlike their counterparts in the East, often resided in public rather than private universities. State legislatures, particularly in western parts of the country, substantially increased their spending on medical education in the early twentieth century; in 1923, states spent fifteen times more money on medical education than they had in 1900. Some states allocated especially large sums and created medical schools as strong as any in the country. Individual donors and philanthropic foundations also augmented state funds.[6] Compared with state funding, the federal government provided very little support for medical schools in this period. The federal government's contributions to the building of medical schools were limited to appropriations for

Howard University and loans for construction administered by New Deal programs.

Despite significant state funding for medical schools, private gifts remained critical. Abraham Flexner emphasized medical colleges' dependence on this form of aid when he spoke before the Council on Medical Education of the American Medical Association in 1924: "East of the Mississippi, medical schools are privately supported; west of the Mississippi, they are mainly tax-supported. In general, it would look easier to raise the necessary sums by taxation than by private subscription; for an infinitesimal tax levy will produce a considerable sum, while $1,000,000 in cash must be raised every time an endowed institution needs an additional income of $50,000. Thus far, however, it has proved easier to interest a small group of private donors than to stir the entire body politic."[7] Although Flexner referenced the privileged few who could make substantial benefactions to medical education, donors who made more modest gifts to medical colleges were also important. As the campaign for Harvard Medical School's 1883 building revealed, small-scale contributions from many community members could raise the necessary funds. At the same time, the number of Americans with extraordinary wealth increased in the late nineteenth century, and in the decades after 1900 many began to turn their attention to medical education. Individuals who made major gifts to medical schools included George Eastman to the University of Rochester, James Buchanan Duke to Duke University, and Samuel Mather to Western Reserve University.[8]

These benefactions had the ability to shape medical schools' policies and buildings, as famously occurred when Johns Hopkins Medical School opened in 1893. The death of Mary Elizabeth Garrett's father in 1884 positioned Garrett among the wealthiest women of the Gilded Age (fig. 3.1). When Johns Hopkins University found itself unable to open its medical school for lack of funds, Mary Elizabeth Garrett and three close friends, all four of whom had personal connections with the young university, inaugurated the Women's Medical School Fund campaign to make Johns Hopkins Medical School a reality and force it to allow coeducation. When the national fundraising effort came up short, Garrett stepped in to fill the breach. Ultimately, she donated more than $350,000 of the $500,000 needed to open the school.[9]

In an example of what some scholars have called coercive philanthropy, whereby a donor uses financial bequests to generate social change, Garrett surprised Johns Hopkins University president Daniel Coit Gilman and founding medical school faculty member William Welch with the conditions of her gift. Drawing on preliminary statements made by

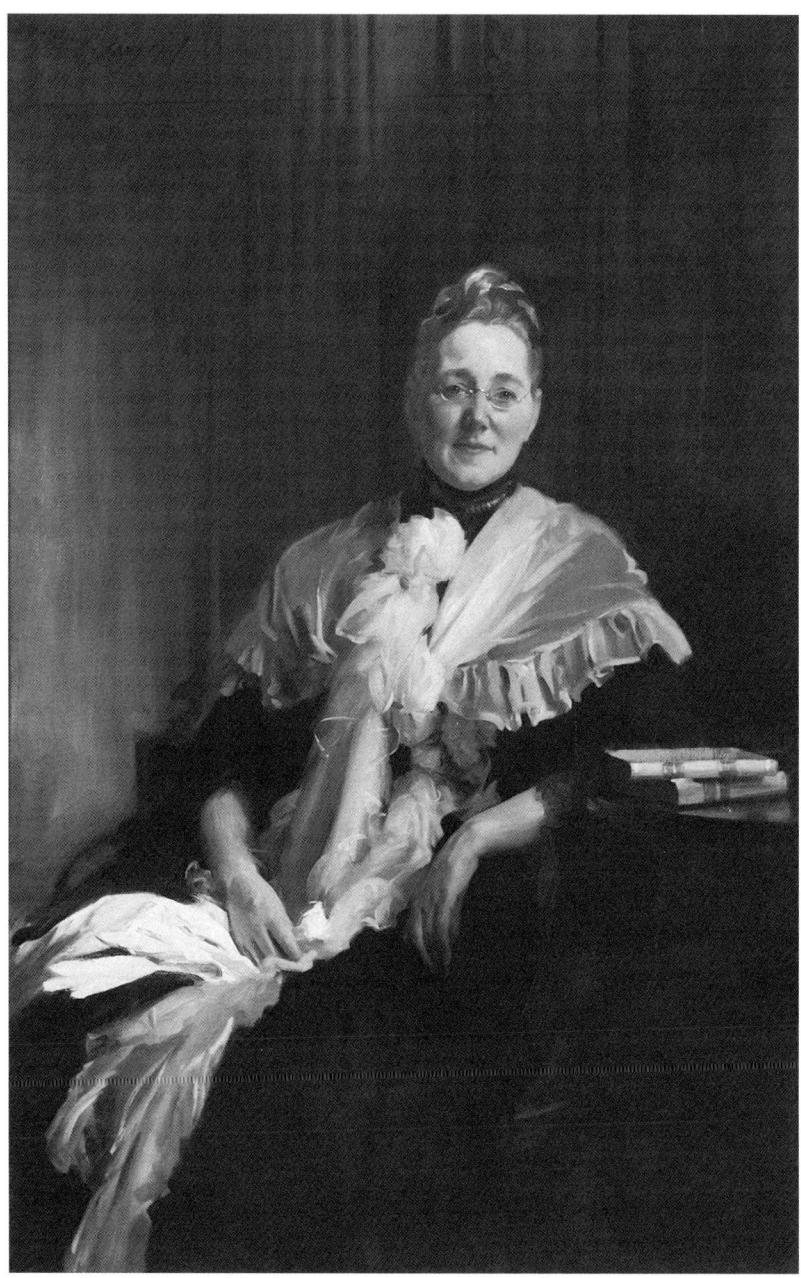

3.1.   John Singer Sargent, *Mary Elizabeth Garrett*, 1904. Oil on canvas, 72 by 40
        inches. The portrait is intimately connected to the Johns Hopkins Medical
        School. Garrett and the trustees of Johns Hopkins University split the
        fee for the portrait, and the original hangs in the William H. Welch Library.
        In 2018 a copy of the painting was installed in the renamed Mary Elizabeth
        Garrett Boardroom in the Miller Research Building, one of several events
        celebrating the 125th anniversary of the medical school's founding.

Gilman and Welch, Garrett startled the men by dictating many of the stringent educational standards for which Johns Hopkins Medical School would become known, as well as the requirement that the medical school admit and educate women on the same terms as their male counterparts.[10] Moreover, she shaped the trajectory of the medical school's campus development when she established how much of the money raised could be spent on buildings and when she stipulated that the school must open less than a year after receiving her pledge—specifications that made complete construction of the medical college impossible.

Garrett not only set an early example for philanthropic gifts for medical education but also indirectly encouraged major philanthropists to follow her lead. Many contributions to medical schools can be traced to an appreciation for the model of education established at Johns Hopkins Medical School and the impact of its faculty and alumni.[11] Launched less than a decade after Garrett's 1892 donation, Harvard Medical School's campaign for its 1906 quadrangle indicated how quickly medical education had become the focus of substantial philanthropic aid. Unlike the series of modest gifts responsible for Harvard Medical School's 1883 building, three large benefactions—from J. P. Morgan, John D. Rockefeller Sr., and Arabella Huntington—accounted for approximately 80 percent of the money raised in the campaign for the 1906 campus. Moreover, while Bostonians funded the earlier undertaking, none of the three major donors to the later effort hailed from the city. Only Morgan highlighted any affiliation with Boston when he dedicated three buildings to his father, who was, as an inscription still bears witness, "a native of Massachusetts[,] a merchant of Boston[,] afterwards a merchant of London." Morgan, Rockefeller, and Huntington based their support of the medical school building campaign primarily on their commitment to Harvard Medical School's mission rather than a direct geographic connection or personal loyalty to the school. They appreciated the breakthroughs in medical research that had occurred in recent years, and they respected Harvard Medical School's reputation as an institution devoted to medical science. Unlike Garrett and the Women's Medical School Fund, none of these philanthropists initiated his or her gift to the medical school. Harvard Medical School faculty members Henry P. Bowditch and J. Collins Warren courted each of them.[12]

Rockefeller subjected the school to the most intensive scrutiny. He sent lawyer Starr J. Murphy to examine the institution. Murphy wrote a detailed report that outlined both the current state of scientific medical education and the training available at Harvard Medical School. Having shown that Harvard Medical School was at the forefront of medical education, offered the possibility of making scientific discoveries, and demonstrated sound financial management, Murphy recommended supporting the campaign.[13] Confident in his investment, Rockefeller donated $1 million. Morgan gave $1,135,000, and Huntington contributed $250,000. The medical school reserved Rockefeller's donation for endowment, while Morgan paid for three buildings and Huntington, a fourth. Rockefeller's gift was conditioned on the medical school raising an additional $765,000, a challenge to which "Boston[ians] responded most spiritedly," according to a 1906 publication, although New Yorkers reportedly gave substantially as well.[14]

J. Collins Warren recalled that, after the fundraising campaign had reached its goal, "it was . . . realized that . . . four of the buildings had been presented by citizens of New York City, [and] none of the new group as yet bore a Boston name." Prominent Bostonian David Sears subsequently made a gift to the building fund that "enabled the Faculty to dedicate the remaining building to the memory of three generations of an honored Boston family."[15] The faculty, however, may have acted generously in this decision; some sources indicate that Sears paid much less for his building than Morgan or Huntington did.[16] The determination to feature a Boston donor underscores the faculty's discomfort with abandoning the primarily local support of the past.

Many motives spurred medical philanthropy. Medical historian Kenneth Ludmerer has summarized a number of them. In some cases, personal circumstances sparked action. The death of Rockefeller's first grandchild from scarlet fever pushed him to found the Rockefeller Institute for Medical Research in 1901. In addition, sizable donations offered fame, immortalization of a family name, and power. At the same time, these gifts attempted to mitigate the negative reputation of the era's "robber barons." Moreover, contemporaneous economic analyses of illness were highlighting the negative financial consequences of disease, which, the argument went, had the potential to hurt not only the worker but also, in turn, the corporation and the nation. Philanthropists' giving also grew out of a belief in the efficacy of scientific medicine—both in the advances already achieved and those yet to be discovered.[17] In addition, historian of Harvard University John T. Bethell notes that competition among philanthropists encouraged action, as was the case with Morgan and Rockefeller during Harvard Medical School's campaign.[18]

For Rockefeller, the gift to Harvard Medical School represented the beginning of what would become an extraordinary legacy of philanthropy for medical education (fig. 3.2). Physician Arthur E. Hertzler, writing in 1938, willingly risked hyperbole: "The Rockefellers have done

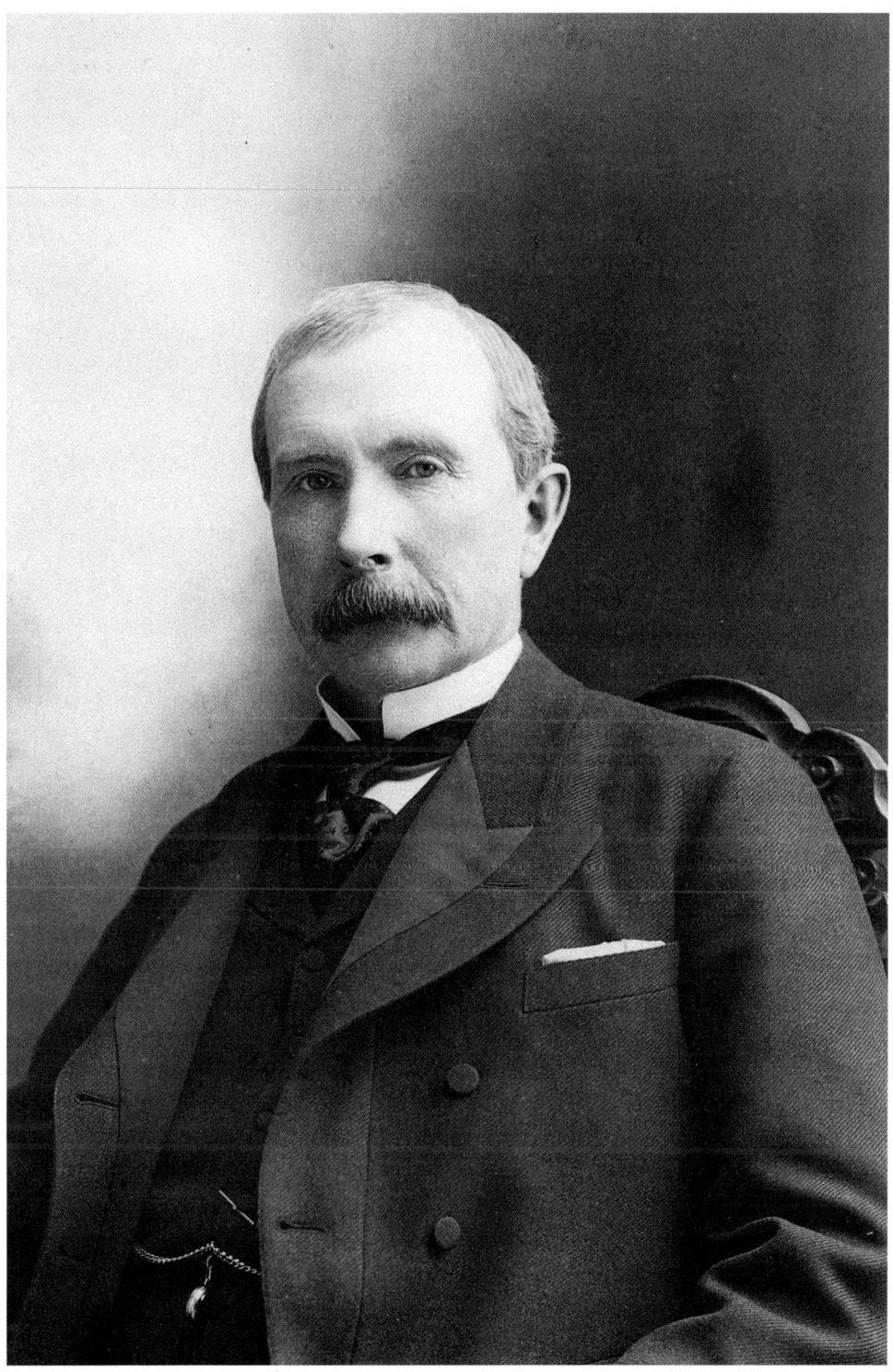

3.2.   John D. Rockefeller Sr., 1895.

more for medical education than all the rest of laymen since the beginning of time. That may be an exaggeration but it will do until someone
comes along with figures."[19] Although private individuals gave more
money overall to medical schools than did philanthropic foundations,
Rockefeller's General Education Board represented the only funding
source with a national program in medical education—including medical
school construction—in this period. Other major foundations, such as
the Rockefeller Foundation and the Carnegie Corporation, supported
medical education, but the GEB's influence dominated the field and the
other foundations followed its lead.[20] Individual donors such as Mary
Elizabeth Garrett could shape the building program of single medical
colleges, but only the GEB's architectural patronage would leave a lasting
mark on American medical schools across the country.

The General Education Board and Its Promotion of the Unified Plans

Compelled by his Baptist faith to begin making charitable contributions
at a young age, John D. Rockefeller in time systematized his giving with
organizations such as the General Education Board. In so doing, he
played a prominent role in the development of the general-purpose foundation at the turn of the twentieth century. General-purpose foundations
provided donors with the opportunity to make gifts to their foundations
and to forgo personal donations to recipients of their choice, which were
an inefficient and time-consuming undertaking, as supplicants hound-
ed benefactors for assistance. Blending their patrons' generosity and
egotism, the foundations attempted to distribute their donors' wealth
efficiently and to alter American society through long-term solutions to
society's challenges. The foundation officers worked with social reformers on broad agendas, such as the "well-being of mankind," and science,
education, and public health became cornerstones of their initiatives.
In 1915, twenty-seven foundations existed, but by 1930 this number had
grown to more than two hundred. Although no single management
method existed, Rockefeller and others took the organizational lessons
they had learned in business and applied them to their philanthropic
foundations. Responsibility for administering these foundations fell
to a board of trustees, which in turn shifted daily operations into the
hands of "philanthropoids," to use a term coined in this period for those
who disbursed the money of others.[21] The creation of this new figure in
American society relates closely to the growing emphasis on specialized
knowledge and the rise of the professions in the late nineteenth and early

twentieth centuries—two interrelated shifts in which physicians as well as architects participated.[22]

In 1903, the US Congress incorporated Rockefeller's General Education Board. Although initially focused on concerns in the American South, the GEB took as its agenda "the promotion of education within the United States without distinction of race, sex, or creed."[23] The GEB's efforts toward this goal took many forms, and in the 1910s medical education became a major initiative. Within Rockefeller's various philanthropies, medicine and education already represented the top two priorities at the time, making this focus for the GEB an alignment of established interests.[24] Moreover, Rockefeller's trusted advisor for both his philanthropic and business investments, Frederick T. Gates, believed deeply in scientific medicine, and he encouraged the GEB to work in this area.[25] Abraham Flexner met with Gates, then chairman of the GEB, the year after the release of his famous 1910 report. Gates asked Flexner to examine clinical teaching at Johns Hopkins Medical School at approximately the same time that John D. Rockefeller Jr. asked Flexner, who was well respected for his surveys, to complete an unrelated project for him. With both men highly pleased with his work, Flexner received the post of assistant secretary of the GEB.[26] In 1913, Flexner began a fifteen-year tenure at the GEB, during which time his role expanded to secretary and then division director, in addition to his joining the board of trustees (fig. 3.3). Flexner became synonymous with the GEB's program in medical education. The program grew dramatically between 1919 and 1921, when Rockefeller gave the board $45 million for US medical schools. By the time the GEB closed its doors in 1960, the board had disbursed slightly more than $94 million to American medical schools. The GEB often required recipients to obtain additional funds even greater than the amount provided by the GEB. The total sum of these outside gifts and the contributions from the GEB resulted in approximately $600 million for medical education.[27]

Even after Flexner's termination from the GEB in 1928 during the reorganization of the Rockefeller philanthropies, his vision for medical education endured, at least within the GEB. Prior to the restructuring, the GEB had focused on domestic medical education, while the Rockefeller Foundation had taken responsibility for medical education abroad, although it sometimes supported GEB efforts within the United States. After the changes, all medical education fell under the purview of the Rockefeller Foundation, which replaced the GEB's focus on institution building with an emphasis on research grants.[28] Nevertheless, the GEB did continue to disburse funds for medical education after 1928; as GEB

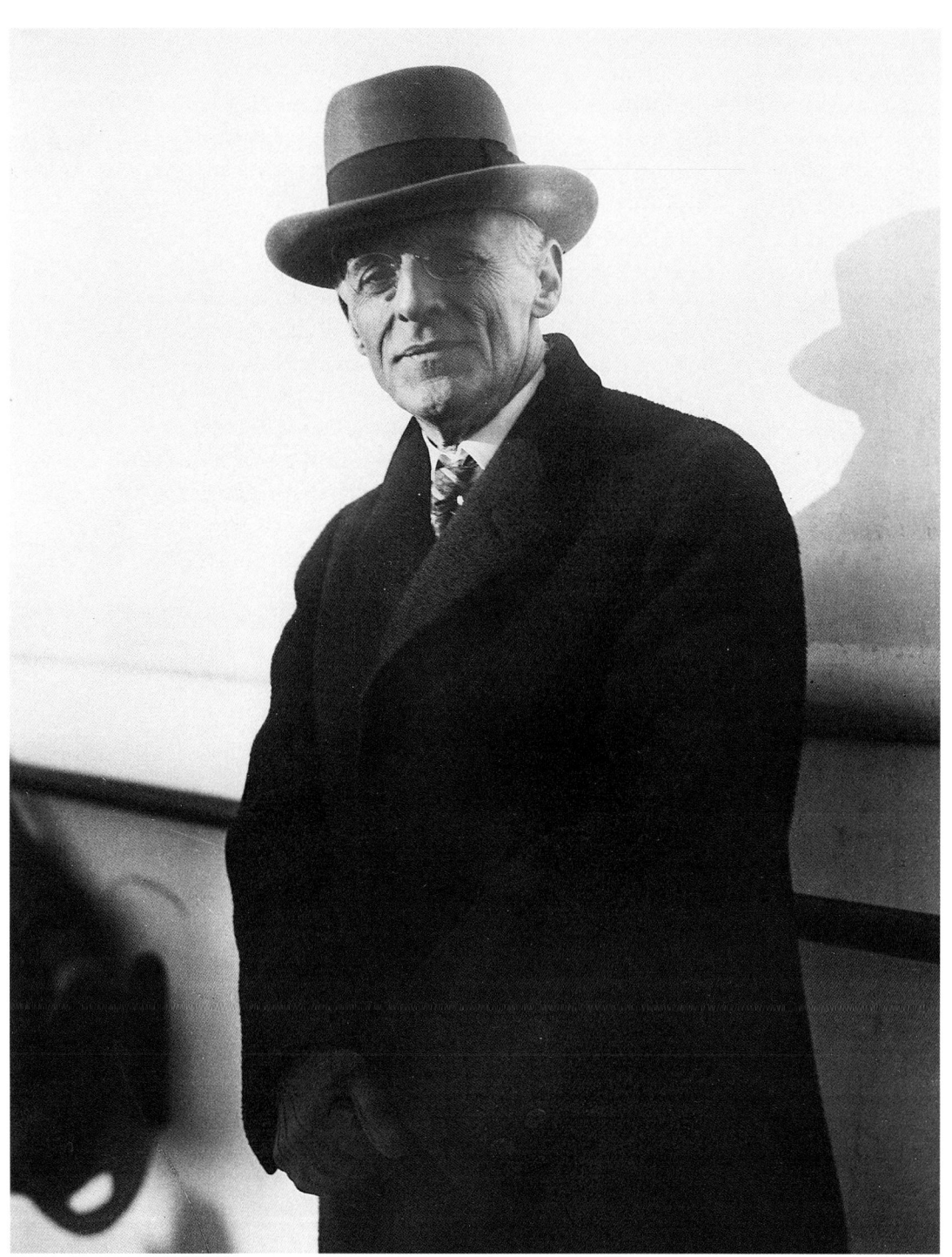

3.3.   Abraham Flexner, ca. 1920.

chairman and then president Raymond B. Fosdick later reflected, "from 1928 to 1960 no new [medical] schools were added to the [General Education] Board's list; the additional sums constituted further grants to institutions which had figured in Flexner's plan."[29]

Charged with wisely investing Rockefeller's resources, Flexner and the other officers at the GEB engaged in "scientific philanthropy," whereby they systematized their practices and carefully screened applicants. In its review of medical colleges, the GEB considered the school's educational standards, investigated its fiscal strength, examined the quality of its leadership, and explored other potential benefactors beyond the GEB. The GEB's administrators wielded significant power when they reviewed applicants and decided whether to recommend them to the board of trustees for support. Although the GEB's managers always kept institutional goals in mind, on a daily basis they worked independently. Through at least 1923, the GEB's board of trustees did not decline a single recommendation of the officers.[30]

With considerable control over the GEB's medical education program, Flexner spent a decade and a half methodically putting in place the vision that he had begun articulating in his 1910 report. From the start, Flexner made Johns Hopkins Medical School his conceptual model and strove to re-create elsewhere its extensive laboratory and clinical experience, university affiliation, and emphasis on research. To this end, Flexner worked to generate a national system of progressive medical schools that would act as standard-bearers for pioneering pedagogy in each region of the country. For example, he singled out Vanderbilt University School of Medicine for substantial GEB aid in order to bring medical education reform to the South.[31] (Personal relationships did not hurt either. Shortly after the GEB extended the first of its many gifts to Vanderbilt University School of Medicine, Flexner began summering on a remote Canadian lake at the property next to the Vanderbilt University chancellor's vacation site.[32]) Furthermore, in direct conflict with Gates, Flexner insisted on making GEB money available to state medical schools rather than reserving GEB gifts for private medical colleges, a shift designed to extend his program in the South and West.[33] In the end, although the GEB funded only about one-third of the medical colleges that survived the modernization of medical training, the board had a powerful influence on schools across the country through its creation of strategically placed pedagogical—and architectural—models of medical education.

When Flexner was preparing his 1910 report, he met with medical educators, examined the available instructional methods, and threw his weight, as well as that of the foundation sponsoring the report, behind the academic system embodied most fully by Johns Hopkins Medical School. Later, as a foundation officer, he maintained a similar relationship with educators. Flexner depended on them for the ideas that fueled the GEB's programs. In choosing which initiatives to support, Flexner impacted the direction of medical training. Simultaneously, however, faculty leaders courted Flexner as their access point to the GEB's money, and some held tremendous influence within the GEB and other major philanthropies.[34]

One of the most frequently cited examples of the way that Flexner shaped medical education was his dedication to the implementation of full-time clinical faculty, whereby clinicians focused on teaching and research rather than on maintaining a private practice. The concept originated with educators, but once Flexner embraced the idea the GEB actively encouraged it by funding this change at several prominent schools. Moreover, through the mid-1920s, the board would aid only those schools willing to adopt a particular definition of full-time clinical status, a policy that opened the board to criticism of meddling in the internal affairs of the schools it supported.[35] Although scholars have recognized the impact of GEB policies on medical education, none has extended this analysis to architecture.

Flexner's 1910 report did reveal attention to architecture and his preferences. Of the six categories Flexner created for assessing individual medical colleges, two were laboratory and clinical facilities.[36] The St. Louis College of Physicians and Surgeons, like many others, earned Flexner's scorn. Flexner reported that "the school occupies a badly kept building, the inner walls covered with huge advertisements. . . . Anatomy was 'over'—only empty tables were found in the dissecting-room, the sole access to which is by way of a fire-escape."[37] Conversely, the University of Michigan's medical school earned praise: "Excellently equipped laboratories are provided for all the fundamental branches. . . . There is a large library, a good museum, and other necessary teaching aids."[38] When pieced together, Flexner's comments indicate that he celebrated clean, well-organized plants with ample laboratory space and affiliated hospitals that housed plenty of patients. Moreover, when discussing the broad principles of reformed medical education, Flexner advocated placing laboratory and hospital in close physical proximity to one another. Locating the two components of medical training—laboratories and hospitals—in the same city was not enough; they should share a campus.[39] These ideas may seem unremarkable today, but as Flexner's caustic reviews made clear, few medical colleges had adopted them by 1910.

Deeply committed to these principles, Flexner appears to have promoted them while he was reviewing schools for his report. At the

University of Nebraska College of Medicine, students completed their two years of preclinical training in Lincoln and their two years of clinical training in Omaha, some sixty miles away—an inconvenient arrangement. The school's leadership, however, was actively charting the college's next steps when Flexner arrived. In its April 1909 *Bulletin*, the school announced an appropriation by the state legislature for $20,000 to purchase land in Omaha for the clinical department at the same time that it described Flexner's visit:

> The plans for the development of the College received material assistance thru the suggestions of Mr. A. Flexner who in behalf of the Carnegie Foundation for the Advancement of Teaching conducted a most rigorous examination of our facilities recently. . . . His comments on various prospective campus locations and on the general plans for the development of the institution were particularly welcome at this stage of progress. The University is indebted to him for many valuable criticisms which will be incorporated in the working out of detailed plans and it also appreciates the words of encouragement he proffered in commendation of the steps already taken and the plans in hand for future progress.[40]

Undoubtedly, Flexner pressed the university to align geographically its medical school's preclinical and clinical training, an opinion he would state publicly in his report the following year.[41] His advice likely contributed to the decision to locate both preclinical and clinical instruction in Omaha. Thus, architecture had from the beginning formed a central part of Flexner's archetype for the modern American medical school.[42]

At the GEB, Flexner's architectural influence operated outside of the organization's official resolutions. No formal architectural requirements existed for recipients of the board's resources. Instead, Flexner shaped schools' building programs when he examined their proposals, encouraged particular requests for financial support, and remained involved in projects even after they received GEB funds.

At the same time, recognizing Flexner as an expert in medical education with a great amount of money to distribute, medical school faculties sought and then implemented his advice—architectural and otherwise—in the hope that making changes he supported would result in GEB aid in the future. In 1914, Syracuse University was deciding whether to obtain control of a local hospital. The medical school's dean brought Flexner into the conversation, and Flexner confirmed the desirability of the college running its own hospital. In a letter to the university's chancellor describing his communication with Flexner, the dean concluded, "There is no better authority in the United States on the question in my opinion than Mr. Flexner. I feel more or less certain that if we can work out this problem successfully it will of itself bring us to the attention of the General Education Board and put us in line for the help that is needed for the development of a first-class medical school."[43] The following year, the university took over the hospital, but no money arrived from the GEB. In the early 1920s, Flexner visited Syracuse's medical college and urged the geographical alignment of all parts of its program.[44] The school began to work toward such a reality, but once again the GEB provided no support. Poor leadership, fiscal mismanagement, lack of local financial resources to augment GEB aid, and Flexner's perception that the medical college remained conservative and unlikely to change stymied efforts to interest Flexner and the GEB. Instead, as Flexner enacted his national agenda, he singled out the University of Rochester among upstate New York schools as the focus of the board's largesse.[45]

The investigation of Flexner's architectural ideas is complicated by a handful of historical circumstances. The GEB typically did not retain files of rejected applications for aid. As a result, the board's archives only partially document the communication that took place between the medical schools and the foundation. Additionally, Flexner committed very few of his ideas about architecture to writing, and his correspondence reveals only traces of his thoughts on this subject. Flexner and others at the GEB relied heavily on oral, confidential exchanges in order to avoid leaving written evidence that could document their efforts to influence universities' internal affairs. When Flexner wrote to Vanderbilt University's chancellor about the reorganization of its medical school, including possible GEB and Carnegie aid, he concluded, "Should you be passing through New York as you go to Canada, come in and we will talk the thing over somewhat more freely than we can write about it."[46] Fortunately, a significant record does remain: the medical schools built with GEB gifts.

GEB support did not necessarily mean direct funds for construction. Faculties often raised money for construction, equipment, and endowment simultaneously. Flexner, however, thoroughly scrutinized each school's proposal, including projected facilities, before extending aid to any part of it.[47] As long as the GEB gift was made during the school's building campaign, I do not differentiate between gifts earmarked for construction, equipment, or endowment. The GEB contributed to fifteen medical schools for their fundraising efforts in conjunction with new structures (table 3.1).[48]

During his time at the GEB, Flexner argued against the institute plan and in favor of the two unified building types: the single-building

Table 3.1.   Medical schools constructed through fundraising campaigns that received GEB support

Medical school	Year completed	Building type
Johns Hopkins University	Multiple	Institute
University of Colorado	1924*	Medical school–hospital
University of Rochester	1925*	Medical school–hospital
Vanderbilt University	1925*; 1938	Medical school–hospital; addition
Howard University	1927*	Single-building medical school
University of Chicago	1927	Partially realized medical school and hospital facilities
Columbia University	1928*	Medical school–hospital
University of Iowa	1928*	Single-building medical school
University of Pennsylvania	1928	Wing for anatomy and chemistry added to existing structure to create a single-building medical school
Yale University	1928	New and renovated space for bacteriology, pathology, and public health near the single-building medical school
University of Virginia	1929*	Single-building medical school connected to existing hospital facility
Western Reserve University	1929	Pathology institute added to campus with single-building medical school
Duke University	1930*	Medical school–hospital
Meharry Medical College	1931*	Medical school–hospital
Cornell University	1932*	Medical school–hospital

Note: List compiled from a review of schools to which the GEB contributed more than $200,000 between 1914 and 1960.

* Complete, new medical school.

medical school with nearby hospital and the medical school–hospital. Earlier, in his 1910 report, Flexner lauded the institute design when he praised Harvard Medical School's facility, to which John D. Rockefeller Sr. had donated personally before the founding of the GEB.[49] In the 1920s, although Flexner was willing to shepherd GEB aid to Johns Hopkins Medical School to reinforce its existing institute design, he also criticized a Johns Hopkins Medical School proposal that envisioned an increase in the number of institutional divisions of the school. Flexner called the idea "reactionary."[50] By the time he wrote this comment, Flexner had already committed GEB resources to the medical school–hospitals under way at Vanderbilt, Colorado, and Rochester. Now convinced that progressive medical education required coordination of departments, Flexner rejected the institute plan.

The development of the Vanderbilt University medical school–hospital project underscores Flexner and the GEB's interest in medical school design when making funding decisions. In February 1921, shortly before the board expanded its gift to Vanderbilt in order to make possible the medical school–hospital on the main university campus, Vanderbilt's chancellor provided Flexner with three potential schemes for the reorganization of the medical school. The materials sent to Flexner included architectural plans for each possibility, all drawn by Coolidge and Shattuck and big enough for easy viewing when hung on the wall.[51] Presumably the generous size would facilitate the examination of the designs by the GEB's officers and possibly also its board of trustees. Although extant documents do not indicate how often GEB officers and perhaps trustees reviewed architectural plans, the GEB's architectural legacy reveals a clear pattern that aligns with Flexner's dissatisfaction with the institute design.

Between 1920 and 1935, the GEB contributed to ten fundraising campaigns for the construction of complete medical school facilities, and all of these schools erected either single-building medical schools with a nearby hospital or fully integrated medical school–hospitals (see table 3.1). More specifically, the GEB served as the primary funder for the prototypical medical school–hospital at Vanderbilt University and helped to ensure the rapid proliferation of the building type. I have identified eight medical school–hospitals constructed in one campaign before 1940. Seven received GEB support, and the medical school–hospital became a central and lasting element of the GEB's medical education program (table 3.2). The GEB's contribution to the 1929 Institute of Pathology of Western Reserve University and the University Hospitals of Cleveland on a medical campus with a single-building medical school does not undermine the overall shift toward unified designs.

The unified plans appealed to Flexner and the GEB for two reasons. First, the designs were economical. They reduced the duplications of space found in campuses with multiple laboratory buildings. For philanthropic foundations, financial support constituted an investment, and Flexner wanted to ensure that the GEB got the most out of the gifts he called upon the board to make.[52] Flexner's condemnation of ornament underscores his commitment to lowering costs. In December 1924, he visited the nearly completed medical school–hospitals at Vanderbilt University and the University of Rochester. In an internal GEB memorandum, he called Coolidge and Shattuck's Vanderbilt medical facility

Table 3.2.   Medical school–hospitals built before 1940 in a single construction campaign

Medical school	Year completed	Architect(s)	GEB funding
University of Colorado	1924	Maurice B. Biscoe, William E. Fisher, and Arthur A. Fisher	Yes
University of Rochester	1925	Gordon and Kaelber; McKim, Mead, and White, consulting architects	Yes
Vanderbilt University	1925	Coolidge and Shattuck	Yes
Columbia University	1928	James Gamble Rogers	Yes
Duke University	1930	Horace Trumbauer	Yes
Woman's Medical College of Pennsylvania	1930	Ritter and Shay	No
Meharry Medical College	1931	Gordon and Kaelber	Yes
Cornell University	1932	Coolidge, Shepley, Bulfinch, and Abbott	Yes

"admirable—simple, tasteful and extraordinarily well arranged." But he did not mince words in his "one criticism": "The architects, in their own phrase, used little or no decoration on the buildings, but felt that the entrances to the hospital and medical school should be somewhat decorative. They are clumsy and ugly. They look like an excrescence."[53] In contrast, Flexner declared to Vanderbilt medical school's dean that Gordon and Kaelber's Rochester "buildings . . . are less ornate on the outside than yours and to that extent I confess I like them better. They have nothing in the way of an entrance half so imposing as your back-door. Mr. Eastman almost murdered the architects, but he succeeded in eliminating every dollar's worth of decoration. Glory be to him!"[54]

Flexner's second reason for supporting the unified designs stemmed from his appreciation for the physical, pedagogical, and intellectual alignment of medical school departments. As early as his 1910 report, Flexner lauded schools with departments "in intimate communication with each other."[55] When comparing the single-building medical schools and adjacent hospital with the medical school–hospital, affiliation of departments only increased in the latter, with its complete integration of both laboratory and clinical facilities, something Flexner specifically encouraged in 1910 when he decried "the isolation of the laboratory sciences, locally or scientifically, from the clinical work."[56] As historian Timothy C. Jacobson has observed, when G. Canby Robinson sent his September 1920 proposal for a more extensive reorganization of

Vanderbilt's medical school to the university's chancellor and the GEB, he emphasized coordination; Robinson "had read Bulletin Number Four [the Flexner Report] and now read it back to its author."[57] Robinson, like other educators in search of funds, may well have developed his program in part to satisfy Flexner's preferences.

At the same time, Flexner did not act alone in encouraging the unified structures, and particularly the medical school–hospital, in the 1920s. Medical journals and other publications disseminated information about the facilities at Vanderbilt University and elsewhere, and architectural firms and medical educators helped to move ideas among schools. Flexner recognized the impact of this network on architectural design, and he personally facilitated the transfer of people and designs from one school to another.

Flexner's involvement with the creation of the medical school–hospital at Vanderbilt University illustrates the ways in which he would encourage the participation of specific individuals and shape the architectural evolution of a project. In November 1919, a few days before the announcement of the first GEB gift to Vanderbilt's medical school, the university's chancellor, James H. Kirkland, contacted Flexner about an architectural firm for the proposed facility, for which only a sketch of a plot plan had been submitted to the GEB in advance of the grant. Kirkland asked Flexner if he and GEB president Wallace Buttrick "approve" the choice of Coolidge and Shattuck.[58] Flexner responded positively on behalf of himself and Buttrick and recommended that Coolidge, Kirkland, and hospital consultant Winford Smith have a conference in the GEB office in New York later in the month.[59] Vanderbilt retained the architectural firm.

Flexner also offered advice on the buildings themselves. In 1920, Kirkland described how Flexner's input had resulted in Coolidge using less expensive materials for the Vanderbilt facility in order to reduce costs. Kirkland went on to underscore the impact of Flexner's opinions, writing, "As you [Flexner] are well aware we have regarded your suggestions as having practically the force of orders. We have so far in every way worked under the consciousness of full agreement with your office."[60] Kirkland seems to have wanted to avoid further demands for economizing from Flexner. Fifteen months later, Kirkland explained to Coolidge that "Mr. Flexner and . . . the officers of the General Education Board . . . have reserved the right to approve our building program, and it is to our interest that we keep this program from developing an excessive expenditure. I am very anxious to prepare my material in such a way and to make my plans so wisely that they will approve everything as offered."[61] Flexner utilized the power of his GEB position at schools other than Vanderbilt. He quickly became a proponent of the medical school–hospital inaugurated in Nashville and helped move the design, as well as the people who could implement it, to other schools.

As the Vanderbilt plans were taking shape, the GEB extended $5 million to the University of Rochester for the founding of a medical school. Intimately involved in both projects, Flexner likely facilitated the communication between the architects for the University of Rochester's medical school, Gordon and Kaelber, and the architects of the Vanderbilt building. In the end, Gordon and Kaelber created a medical school–hospital for Rochester modeled on the Vanderbilt design.[62] Shortly after the completion of the University of Rochester medical facility, Flexner asked that university's president for assistance in determining whether Gordon and Kaelber would be interested in traveling confidentially to Nashville for early planning of the new Meharry Medical College, ultimately located two miles from Vanderbilt's medical school.[63] Gordon and Kaelber subsequently became the architects for the Meharry project, for which they designed another medical school–hospital with a footprint similar to that of the Vanderbilt and Rochester facilities.

For medical colleges, GEB aid proved particularly critical for the construction of the medical school–hospital. With the institute type, schools could add structures over time when funds became available, as Johns Hopkins University did when developing its medical campus. With the single-building medical school separate from the hospital, medical colleges could also stagger construction, as happened at the University of Nebraska when it opened a medical school in Omaha in 1913 and a nearby hospital in 1917. The medical school–hospital, however, required the completion of all of the laboratory and clinical facilities at once. Although a school such as Woman's Medical College of Pennsylvania could build a very modest medical school–hospital, medical school–hospitals inevitably cost more to erect than any one of their constituent parts. The GEB's particular form of patronage could help guarantee the great sum required at one time to construct a medical school–hospital; beyond the often substantial gifts provided by the GEB, the board typically augmented its support by requiring schools to obtain significant additional donations in order to secure GEB aid. Moreover, with Flexner in the lead, the Rockefeller Foundation and the Carnegie Corporation cooperated with the GEB on big medical school projects, such as the construction of Vanderbilt University School of Medicine and Hospital in 1925 and Columbia-Presbyterian Medical Center in 1928.[64] Flexner's vision for American medical education so permeated the Rockefeller philanthropies that the Rockefeller Foundation not only made coordinat-ed grants with the GEB but also encouraged Flexner's initiatives through its journal, *Methods and Problems of Medical Education.*

Methods and Problems of Medical Education highlights the convic-tion in this period that designs of buildings and methods of instruction were so intertwined that they must be studied together. The journal, published at irregular intervals between 1924 and 1932, provided readers with the opportunity to examine "brief descriptions of clinics, labora-tories, and methods of teaching in different parts of the world . . . [as] it is hoped that the material may be of assistance to those planning improvements in buildings and [teaching] methods." Recognizing that recent architectural plans and descriptions of pedagogical experiments were not widely available, the officers of the Rockefeller Foundation sought broad dissemination of the journal. Articles had no copyright restrictions, and reprints required no authorization.[65] The Rockefeller Foundation sent the journal free of charge to all medical schools, both national and international, as well as to other interested parties.[66]

The journal's readership grew quickly. In 1925, 460 medical schools around the world received complimentary copies of the journal.[67] Two years later, the Rockefeller Foundation reported "an unexpectedly large demand for [*Methods and Problems of Medical Education*] on the part of libraries, architects, teachers, and editors of medical publications."[68] Underscoring physicians' interest in *Methods and Problems of Medical Education*, leading American medical journals reviewed the publication. Articles in the *Journal of the American Medical Association* repeatedly praised *Methods and Problems of Medical Education*, and twice contributors to the *New England Journal of Medicine* lauded the Rockefeller journal.[69] Authors also included images and architectural plans from *Methods and Problems of Medical Education* in original articles published in other journals.[70] Among the architects who utilized the journal as a resource were Dwight James Baum and John Russell Pope, who received three issues on the facilities at Vanderbilt Uni-versity, University of Chicago, and University of Rochester, respectively, while they were designing Syracuse University's 1937 medical school.[71]

The officers of the Rockefeller Foundation solicited articles for *Methods and Problems of Medical Education* with a preference for new buildings, although the publication did occasionally include "ideal" historical structures.[72] With regard to the articles related to American schools, faculty members wrote the articles. These pieces followed a fairly consistent format, which suggests either that the authors received clear guidelines from the Rockefeller Foundation or that the foundation heavily edited submissions. The articles usually focused on a particular preclinical laboratory department, such as anatomy, or on a specific clinical department, such as pediatrics. By the time of the journal's termination, it had distributed a total of 448 articles with more than 3,000 illustrations.[73] With its considerable number of pictures of buildings and reproductions of architectural plans, *Methods and Problems of Medical Education* offers the only compilation of images and plans of early twentieth-century American medical schools.

Methods and Problems of Medical Education supported Flexner's architectural vision for American medical colleges. Of the twenty-one issues ultimately published, four dedicated the entire issue to one school.[74] Each of these four schools—at the University of Rochester, Vanderbilt University, and the University of Chicago, as well as Albany Medical College—received some amount of GEB funds, and all of them displayed one of the unified plans encouraged by Flexner. The issues on Rochester and Vanderbilt detailed the medical school–hospital type. The journal highlighted the schools that the GEB aided financially and endorsed the architectural innovations in which the GEB had the greatest interest. These criteria had their limits, however. Meharry Medical College received substantial GEB funds to construct a medical school–hospital with an unusual design. Nevertheless, the publication failed to provide any coverage of this, or the nation's one other, Black medical college, an omission that reinforced the marginalized position of Black medical schools within the GEB's agenda. Far from the impartial source the Rockefeller Foundation claimed it to be, the journal functioned as an extension of the GEB program for medical education.[75]

Flexner's attention to architecture left a lasting impact on medical training. Even before he completed his 1910 report, Flexner urged medical schools to locate near hospitals, a call he continued and that contributed to the development of the large medical school and hospital complexes that still form the nucleus of medical education today. Once at the General Education Board, he promoted the unified plans and particularly the medical school–hospital through his leadership and by setting the architectural standards for the GEB and the Rockefeller Foundation's *Methods and Problems of Medical Education*. Like many of the country's medical educators, Flexner believed that, in contrast to the institute plan, the unified designs and especially the fully integrated medical school–hospital produced a better type of medical practitioner: physicians whose integrated learning taught them to understand the branches of medicine as parts of a whole. The GEB's contribution to the dominance of the unified plans in the United States represents a significant legacy of the philanthropic foundation.

The General Education Board's Rejection of Medical Schools for Women

GEB support for medical education centered on a small number of schools; more than two-thirds of GEB aid went to seven medical colleges. Hardly the neutral foundation it purported to be, the GEB worked to generate a form of medical education more closely aligned with research than medical practice. Although GEB resources could ensure that a school remained open, their absence did not necessarily mean the school would close; with enough determination, medical colleges could continue without GEB funds. Instead, GEB policies controlled which schools would lead, how they would be administered, and what ideals would predominate.[76]

In his 1910 report, Flexner set apart for special consideration the education of African Americans and women. Not only did this action signal the marginalization of these groups within medicine, but Flexner's analysis also failed to recognize Black women physicians by conceptualizing women as white and African Americans as men.[77] Flexner rendered Black women physicians invisible despite the fact that Black women did become physicians in this period. Black women primarily trained at Meharry Medical College and Howard University College of Medicine, by 1923 the nation's only two medical colleges for Black students, and at Woman's Medical College of Pennsylvania, the one medical school for women that remained open in the wake of medical education reform.[78] Black women succeeded in becoming physicians despite the discrimination they experienced from the medical profession, which marginalized Black women on account of both their race and sex.[79]

For educating women in medicine, Flexner championed coeducation. Citing the weaknesses of the schools for women and the availability of coeducational training, Flexner saw no need to help finance the single-sex medical colleges for women; instead, he encouraged donors interested in supporting women's medical education "to develop coeducational institutions, in which their benefits would be shared by men without loss to women students."[80] Flexner followed these prescriptions when he formulated how the GEB would distribute its resources.[81]

Only one women's school, Woman's Medical College of Pennsylvania, survived the transformation of medical education (see fig. 2.23). Founded in Philadelphia in 1850 as the nation's first medical school for women offering the MD degree, the predominantly white institution strove to remain at the forefront of medical education so that opponents of women in medicine could not claim that women's training was subpar.

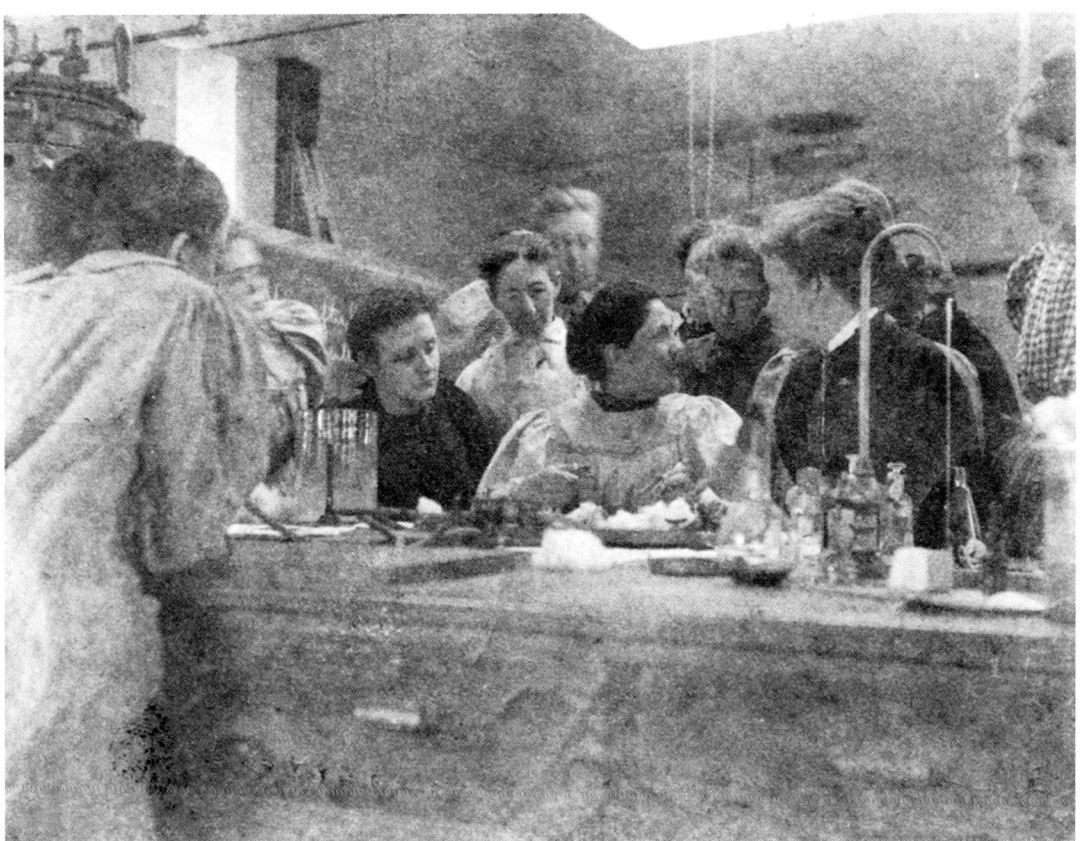

3.4.   Lydia Rabinowitsch (*seated center, light clothing*) and her students at Woman's Medical College of
        Pennsylvania, where she taught from 1895 to 1898 and introduced bacteriology.

When the laboratory became the benchmark of progressive scientific
instruction, Woman's Medical College took note and in the 1880s and
1890s likely offered more laboratory courses than the vast majority of the
country's medical colleges (fig. 3.4).[82]

    Despite the early commitment to modern medical education made
by Woman's Medical College, Flexner rebuffed the college's requests
for aid. In 1909, the school's dean contacted Flexner and requested his
assistance in obtaining foundation funding for the college, but he did
not soften his position on single-sex training for women.[83] By the spring
of 1921, Woman's Medical College was sitting on the edge of financial
disaster. The school's unpaid bills ran to $25,000, while its hospital re-
corded a $20,000 deficit. At the same time, the school was using special
funds, such as scholarship trusts, to meet operating expenses.[84] In this
difficult financial moment, the school's attempts to interest the GEB
in its work at last resulted in an inspection by Flexner. The outcome of

his trip dismayed the leadership of Woman's Medical College. By the school's own report, "as soon as he [Flexner] found that no provision had ever been made for meeting as they arose the deficits in operation which continually occurred, he stated that no application of any kind would be entertained from an institution so managed, either by the Rockefeller [GEB] or any other Foundation. A thorough reorganization thus became a condition precedent to the securing of outside aid of this sort."[85] The college immediately began to overhaul its financial and administrative practices. It created a new accounting system and a centralized administration for the medical school and hospital, with Sarah Logan Wister Starr at its head.[86] In this and other endeavors, Starr worked to create changes that she hoped would result in GEB support.[87] Aid did not materialize, however. Flexner saw no reason to fund single-sex medical colleges for women, and the school demonstrated financial vulnerability and mismanagement. Furthermore, Woman's Medical College was not part of a university, it did not have a research program, and it had few full-time faculty members.[88]

Exacerbating these circumstances, the leaders of Woman's Medical College struggled to establish connections with officers of the major philanthropic foundations. They understood the importance of using their colleagues and acquaintances to interest philanthropists and their staff.[89] Yet, confusion existed about how to engage the members of the philanthropic hierarchy. Ellen Culver Potter, Woman's Medical College alumna and, at points, faculty member and acting president, reported in 1936 that the college's Board of Corporators had charged her with determining potential sources for substantial financial gifts. She described what she had learned about how to recruit support: "My contact with other organizations indicates that the general practice is to 'explore' the proper methods of approach to the persons higher up, selling the ideas to the person lower down so that one gets friends at court." She clarified that "after the exploratory process, the method of approach then is taken up by the Corporation or Board of Directors."[90] Prominent educators and administrators such as Vanderbilt's Chancellor Kirkland had honed this technique and the necessary relationships more than a decade earlier. Unfortunately for Woman's Medical College, men ran the major philanthropic foundations and all of the country's medical schools except for Woman's Medical College. No precedent existed for close working relationships between medical women and foundation officers, which made it that much more difficult, if not impossible, for the predominantly female leadership at Woman's Medical College to cultivate contacts within the dominant philanthropies. Without direct access to the foundations and without an influential "friend at court," such as Flexner, Woman's Medical College remained handicapped. The school continued to depend on relatively small donations and the help of its alumnae in raising funds.

In the mid-1920s, Woman's Medical College undertook a $1.5 million campaign to build and endow a medical school and a hospital, but obtaining this sum proved impossible. Instead, Woman's Medical College procured a $600,000 loan in order to erect a medical school–hospital with an estimated construction cost of just under $870,000.[91] Typical of the school's grassroots fundraising efforts, a house-to-house canvass supported the equipment fund for the facility.[92] The debt accrued in constructing the plant remained a burden for the school, however, as it struggled to survive the Great Depression and to stay abreast of the expensive requirements established by the American Medical Association for medical education. In 1946, concerns about the school's finances, which still included its mortgage, nearly resulted in the absorption of Woman's Medical College by Jefferson Medical College, but the treasurer of the board proclaimed Woman's Medical College financially secure. Faculty, students, alumnae, and others rallied in defense of Woman's Medical College, and the school maintained its autonomy for the time being.[93]

Flexner denied aid to many schools in addition to Woman's Medical College. As we have seen, events at Syracuse University, for example, followed a trajectory similar to those at Woman's Medical College when the leadership in upstate New York failed to interest Flexner in their program. Unable to find other donors, the school stayed in its antiquated and overcrowded 1896 building until New Deal funding provided a solution. Syracuse University received a loan for $825,000 from the Public Works Administration to construct and equip a medical school.[94] The relatively modest single-building medical college designed by Dwight James Baum and John Russell Pope opened in 1937.

The economies practiced in constructing the medical school at Syracuse, however, paled in comparison to those undertaken at Woman's Medical College. Woman's Medical College built a combined school and hospital, occupied in 1930, for approximately the same amount of money that Syracuse University spent to erect a medical college alone later in the decade. To realize its school with so few funds, the faculty at Woman's Medical College focused on facilities for teaching rather than significant dedicated research space, despite their long-standing interest in conducting more research.[95]

At Woman's Medical College, some research areas doubled as office, teaching, or preparation space, and no department had more than one

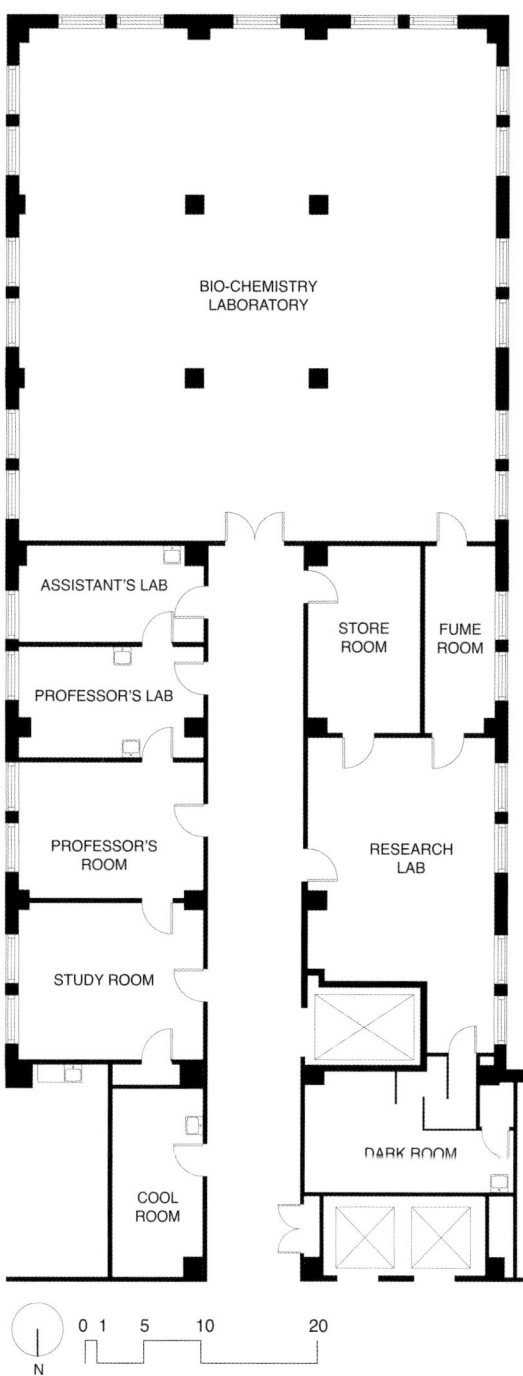

BIO-CHEMISTRY
LABORATORY

ASSISTANT'S LAB

STORE
ROOM

FUME
ROOM

PROFESSOR'S LAB

PROFESSOR'S
ROOM

RESEARCH
LAB

STUDY ROOM

DARK ROOM

COOL
ROOM

0 1   5   10   20

N

3.5.   Woman's Medical College of Pennsylvania, 1930, Ritter and Shay, architects, plan, first floor, department of chemistry, redrawn. This wing connects to the hallway in fig. 3.7.

room exclusively for research. A report published shortly after the building opened contained a written description and an architectural plan of the chemistry department (fig. 3.5). In a slight departure from the plan itself, the text asserted that the three rooms between the study room and the large teaching laboratory provided an office for the assistant professor, an office for the professor, and a private laboratory for the professor, this last area being the department's lone space designated solely for research. On the opposite side of the hallway, the "research lab" offered eight workstations and contained specialized equipment, but preparation for laboratory courses also took place in this room.[96] Despite the limited space for research, the various departments initially seemed pleased with the building, which was a dramatic improvement over their previous home. Those pursuing research felt that a lack of equipment, personnel, and funding, not the building itself, held back their investigative work.[97]

In 1935, the Council on Medical Education and Hospitals of the American Medical Association reviewed Woman's Medical College as part of its broader examination of all of the medical schools in the United States and Canada. The council withdrew Woman's Medical College from its list of approved medical schools after identifying a series of deficits, including a lack of full-time heads of preclinical departments. As part of its efforts to earn back the council's approval, the school expanded its full-time preclinical faculty to twelve women and two men by 1937. With the growth of the faculty, substantial research in the fundamental sciences began to develop at the school for the first time.[98]

The building's minimal provisions for research could not sustain the enlarged investigative program, however. In 1937, the acting professor of anatomy, Hartwig Kuhlenbeck, described a department designed principally for teaching, and he hoped that research facilities would be provided in the future.[99] Although Kuhlenbeck ultimately saw his wish fulfilled, he no doubt would have desired swifter action. Not until 1960 did the school obtain its first major addition: a wing dedicated primarily to research space. The expansion enabled significant growth in the school's investigative undertakings.[100]

Even with the requirements established by the American Medical Association, the standardization that accompanied medical education reform did not create identical medical schools. Faculty at elite university schools with deep endowments engaged in research at a level all but impossible to maintain at less wealthy institutions. As Joe Holoubek wrote of his experience at the University of Nebraska between 1934 and 1938, "there was only one goal of the school—to train young men from Nebraska to be country doctors in Nebraska. . . . Research at the medical school was almost non-existent."[101] Students like Holoubek may have had little exposure to research, but they were well equipped to practice medicine:

> We received a thorough training in anatomy and all of the basic sciences. We received very thorough training in the value of house calls and seeing the patients in their home environment so that we could better understand their needs. Even though I ended up a big city specialist, I have always made it a point to see a patient at home when necessary. During my internship [at the University of Nebraska] I had a [thorough] training in every specialty. . . . In short, I was well prepared to do general practice out in the hills of Nebraska far from a hospital.[102]

Although white, Protestant men enjoyed nearly unrestricted access to the full spectrum of American medical colleges, women did not share this luxury as students, residents, or faculty. In 1938, Holoubek became engaged to Alice Baker, whom he had met when both had summer fellowships at the Mayo Clinic in Rochester, Minnesota. Holoubek described "the problem that Alice and I had trying to obtain residencies together so that we could get married." First among their challenges was the fact that "very few hospitals wanted to have a female physician—particularly one who was to be married." In the end, Baker's personal physician offered her the last spot he had in internal medicine; when he learned of her desire to marry, he gave Holoubek a position as well—on the condition that they would together receive one salary.[103]

The careers of two women hired by Woman's Medical College shortly after it enlarged the preclinical faculty reveal the discrimination women scientists faced in the United States in this period, as medical historian Steven Peitzman has explained. Phyllis Bott, a biochemist and physiologist, earned her PhD in 1930 from the University of Pennsylvania. After two years at Princeton as a research fellow, Bott returned to Penn and built an impressive record over the next eight years. Nevertheless, Bott was not promoted above the rank of research associate. Upon arrival at Woman's Medical College in 1941, Bott received appointment to the faculty. She published several significant papers and in time became full professor. Similarly, Linda Bartels Lange became professor of bacteriology at Woman's Medical College in 1937 after twenty years at Johns Hopkins University, during which time she had not been advanced beyond the rank of associate professor. Peitzman underscores the significance of Woman's Medical College for female scientists in the 1930s: "Remarkably, after the new appointments beginning in 1935, the tiny Woman's Medical College became one of the leading employers of female medical science faculty, and certainly *the* leader among United States medical schools."[104]

In fact, across the Woman's Medical College faculty, women dominated. Among the college's senior faculty, women typically outnumbered men two to one at this time. By comparison, in 1930 the five-hundred-person medical faculty at the University of Pennsylvania included just eight women, all of whom held junior posts. Among the nation's medical schools, only at Woman's Medical College did women hold the deanship and a majority of the faculty positions, most of which were full time.[105] (Chapter 5 discusses women medical students, who faced hostility similar to that experienced by their faculty counterparts in coeducational institutions, where they constituted small percentages of the student body.)

Woman's Medical College may have provided female medical scientists and physicians with an unparalleled opportunity for advancement, but it extended this opportunity only to white women, not to African American women. Historian Vanessa Northington Gamble has examined the experiences of African American alumnae of Woman's Medical College through the class of 1925. The Woman's Medical College faculty refused to accept Black women, including its own graduates, as interns at the school's hospital; the leadership at Woman's Medical College assumed that the school's African American alumnae would spend their careers in Black hospitals and clinics. Between 1867 and 1925 Woman's Medical College graduated eighteen Black women—more than any other predominantly white medical school, but the college's policies promoted the separation of women physicians by race.[106]

Even if Woman's Medical College demonstrated that white women could succeed as both faculty leaders and investigators, these women did not have access to the resources that their white, male colleagues enjoyed at some institutions. The college's research space and budgets were small, and its resources hardly rivaled those of the elite medical schools for white men affiliated with major universities. Unlike, for example, at the medical schools at Johns Hopkins, Harvard, or Vanderbilt, the facilities at Woman's Medical College were not designed to create medical scientists. The white women—and some men—who forged investigative programs at Woman's Medical College in the 1930s and 1940s did so despite the building. Although the structure's design failed to encourage research, it did emphasize the specialties most closely associated with and most frequently practiced by women physicians: obstetrics, gynecology, pediatrics, and public health.[107]

Martha Tracy, an alumna of Woman's Medical College and the school's dean from 1917 to 1940, affirmed in a 1926 report that the school's objective was to prepare medical students to care for patients rather than undertake research. Tracy did not deny that women could carry out investigative projects in the basic sciences, but she felt that instruction in research might better be completed elsewhere or in subsequent years— scenarios that Tracy must have known were unlikely. Instead, Tracy described the college's goal "to give to the woman student of medicine a sound training for practice in the special fields which in the majority of instances are hers: a training which for her purposes shall be second to none in the United States." She went on to explain, "This cannot be done by imitating at all points the best University Schools. It will be done by expressing an individuality which shall be recognized in the product of this college; fundamental facts of the medical sciences, understandingly applied by physicians who are better gynecologists, better obstetricians, better pediatricians than is the average practitioner."[108] At the same time, Tracy called for an expansion of the school's work in preventive medicine (a field of study whose scope and content overlapped with public health and hygiene in this period) and explained the need for a new facility for the medical school and its hospital.[109] Tracy made her prophecy of a practical medical education focused on the specialties most closely aligned

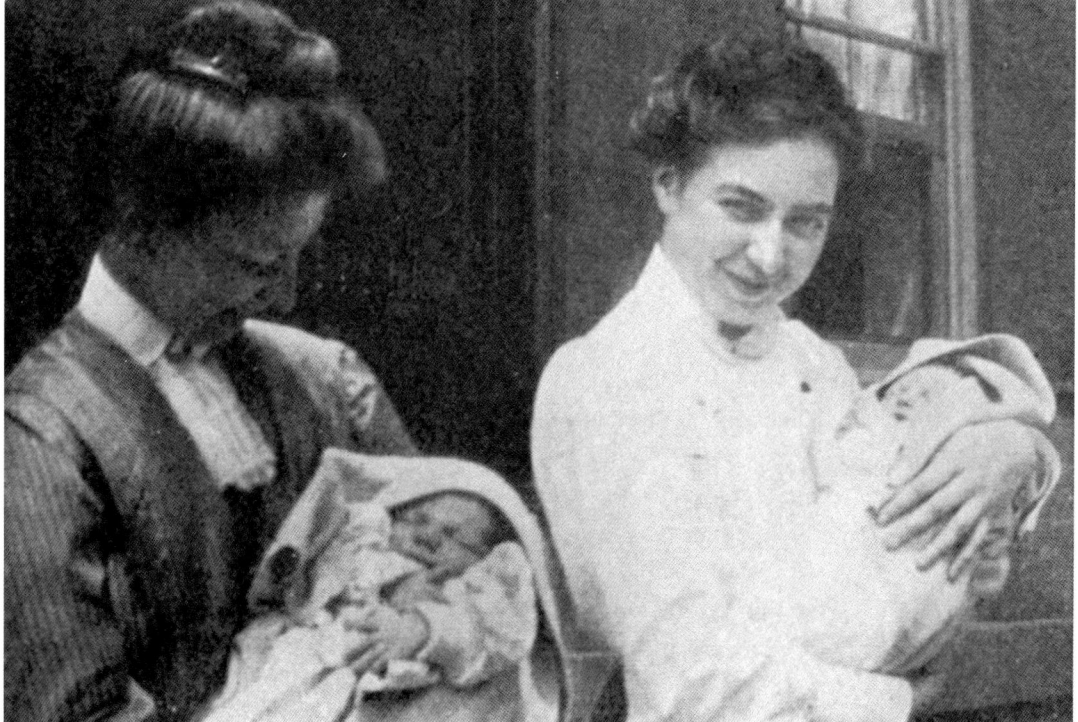

3.6.   Woman's Medical College of Pennsylvania senior students with babies from deliveries they attended, ca. 1911.

with women a reality. According to historian Regina Morantz-Sanchez, Woman's Medical College provided superior programs in obstetrics, gynecology, and preventive medicine to its twenty to fifty students who graduated annually between 1920 and 1968, the year the college became coeducational; that range represented between one-fifth and one-third of female medical graduates nationwide.[110]

Although Woman's Medical College trained women in all areas of medicine, the college emphasized obstetrics and gynecology, preventive medicine and public health, and pediatrics out of a conviction that most women physicians would practice in these areas due to personal choice or societal and professional limitations (fig. 3.6).[111] Women physicians enthusiastically participated in Progressive Era reform efforts centered on women and children, an extension of the role they had claimed in the nineteenth century, when women called for access to medical education in part to integrate science into family life. As public health became professionalized in the early twentieth century, women physicians figured prominently in the movement despite the prevalence of men in the field's leadership positions. Women physicians had long engaged in preventive

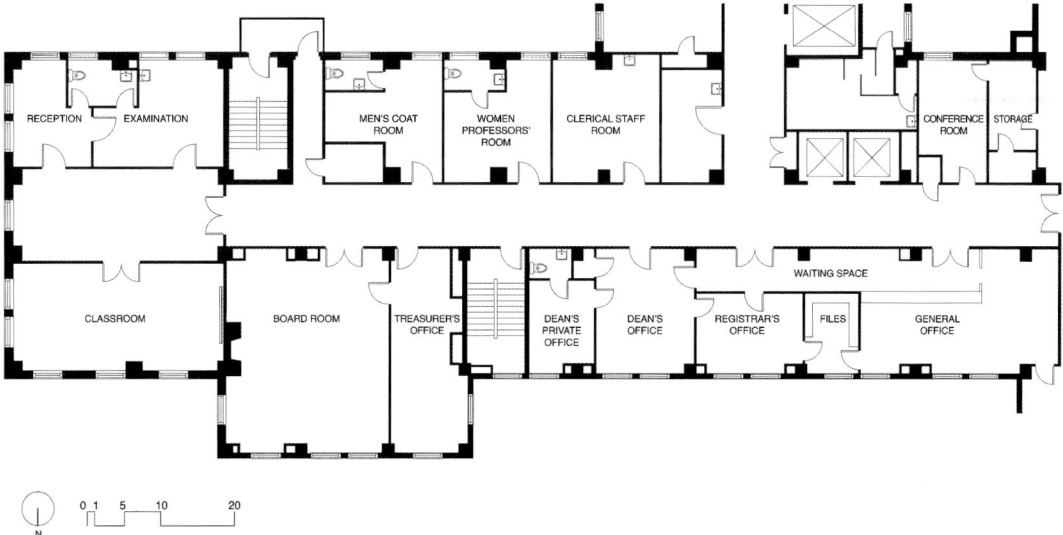

RECEPTION EXAMINATION   MEN'S COAT ROOM   WOMEN PROFESSORS' ROOM   CLERICAL STAFF ROOM   CONFERENCE ROOM   STORAGE

WAITING SPACE

CLASSROOM   BOARD ROOM   TREASURER'S OFFICE   DEAN'S PRIVATE OFFICE   DEAN'S OFFICE   REGISTRAR'S OFFICE   FILES   GENERAL OFFICE

0 1 5 10   20

N

3.7.   Woman's Medical College of Pennsylvania, 1930, Ritter and Shay, architects, plan, first floor, administration hallway with preventive medicine suite accessed through double doors at far end (*left*), redrawn. On the original plan, the "classroom" is labeled only "Preventive Medicine," but the black board on the interior short wall indicates its purpose. For the wing at the top of the plan, see fig. 3.5.

medicine and public health work and adopted these efforts as their particular domain.[112] At Woman's Medical College, preventive medicine and pediatrics developed more slowly than obstetrics, but both received increased attention in the early decades of the twentieth century.[113]

Some women surely chafed at the idea that their womanhood uniquely suited them for certain specialties, but Woman's Medical College publicized its commitment to these occupations.[114] Constantly campaigning for funds, the college attempted to capitalize (literally) on the public's expectations about women in medicine.[115] During the campaign for the 1930 building, one pamphlet, for example, provided "twenty-one reasons" to support Woman's Medical College, including the strength of its existing programs in obstetrics, gynecology, and pediatrics, as well as its plans for expanded training in preventive medicine.[116] Solicitations of this type did more than petition for donations; they also reinforced gendered perceptions of women physicians.

Even as the Woman's Medical College leadership stripped the 1930 medical school–hospital to its barest necessities, Tracy and her colleagues retained within the design their particular vision for the college. A suite dedicated to preventive medicine and composed of a classroom, examining room, and reception room sat prominently, if awkwardly, at the end of the first-floor administration hallway just beyond the board room (fig. 3.7). Moreover, although the program in preventive medicine would falter in the 1940s, its revival in the 1950s brought with it the opening in 1954 of the Martha Tracy Memorial, a small wing attached to the clinical section of the building for the preventive medicine department.[117]

Obstetrics and pediatrics also received close attention. In 1927, three years before Woman's Medical College transferred to its new facility, the school's Amy S. Barton Dispensary, an outpatient clinic, moved to the college's future neighborhood. The superintendent of the hospital described the dispensary's carefully chosen location as a "house . . . in excellent repair, in the heart of the most thickly settled portion of the [neighborhood] . . . fifteen minutes by direct carline from the College." As for the dispensary's work, she explained that "in addition to the maternity outpractice we are planning to make of this a health center for the district and are arranging for a daily diagnostic clinic, pre-natal, post-natal, children's clinic, etc."[118] Maternity care and the treatment of children featured heavily in the plans for the college's relocation.

Circumstances could not have been more different as events unfolded in Nashville regarding Vanderbilt University's 1925 medical school–hospital. In the final tally, the officers of the General Education Board decided that the school would forgo dedicated space in the building for certain specialties, including obstetrics, gynecology, and pediatrics, with the hope that a local donor could be interested in supporting construction for these specialties. When the hospital opened, pediatrics, obstetrics, and gynecology faculty struggled to make do with borrowed space from medicine and surgery, a situation that also left medicine and surgery compromised. No donors materialized, and in order to protect its already sizable investment in Vanderbilt's medical school, the General Education Board funded the 1938 expansion of the hospital that remedied the deficits.[119] At this majority-male institution, the instruction of physicians in the specialized care of women and children initially received relatively little attention.

Medical students' obstetrical training highlights the focus on women and children at Woman's Medical College. Physicians educated in the early twentieth century learned to deliver babies in part in patients' homes. Francis D. Moore, Harvard Medical School class of 1939, recalled the circumstances of being "on District": "Medical students (externes) were assigned an area of Boston (a district) in which, under the watchful eye of first-year house officers (internes) from the obstetrical hospital (the Boston Lying-In), they were to deliver the babies of very poor women."[120] Although the specifics, including oversight and other members of the team, differed from school to school, two common themes among physicians' recollections were the intense poverty of the women they served and their own lack of experience. In Nebraska, Holoubek recounted that "one cold, winter night we were called to [a] shack in south Omaha. They had heat in one room and not in the other, where the obstetrical patient had her bed." He explained, "Two medical students would go with two nurses, one very experienced. . . . We were told that if we would use the instruments she handed us, everything would work well."[121] In Boston, Moore described attending to a mother who "had been there before. Between uterine contractions she often told the sweating young externe what to do next." If the students needed assistance, Moore wrote, "our instructions were to give the husband a nickel. He was to go to a pay phone and call the interne, who would drive over to help us in his rickety jalopy, or maybe take the streetcar."[122] Within the relatively similar events described by medical students, a seemingly significant difference existed. At Harvard, Moore "delivered the requisite 12 such babies," and, at Nebraska, Holoubek remembered "about six home deliveries."[123] The students at these entirely or predominantly male medical colleges in the 1930s delivered far fewer babies in patients' homes than the students at Woman's Medical College, where Mary Bruins Allison, class of 1932, reported, "we did twenty deliveries at homes."[124]

The design for the 1930 medical school–hospital for Woman's Medical College may have also emphasized the school's commitment to women and children. A full analysis of the building cannot be undertaken since complete architectural plans no longer exist (the maternity department plans are among the missing sections). Notably, however, the children's ward received prime billing, with an easily accessible location steps away from the main entrance.[125]

Unable to find a major funder, Woman's Medical College of Pennsylvania kept its doors open against tremendous odds. Its very modest 1930 facility formulated in brick and stone what it meant to be a woman in medicine in the early twentieth century. Nationally, white and Black women rarely received the support necessary to distinguish themselves as research scientists. White women might obtain an appointment at Woman's Medical College, but here research facilities and other resources were minimal. Without the opportunity to participate in a strong investigative program, white and Black women were hampered, especially after the interwar period, which witnessed a growing focus on research as the primary litmus of individual and institutional success.[126] Moreover, societal, professional, and sometimes personal expectations concentrated the women's energies in obstetrics, gynecology, pediatrics, and preventive medicine. Nevertheless, Woman's Medical College trained a significant number of Black and white women in the full spectrum of modern medicine and with superior instruction in certain specialties. It also gave students a virtually unique chance to learn in an environment rich with female role models, with many white women on the faculty, including top leadership positions.[127] Black students, however, endured racism at the college.[128] Even as white students and faculty discriminated against African American women training at the school, Woman's Medical College helped to expand the demographics of American physicians. In addition to African American women, the college admitted international and Jewish women. Furthermore, Woman's Medical College developed a reputation abroad for its estimated 230 graduates who became medical missionaries, and the school saw celebrated work emerge from its graduates and faculty, such as Catherine Macfarlane and Virginia M. Alexander (the faculty denied this Black alumna an internship due to her race and then later appointed her an assistant physician at the college hospital).[129] A careful reading of the 1930 building underscores both the constraints of and the opportunities to be gained from training and working at Woman's Medical College.

The General Education Board's Limited Support for Black Medical Schools

In his 1910 report, Flexner singled out Black medical colleges for separate consideration, a decision that reinforced the racial divide within the medical field.[130] Flexner counseled prospective donors to concentrate their efforts by investing in just two of the country's Black medical schools—Meharry Medical College and Howard University's medical school—while allowing the nation's other five schools for African American students to close. In addition, Flexner asserted that African American physicians should serve only African American patients, and he called for "schools to which the more promising of the race can be sent to receive a substantial education in which hygiene [public health] rather than surgery . . . is strongly accentuated."[131] African American physicians found themselves restricted with regard to where they could train and what they were encouraged to practice. Medical school buildings reflected and promoted the idea that medical colleges for Black men and women differed from medical schools for white students.

Flexner's work at the GEB fit squarely within the many Progressive Era campaigns carried out by foundations sponsored and run by white northerners to improve the health and education of Black and white southerners. In this period, for example, the Julius Rosenwald Fund positioned itself as a leading supporter of African American education and health and counted among its programs the creation of rural schools for Black children and scholarships for African American physicians and nurses. The Rockefeller Sanitary Commission in association with the US Public Health Service also launched a highly effective campaign to eradicate hookworm in the South. Outside of its work in medical training, the GEB invested heavily in southern public school systems to improve the education of Black and white students in urban and rural areas. With its size, the breadth of its work, and its decades of activity, the GEB dominated philanthropic efforts to improve schooling in the South and for African American young people. Analyses of the motives and outcomes of undertakings organized by white philanthropists for the benefit of Black southerners have figured prominently in historical investigations of medical training.[132]

The officers at the GEB and other philanthropies created programs in medical education rooted in racist beliefs that constrained Black physicians and contributed to racial disparities in health care. As expressed in his report, Flexner promoted for African American physicians a circumscribed function that centered on public health. Moreover, the country had just seven medical colleges for Black students in 1910, all of which were struggling to keep pace with education reforms, but Flexner advocated supporting only two, a prescription that curtailed still further the options African American students had for medical training and the availability of Black physicians. Seemingly recognizing that his proposal would worsen the shortage of Black physicians, Flexner explained that, although Black doctors would serve only Black patients, white physicians would treat both Black patients and white. Under segregation, however, the care of Black patients by white physicians was deeply unequal, and at the time of Flexner's report approximately 9 million Black Americans lived in the segregated South.[133] Compounding these directives, GEB officials considered African American physicians less intelligent than their white counterparts and thus unable to become research scientists.[134] In the end, philanthropic leaders intended that separate medical schools for Black and white students would provide different training, the former focused on hygiene and sanitation and the latter committed to scientific medicine and research.[135] Flexner and his colleagues at the GEB and elsewhere treated the Black medical schools paternalistically, and they refused to encourage racial integration in medical training.[136]

At the same time, Flexner's dedication to Howard University and Meharry Medical College extended through more than one phase of his career and merged his professional and personal activities. As an officer at the GEB, Flexner channeled the board's funds to Howard's medical school and Meharry. Later, after he no longer worked at the GEB and had less involvement in medical education, Flexner became a trustee of Howard University and continued to fundraise for Meharry, where he even led the national fundraising campaign begun in January 1941 to raise the matching funds required by the GEB as a condition of its gift for the school's endowment.[137] Flexner also consistently petitioned the American Medical Association's Council on Medical Education to acknowledge local variations in its treatment and assessment of medical schools in the South, regardless of whether they enrolled Black or white students, due to the region's less developed education system, and he emphasized the need to ensure that southerners, and specifically African American southerners, had access to medical education.[138]

Karen Kruse Thomas has further complicated our reading of Flexner by arguing that "Flexner's hope that black schools would prepare many competent sanitarians rather than a handful of surgeons was well founded in the greatest practical and humanitarian needs of the South, where far more deaths and illness would be prevented by the application of public health methods than by the slice of a scalpel."[139] Whether we label Flexner a racist, an ally, a pragmatist, or—most accurately—all three, Flexner's national vision for medical education included specific restrictions on where African Americans would study and the positions they would fill. The medical school buildings at Howard, Meharry, and Vanderbilt reveal much about how the General Education Board invested its money and the divergent roles the board envisioned for Black and white physicians.

True to the agenda put forth in his 1910 report, Flexner provided GEB aid to just two Black medical colleges: Howard University College of Medicine and Meharry Medical College, which by 1923 were the only medical schools in the country for Black students.[140] In the 1938–1939 academic year, Meharry and Howard enrolled 87 percent of African American medical students, with the remaining 13 percent attending schools outside of the South.[141] Compared to Meharry, Howard's medical school received a relatively small share of GEB resources, just shy of $588,000. The federal government allocated funds, however meager, to Howard University, and the GEB thus saw Howard's medical school as primarily the responsibility of the federal government. The GEB placed Meharry in a different category as an independent medical college without the support of the government or a university. In the end, the GEB extended a total of more than $8.6 million to Meharry Medical College.[142]

In the late 1920s, Howard University College of Medicine and Meharry Medical College undertook the construction of new facilities to

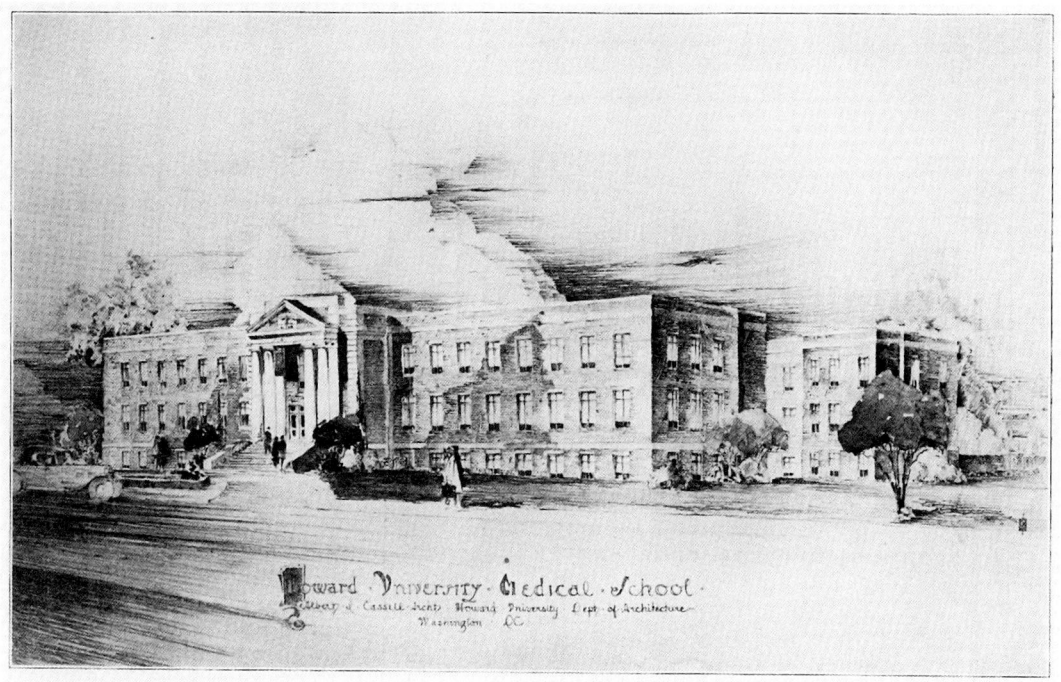

3.8.   Howard University College of Medicine, 1927, Albert I. Cassell, architect.

keep pace with medical education reform. Howard opened its new building in 1927 (fig. 3.8). To construct and equip the structure, the federal
government provided the bulk of the funding, $370,000, with the GEB
contributing $130,000. Four years later, Meharry completed a combined
medical school–hospital (fig. 3.9). For this project, the GEB gave far
more: two gifts totaling nearly $1.6 million toward the approximately $2
million facility, including site, medical school–hospital, nurses' home,
power plant, and equipment.[143] Flexner initiated the plan for Meharry
before he left the GEB in the spring of 1928. Even after his position at
the GEB ended, Flexner worked hard to ensure the plan's success and
personally encouraged George Eastman, pioneer in photography and
founder of Eastman Kodak Company, to contribute to the building.[144]
In the end, Eastman gave $200,000 to construct and equip the school's
dental department, a welcome gift toward the $500,000 on which the
GEB conditioned its support.[145]

Restricted by the inability of philanthropists and the federal government to conceptualize African American physicians as medical scientists, Howard University College of Medicine and Meharry Medical
College did not receive enough funding to construct significant dedicated research space. For example, the Howard building included ten

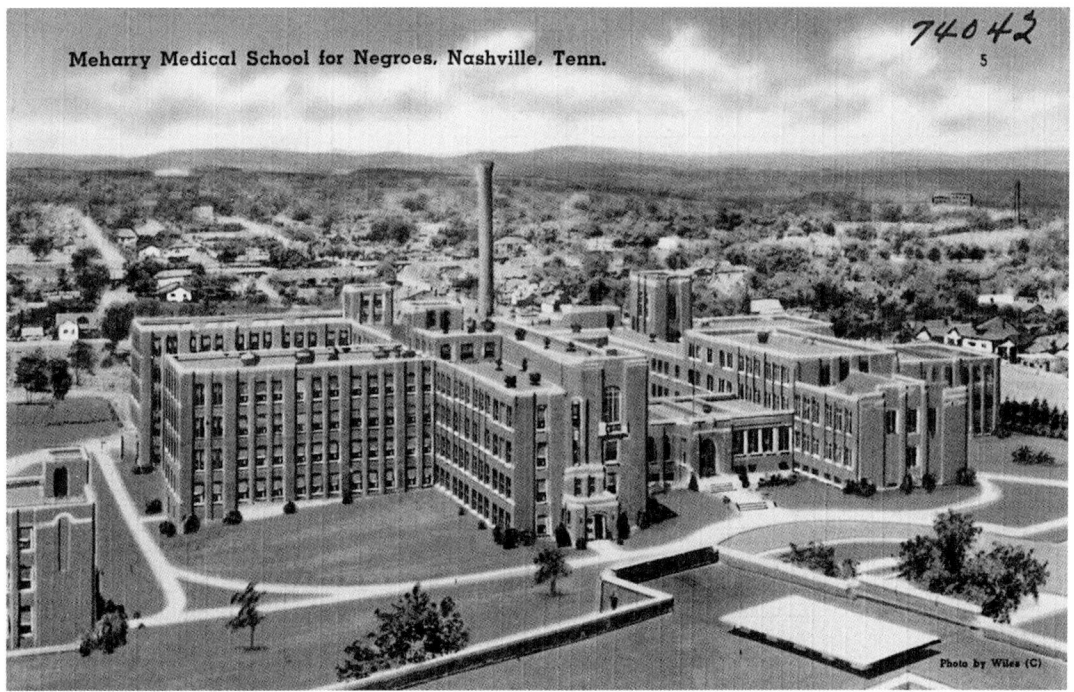

Meharry Medical School for Negroes, Nashville, Tenn.

3.9.   Meharry Medical College, 1931, Gordon and Kaelber, architects.

teaching wings, each typically composed of a classroom, a large teaching laboratory, an office, and a small research laboratory, which gave the school ten rooms specifically for research (fig. 3.10). Meharry contained a comparable number of small laboratories that could have served research purposes, although on the architectural plans only one is labeled for research. At Meharry, the negative attitude of its white president, John J. Mullowney, about the school's predominantly African American faculty undertaking research further discouraged original investigation at the college. The new leadership installed at the GEB at the end of the 1920s became critical of Mullowney's stance against research, as well as his financial policies, and in 1938 the GEB's officers facilitated his replacement.[146] Despite the GEB officials' shifting opinion on research at Meharry, the college's 1931 plant included very little research space.

Just two miles from Meharry, Vanderbilt University School of Medicine occupied its 1925 medical school–hospital designed for white students. There, the physiology wing alone contained five rooms for research (fig. 3.11). For Flexner and the General Education Board, Nashville represented a critical southern outpost in the board's plan to improve medical training nationwide, and it spent more money in Nashville than in any other city in the country. But the board did not give equally to

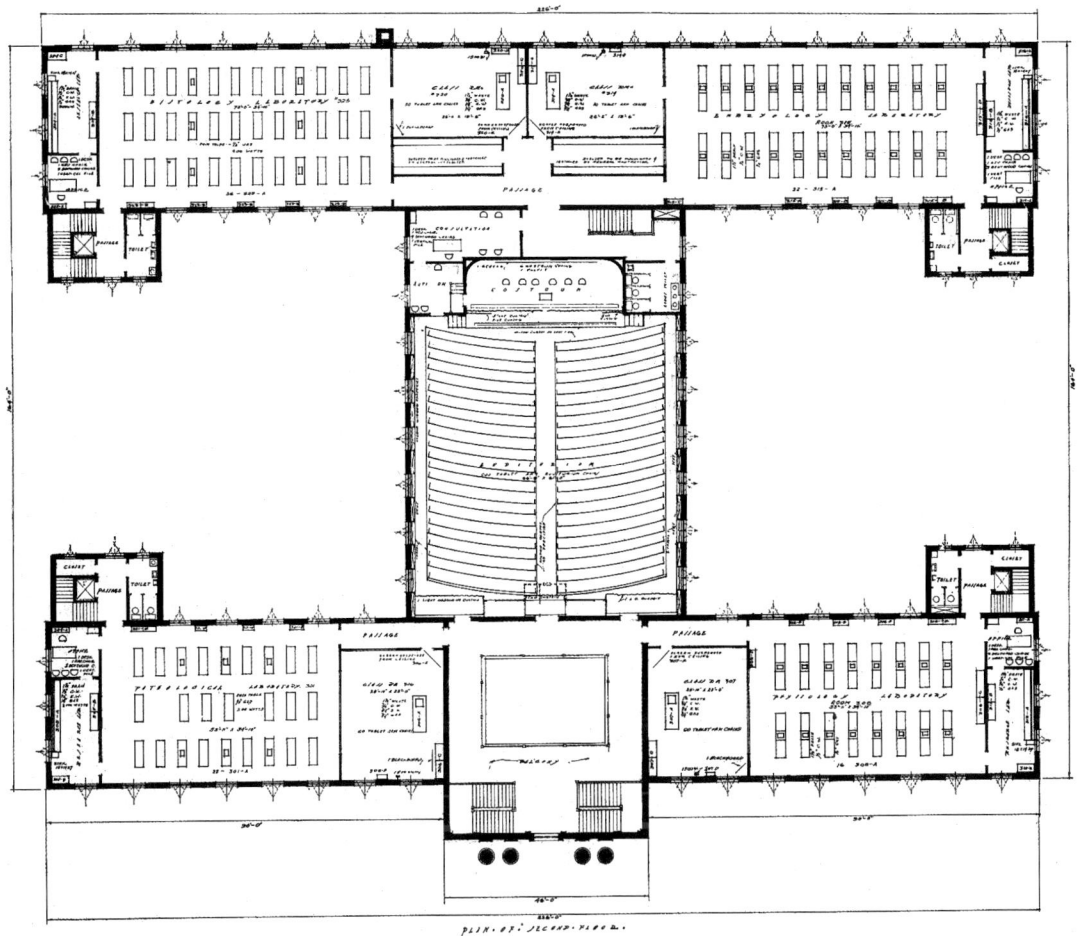

PLAN OF SECOND FLOOR, SHOWING EQUIPMENT AND AUDITORIUM WHICH IS TO HAVE A SEATING CAPACITY OF FIVE HUNDRED

3.10.   Howard University College of Medicine, 1927, Albert I. Cassell, architect, plan, second floor. The end of each wing contains a rectangular research laboratory connected to an approximately square office.

Black and white institutions. It allocated more than twice as much aid for Vanderbilt as it did for Meharry.[147] Vanderbilt's 1925 medical school–hospital, nurses' home, and power plant cost at least 75 percent more to build and equip than the same structures completed in 1931 at Meharry, and the white faculty and students enjoyed at least 55 percent more cubic feet in Vanderbilt's medical school–hospital than did their Black neighbors in Meharry's medical school–hospital.[148] This discrepancy in size existed despite the fact that the GEB officers, Mullowney, and the architects designed Meharry for approximately 225 medical students as well as at least 310 additional pupils in dentistry, pharmacy, nursing, and dental hygiene, while the Vanderbilt plant could accommodate up to 200

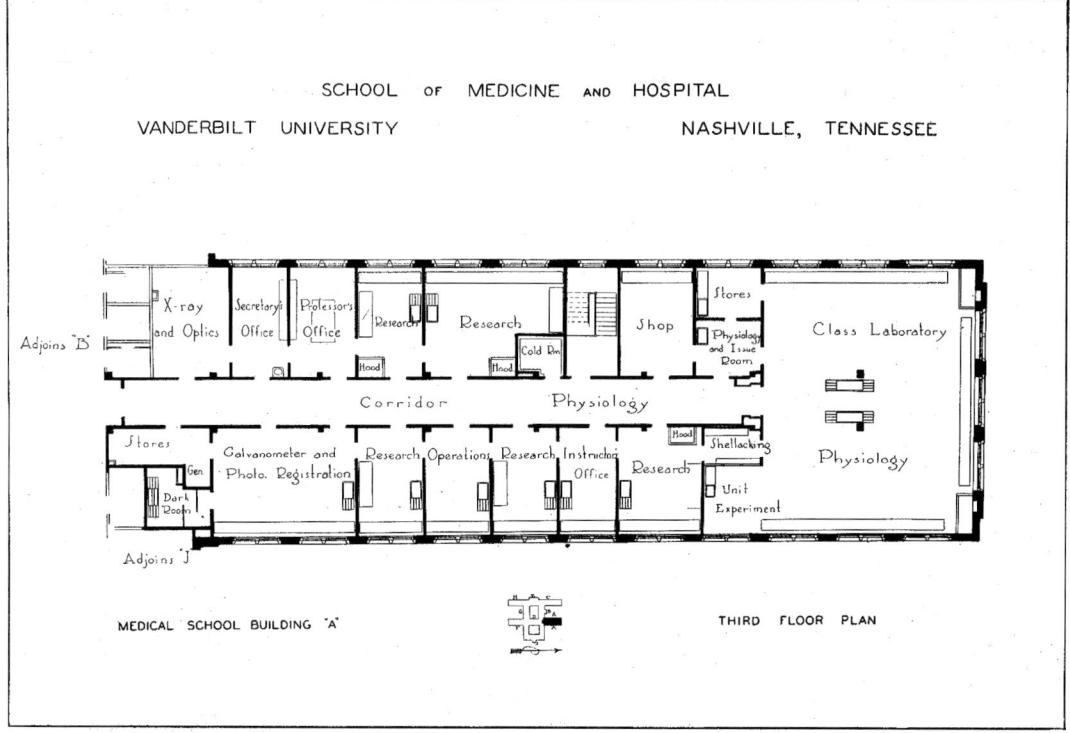

3.11.   Vanderbilt University School of Medicine and Hospital, 1925, Coolidge and Shattuck, architects, plan, third floor, physiology wing.

medical students along with the nursing students.[149] Vanderbilt's structure not only cost more per cubic foot but contained more space for fewer students. In addition to greater research facilities, Vanderbilt students and faculty had access to more clinical facilities than their counterparts at Meharry. Meharry's hospital accommodated 140 beds to Vanderbilt's 208 beds, a number Robinson classified as "too small to offer ideal conditions for clinical teaching and research."[150] By committing significantly less money to Meharry, the GEB, along with the other philanthropists and foundations that followed its lead, ensured that Meharry would focus its efforts on constructing accommodations for teaching and could not afford to create research space on par with premier white institutions.

By the 1920s and 1930s, nearly all medical schools were professing a dedication to research, but few matched the buildings, equipment, budgets, and faculty of the medical schools at Johns Hopkins University, Harvard University, or Vanderbilt University. For African Americans, however, who had very limited opportunities to study or teach at schools other than Howard and Meharry, the lack of research at the

Black medical colleges resulted in a distinct disadvantage in a period that increasingly recognized research as the primary barometer of personal and institutional success.[151] Reinforcing this reality, the GEB fellowships for faculty from Howard University College of Medicine offered only remedial training, while the board's fellowships for faculty from predominantly white medical schools aimed to create research-focused medical scientists.[152]

In the competition for funding in the early twentieth century, medical schools with financial stability, university affiliation, and a superior academic program, which included a commitment to research, tended to receive the most gifts. The GEB actively participated in this trend. In its distribution of funds, the GEB preferred the stronger schools and encouraged medical schools to undertake research.[153] No doubt an established investigative program with the possibility of future medical advances helped to stir the enthusiasm and loosen the purse strings of the GEB and other donors. The Black medical schools, however, existed outside of this overall trajectory. The GEB and other benefactors focused their aid on what they perceived to be the two best medical colleges for Black students but failed to conceive of these schools as locations for research.

Even if the medical schools at Howard and Meharry did not receive the financial support necessary to inaugurate substantial research programs, they did educate their students in all areas of medicine, including surgery, which Flexner had labeled unnecessary for African American physicians. Both schools, however, joined Flexner in emphasizing training in public health for Black doctors. As Lynn E. Miller and Richard M. Weiss have shown, before the release of the Flexner Report the leadership at Howard and Meharry had highlighted the need for Black physicians to work in public health.[154] This focus may have represented, at least partially, the same tactic adopted by Woman's Medical College of Pennsylvania when it attempted to capitalize on the expectation that women physicians would pursue particular specialties. Miller and Weiss explain that "promoting a public health role for black doctors . . . may have been intended [by officials at Black medical schools and by Flexner] to carve out a niche for black physicians that would help convince both blacks and whites to care about preserving black medical schools."[155] Flexner and the leaders of Black medical schools may also have believed that Black doctors trained in public health could fill critical needs. In particular, Flexner and officials at Meharry and Howard highlighted the tuberculosis epidemic. One of the nation's top three causes of death at the time, tuberculosis claimed the lives of Black Americans at far higher rates than white Americans, a disparity that was increasingly

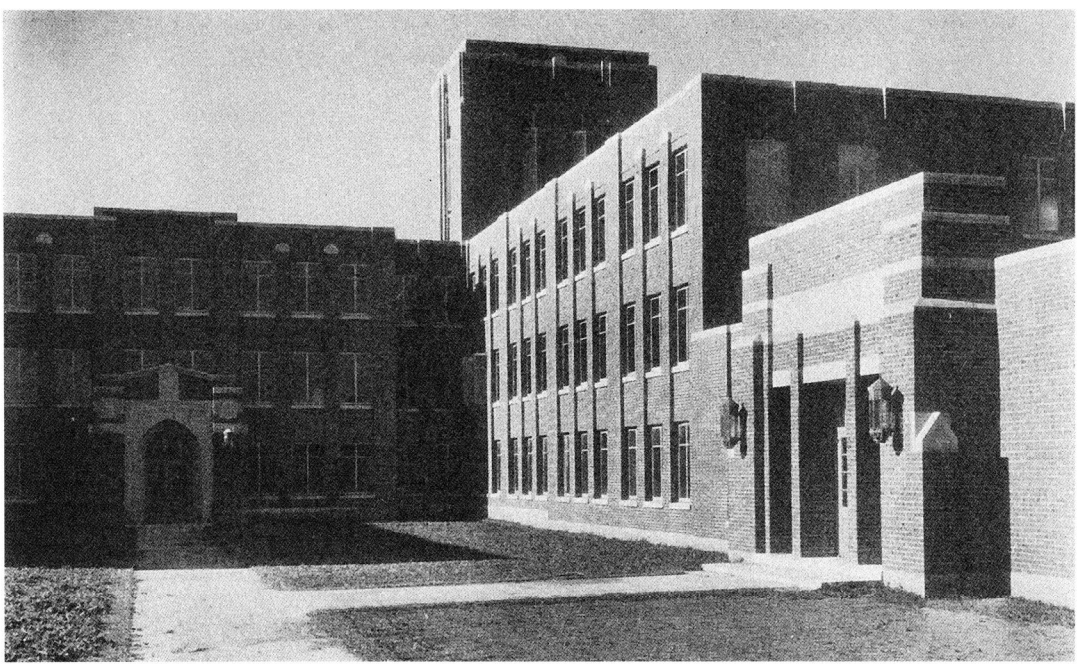

3.12.   Meharry Medical College, 1931, Gordon and Kaelber, architects. View from Heffernan Street (now
         Meharry Boulevard) of the entrance to the medical school (*left*) and the entrance to the Public Health
         Lecture Room (*right*), ca. 1931.

understood to stem in part from inadequate nutrition and unsanitary living arrangements.[156]

However, for Black medical schools, the narrative of the African American physician as public health guardian was constraining. In 1912, when a Howard medical school faculty member attempted to demonstrate the school's need for philanthropic support by comparing that school to Harvard Medical School and Johns Hopkins Medical School, Flexner admonished him and called the argument "presumptious [*sic*]." Flexner instead advocated a "simple and unpretentious" plan that would begin by building up the school's departments in the basic medical sciences.[157] Shortly after receiving Flexner's response, Howard's medical school leaders submitted to the General Education Board a funding appeal that made no mention of the elite, predominantly white schools. Instead, they described the function of the medical college in familiar terms that emphasized the role of Howard medical graduates in improving the public health of African Americans, who, they wrote, suffered an "appalling death rate . . . from communicable and preventable diseases."[158] As Howard R. Epps argues, "the threat of disease gave white philanthropists incentive to donate, but not grants of the magnitude

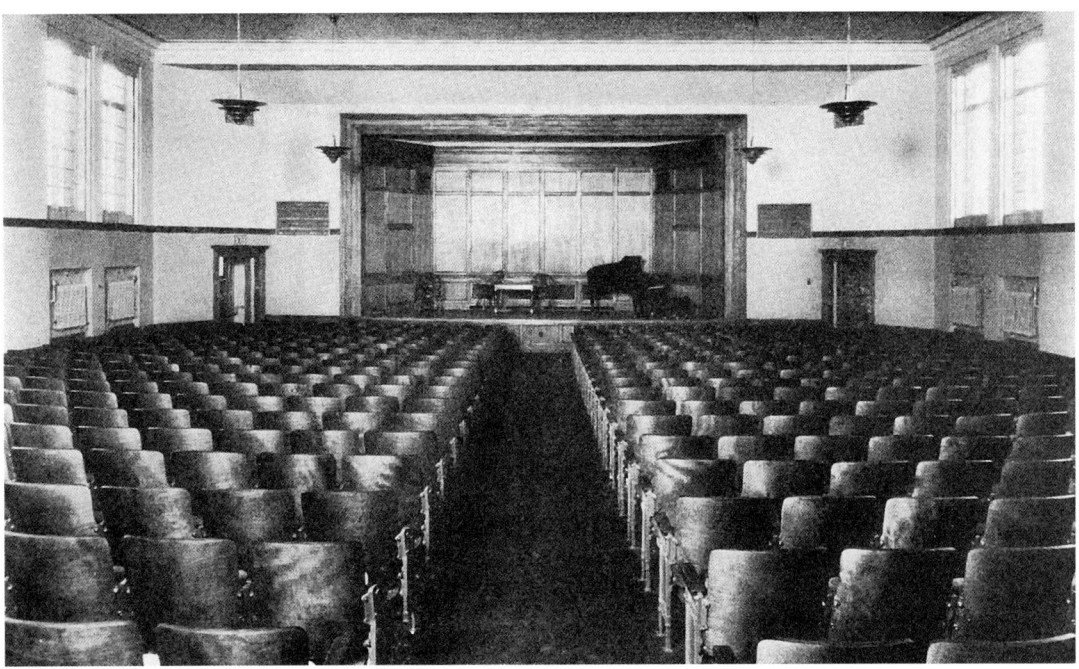

3.13.   Meharry Medical College, 1931, Gordon and Kaelber, architects. Interior of the Public Health Lecture
          Room, ca. 1931.

Howard needed" to match the country's strongest schools.[159] Meharry
also desperately required philanthropic aid and faced the same circumscribed mandate.[160]

Not surprisingly, Howard's and Meharry's dedication ceremonies for
their medical buildings underscored both schools' commitment to public
health. The first day of dedication exercises for Howard University's
1927 medical school included a public health meeting, and at least two
of the addresses given on the second day centered on major public health
issues.[161] Similarly, the dedication program for Meharry's 1931 facility
highlighted "the problems of public health work, and the opportunity for
service open to Meharry graduates in this field of medical endeavor."[162]
Although the building at Howard did not specifically promote public
health, a late change in the design made public health a prominent feature of the Meharry Medical College structure.

Initially, the 1931 Meharry Medical College contained no provisions
for public health, but by the time the facility was completed it included
a large, six-hundred-seat "Public Health Lecture Room" with a separate
exterior entrance for direct access to the street, along with restrooms and
coat rooms to accommodate visitors (figs. 3.12 and 3.13).[163] While raising
the money required to obtain the GEB grant, Meharry president John J.

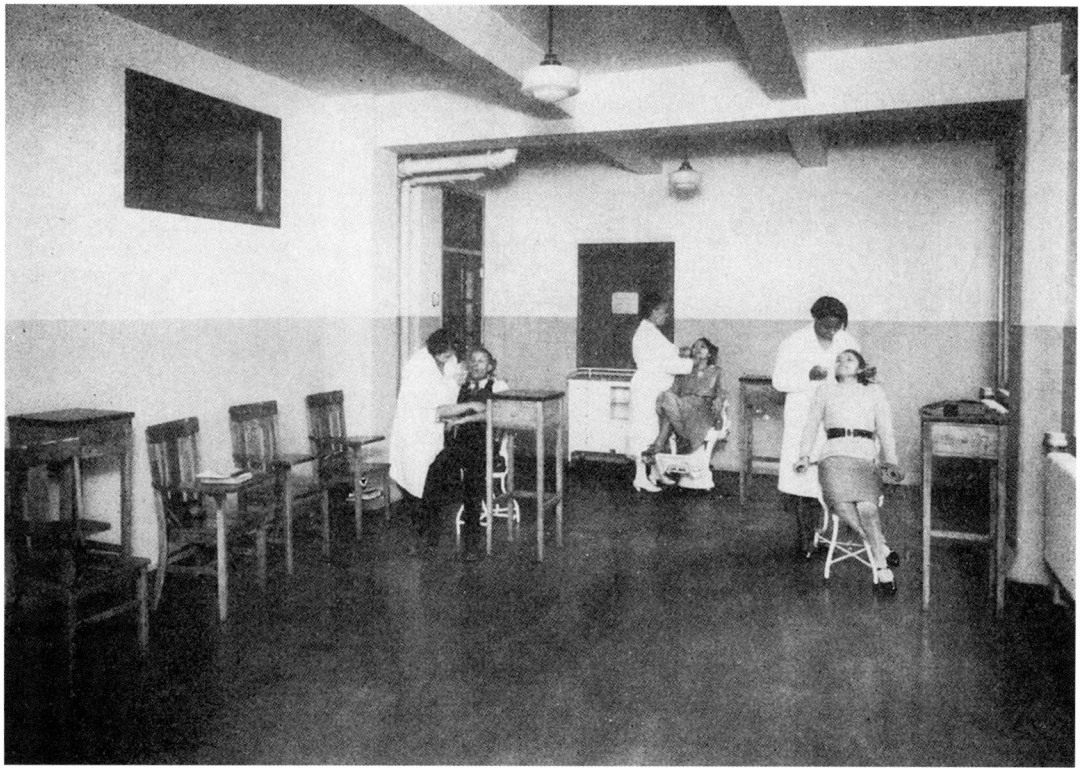

3.14.   Students in dental hygiene, Meharry Medical College, ca. 1931.

Mullowney itemized the lecture hall as an appropriate gift for an interested benefactor. In his pitch to George Eastman, Mullowney described
the "Assembly Room," projected to cost $40,000, as valuable only for
students.[164] Eastman did not supply the needed sum, but philanthropist
Edward Harkness did make a $50,000 gift, which may have been ear-
marked for the auditorium.[165] Shortly after the facility opened, the college
explained that the auditorium served both the school and the public, to
whom Meharry offered "lectures on Hygiene, Public Health, and similar
subjects."[166] Whether Mullowney or the donor orchestrated the shift in
function to include instruction to the community is unknown. Regardless, the "Public Health Lecture Room" reinforced the expectation that
Meharry would participate in public health outreach.

Although the Meharry building expressed a particular commitment
to educating the community in matters of public health, no section of
the structure was set aside for the school's public health department or
any research its members might undertake. In justifying to an officer of
the GEB the college's proposed $3,000 yearly budget for public health
and preventive medicine, Mullowney described lectures and films related

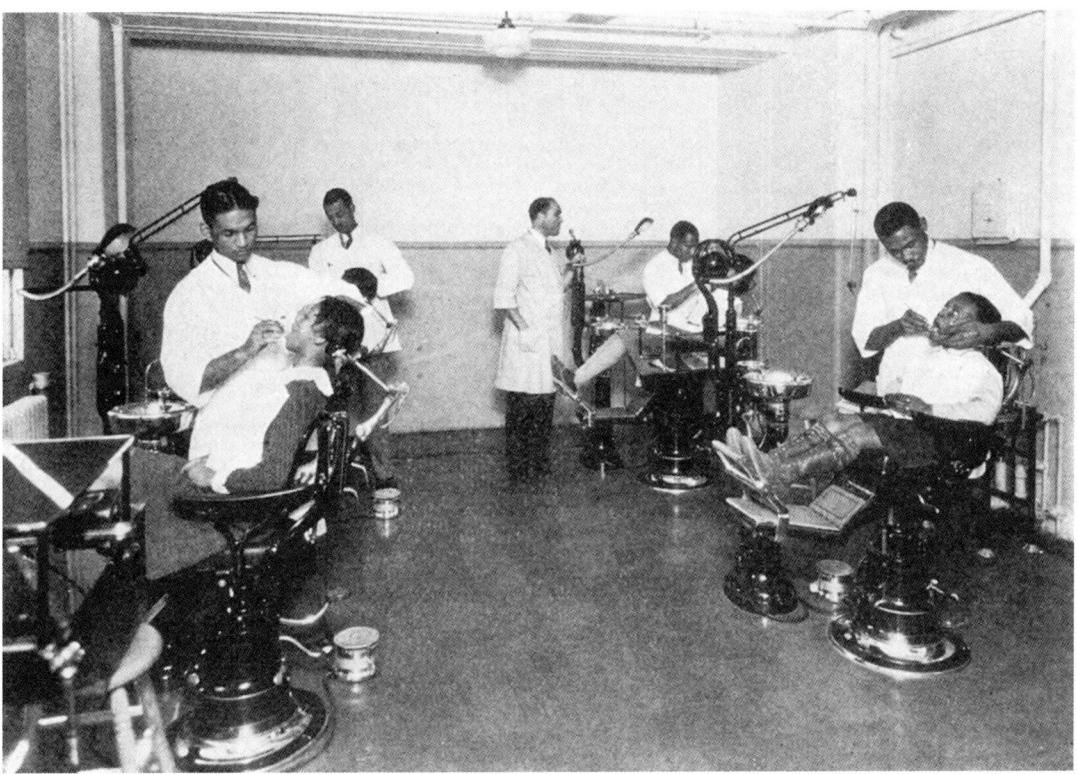

3.15.   Children's dental clinic, Meharry Medical College, ca. 1931.

to public health. He mentioned no funding for research and no full-time faculty member to head the department, despite the fact that every Meharry student had to conduct a sanitary survey or write a thesis in public health, a curricular element designed to ensure that all students obtained depth of knowledge in public health matters.[167] At the laying of the cornerstone for the facility, Mullowney celebrated the school's soon-to-be expanded program in dentistry, with its new course in dental hygiene made possible by Eastman's gift. Mullowney lauded the dental hygiene department as "the first of its kind in the South" and connected dentistry to public health when he noted, "There is already demand, particularly in Public Health work, for Dental Hygienists, and in the schools" (fig. 3.14).[168] Similarly, the college celebrated the opening of one of the South's first dental clinics for children in the 1931 building (fig. 3.15).[169] The school's other clinics, which included the South's first prenatal clinic for Black women and free clinics for people with tuberculosis and children with congenital syphilis, further reinforced the public health focus.[170] Meharry's design, curriculum, and clinics reveal a commitment to training students for a variety of fields in matters related

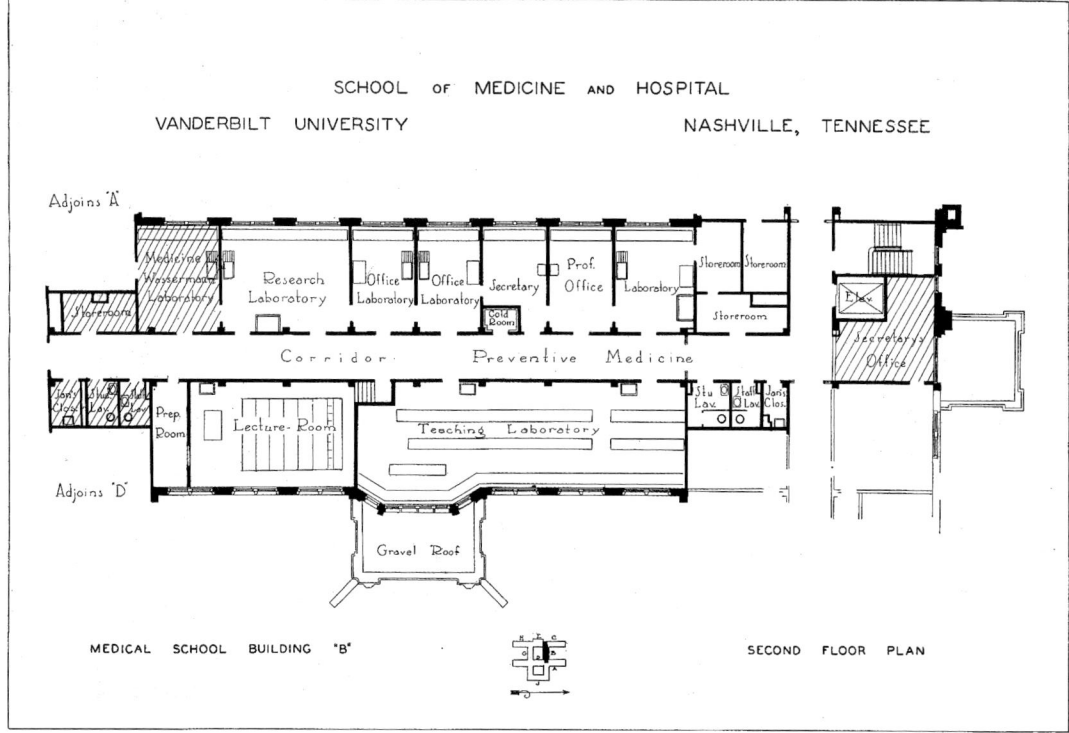

3.16.   Vanderbilt University School of Medicine and Hospital, 1925, Coolidge and Shattuck, architects, plan, second floor, corridor for Department of Preventive Medicine and Public Health.

to public health and providing public health outreach, but outside of the medical students' theses and sanitary surveys, no emphasis on investigation in public health existed.

As at Meharry, Vanderbilt's medical school–hospital plant also failed to contain facilities for public health in its initial design. With a bigger building than Meharry, however, Vanderbilt had enough square footage for its preventive medicine and public health department to "borrow" space from the library and the anatomy department.[171] The result was a corridor dedicated to teaching and research in this subject (fig. 3.16).

Aware that public health lagged in the South in comparison to the North, GEB officers had an interest in funding preventive medicine and public health at Vanderbilt, an interest that no doubt encouraged the medical school leadership to find room for the preventive medicine and public health program.[172] Beginning in 1925, the GEB extended $10,000 a year for five years to Vanderbilt's preventive medicine and public health department, which was under the full-time leadership of the highly experienced Waller Leathers.[173] By 1929, the department had research under way related to multiple topics of local and state concern.[174] The year before the opening of Vanderbilt's 1925 medical building, Flexner asserted that this modern medical college would "create a new standard and ought to make a profound impression in the field of medicine *and* public health throughout the South."[175] GEB officials set national goals for Vanderbilt's department, too. Recognizing the inadequacy of training in preventive medicine in medical schools throughout the country, the officers of the GEB also supported Vanderbilt's program in the hope that it would develop a course of study in preventive medicine that would function as a prototype for other schools.[176] Apparently it achieved this goal. In 1929, the leadership of the public health department at Albany Medical College in New York State reported, "It is hoped gradually to correlate the work in public health with the other teaching branches in the College in a way similar to that which has been adopted by . . . W. S. Leathers at the Vanderbilt University School of Medicine."[177] The GEB later reaffirmed its commitment to public health at Vanderbilt by including facilities for preventive medicine and public health in the 1938 addition to the medical school–hospital that it funded.[178] Flexner called on African American physicians to focus on public health and serve African American communities, a vision promoted by Meharry's design, curriculum, and clinics. In contrast, at Vanderbilt, where faculty and students were white, Flexner worked to create a public health research program and pedagogical innovator.

The divergent agendas codified by the Vanderbilt and Meharry medical school–hospitals are masked by the buildings' similar footprints, a confluence of design that stems from Flexner's involvement with the Vanderbilt, Meharry, and University of Rochester medical facilities. With Flexner moving people and ideas around behind the scenes, the Rochester architects and medical educators based the design for Rochester's medical school–hospital on the facility at Vanderbilt, and Meharry later employed Rochester's architects for its 1931 building.[179] The result was a second Nashville medical college with the distinctive grid-like footprint first found at Vanderbilt.

The apparent resemblance between the schools, however, belied serious disparities. In addition to Meharry's smaller size, relative lack of research space, and different relationship to public health than its counterpart across town, the building supported the education of five groups of medical personnel—physicians, dentists, dental hygienists, nurses, and pharmacists—to Vanderbilt's two—doctors and nurses. In housing the facilities for training these five types of medical personnel in one structure, Meharry was almost certainly unique among American medical colleges, an observation about the edifice frequently repeated when it opened.[180] Compared to white Americans, Black Americans had relatively few opportunities to train in medicine, dentistry, nursing, or pharmacy. Recognizing this inequality, Meharry educated its students in a number of medical fields, as did Howard University, which, in addition to medicine, offered programs in dentistry, pharmacy, and, after 1934, dental hygiene. Beginning in 1933, Howard also provided training in the basic sciences to students enrolled in the nursing course at Freedmen's Hospital.

The architects for Meharry accommodated the variety of students by dividing the building into mostly separate zones for medicine, dentistry, and pharmacy. This design greatly reduced the ability to move from laboratory to bedside along a single corridor in the fashion that was so lauded at Vanderbilt. Nevertheless, Meharry's president appears to have been pleased with the results. In 1936, Mullowney discussed the structure's efficiency. He emphasized the coordination of medicine and dentistry and highlighted the economy of the two departments sharing not only the basic science laboratories but also many of the faculty and a lot of the equipment. From a pedagogical standpoint, he underscored the usefulness of physical proximity when medical and dental students were undergoing instruction in systemic diseases.[181]

The officers of the GEB never planned to create two identical institutions at Vanderbilt and Meharry for the South's white and Black medical communities. Like the other philanthropists and foundation managers who supported the construction efforts at Vanderbilt and Meharry, GEB officials understood the schools to be fulfilling distinct objectives in the reform of American medical education, a reality reflected and promoted by the buildings themselves. Of course, intention and outcome are not always the same. On the one hand, Vanderbilt did produce far more research than Meharry. Robert Collins has identified five significant discoveries in the first ten years after Vanderbilt reorganized and opened its 1925 facility.[182] On the other hand, Flexner and his colleagues at the Carnegie Corporation, Rockefeller Foundation, and Julius Rosenwald Fund wanted southern graduates of Howard, Meharry, and the white southern medical colleges to remain in the South and care for the rural and poor communities of the region, but in practice they had no way to ensure this outcome. Even Meharry, the medical college with the greatest number of Black southerners, saw most students settle in cities, and many moved north.[183] In choosing to practice in the nation's wealthier areas, Black physicians acted no differently than their white counterparts.[184] It is also hard to quantify what the dissimilar training environments at Meharry and Vanderbilt meant for students' long-term careers. We do know, however, that African American medical leaders recognized that the standards of the Black medical schools impacted the "quality and reputation" of Black physicians.[185]

Despite immense challenges, the two Black medical colleges provided opportunities for African American men and women largely unavailable elsewhere. The funds Meharry and Howard received from the General Education Board and other donors did not allow them to construct buildings on par with those at the elite medical colleges with predominantly or entirely white student bodies, and the absence of significant investigative programs became a growing handicap for both schools in the increasingly research-focused environment of the 1920s and 1930s. Nevertheless, even as they emphasized public health outreach, Howard and Meharry educated their students in the full complement of medical practice, and they broadened the demographics of physicians in the United States by training African American men and a smaller number of African American women—groups with very limited options for studying at other institutions. Moreover, Howard and Meharry offered Black physicians faculty positions, which were all but impossible to obtain elsewhere.[186] In time African American medical educators held leadership roles as well. Howard University's medical school welcomed its first Black dean in 1929, and Meharry inaugurated its first Black president in 1952. As historian Darlene Clark Hine explains, both schools enabled African Americans to join the professional class.[187] Howard and Meharry also produced distinguished medical graduates such as W. Montague Cobb (Howard, class of 1929) and Dorothy Lavinia Brown (Meharry, class of 1948).

Architects and the Prominence of Shepley, Rutan, and Coolidge

Although Charles S. Minot, the Harvard Medical School faculty member who conceived and promoted the unit system, believed that an architect's interest lay primarily in the structure's exterior, the architect's function actually went much further.[188] As we know, donors shaped the general forms of the buildings they helped to fund through the terms and size of their gifts and their oversight. They were not, however, typically engaged in the details of the design process, which required close and extended collaboration between medical educators and architects.

At established schools relocating to new facilities, department representatives and building committees ensured that the faculty remained involved in the design. For example, the faculty at Woman's Medical College of Pennsylvania participated in all phases of the development of the 1930 medical school–hospital in Philadelphia. Beyond generating the program for the building, they prepared preliminary plans for laboratories.[189] As the project moved forward, department chairs met frequently with the architects regarding the arrangement of rooms and equipment, and when the structure neared completion, one member of each department remained in the city over the summer to make last-minute decisions.[190] To the college's building committee fell seemingly endless questions, such as choosing "the tiles for the bathrooms and the tints which will be used on the walls of the private rooms and wards in the hospital."[191] In this case, the architects, Ritter and Shay, and the faculty reflected positively on each other's work.[192]

Of course, the relationship between faculty and architects was not always smooth, and building committees could prove inefficient and even inconclusive at times. Architects Shepley, Rutan, and Coolidge expected Harvard Medical School's 1906 quadrangle to include inscriptions of famous scientists on the exterior of the four laboratory buildings, but lack of consensus among faculty representatives with regard to appropriate honorees resulted in permanently blank panels. Architect Charles Coolidge expressed disappointment that the rather austere exterior did not receive the planned embellishments.[193] Discord undoubtedly developed between faculty and architects on more substantive issues as well.[194]

When the planning of the facility preceded the inauguration of the college, the dean played a particularly prominent role in designing and equipping the structure. In 1927, Wilburt C. Davison left Johns Hopkins Medical School for Duke University, where he assumed the deanship of the medical school that would open three years later. When Davison arrived at Duke, the initial plans for the medical school–hospital had already been completed by the firm of architect Horace Trumbauer, which included pioneering African American architect Julian Abele and which was also responsible for the expansion of Trinity College into Duke University. With the medical facility's Gothic style and multicolor stone already determined, focus turned to the organization of the interior. Davison and Winford H. Smith, director of Johns Hopkins Hospital and a popular hospital consultant, decided to follow the plans of Vanderbilt, Rochester, and others in this latest medical school–hospital and to correlate physically the departments related by medical practice.[195]

Many modifications remained to be made, however. Duke University's president convinced the trustees of the Duke Endowment to add an additional floor to the hospital in order to augment the space for private patients and enlarge the hospital's income. Davison, as the medical school's dean, proposed the unusual bend in the medical school–hospital

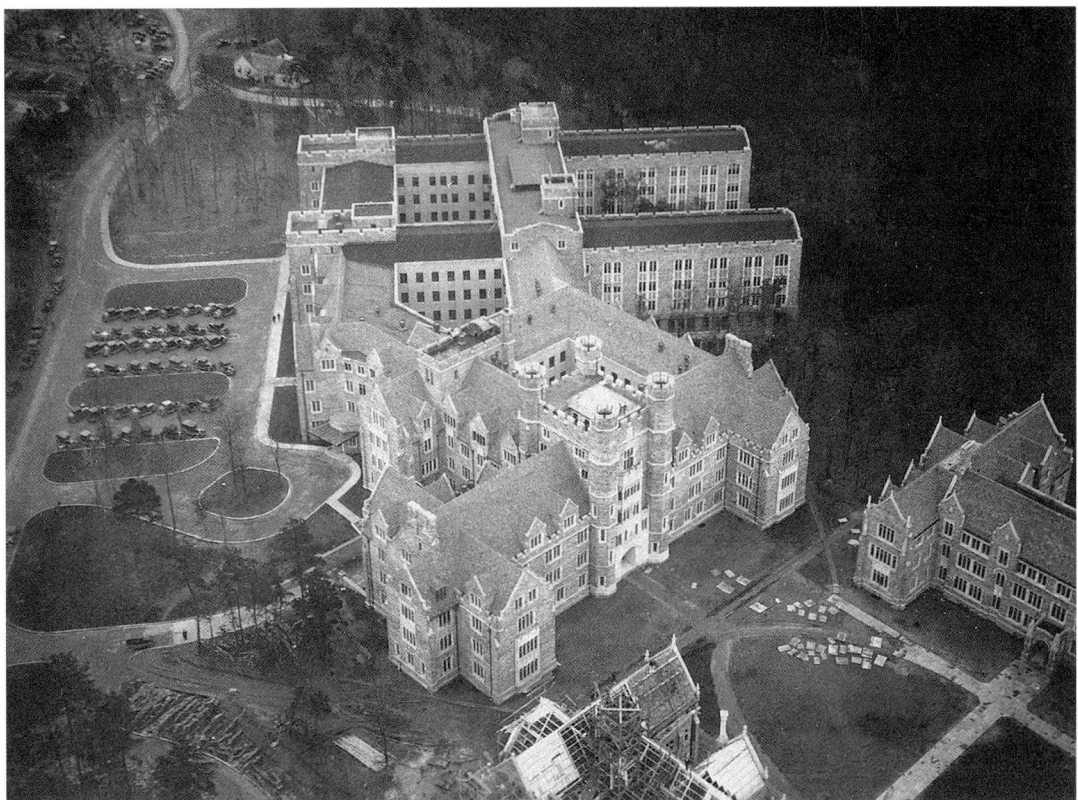

3.17.   Duke University School of Medicine and Hospital, 1930, Horace Trumbauer, architect.

to increase light and utilize a variation in grade to expand a section of
the hospital to seven stories (fig. 3.17). In August 1929, just a few months
before Davison began recruiting the first faculty, he took to climbing
the scaffolding of the unfinished building with the university's chief
engineer in a late effort to incorporate ideas obtained from administrators
at other hospitals. Before long, Davison was devoting his attention to
equipment. He derived his equipment lists from the inventories provided by the faculties at the Hopkins, Vanderbilt, and Rochester medical
schools, and he consulted with his department heads as rooms were
assigned, final alterations made to the building, and equipment chosen.
Davison continued to review each detail and spent an agonizing week
checking the 1,447 doors in the medical school and hospital for size and
opening direction, determined that no three-foot, six-inch bed would
be faced with a doorway three feet wide, a situation that had sometimes
occurred at Johns Hopkins's Harriet Lane Home, a medical facility for
children. Davison, along with the medical librarian and her mother,
applied the same meticulousness to collecting books for the library.[196]

The intensive involvement of faculty and deans in planning medical school buildings did not diminish the role of architects, particularly those who specialized in medical facilities. The publications of Edward F. Stevens, Henry R. Shepley, and Maurice B. Biscoe reveal that architects were well versed in the modern educational programs incorporated into and advanced by their designs.[197] When architects described a close relationship between pedagogy and design, they joined with medical educators in asserting that medical school buildings would participate actively in training physicians according to the principles of reformed medical education. A 1933 article in *Architectural Forum* underscored the depth of knowledge related to facilities for medical training provided by at least some architects. By this time, Vanderbilt University's medical school dean, G. Canby Robinson, had relocated to New York City, where he reunited with the architects of Coolidge, Shepley, Bulfinch, and Abbott, the firm responsible for Vanderbilt's 1925 medical school–hospital, in the creation of New York Hospital–Cornell Medical College. The writer of the *Architectural Forum* article explained, "As a matter of fact, the space requirements and details of the different departments of a teaching hospital were so well known both to the architects and to Dr. Robinson that they could be assumed."[198]

Although architects worked closely with medical educators, in a 1926 article Shepley distinguished the function of the architect from that of the educator when he examined design challenges not typically discussed by physicians. Shepley concluded his article by investigating "problems architects meet," and he emphasized the medical school–hospital's varied mechanical and physical requirements. Although specialists in engineering might be brought in for the school's mechanical components, as occurred with Shepley, Rutan, and Coolidge's Harvard Medical School and Coolidge, Shepley, Bulfinch, and Abbott's New York Hospital–Cornell Medical College, Shepley still had general advice for architects on this topic. He encouraged architects to group departments and individual rooms based on their need for "expensive and bulky services," including the ventilation of chemicals, plumbing for waste and corrosive chemicals, refrigeration of both food and cadavers, and pressure steam for cooking and sterilization. When Shepley turned his attention to the physical demands of a medical school–hospital, he highlighted the diverse room types—from private hospital rooms to laboratories—that created spaces of many sizes. He cautioned his fellow architects, "If departments whose units are incapable of conformity are superimposed, the result will be a chaotic building both in appearance and construction," and he advised early consideration of this problem.[199]

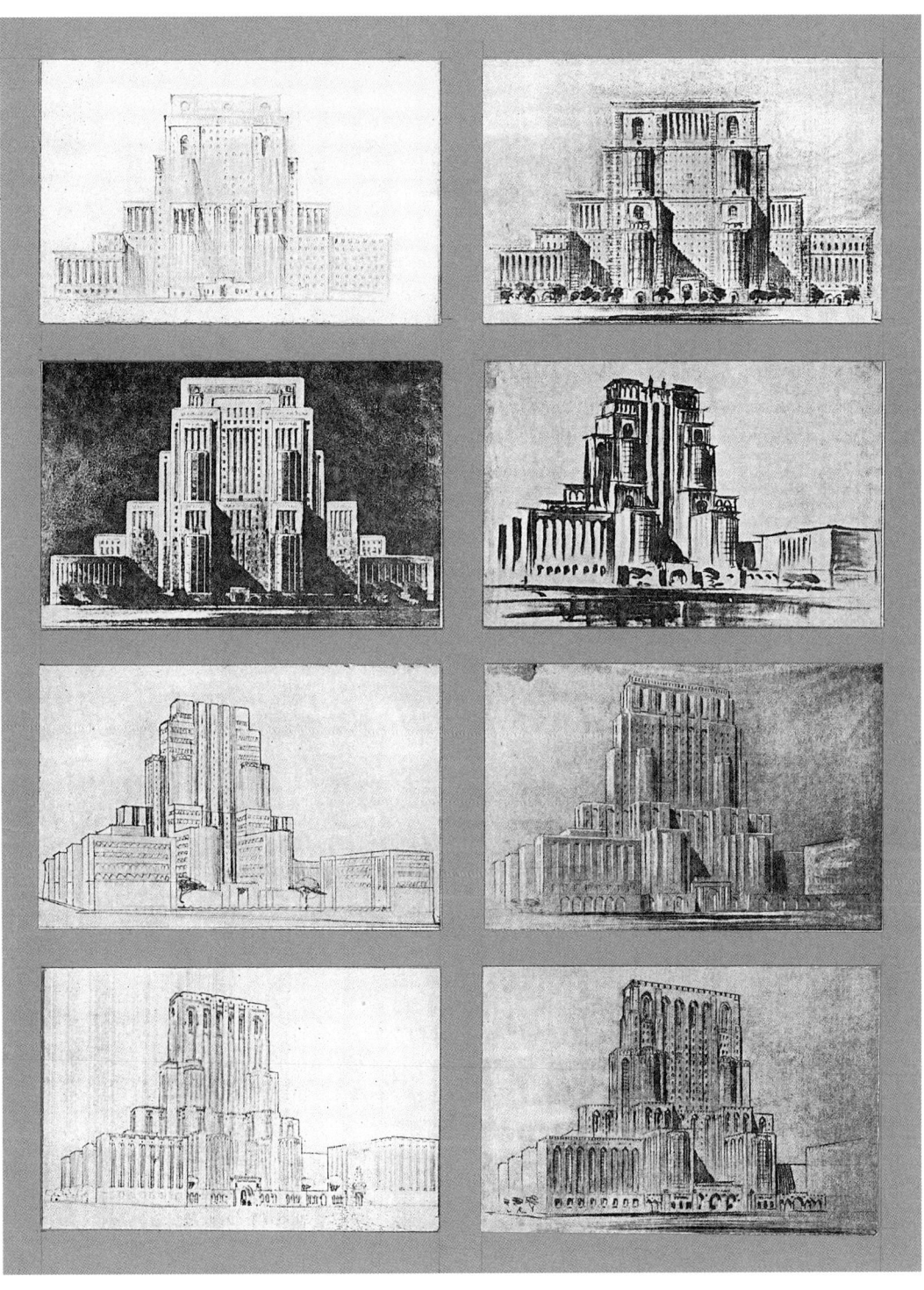

3.18.　New York Hospital–Cornell Medical College, 1932, Coolidge, Shepley, Bulfinch, and Abbott, architects. Study sketches by Harry Wijk and Herman Voss for Henry Shepley.

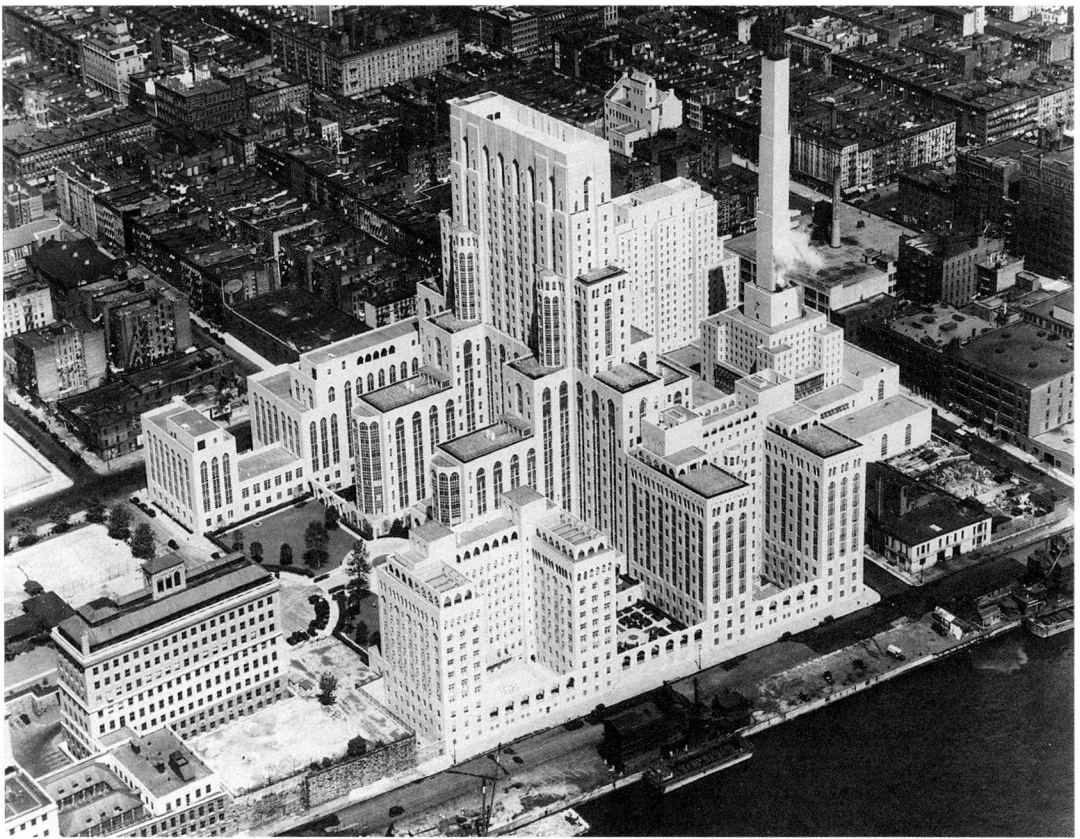

3.19.   New York Hospital–Cornell Medical College, 1932, Coolidge, Shepley, Bulfinch, and Abbott, architects.

Of course, as Shepley hints, a medical school's exterior mattered, too. Although the design process focused first on the building's "rightness of plan, orientation of parts and masses," the exterior still received careful consideration. Coolidge, Shepley, Bulfinch, and Abbott completed many studies before choosing an exterior for New York Hospital–Cornell Medical College (figs. 3.18 and 3.19).[200] The effort paid off. In 1933, the Architectural League of New York gave Shepley a Gold Medal for "the orderly arrangement of the many and varied parts of an unusually complex problem, and the excellence of the plan and originality of the design." Lewis Mumford called it "the last smile of skyscraper romanticism."[201] In the architect's hands, pedagogical, mechanical, structural, and aesthetic considerations had to coalesce, all, with any luck, within the given budget. Determining the architect, therefore, represented a major step in the building process.

Institutional connections frequently affected the selection of architect. Medical school leaders often hired architects with whom their university had an established relationship. For example, Albert Cassell had designed a number of buildings on Howard University's campus and was employed as both the head of the architecture department and the university architect when he received the medical school project.[202] Similarly, Dwight James Baum and John Russell Pope had ties to Syracuse University and a local hospital before they got the commission for the 1937 medical college there. Baum had completed his architecture training at Syracuse University in 1909, and in the late 1920s Baum and Pope designed a campus plan for the university, the university's Hendricks Chapel, and Syracuse Memorial Hospital, the last located next to the proposed site for the medical school. When the medical college opened, Baum and Pope organized the floor heights and hallways in such a way that the school could attach directly to an expanded Syracuse Memorial Hospital in the future, an extension that never came to pass.[203] At Johns Hopkins, George Archer had worked on the hospital design before the university called on him for the early medical school buildings.[204]

Personal affiliations could also determine which architect obtained the job. In the case of Columbia-Presbyterian Medical Center, Edward Harkness played a critical part in the organizational and physical alignment of Presbyterian Hospital with Columbia University's College of Physicians and Surgeons, and Harkness and his mother gave substantial sums for the Columbia-Presbyterian project.[205] Harkness's personal architect, friend, and fellow Yale graduate James Gamble Rogers secured the commission for Presbyterian Hospital and then for the medical school.[206] Rogers went on to create additional buildings at the medical center. Similarly, the firm of Horace Trumbauer had already designed a residence for James B. Duke in New York City, an addition for his Newport summer home, and an unrealized house for his New Jersey estate when the firm earned the commission at Duke University, including the medical school–hospital there.

The choice of architect at some schools, such as Columbia University, appears to have generated little discussion, but at other schools the decision became protracted. At the end of the nineteenth century, as a result of the influence of the École des Beaux-Arts, American universities frequently hosted competitions for master plans.[207] In 1909, the University of Nebraska decided to hold a competition for the master plan of its medical campus in Omaha. The committee in charge of the design for the campus generated a specific set of guidelines for entrants in the competition to follow. In addition to stipulating the size and placement of the buildings and the preferred architectural style and material, the committee provided a sketch of a plot plan for competing architects (fig. 3.20).[208] The competition, however, did not go smoothly.

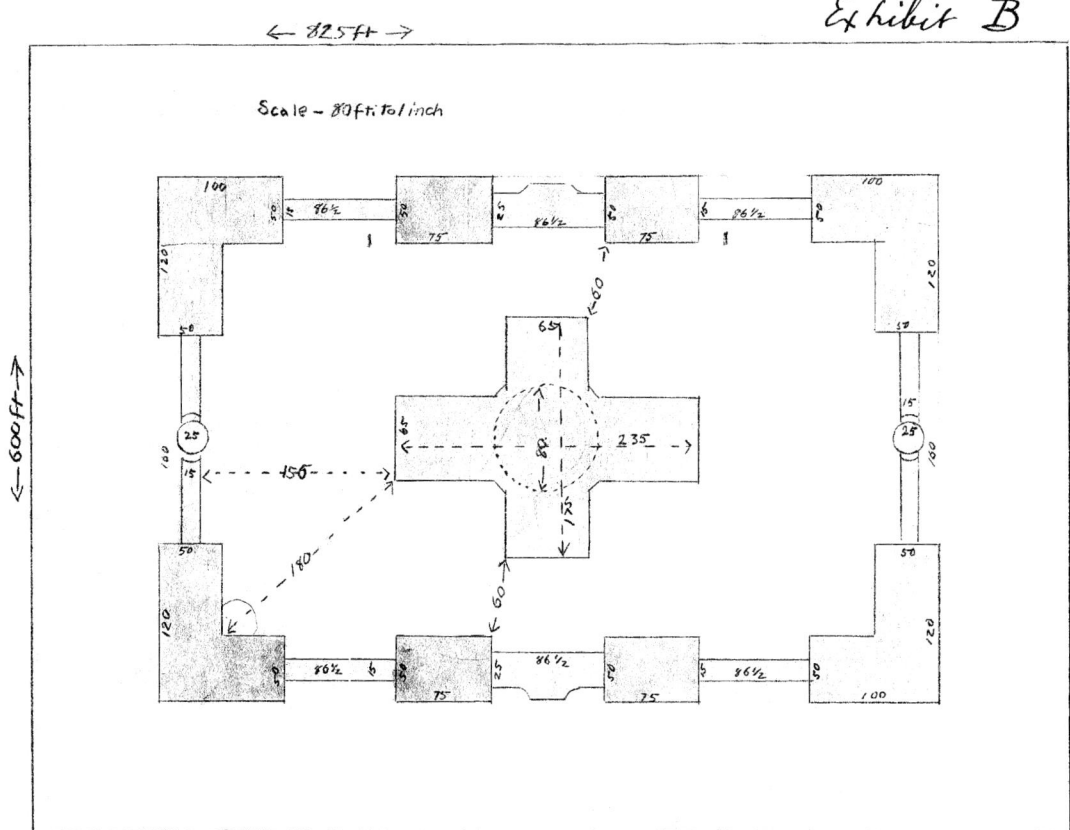

3.20. University of Nebraska College of Medicine sketch for architects in competition to design master plan of new campus, 1909.

As the university's chancellor recounted, "The committee on awards . . . first decided to reject all of the plans submitted. It was found that the plan of Shepley, Rutan and Coolidge was far superior to any of the others, but that it did not fit the ground. This, however, seemed to be the fault of the Omaha committee in preparing a description of the plot." The committee members considered a second competition, but constraints of time compelled them to "withdraw their first report and award the prize to Shepley, Rutan and Coolidge, asking them, in consideration of the award, to do some extra work and make the plan coincide with the plot of ground."[209] As so often happens, the university only followed the master plan in part, but it did choose Shepley, Rutan, and Coolidge to design one building, the first, on the new campus.

The committee's conclusion that Shepley, Rutan, and Coolidge had created the best plan comes as no surprise. The firm's 1906 Harvard

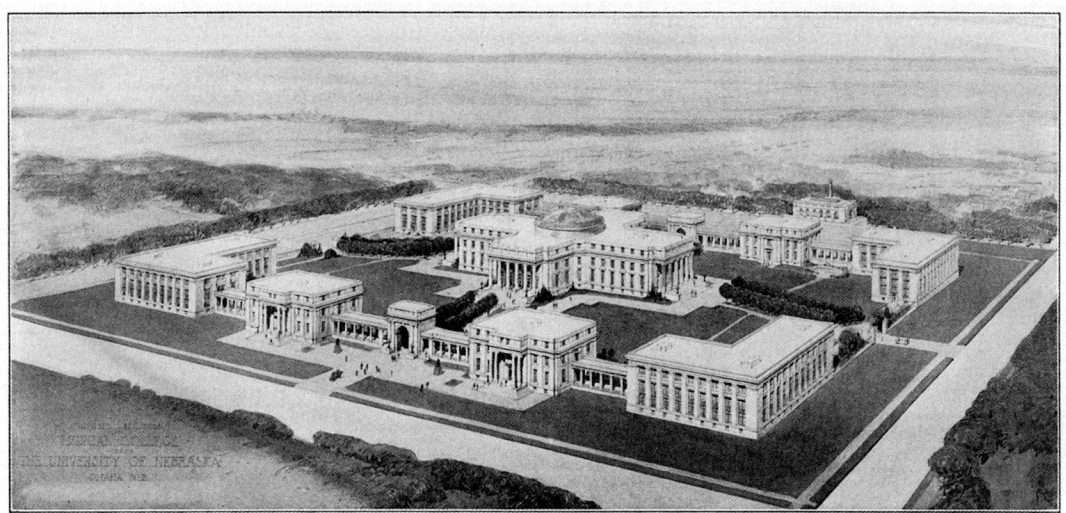

3.21.   Master plan for University of Nebraska College of Medicine in Omaha, 1909, Shepley, Rutan, and
Coolidge, architects.

Medical School quadrangle had recently been lauded in a publication of
the Nebraska medical school and in a lecture given by Harvard Medical School faculty member Charles S. Minot at the Nebraska medical
college.[210] Shortly after the competition, Shepley, Rutan, and Coolidge's
master plan was published with a description that enthusiastically—and
overly optimistically—compared the Nebraska project to the prestigious
Massachusetts school: "the proposed group . . . will give Omaha one
of the finest institutions of its kind in the country, even a more artistic
and beautiful group than that of Harvard" (fig. 3.21).[211] Not long after
the first building opened, a reviewer tempered expectations: "in time an
attractive campus planned somewhat after that of the Harvard medical
school will be built."[212]

Earlier in the first decade of the twentieth century, Harvard University leaders had contemplated holding a competition for their 1906
medical campus.[213] No competition appears to have occurred, but university officials explored at least three options for architect, all from Boston:
Shaw and Hunnewell, Edmund M. Wheelwright, and Shepley, Rutan,
and Coolidge. The decision centered on the firm's size, organization,
and ability to manage a considerable assignment, the firm's experience in
hospital design, and its familiarity with educational and medical buildings.[214] Shepley, Rutan, and Coolidge received the job.

Shepley, Rutan, and Coolidge could offer Harvard Medical School
expertise in both hospital and school facilities, and the firm had the

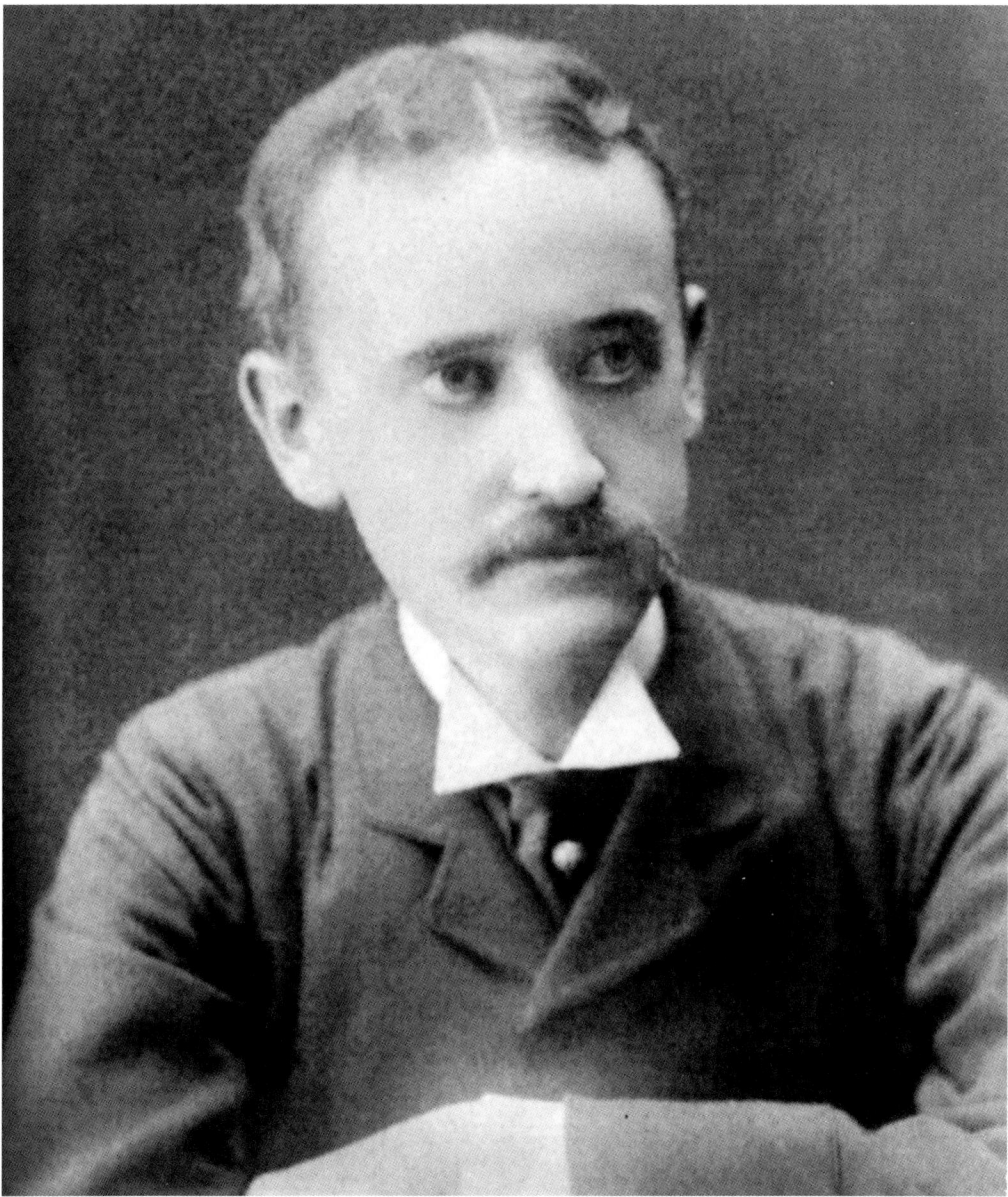

3.22.   George F. Shepley.

staff and organizational capacity to complete big projects. When Henry Hobson Richardson died in 1886 at the age of forty-seven, three of Richardson's assistants, George F. Shepley, Charles H. Rutan, and Charles A. Coolidge, formed the firm that continues today, although with a number of name changes (figs. 3.22, 3.23, and 3.24).[215] Even before Richardson's death, the environment in the studio he attached to his

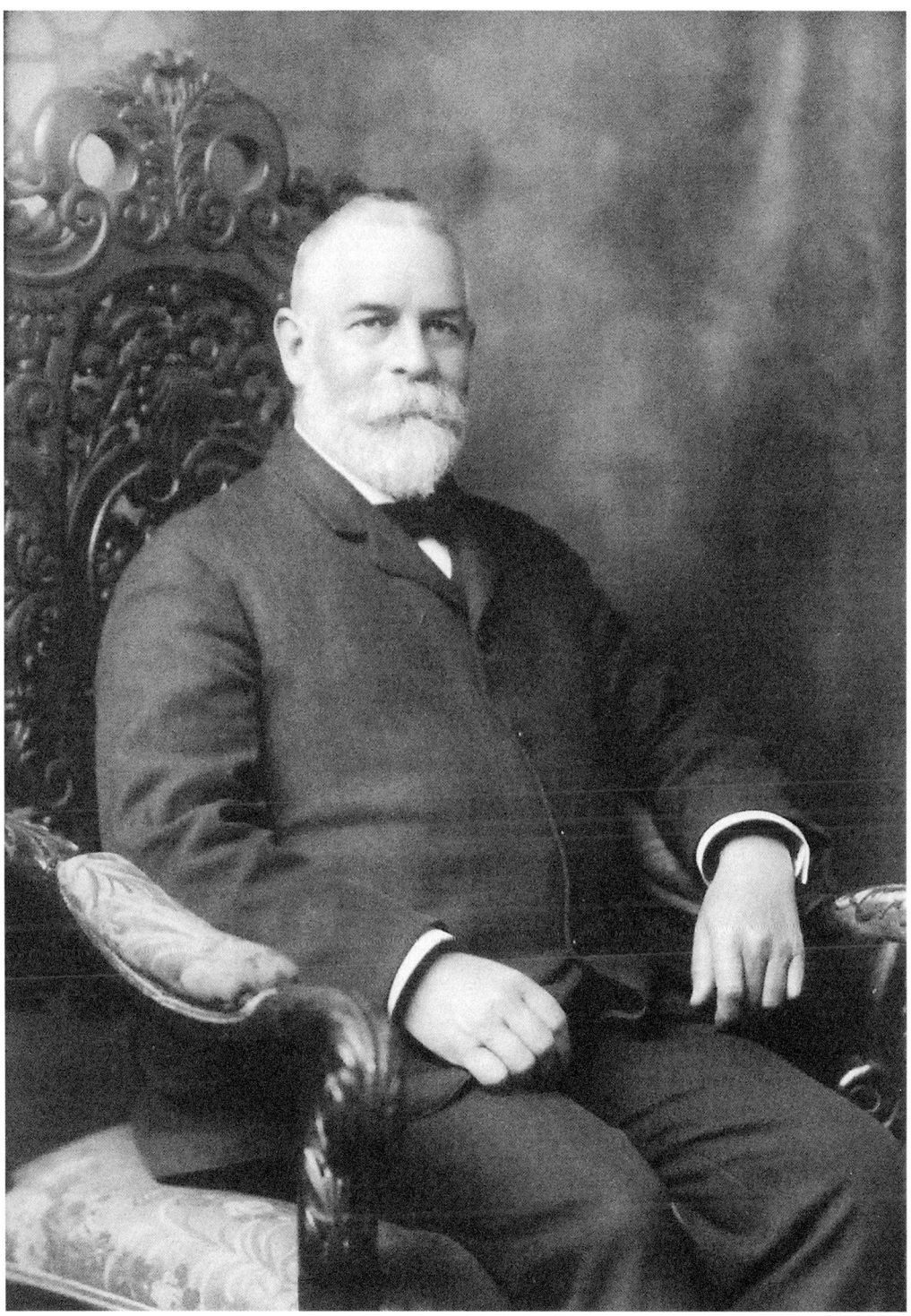

3.23.   Charles H. Rutan.

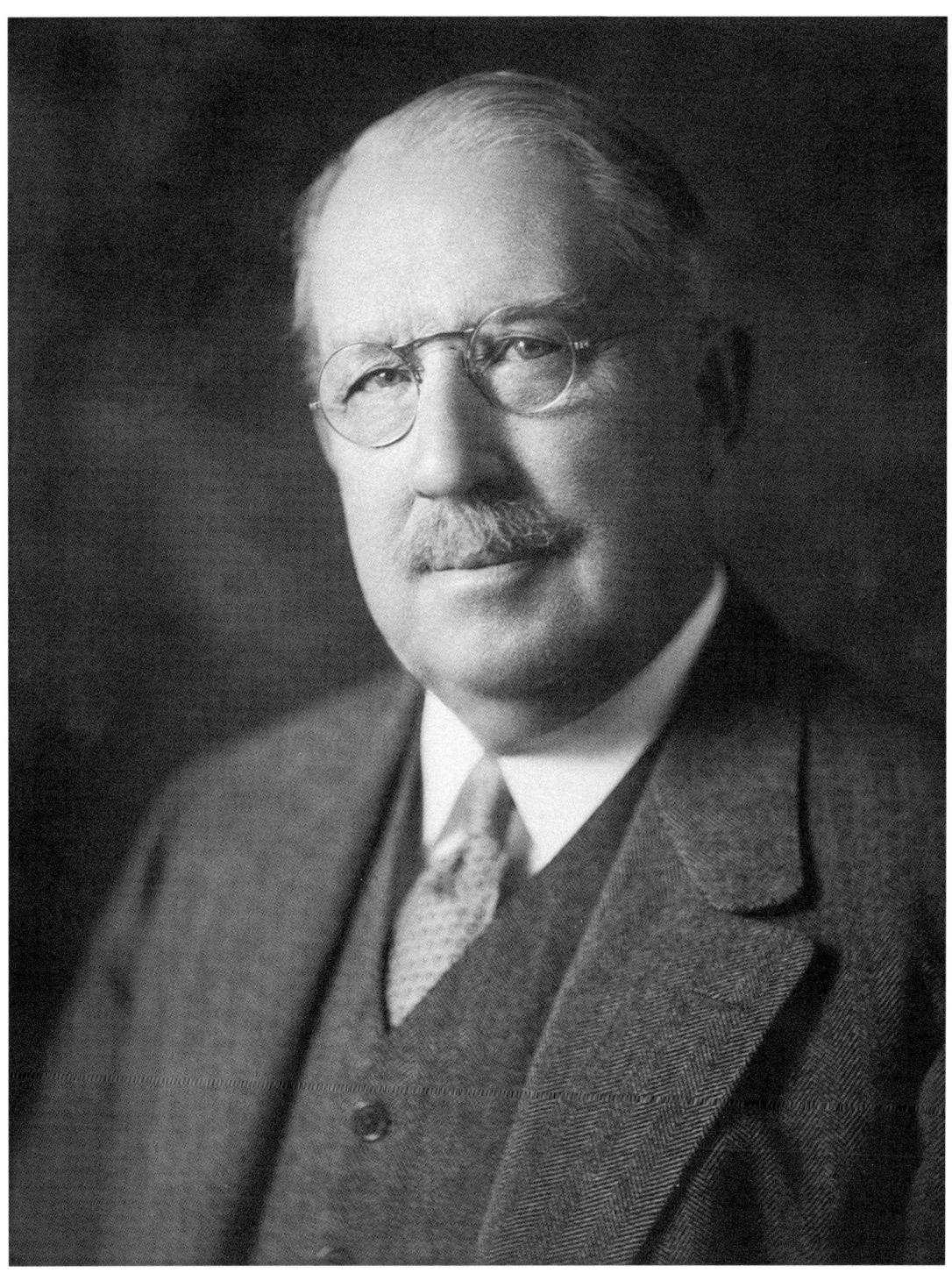

3.24.   Charles A. Coolidge.

home in Brookline, a suburb of Boston, had become less casual and more businesslike. Shaped by his training at the École des Beaux-Arts in Paris, Richardson had initially modeled his firm's work environment on the atelier he had experienced in France. In a congenial, fraternal atmosphere, young architects, many trained at MIT, learned from Richardson and honed their practice while they served as his draftsmen. As Richardson's commissions grew in number and size, however, the environment quickly shifted. Deadlines became tighter and the pressure more intense. Draftsmen could no longer comb Richardson's study with its books and artifacts, nor could Richardson afford to spend part of the day mentoring a young draftsman on a single design element. Instead, Richardson worked directly with his head draftsman to develop his concepts and sketches while a team of younger draftsmen generated working drawings and copies.[216]

After Richardson's death, the firm continued the trend toward more of a business structure. Shepley, Rutan, and Coolidge moved out of Richardson's home and into the Ames Building, designed by the firm, in downtown Boston. The prominent commercial building was the tallest in Boston at the time of its construction in 1889 and remained the firm's home for almost one hundred years. Unlike under Richardson, no individual in the firm dominated; the designers behind specific projects remained anonymous, with credit given only to the firm.[217] Shepley, Rutan, and Coolidge also expanded, opening branches in Chicago and St. Louis in the early 1890s.

During the last decades of the nineteenth century, the practice of architecture shifted with the establishment of university training, licensing laws, certification of architects, and professional societies. In the country's major cities, large architectural firms opened with systematically organized staff and offices, which were frequently located in commercial buildings designed by the firms. Capable of carrying out expensive and sizable projects, these firms specialized in major commercial and institutional commissions.[218] In the early twentieth century, the growing complexity of hospital design resulted in an increase in the number of architectural firms that specialized in hospitals, including Stevens and Lee, York and Sawyer, and James Gamble Rogers.[219]

Shepley, Rutan, and Coolidge had a reputation for academic, civic, and medical facilities. By 1900, the firm had created a campus plan for Stanford University and the university's Inner Quadrangle had been built. Shepley, Rutan, and Coolidge had also designed Harvard University's Conant Hall and Perkins Hall (1893), continuing a relationship with Harvard that was begun by Richardson and would extend well into the next century. The firm's early civic commissions included Boston's Chamber of Commerce Building (1892) and the Chicago Public Library (1897), while its preeminence in medical design grew out of its work on hospitals, research facilities, and medical schools.[220]

Around the turn of the twentieth century, architectural firms, medical schools, and philanthropies became big businesses. They expanded in scale and complexity at the same time that they celebrated the rising professionals—architects, physicians, and foundation officers—who ran their organizations. Warmly received by medical school leaders and officials within the Rockefeller philanthropies, iterations of Shepley, Rutan, and Coolidge designed a record eight medical schools between 1906 and 1932. With seven of these schools in the United States, the firm could claim responsibility for approximately 10 percent of the country's seventy-seven schools that offered the MD degree in 1933. Shepley, Rutan, and Coolidge and its successors were the leading architectural firm for medical schools in this period.

In 1906, having met Harvard University's criteria of size, management, and expertise, Shepley, Rutan, and Coolidge designed for the esteemed Ivy League institution the firm's first medical school. In quick succession, several organizations granted the firm commissions for structures located in the neighborhood around Harvard Medical School: the Carnegie Nutrition Laboratory (1908), Harvard Dental School (1909), Children's Hospital (1914), Boston Lying-In Hospital (1922), and Harvard Medical School's Vanderbilt Hall (1927). All fueled Shepley, Rutan, and Coolidge's growing reputation for medical and educational buildings, a reputation that also benefited from the firm's long-standing relationship with the Rockefeller Institute for Medical Research.

At the same time that John D. Rockefeller Sr. was donating personally to Harvard Medical School for its 1906 facility, he was also funding—and building with Shepley, Rutan, and Coolidge—his own organization for medical advancement: the Rockefeller Institute for Medical Research, in New York City. Incorporated in 1901, the institute by February 1903 had need of an architect for a master plan and its first building. As John D. Rockefeller Jr. explained, a committee at the Institute "naturally thought of Messrs. Shepley, Rutan and Coolidge, who planned the Harvard Medical Buildings," and it contacted him for advice (presumably due to his family's involvement with the Harvard Medical School project that would break ground that summer). Rockefeller Jr. in turn wrote to Harvard University president Charles W. Eliot for his opinion of Shepley, Rutan, and Coolidge.[221] Apparently Eliot encouraged retaining the firm, and a relationship began between Shepley, Rutan, and

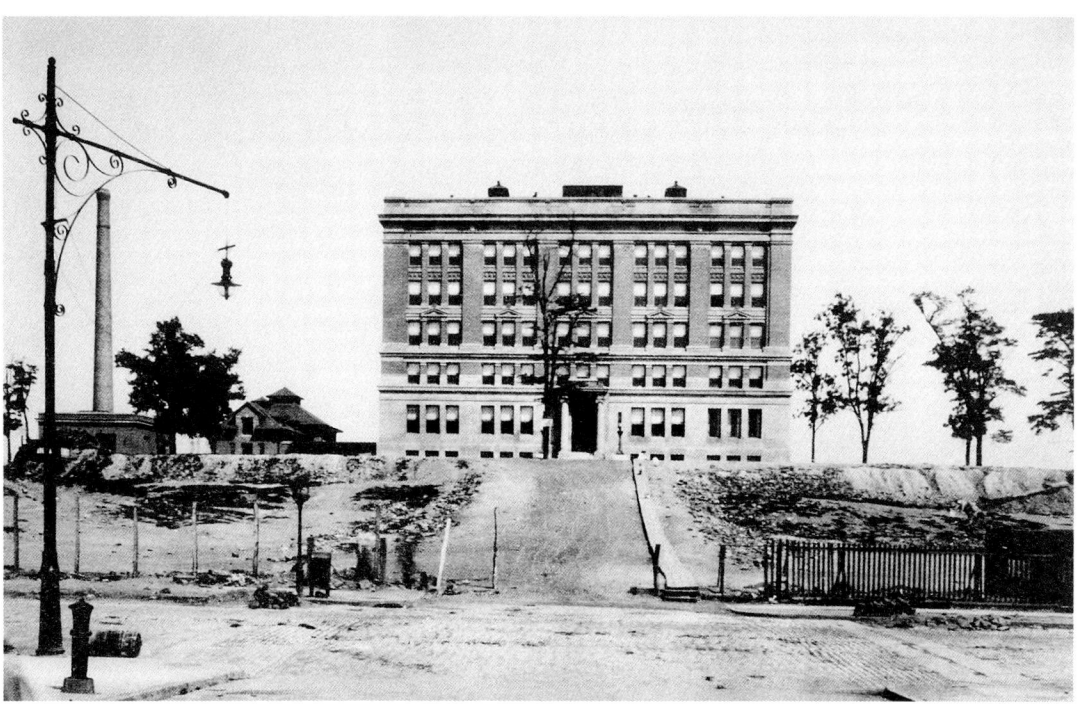

3.25.   Founder's Hall, Rockefeller Institute for Medical Research, 1906, Shepley, Rutan, and Coolidge, architects, nearing completion. Photograph 1905.

Coolidge and the Rockefeller Institute that lasted half a century. After it finished Founder's Hall at the Rockefeller Institute in 1906 (fig. 3.25), Shepley, Rutan, and Coolidge undertook more than two dozen projects of all sizes for the institute's New York City campus, in addition to more than twenty-five projects of varying scale for the organization's Princeton, New Jersey, site. This ongoing association ensured that Shepley, Rutan, and Coolidge and later iterations of the firm remained highly visible within the Rockefeller network, a position augmented by the more than one dozen commissions undertaken by the firm at the University of Chicago, which John D. Rockefeller Sr. helped to found and which he heavily supported. These works included the William Rainey Harper Memorial Library (1912) and the medical campus constructed in the mid-1920s.[222]

Shepley, Rutan, and Coolidge and its successors, Coolidge and Shattuck (1915–1924) and Coolidge, Shepley, Bulfinch, and Abbott (1924–1952), designed eight medical schools between 1906 and 1932: for Harvard University (1906), University of Nebraska (1913), Peking Union Medical College (consulting architects, 1921), Western Reserve University (1924), Vanderbilt University (1925), University of Chicago (1927),

University of Virginia (1929), and Cornell University (1932). All but the University of Nebraska and Western Reserve University received funding at the time of construction from at least one of four Rockefeller sources: John D. Rockefeller Sr., the General Education Board, the Rockefeller Foundation, and the Rockefeller Foundation's China Medical Board. The medical schools furthered the association between the firm and the extended Rockefeller circle.

Not all medical schools that received funds from the General Education Board at the time that they built new facilities retained Shepley, Rutan, and Coolidge and its subsequent iterations as architects (see table 3.2), but key figures within the Rockefeller organizations did endorse the firm. In 1916, Simon Flexner, brother of Abraham Flexner and the first director of the Rockefeller Institute for Medical Research, suggested hiring Charles A. Coolidge for the Peking Union Medical College project and personally recruited him due to the positive experience of working with Coolidge on the Rockefeller Institute.[223] In 1919, Abraham Flexner and General Education Board president Wallace Buttrick affirmed to Vanderbilt University's chancellor that "Mr. Coolidge is, we think, probably the best person in the country" to design that school's medical facility.[224]

Flexner particularly appreciated architects who could create economical structures, as he revealed when he explained to George Eastman his reasons for recruiting Gordon and Kaelber for Meharry Medical College: "I . . . brought into the conference on plans the architects who did the Rochester job, for I felt that their experience would be most valuable in avoiding useless expenditures."[225] Economical buildings mattered to Flexner because he wanted to stretch the GEB's investments as far as possible. For this reason, only a few months after praising Coolidge to Vanderbilt University's chancellor, Flexner began to criticize repeatedly the work of Coolidge and hospital consultant Winford Smith on the grounds that "both men may plan details on a more elaborate and expensive basis than is really essential," particularly for Nashville, where standards differed greatly, at least according to Flexner, from those of New York City. In the end, he suggested that the chancellor consider dropping Coolidge and Smith.[226] The chancellor did not change architects, but losing Flexner's favor may have reduced the firm's future commissions in medical education.

Fortunately for Shepley, Rutan, and Coolidge, the firm also enjoyed the support of respected medical leaders. Winford Smith, director of the Johns Hopkins Hospital from 1911 to 1946, was a prominent consultant on academic hospital design, and his projects included hospitals for Vanderbilt University, Duke University, Cornell University, Yale University, University of Chicago, University of California, and Peking Union Medical College. Smith first proposed to Vanderbilt's chancellor that the university retain Coolidge and Shattuck for its medical facility and reportedly asserted that the firm "had more experience in designing modern teaching hospitals than any firm he knows of."[227] In addition, G. Canby Robinson, the medical school dean during the construction of Vanderbilt's and Cornell's medical school–hospitals, praised his experience with the firm and particularly Henry R. Shepley, son of the firm's founder, George Shepley, and the architect primarily responsible for designing both buildings. Robinson later recalled that when he and Shepley started working together on the Vanderbilt project, "we began a period of happy association that was to last a number of years. I endeavored to tell him what use each part of the plant was to have and the activities that would go on there; he showed great skill, ingenuity, and good taste in designing the suitable structures. He was the anatomist [the expert in form] and I the physiologist [the expert in function] . . . and we pooled our concepts and understanding in a very congenial way."[228]

Shepley, Rutan, and Coolidge and its later iterations profited from the approval of respected physicians, heads of top universities, and individuals within the Rockefeller community, but many factors fueled its dominance. On top of actively seeking commissions, as when it entered the University of Nebraska competition, the firm increased its visibility and authority through the publications its architects wrote on the design of medical colleges.[229] The firm's projects for elite medical schools, such as multiple structures at Harvard Medical School, further cemented its reputation. Additionally, the firm's popularity likely received a boost from its familiarity with the celebrated unit system developed by the Harvard Medical School faculty in conjunction with members of the firm. Even more, the experience of Shepley, Rutan, and Coolidge and its successors with all three major medical school types enabled it to offer its clients unparalleled depth of knowledge regarding medical college design.

———————————

Constructing progressive medical schools required the alignment of physicians, donors, and architects. The General Education Board's national program for medical education channeled substantial sums into medical schools, an agenda that accelerated the rate at which medical colleges reorganized and rebuilt both directly—by funding new buildings—and indirectly—through competition and emulation. The GEB's program, however, did more than enable medical colleges to modernize; it also shaped the development of American medical school design through the work of Abraham Flexner. Flexner encouraged the geographic co-ordination of medical schools and hospitals and promoted the unified medical school types, particularly the medical school–hospital. At the same time, he ensured that the coeducational Black medical colleges and the predominantly white school for women did not enjoy the same financial and physical resources as the schools predominantly or entirely for white men, one outcome of which was the privileging of white men within the medical profession, a topic to be addressed in chapter 5.

Among architectural firms, Shepley, Rutan, and Coolidge and its successors attained prominence in this period for their medical school projects. Responsible for an unparalleled eight medical schools, they had experience with all three medical school types. The firm's endorsements from members of the Rockefeller circle, prestigious physicians, and leaders of esteemed institutions, particularly Harvard University, helped to generate its unmatched reputation in medical education.

As doctors, foundation officers, and architects worked together to develop ever-bigger medical schools, they intertwined their rising professional reputations and the increasingly large organizations they ran. Medical colleges may have abandoned their for-profit, proprietary roots, but the business of medical education only grew. The dedication to experiential learning and original research made medical training incredibly expensive, and schools required constant fundraising and careful management to keep the doors open. Together physicians, donors, and architects in the early twentieth century created the nuclei of today's enormous medical centers.

4

SCHOOL BUILDINGS AND THE MARKETING OF MODERN MEDICAL EDUCATION

PHYSICIANS RECOGNIZED THAT REFORMED MEDICAL TRAINING needed public support to succeed. Medical schools relied heavily on their local and regional neighbors for patients and students and—to varying degrees—funding. Buildings became signposts in the city (medical schools were almost always in urban areas) that proclaimed the ambitions of progressive medical educators. In his study of research laboratories, Thomas R. Gieryn has argued that "through their very existence, outward appearances, and internal arrangements of space, research buildings give meanings to science, scientists, disciplines, and universities—for those who work inside and for those who just pass by."[1] Medical educators, donors, and architects in the early twentieth century would have agreed.

Although work as a physician had failed to guarantee wealth, status, or cultural authority for most of the nineteenth century, physicians ranked near or at the top of American professions in analyses of occupational prestige issued in 1925 and 1934.[2] This dramatic change grew out of many factors, but the schools constructed in the early twentieth century were a driving force. As educators, architects, and donors realized, the schools created a new image not only for medical education but also for the American physician.

Medical educators were not alone in their use of architecture as a tool to publicly reinvent an organization or profession. Architectural historian Paula Lupkin discusses the 1869 New York YMCA building, which she describes as "the first modern YMCA." Lupkin states that the organization's leadership believed that a physical structure would generate permanency for the association and improve its status in the eyes of its members, the press, and the general public.[3] Another scholar, Karen Kingsley, assigns a critical role to architecture in the reinvention of the field of nursing at the turn of the twentieth century. She affirms that nursing, like many other groups, relied on architecture to generate an image of itself both for its members and for society at large. As nursing evolved into a trained vocation, the construction of nurses' homes physically separate from the hospital just before and in the decades after 1900 helped redefine the identity of the nurse.[4]

Medical educators working to promote the profession and the latest training capitalized on the visibility of the medical school construction process and the final structures. They used the schools as an opportunity to court the public and to introduce laypeople to the remodeled curriculum and the scientific medicine it celebrated. At the same time, educators and architects designed the buildings to present medical education as established, as authoritative, and, particularly to those in the public concerned about animal experimentation and human dissection, as acceptable. This effort proved successful in a broad sense, but on a smaller scale the construction of a medical school could painfully disrupt the local community.

Medical Schools and the Decision to Relocate

The reformed medical school ideal demanded that medical colleges partner and physically coordinate with both hospitals and universities. Although nineteenth-century medical schools and hospitals sometimes clustered near one another in the city, proprietary schools generally had minimal, if any, administrative or direct physical relationship with hospitals and universities. The new emphasis on hospital and university affiliations urged medical schools contemplating modern structures to relocate rather than to renovate or rebuild on their current site.

As discussed in previous chapters, medical educators, architects, and donors saw many benefits of aligning preclinical and clinical training. The decision to place the medical school near the university drew on parallel themes. Just as the physical coordination of preclinical and clinical facilities on the same campus was believed to foster a cross-pollination of ideas, locating the medical college next to the university offered the opportunity for "a constant interchange of ideas" between the professional and undergraduate schools.[5] Architect Henry R. Shepley also argued that because "satisfactory clinical material will always present itself to a modern general hospital provided it is accessible by street car or motor bus lines . . . , no real obstacle [exists] to conducting medical education as an integral part of a general hospital on or adjoining a university campus."[6]

Shepley's words accurately described the situation at Duke University. During the 1927–1930 construction of the medical school–hospital contiguous with the university in Durham, North Carolina, many questioned whether a hospital in such a modest city would have enough patients. The concerns proved unfounded. Patients quickly filled the hospital's beds, and 75 percent of those seeking medical care traveled more than twenty miles to reach the facility.[7] Not every medical college could fully meet the geographical ideal of aligning with a hospital and university, but the desire to realize this goal at least partially pushed most medical schools to move. The need to relocate, along with the physical requirements for modern medical training and educators' belief in design as a pedagogical tool, encouraged the construction of purpose-built schools.

New buildings did more than satisfy the tenets of reformed medical education. For donors, they provided the opportunity to construct a monument to their largesse. For university and medical school administrators, a structure could help to recruit students and patients, stimulate financial pledges and media attention, and inspire public enthusiasm for modern training, scientific medicine, and progressive physicians. Medical educators, university officials, hospital administrators, and major donors often invested tremendous energy in choosing the site for the medical school and its affiliated hospital(s). Local conditions inevitably inflected the decisions, but certain factors remained consistent regardless of the city, medical college, university, or hospital.

In the mid-1910s, the leadership at Western Reserve University School of Medicine was looking to move the college. A faculty committee tasked with investigating potential locations affirmed that in an ideal scenario the school and hospitals would be sited on one expansive plot near the university.[8] Determining adequate size, however, was difficult, since they had to allow for future needs. After examining other schools, all of which had failed to reserve enough land for long-term development, a committee at Western Reserve recommended a "provision of 100% for growth," a seemingly generous margin, but one it described as "narrow rather than . . . wide."[9] Faculties recognized that medicine was evolving and expanding rapidly and, in the absence of precise data, more room was better.

Because the plots were intended to house hospitals in conjunction with medical schools, the conditions for the sites mirrored in many ways those of any hospital. Architectural historian Jeanne Kisacky has shown that, by the 1920s, hospitals planning new construction were considering the distribution of other hospitals, density of population, public transportation routes, and major roads in order to ensure patient supply.[10] Teaching hospitals differed from nonacademic hospitals, however, because the goal was not simply to fill the beds but to introduce medical students to a spectrum of cases. And in this effort, larger populations helped. Medical school administrators faced a difficult decision when their affiliated university resided in a small city or rural town.

American colleges have long romanticized the idea of rural education as a means of removing students from the supposed distractions and vices of the city and surrounding them with the presumed purity of the natural world.[11] But medical schools did not share this notion. For medical schools in need of rich clinical material, limited populations were a liability. As Isadore Rosenfield and Edgar C. Hayhow explained to readers of *Modern Hospital* in 1927, "A university or teaching hospital must be within reasonable distance of the university, but if the university is in a neighborhood that lacks sufficient clinical material, its hospital must sometimes be in an urban district."[12] In 1913 the University of Nebraska unified its medical program in Omaha, where its clinical training took place, rather than in Lincoln, home of the university and the preclinical departments. The greater Omaha area offered fully equipped hospitals, but even more critically it provided access to a far larger population than Lincoln.[13] Similarly, Cornell University is in rural Ithaca in upstate New York, but its medical school is downstate, in metropolitan New York City. The University of Michigan managed to keep its medical college in the very small city of Ann Arbor, home of the university, despite calls to relocate the medical college to more populous Detroit. This choice caused controversy, however, and deep anxiety for the medical school leadership through at least the 1910s.[14]

Even in a sizable city, aligning a medical school and hospital with a university was difficult. Lack of available land adjacent to the university, for example, could thwart schools' efforts. When Columbia University's College of Physicians and Surgeons prepared to move, it considered a one-block plot near the university in New York City's Morningside Heights, but the small site would have accommodated only the medical school and not a hospital.[15] The school ultimately decided to coordinate with the Presbyterian Hospital on a much larger site fifty blocks north of the university. When faced with a shortage of patients or land, medical schools chose physical proximity with the hospital rather than the university, and many did not build on the university campus. In a report for the American Medical Association undertaken in the late 1930s, Herman G. Weiskotten and his collaborators reported that just twenty-three of sixty-six four-year medical schools, or approximately 35 percent, resided on the university campus. However, they found that among the fifty-seven university-affiliated medical colleges 68 percent "were located so that

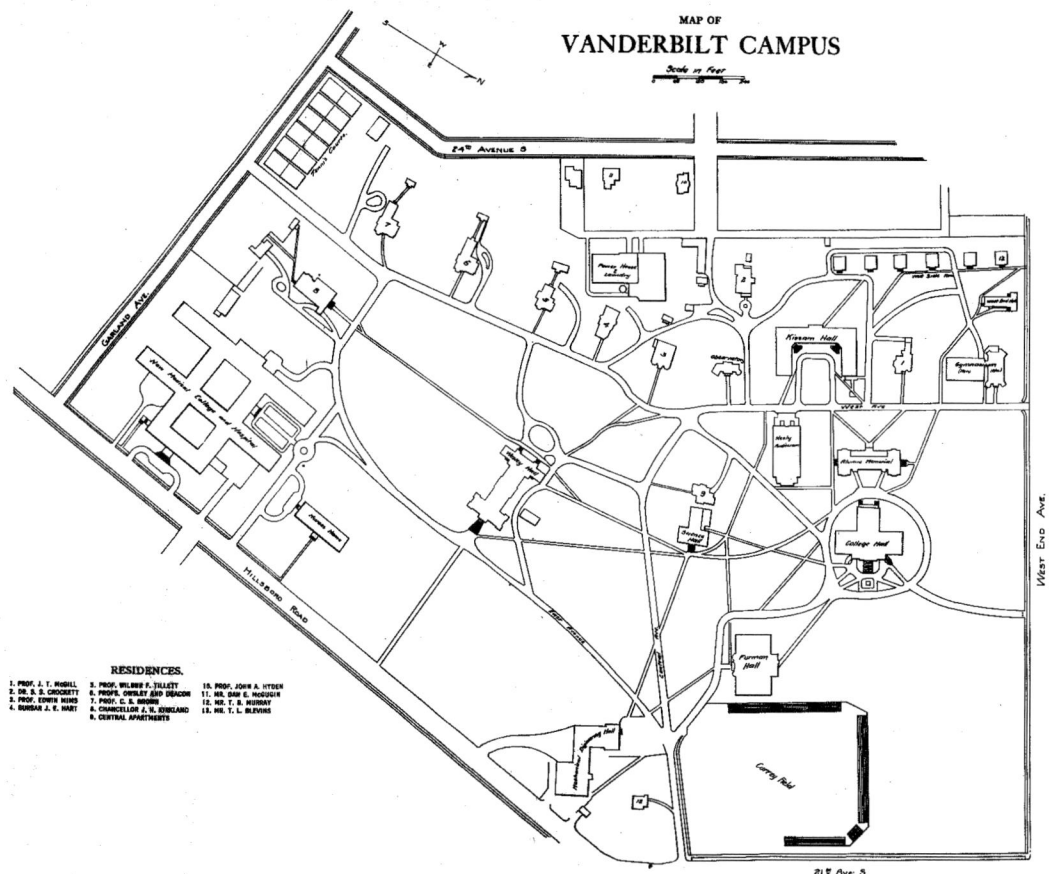

4.1.   Vanderbilt University campus map, ca. 1923, with projected medical school–hospital at far left.

the university and the medical school exercised an undoubted influence on each other," results they called "surprisingly satisfactory" considering the relatively recent coordination of medical schools with universities.[16]

Some universities, such as Vanderbilt, Syracuse, and Michigan, did manage to create an arrangement in keeping with the ideal: a medical school in physical contact with both the university and the hospital. In Vanderbilt's case, the perceived benefits of siting the medical school and the hospital together on the main Vanderbilt campus outweighed the cost savings of using the existing clinical facilities located two miles from the university, whose campus had no clinical facilities.[17] At the university campus, the leadership examined two potential sites for the medical complex. They ultimately chose a plot along Hillsboro Road on the campus's southeast corner for the medical school–hospital, which would significantly exceed in size all other university buildings (fig. 4.1). Although challenging for construction due to its slope, the location was preferred by administrators. It offered patients easy access to the Hillsboro Road streetcar line, whereas the proposed site on the west side of campus necessitated a quarter-mile walk to reach public transit.[18] More so than universities, hospitals needed to ensure that they sat on or as close as possible to transportation lines. Once the Vanderbilt medical facility was constructed, its design reinforced two distinct connections: the medical school with the university and the hospital with the community. Medical school dean G. Canby Robinson explained that "the laboratories and the general student activities are conducted in the northern portion of the building adjoining the other schools and buildings of the University, while the hospital wards extend toward the south, and are separated from the main activities of the university campus."[19] Highlighting this bifurcated orientation, the medical school entrance in the north court faced the university, and the patient and service entrances opened onto the more public Hillsboro Road, with its automobiles and streetcars.

When medical school leaders chose not to coordinate with the university, they carefully considered neighborhood characteristics when finding a new site. The same was true for schools that had no university parent, such as Meharry Medical College and Woman's Medical College of Pennsylvania. Shifting racial demographics played a part in the 1930 relocation of Woman's Medical College from North College Avenue and Twenty-First Street in downtown Philadelphia to East Falls, north of the central part of the city. The impetuses for the move are familiar: the college occupied an antiquated medical school for which adequate renovations were not feasible, and it had no room to expand.[20] In discussing the school's future site, officers of the college emphasized transportation access, distance to other hospitals, availability of potential patients, and space for growth (fig. 4.2).[21]

Woman's Medical College officials, however, also responded to the racial composition of its current and proposed neighborhoods. Like many other northern cities in the early twentieth century, Philadelphia experienced the arrival from the South of large numbers of African Americans seeking work.[22] In language that is difficult to read today, one description of the move explained that "the [downtown] neighborhood had become an almost impossible one for a Woman's College for during fifty years the population had changed from the sturdy well-to-do German to the lowest type of negroe [sic]."[23] Further underscoring the anxiety about the college's women, who were predominantly white, in a neighborhood with Black residents, another correspondent described the college's decision "to secure a campus . . . in an environment other than a negro neighborhood such as the one which now surrounds us on every side.

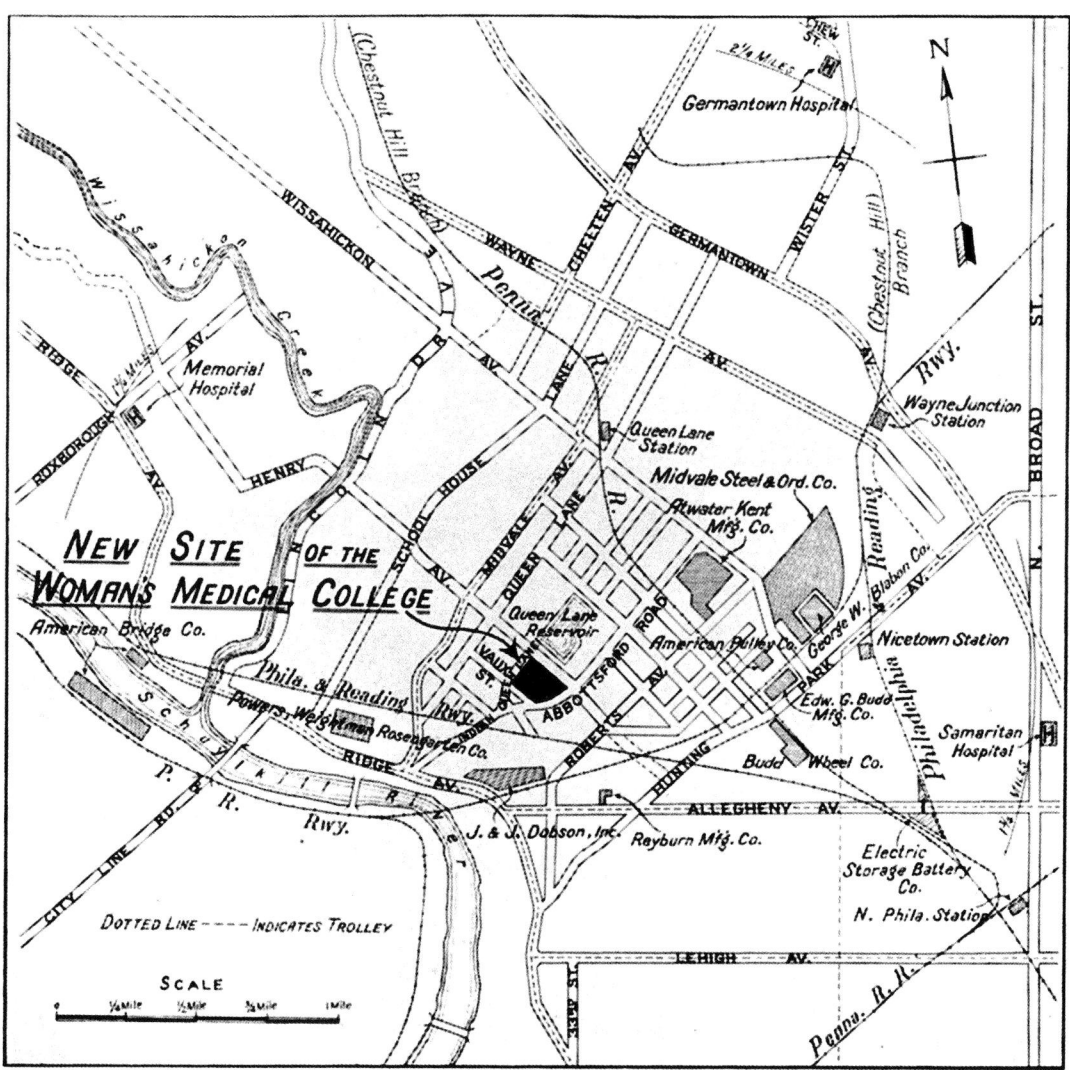

Transportation routes, large industrial plants and the residential districts in the neighborhood of the new site.

4.2.   Neighborhood map, ca. 1926, showing transportation lines, hospitals, industrial plants, and residential districts in the area of the proposed Woman's Medical College of Pennsylvania.

Not only our students, but most of the members of our faculty and staff and corporation are women, and all are convinced that a removal from this neighborhood is imperative."[24] A letter to an alumna addressed the perceived problem from the perspective of housing: "the character of the neighborhood has entirely changed so that the students are no longer able to find suitable living quarters."[25] In contrast, a description of the new site proclaimed it "peculiarly adapted in size, altitude, conformation, and environment, to meet every requirement of the college and its hospital, both as a place of residence of its women students, and as a place of maintenance of hospital service; being accessible on one side to a high class and permanently developed residential community, and on the other side to a large and rapidly spreading industrial area."[26] Not coincidentally, most of the college's small leadership circle lived in the affluent areas of Germantown and Chestnut Hill near the future site.[27]

Harvard Medical School faculty examined neighborhood characteristics of a different type when choosing the location for its 1906 Longwood facility. As with the school's 1883 structure on Boylston Street near Copley Square, the growing concentration of other institutions in the area contributed to the choice of land. Institutions near the Longwood site included the Boston Medical Library (1900), Tufts College Medical School (1900), Isabella Stewart Gardner Museum (1902), Simmons College (1904), and Museum of Fine Arts (1909).[28] The Longwood location also appealed to Harvard officials because it satisfied the conditions of the Peter Bent Brigham will. Brigham had died in 1877 and left a fund for the construction of a hospital in the city of Boston after his bequest had matured for twenty-five years. The Harvard medical faculty kept this trust in mind as they considered future homes for the school. By choosing a site in Boston rather than in Cambridge, closer to the Harvard campus, the medical school administrators made it possible for the Brigham hospital facility and Harvard Medical School to align physically, an outcome Harvard Medical School leaders could shape through personal connections. In the end, the Peter Bent Brigham Hospital incorporated in 1902, its trustees purchased part of the medical school's property in 1907, and the hospital opened on New Year's Day 1913. More than physical coordination resulted. A gentlemen's agreement permitted Harvard Medical School to nominate the hospital's department heads. By enabling Harvard to offer physicians simultaneous appointments in the medical school and the hospital, the arrangement allowed the medical school to start recruiting clinical physicians from around the country.[29]

The Peter Bent Brigham Hospital was not the only medical establishment that decided to build near, and in some cases affiliate with, the medical school. By 1920, new hospital and medical facilities in the area included Hospital of the Good Samaritan (1905), New England Deaconess Hospital (1907), Carnegie Nutrition Laboratory (1908), Harvard Dental School (1909), Collis P. Huntington Memorial Hospital (1912), Forsyth Dental Infirmary for Children (1914), Children's Hospital (1914), Infants' Hospital (1914), Angell Memorial Animal Hospital (1915), and Massachusetts College of Pharmacy (1918) (fig. 4.3). Not only did Harvard Medical

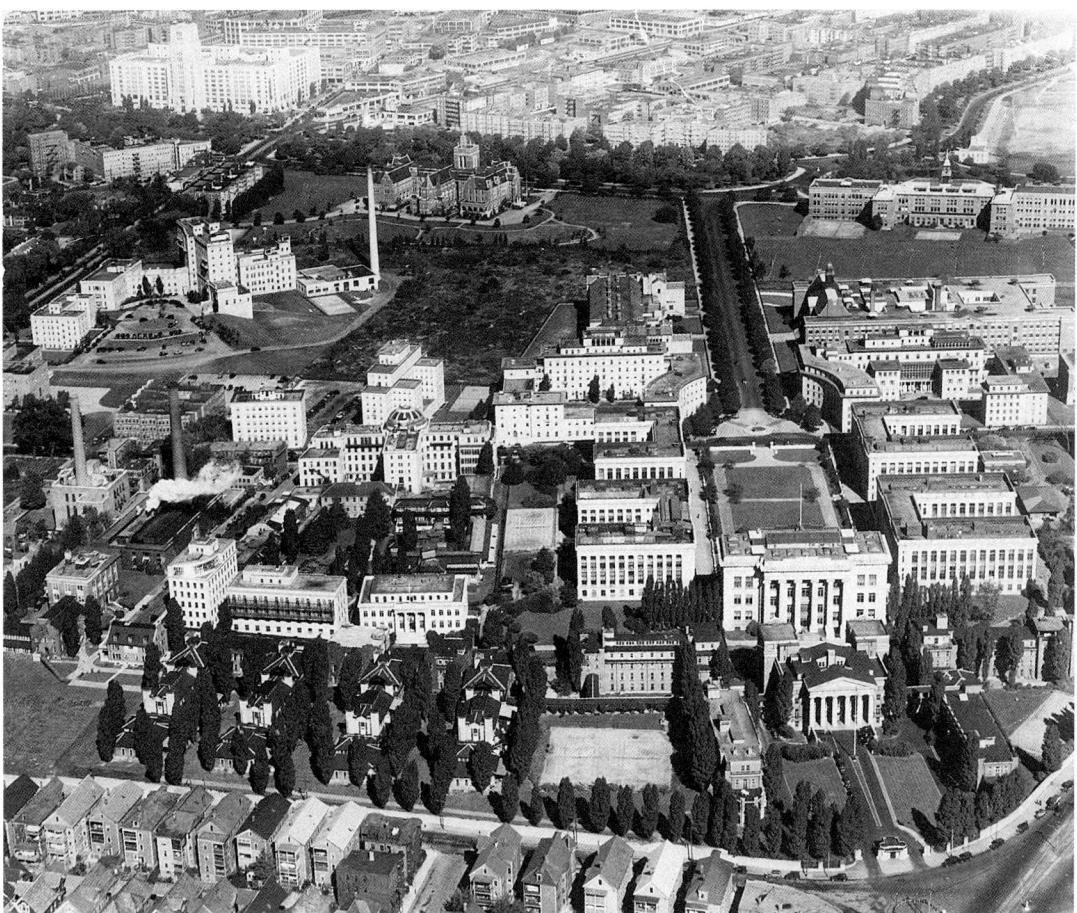

4.3.   Aerial view of Harvard Medical School and the Longwood Medical Area, 1934. The Harvard Medical
School quadrangle (*center right*) is surrounded by institutions, many of which are medical, and sits at one
end of Avenue Louis Pasteur.

School faculty respond to the institutional character of the neighborhood
when they chose the site, but the school in turn also became an impetus
for institutional—and particularly medical—development in the area.[30]

Medical school administrators carefully examined urban environments in the protracted discussions that often accompanied the purchase
of a plot of land. In each case, the standard concerns were inflected by
local conditions: for Woman's Medical College, a move to what its leaders considered a superior neighborhood for the women of the college and,
for Harvard Medical School, a relocation that promised ready hospital
access within a district that was home to an increasing number of institutions. As much as medical schools responded to the urban environment,
however, they also shaped it.

Altering the City to (Attempt to) Meet Aspirations

Harvard Medical School's impact on the city of Boston involved more than its encouragement of an institutional center in the Longwood area. The medical school leadership also organized the construction of a wide boulevard leading from the medical school quadrangle toward downtown Boston and terminating at the Back Bay Fens, the first component of Frederick Law Olmsted's plan for the Boston Park System. Executed in 1895, the Back Bay Fens was the original impetus for institutional growth in the area.[31] When the medical school leadership sought a landscape architect to design the boulevard, they turned to Olmsted Brothers, a successor firm to the office of Frederick Law Olmsted.[32] Based in nearby Brookline, Olmsted Brothers enjoyed a national reputation and had close ties to Harvard University and to Shepley, Rutan, and Coolidge.[33]

The boulevard, named Avenue Louis Pasteur, eliminated a row of residential homes along the far side of the street opposite the medical school and created a stately approach that intensified the experience of the impressive marble quadrangle (fig. 4.4; see also fig. 4.3). The plan to construct a road through the unimproved land between Longwood Avenue at the base of the medical school and the Back Bay Fens developed early and resulted in the orientation of the school toward the park at the boulevard's terminus. The road connected the school with the public green space rather than with the dense housing on the opposite side of the medical institutions.[34] A letter to medical school benefactor J. P. Morgan describing the projected road further considers the relationship between the medical school and the neighborhood:

> The Medical School fronts on a narrow and unimportant street. . . . The proposed street [Avenue Louis Pasteur] would make a dignified, handsome, and proper approach to it. Without such a park avenue it is possible that all the region between the Fens [the park] and the Medical School will be covered with cheap tenements which will injure the appearance of the Medical School and depreciate the value of the property. If the proposed street can be built, it is possible that all this region will be occupied by institutions of various kinds, and that the whole district will be changed and improved.[35]

In the end, of course, the institutions came, and the prominence of Harvard Medical School only became more pronounced. Oscar C. Tugo Circle was dedicated in 1921 where Avenue Louis Pasteur abuts the medical school quadrangle, and shortly thereafter the Boston Lying-In Hospital (1922) and Vanderbilt Hall (1927) were completed. The buildings, sited

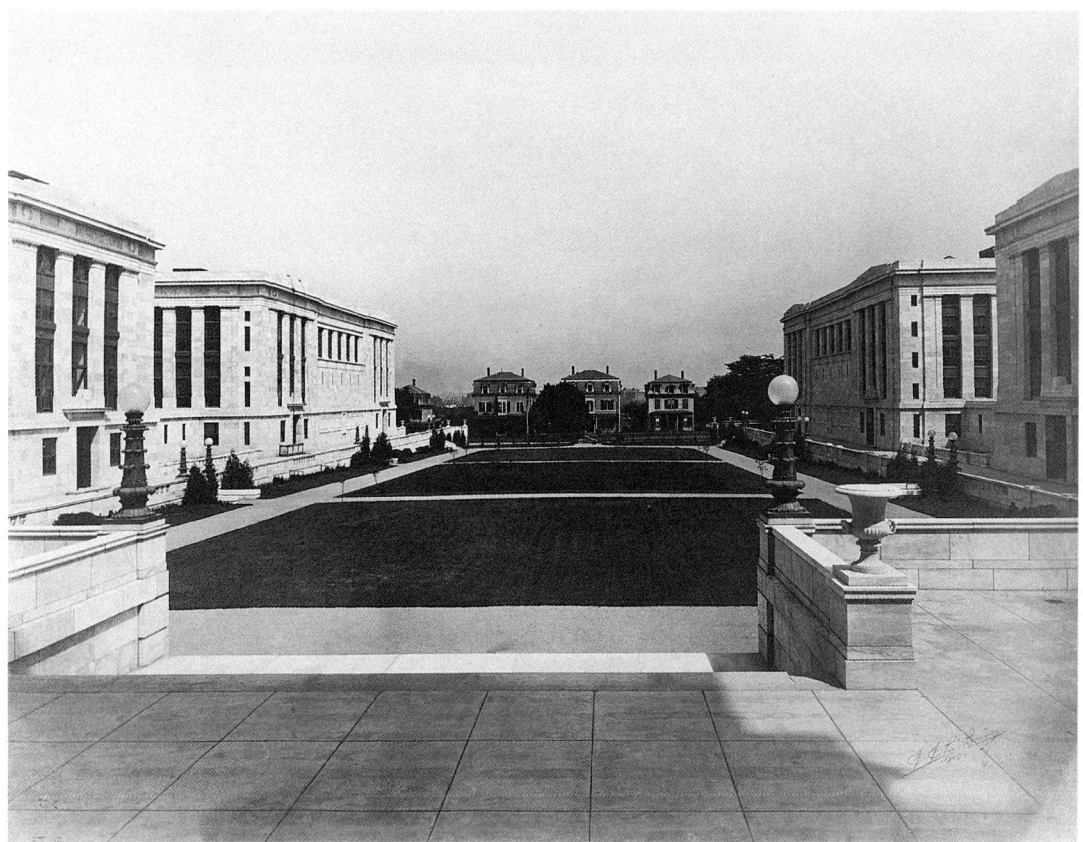

4.4.   View from Harvard Medical School quadrangle before the construction of Avenue Louis Pasteur, ca. 1907.

opposite one another, curved around two sides of the circle and drama-
tized the transition from the avenue to the quadrangle. Moreover, a city
ordinance decreed that no buildings along the avenue could exceed the
height of the medical college.[36] The central place of Harvard Medical
School within the growing neighborhood was thus ensured.

Harvard Medical School left an indelible mark on the city of Boston, but it occupied an undeveloped stretch of land. Medical schools
generally desired open land for obvious reasons. It typically cost less than
developed sites, and it did not require the demolition of current buildings. Sometimes, however, the creation of a medical complex involved
the purchase and removal of an existing neighborhood. In the case of
Meharry Medical College, General Education Board officials demanded
and then closely managed Meharry's move to North Nashville, a relocation that failed to meet the ultimate goal of the board and compromised
the school's early relationship with its new neighbors by disrupting an
established community of Black residents.

As discussed earlier, the General Education Board involved itself deeply in the affairs of Meharry Medical College. Historian Darlene Clark Hine has characterized the years 1920 to 1938 as Meharry's "period of paternalistic white control."[37] When the school faced financial failure just before 1920, Hine explains, the GEB and the Carnegie Foundation provided Meharry with a combined $300,000, but many requirements accompanied this gift. The school had to reorganize in accordance with modern educational standards, occupy the site of the former Walden College, raise an additional $200,000, and replace the retiring president with a person whose credentials were shared with the GEB before his appointment. Hine concludes, "By 1920 the philanthropic foundations had essentially acquired a medical college and would[,] through the man selected to be the president [John J. Mullowney], exercise tremendous power over the lives and destinies of black doctors, students, faculty, and by extension the black masses."[38] In the 1930s, GEB officers facilitated the appointment of Edward Lewis Turner to replace Mullowney as president.[39] The GEB required Meharry to adhere to terms never imposed on white schools.[40]

When the General Education Board decided to lead the effort to rebuild Meharry Medical College in the late 1920s, it continued its pattern of control over the school. With the support of the Julius Rosenwald Fund, which contributed $250,000 to the new structure, the GEB determined the school's location. The board insisted that the school relocate next to Fisk University in the hope that geographic proximity would prompt the two organizations to merge. A merger would allow the schools, both of which received GEB funds, to share their facilities and at the same time give Meharry Medical College the university affiliation necessary to become, in the words of one foundation official, "a strong outstanding school."[41]

The GEB's choice of location for Meharry also fit its broader interests. In addition to its activities in Nashville, the GEB promoted the affiliation or merger of Black institutions of higher education in Atlanta and New Orleans.[42] Moreover, in the 1930s and 1940s the GEB encouraged regional collaboration among colleges and universities, including the Joint University Library for Nashville's Vanderbilt University, George Peabody College for Teachers, and Scarritt College.[43] When Meharry Medical College relocated in 1931, its library resided in Fisk University's library, which had opened the previous year and was constructed with GEB funds.[44] Even after Meharry's medical library moved to the medical school in 1939, the Fisk and Meharry libraries continued to share a director.[45]

Often bypassing Meharry's president, John J. Mullowney, the officers of the General Education Board worked closely with Vanderbilt chancellor James H. Kirkland and at times Vanderbilt medical school dean G. Canby Robinson to make preliminary plans for the new Meharry facility, procure the land, and obtain city permission to close a street that would bifurcate the school's ultimate site.[46] With their eye on encouraging an alignment between Fisk and Meharry, the General Education Board's officers clearly thought proximity was critical. They appear not to have seriously considered two open parcels of land in the general vicinity of Fisk.[47] Instead, they gave careful study to placing Meharry on the Fisk campus. The officers abandoned this plan, however, after Robinson, Mullowney, and the Meharry treasurer spent at least an hour on the Fisk campus. Robinson first wrote Flexner, who heard from Mullowney a few days later, about a different site. Robinson described "watching the circulation of the student body and its character" and deciding that they should forgo the Fisk campus location due to the site's student foot traffic and remoteness from the streetcar line. Robinson suggested as an alternative the land directly across Eighteenth Avenue North from Fisk (where the Meharry facility eventually sat) and noted, "There is very little on this lot of any great value."[48] Kirkland concurred: "Nearly half of the property is vacant, and is owned by Fisk University. I presume they have no plans for utilizing it. This would be favorable to your purposes. The rest of the property is occupied by small houses . . . mostly of inferior quality." Kirkland noted that the challenge would be purchasing the land from approximately twenty-five different owners.[49]

Kirkland's words proved prophetic. Despite the fact that "the city had not extended to this district the usual facilities of sewer, water, gas, and lights," residents regarded it as home.[50] Kirkland described the discouraging experience of the realtor, W. W. Dillon Jr., who met with the various Black homeowners:

> He has talked with possibly a dozen property owners. . . . Not a single one of them is willing to sell, even under very unusual inducements. It seems that the people on this street have lived there many years, some of them for twenty or thirty years. The houses are old because they have been occupied so long. . . . Some of these people have been paying for their property during a long term of years. Some of them are old people and attached to their homes. Within the last few years they have gotten Hefferman [*sic*] Street paved, and it is now a good street. They have worked for this improvement, and for that reason feel unwilling to go into another street where such improvements might be lacking. Mr. Dillon's opinion is that it will be utterly impossible to secure the property.[51]

This description reveals an established neighborhood whose inhabitants did not want to be displaced.

Nevertheless, the project went forward, with General Education Board officials driving its development. Mullowney emphasized the need to obtain purchase options on the land swiftly, "for soon as this becomes public talk, real estate will go sky high."[52] The GEB's officers moved quickly and continued to sidestep the Meharry administration to work largely with Kirkland. Dillon began by acquiring options on land a half block away from Heffernan Street along both sides of Alameda Avenue (later closed) and promised the owners that their property would "be used for some enterprise of importance to the Negro race."[53] An eventual "rumor that a hospital building is to be erected" enabled him to secure the land fronting on Heffernan Street originally thought unprocurable.[54] In a series of events that underlined the GEB's control, board officials did not request that Meharry Medical College make a formal application to the GEB for new facilities until after the GEB had the purchase options for the site all but in hand. In addition, although the properties were put in Meharry Medical College's name, GEB officials appear to have managed the purchases and then turned the deeds over to Meharry rather than allow Meharry's leaders to facilitate the transactions.[55]

One homeowner, however, refused to sell for anything less than an extraordinary price, and without this plot the architects would have had to site the medical school–hospital and the nurses' home closer to one another than they preferred. To provide the additional land that would enable more generous spacing between the structures, Meharry officials decided, at the suggestion of the architects and with the support of the GEB's officers, to use funds intended for construction of the medical school–hospital to buy the remaining lots at the corner of Eighteenth Avenue and Albion Street.[56] This expansion of the Meharry property meant that the neighborhood now lost a store as well as many residences (fig. 4.5).[57]

One General Education Board official went so far as to raise the possibility of the GEB not only buying the land but also building the medical facility before turning the property over to Meharry.[58] In the end, however, Meharry received the deeds for the land well before the cornerstone was laid, even if the GEB paid for the property through the bursar's office at Vanderbilt.[59] Clearly the GEB officers, who grew increasingly doubtful about Mullowney's abilities in the late 1920s, preferred working with the Vanderbilt leadership rather than with the white president the board had earlier approved for Meharry.[60]

Ultimately, however, the General Education Board's plans were only partially realized. Meharry sat across the street from Fisk University, just

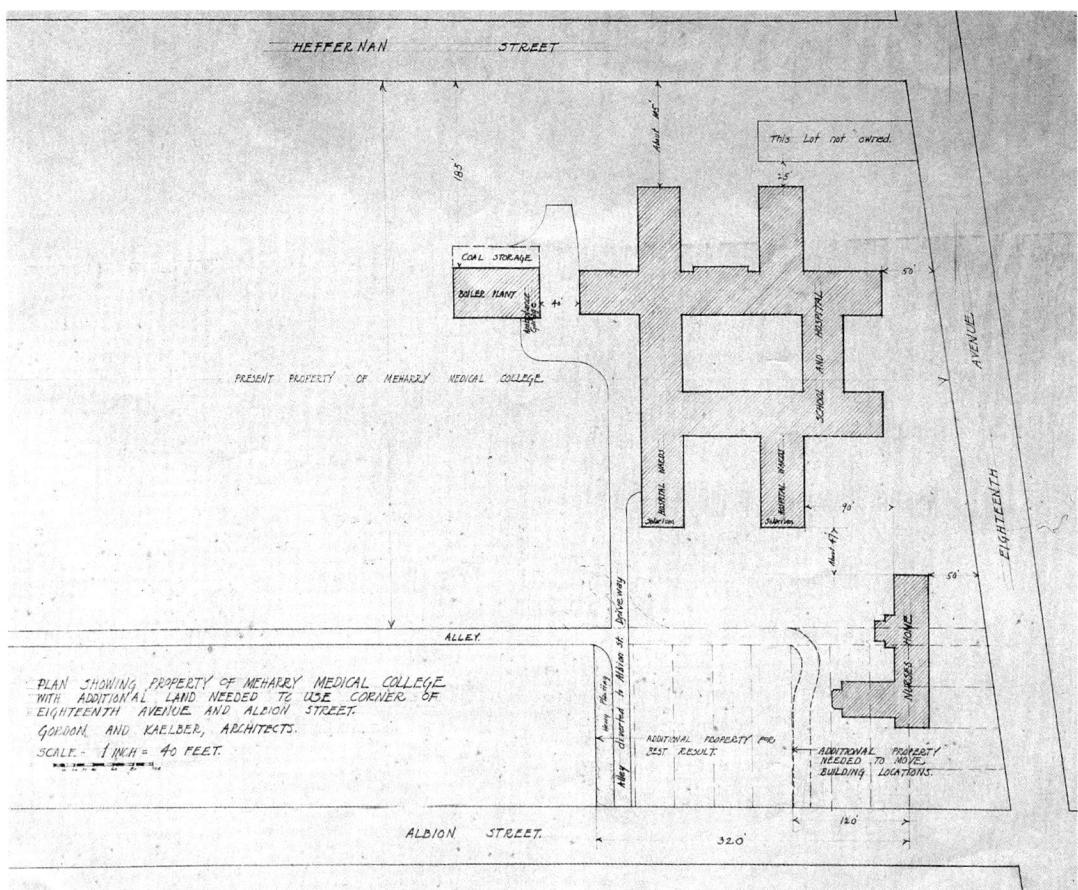

4.5.   Plot plan showing siting of Meharry Medical College buildings with additional land, ca. 23 May
1929, Gordon and Kaelber, architects. Plan indicates the one property not sold to the college near the
corner of Heffernan Street (now Meharry Boulevard) and Eighteenth Avenue (now Dr. D. B. Todd Jr.
Boulevard). It also shows the additional land required at the corner of Eighteenth Avenue and Albion
Street in order to have optimal space for the buildings. Before its closure, Alameda Street ran parallel to
and midway between Heffernan Street and Albion Street.

as the GEB officers had wanted, but the merger desired by the GEB
never took place. Meharry and Fisk's decision not to combine despite
intense pressure from the GEB highlights the limits of philanthropic
control and the power retained by local institutions, even Black universities and medical schools that received paternalistic treatment from
the GEB. In addition, Meharry Medical College struggled to establish
a positive relationship with the North Nashville neighborhood. In his
history of Meharry Medical College, James Summerville notes that the
arrival of Meharry on the site of a formerly residential block meant that
"the change in character of the area was resented by many residents.

Meharry came into its new home suspected, distrusted, and disliked by many of its neighbors."[61] As discussed in more detail at the end of the chapter, the African American community registered its doubts about Meharry by seeking treatment elsewhere, even though that often meant enduring the degrading experience of segregated medicine at the city's hospitals designed primarily for white patients.

Even when no neighborhoods were displaced, the construction of a medical school might be met with anxiety, particularly among local physicians who felt they had much to lose from the founding or reorganization of a medical school and hospital. Jacob D. Goldstein, University of Rochester medical school class of 1929, recalled, "The arrival of the Medical School was not accepted as an unmixed blessing by all the physicians in the Rochester area. Many feared that they would lose patients from their offices and from their favored hospitals. Inevitably this did occur, and to some extent medical students contributed to the problem. Patients being in short supply, we were not always prompt in returning them to the doctor of record. The more interesting the patient or the problem, the more likely we were to delay their return."[62] According to Kenneth Ludmerer, the practice among new and reorganizing medical schools to recruit the faculty leadership from around the country rather than from the nearby region also fueled discord. Although the tensions between medical faculty and area practitioners remain to this day, by 1930 the period of greatest friction had ended.[63]

Medical school officials recognized that their institutions depended on maintaining a positive relationship with the local community. Faculty and administrators generally sought the support and trust of their neighbors, even if this proved challenging at times. School leaders took courting the public seriously, and the structures' exteriors participated actively in this effort.

Modern Buildings with Historicist Exteriors

Educators and architects recognized that a building created a public face for the medical college. Although educators and architects may have written most extensively about the pedagogical components of the reformed medical school, this does not diminish the effort that went into the facilities' exteriors. In general, educators and architects chose exteriors with historical references to project the image of an established institution and profession.

The transformation of the medical school was indivisible from the advent of the American university in the late nineteenth century, and in many senses medical school construction followed general trends in campus architecture. The new universities, like medical schools a few decades later, began receiving unprecedented financial support in the late nineteenth century. John D. Rockefeller, for example, gave some $30 million to the University of Chicago, while Leland Stanford contributed approximately $20 million to the university named for his son. These gifts amounted to ambitious architectural undertakings.[64] A Columbia University trustee published an article in 1914 in which he encouraged universities to develop "a fine architectural effect which will represent to its students the ideals and purposes of a university and command the attention and the admiration of the public."[65] Medical school leaders would no doubt have echoed those sentiments. To achieve this "fine architectural effect," the architects at many universities took inspiration from the system of planning synonymous with the École des Beaux-Arts and the City Beautiful movement and fueled in large part by the 1893 World's Columbian Exposition in Chicago.[66] Perhaps no medical college embodied this planning method more fully than Harvard Medical School (see fig. 1.16). American university leaders and architects, however, chose a variety of architectural styles, from the classical to the medieval, for their buildings.[67] Particularly when the medical school sat on or next to university property, medical colleges often matched the dominant style of the university. Despite the increasing acceptance of the International style and other modern architectural movements in the United States in the 1930s, colleges and universities rarely adopted these styles.[68] Similarly, Jeanne Kisacky explains that "American hospital designs remained remarkably unaffected" by the spread of modernist architecture in the 1930s.[69] Within this context, it is not surprising that far more American medical schools occupied buildings in historicist styles between 1893 and 1940 than did not, although some medical schools embraced the art deco style to varying degrees beginning in the late 1920s. Rather, what is noteworthy are the associations these styles offered medical educators.

In the case of the Gothic revival, architects and medical educators persisted in using the style despite many critics. Some denounced the style for its relatively high cost. Architect Charles Coolidge and Vanderbilt University's chancellor at least briefly considered a colonial revival exterior for the university's 1925 medical school–hospital. Coolidge weighed the style's expense and aesthetics along with the opinions of members of the General Education Board. The colonial revival style would require $62,000 less than the collegiate Gothic. Despite the additional expenditure, however, GEB president Wallace Buttrick preferred the Gothic revival, but Coolidge was "terribly afraid of . . . Flexner."[70] Presumably Coolidge recognized Flexner's insistence on reducing the construction budget. Coolidge added that "the Colonial building will do the work as well as the Gothic and whereas it is a plain building it will not be ugly."[71] In the end, the chancellor and Coolidge decided to construct a Gothic revival medical school–hospital in adherence with the architectural policy adopted for the university campus in 1907.[72] Similarly, a number of science faculty at the University of Chicago suggested building in the classical revival style rather than the Gothic revival due to the cost savings.[73]

Scientists, hospital planners, architects, and physicians also condemned the Gothic revival for hospitals and laboratories due to lack of light. Hospital consultant Winford Smith wrote directly of his disapproval of the Gothic revival style for hospitals: "it is more extravagant in the cost of construction and more difficult to obtain desirable fenestration."[74] In 1919, the president of the University of Chicago met with hospital representatives, architects, and a medical educator involved in planning the university's new medical school and hospital. Afterward the president asserted, "It is questionable whether a hospital can advantageously involve the Gothic forms."[75] Four years later, a University of Chicago physiologist reportedly criticized the Gothic revival edifice that housed his department and argued instead for "a factory type building where they can have all the light they need."[76] Likely the physiologist imagined a steel-frame structure devoid of ornamentation and punctuated with large windows for easy illumination of interior spaces. In fact, most medical schools utilized steel framing in this period, but exteriors with historical references remained the norm. At Chicago, despite the many protests, the desire to maintain a consistent architectural style across the university resulted in the construction of a Gothic revival medical complex.[77]

At Duke University, the donor's wishes won the day for collegiate Gothic (see fig. 3.17). Duke's first medical school dean, Wilburt C. Davison, recalled that "Mr. Duke had approved the Gothic architecture of the West Campus: [stating] 'I have seen the Princeton buildings and they appeal to me.'" Davison went on to explain that Princeton's buildings "are beautiful to behold, but difficult to adapt for a medical center. . . . We . . . persuaded . . . the architect, and . . . the builder, to widen the medieval windows so that they could admit more light."[78] Likely Princeton's Gothic revival architecture attracted James B. Duke at least in part because of the connotations of permanency and venerability that had formed around the Gothic revival on American campuses beginning in the middle of the nineteenth century.[79] For recently reformed medical schools teaching the latest medical science and eager to gain respectability, the associations of the Gothic presented the public with the image of an established, enduring, and reputable institution.

Not all schools embraced the Gothic revival style, however. Some, including Harvard Medical School, chose classical revival (see fig. 1.16). During the dedication proceedings of the 1906 Harvard Medical School, the Johns Hopkins Medical School dean, William Welch, gave an address and linked the quadrangle's classicizing style to the medicine of ancient Greece: "This design is adapted from the Greek, and it is peculiarly fitting that the medical sciences should be housed in a style which suggests the spirit of ancient Greece, where first flowed the springs of medical science and art."[80] If classical revival created for some a connection to medicine's origins, it also, like Gothic revival, would have aligned the medical schools with esteemed institutions across the urban landscape, such as art museums, libraries, churches, and schools. Still other medical colleges, such as Woman's Medical College of Pennsylvania, utilized the colonial revival style, a choice that reflected familiar themes of economical construction and associations with respected institutions, including universities (see fig. 2.23). By linking the medical college to other organizations dependent on the public for financial support, historicist exteriors also reinforced for the community the medical school's reliance on philanthropic gifts.

At first glance, the decision to embrace historicist designs may seem surprising when we consider the pioneering medical training the buildings housed. Architectural historian Annmarie Adams argues, however, that historicist exteriors in interwar hospitals did not diminish the buildings' overall modernity. These facilities enabled aseptic techniques, embraced fireproofing and noise management, and responded to new social structures and urbanization. Adams concludes, "Modernism . . . literally meant clothing modern plans in historic dress in order to smooth the effects of social change. Historicism, in fact, was an important part of making the hospital modern, especially in its role of cushioning some of the less pleasant effects of urban life."[81] Similarly, medical schools cloaked reformed methods of medical education, cutting-edge scientific equipment, and advanced building techniques and mechanical equipment in historicist exteriors that softened, at least visually, the impact of scientific medicine.

Once one entered the medical school, the historicist styling quickly receded. In the hospitals Adams investigates, the lobbies recalled hotel entrance areas with rich materials and historicist ornament, while the

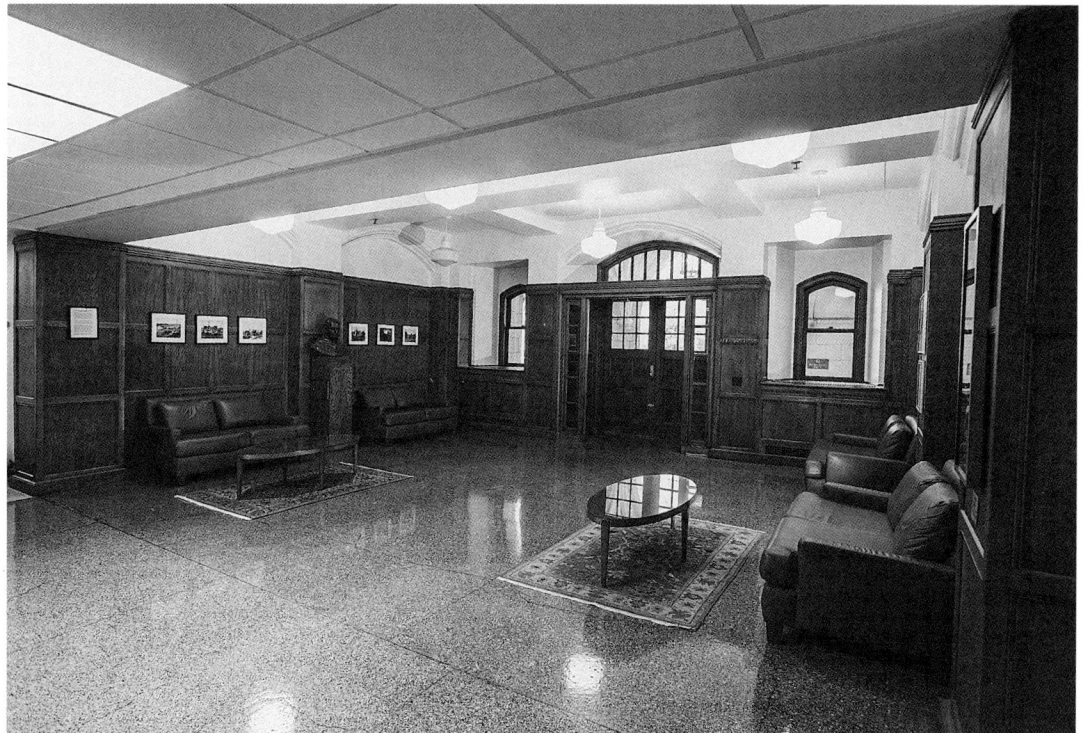

4.6.   Vanderbilt University School of Medicine and Hospital, 1925, Coolidge and Shattuck, architects,
              medical school entrance. Photograph 2019. The wood paneling in Vanderbilt's medical school entrance
              lobby matched that in the hospital entrance. Although the lobby remains wood paneled, some changes
              have been made. The architectural plans indicate that the sidewalls each originally contained a door
              and window leading into administrative offices.

rest of the hospital typically contained more practical and less expensive
materials and often avoided historicist decoration, particularly in places,
such as the operating room, that strove to convey the image of sterile
and aseptic medical practice.[82] Likewise, in medical schools, historicist
decoration and costly marble surfaces or wood paneling rarely extended
past the more public or communal spaces: lobbies and sometimes also
the boardroom, library, lounge, or museum (fig. 4.6).

Although medical libraries in general might include historicist
elements, a subset of the library—the medical history library—consistently maintained a historicist character. Historian John Harley Warner
explains that in the late nineteenth and early twentieth century, elite,
scientifically minded male physicians increasingly devoted their energies
to the history of medicine and the collecting of books. They saw these
efforts as not only a humanizing force that would encourage the development of refined physicians but also a means of fostering cohesion as

an antidote to growing specialization across the profession. To these men the art of healing, as manifest in history and books, represented a critical ancillary rather than a challenge to medical science. In the 1920s and 1930s, the deaths of men of this bibliophilic generation, perhaps most famously William Osler, resulted in an explosion of gifts of personal collections to medical schools and the rapid founding of medical history libraries. By the middle of the century, literally every medical college in North America boasted at the minimum an alcove or room dedicated to medical history, with one or more bequests often the core of the collection. The men responsible for the creation of medical history libraries wanted the spaces to cultivate a physical connection between progressive medicine and the past, and for this they turned to historicist styling, as seen in Yale's Medical History Library, opened in 1941, a library Warner designates as typical in its emphasis on historicism if not its generous size (fig. 4.7). The result was private, club-like spaces, and Warner labels the social events organized by physicians to champion books and medical history "virtual gentlemen's clubs." This celebration of the profession's elite members as male—and, I would emphasize, also white—reinforced the demographics of medicine's upper ranks, a hierarchy in medicine that continues today.[83] Chapter 5 returns to discussion of the privileging of white men in the modern medical school.

Unlike the lobbies and spaces for medical history, the laboratories that consumed so much of medical schools' square footage remained devoid of historicist elements, which had no part in the execution of scientific medicine. Good laboratory design required a well-lighted, open space with rows of benches or dissecting tables, carefully planned work areas, and new features such as hoods and gas. Although these rooms included expensive technology, such as ventilation systems, other building costs could be aggressively conserved. Descriptions mention exposed pipes, brick, and radiators; concrete floors; and walls of painted terra-cotta tiles. The absence of suspended ceilings in the laboratories may also have reflected a desire to make maintenance of mechanical systems easier and to facilitate mechanical reconfiguration.[84] Medical school exteriors typically did not look modern in a stylistic sense, but the buildings functioned as the spaces of modern institutions that codified physically the transformed pedagogical program, produced physicians fully inculcated in the latest conceptions of medical practice and professional identity, and celebrated scientific medicine even as the medical history library insisted that this pursuit be balanced by at least a nod to the art of healing.

If historicist styles supported rather than undermined the modernity

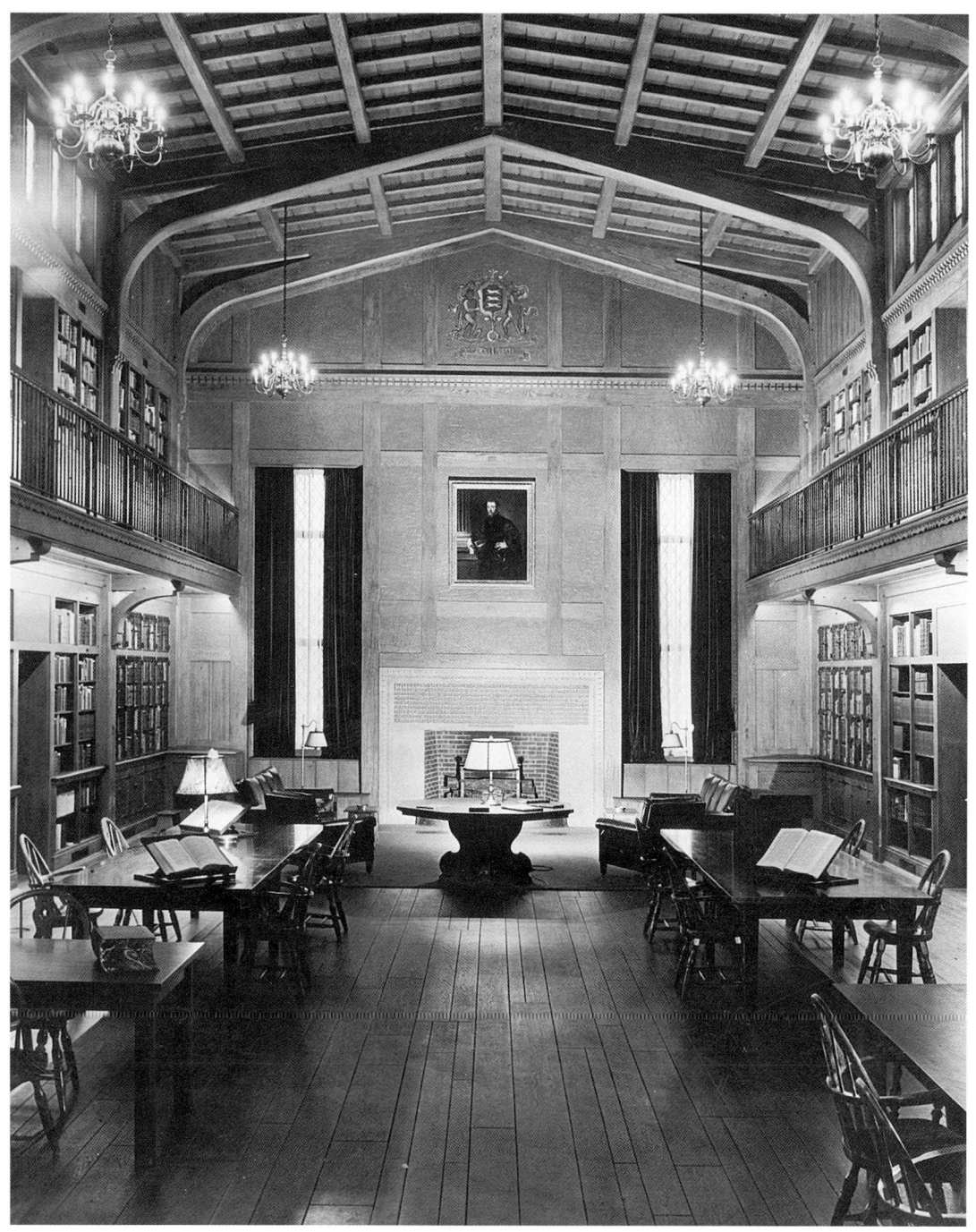

4.7.　　Yale University School of Medicine, Medical Historical Library, 1941, Grosvenor Atterbury, architect.

of reformed medical schools, then the adoption of the art deco style by some medical colleges appears less like a break with convention. Annmarie Adams has explored the international use of art deco design for a wide variety of hospitals and other medical buildings, including medical schools, in the interwar years. She argues that the art deco style created advantageous associations for the profession; visual parallels with art deco department stores, for example, suggested to the public that it was fashionable to enter art deco medical spaces. Adams discusses Columbia-Presbyterian Medical Center and Bard Hall, Columbia's medical student dormitory, and asserts that the art deco style had much to offer the medical center, most significantly an association with modernity (see figs. 2.22 and 5.9). Adams concludes that "Art Deco design dignified, glamorized, and demonstrated interwar medicine to a broad public audience by relying on a general association with urbanism, progress, modernity, and even fashion."[85] Likely hoping for similar associations, some architects and medical educators included more muted or limited art deco styling in their medical college buildings. Gordon and Kaelber, for example, created a progressive iteration of the collegiate Gothic at Meharry Medical College, where the "Public Health Lecture Room" entrance in particular conveys the impact of art deco design (see fig. 3.12). When the art deco style became popular in North America in the late 1920s, more than fifteen years had passed since the publication of the Flexner Report and more than three decades had elapsed since Johns Hopkins University opened its medical college. Perhaps the relatively established state of reformed medical education and the profession's rising cultural authority gave some medical school administrators the confidence to move away from revival styles and instead to embrace a more modern one.

Beyond the buildings themselves, medical colleges also strove to make their campuses attractive landmarks for the community. Institutions with enough resources could hire a landscape architect to further enhance their properties, as Harvard did when it retained the Olmsted Brothers for its Longwood quadrangle. But even medical colleges with smaller budgets could maintain visually pleasing grounds. In 1929, University of Nebraska medical students expressed their appreciation in the yearbook for the work undertaken over the previous decade and a half by Richard C. Darcy. When the University of Nebraska unified its medical program in 1913 by transferring preclinical studies from Lincoln to the new campus in Omaha, Darcy also made the move and became operating superintendent responsible for maintaining the school's buildings and grounds. He brought to his position unusual experience from his training in floriculture

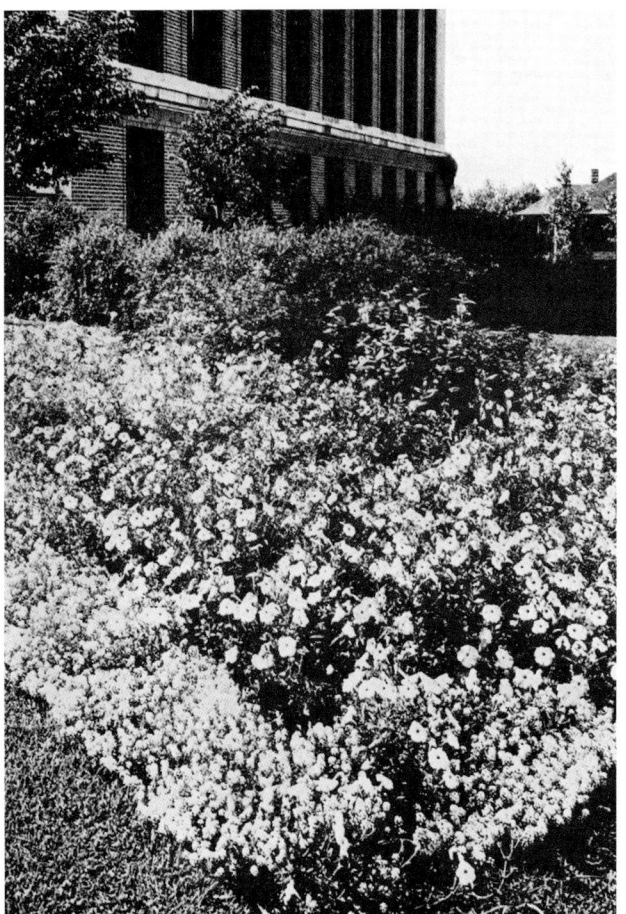

4.8.   Grounds of the University of Nebraska medical
campus, ca. 1929.

and time spent running a distinguished flower farm in his native England. The students proclaimed, "With the growth of the College, Mr. Darcy has devoted more of his time to the grounds and has won an enviable reputation for the beauty of his flowers and the attractive setting of his trees and shrubs. He has made the campus one of the beauty places of Omaha."[86] The yearbook's photographs prove the accuracy of these remarks (fig. 4.8).

Almost every medical college in the country rebuilt its school between 1893 and 1940. This construction effort meant larger, consistently purpose-built facilities designed to mark the urban fabric with the transformed image of medical education. In June 1906, the annual meeting of the American Medical Association convened in Boston, and attendees had the chance to experience the five buildings of Harvard Medical School's nearly finished quadrangle (fig. 4.9). Harvard president Charles W. Eliot reflected on the guests' impressions to faculty member J. Collins Warren: "The great throng of interested persons found them spacious, handsome, well set, and of noble aspect. They are pronounced good, not only for our School but for the course of medical education and progress in general."[87] Warren agreed: "I think we have produced the desired effect upon the minds of our visitors. . . . Some are wondering if we shall have room for all the students who will want to come next year. The buildings seemed to say to others that medicine was being put upon an altogether new plane."[88] For Eliot and Warren, the impressive structures had achieved the intended results by embodying for the visitors reformed medical education, scientific medicine, and the shifting professional identity of physicians.

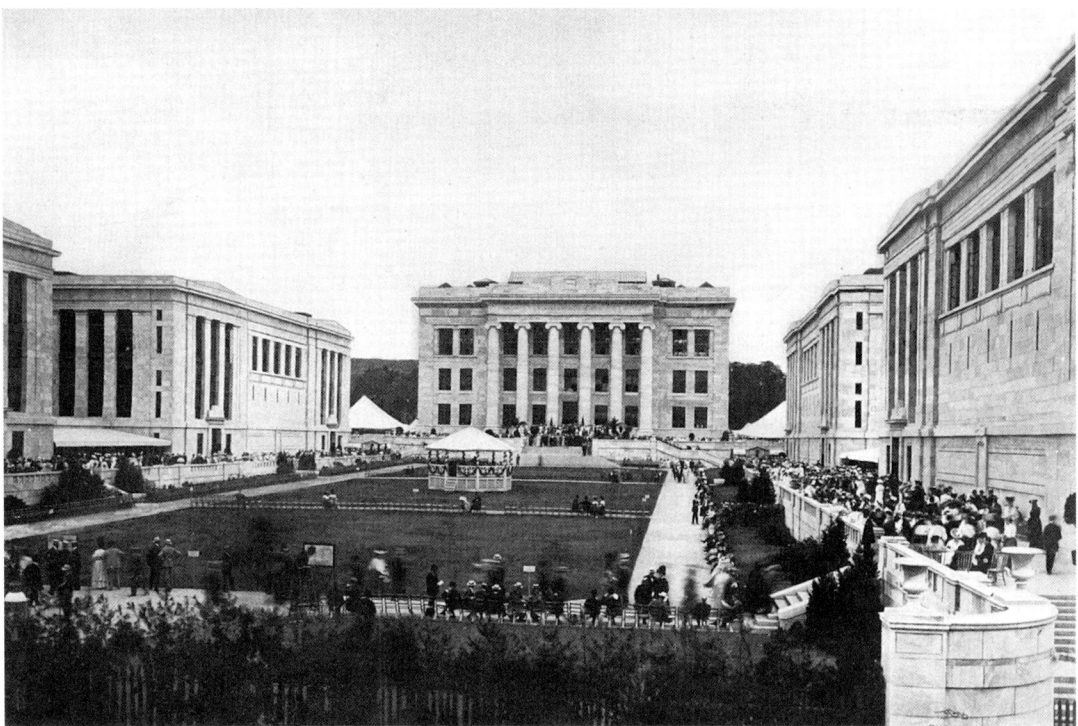

4.9.   American Medical Association annual meeting event at Harvard Medical School, June 1906.

For medical schools designed for marginalized members of the profession, specifically Meharry Medical College, Howard University College of Medicine, and Woman's Medical College of Pennsylvania, the promotional opportunity afforded by new facilities became even more pronounced. The first purpose-built school for Woman's Medical College opened in 1875, and as Steven Peitzman explains, the edifice "symbolized the progress and status of the College and of Philadelphia's medical women. The large brick structure proclaimed that women's medical education was no transient or trifling fancy."[89] Similar to the construction of a women's dormitory, which announced the permanency of a college's female students, the medical schools built for the coeducational Black medical colleges and the predominantly white school for women declared to the community the stability and progress of these schools and in turn an ongoing role for their students and graduates.[90]

A number of considerations, including changing racial demographics, prompted the leadership of Woman's Medical College to move the school to East Falls in 1930; another factor was the importance of visibility to advancing the school's mission. In certain ways, the relocation left the school somewhat isolated. It removed the college from center

Philadelphia, from the heart of the city's medical community and its medical societies, and from the implied and actual competition with the sizable medical colleges and hospitals in the downtown area.[91] But for whatever the school may have given up by leaving the city's core, the women could point to the prominence provided by the East Falls location. By the late 1920s, the college's downtown building no longer stood out. As one faculty member observed, "anyone wanting to find the Woman's Medical College had to be first directed to Girard College and then told to 'look behind it.'"[92] Conversely, its new home, a local reporter explained, occupied "one of the highest points in the city."[93] Dean Martha Tracy elaborated, indicating that in East Falls the school enjoyed a "magnificent site visible from the East River Drive, from Allegheny and Hunting Park Avenues and other much travelled railroad and motor routes."[94]

Woman's Medical College of Pennsylvania, Howard University College of Medicine, and Meharry Medical College, in keeping with the schools composed exclusively or predominantly of white men, chose revival styles for their buildings, completed in 1930, 1927, and 1931, respectively. The historicist exteriors aligned the marginalized schools with the same associations of permanence and venerability that drew the leaders of the white and male schools to these styles. For Black medical colleges, the exteriors may also have been understood as a challenge to racial hierarchies. In his research on Black educational institutions founded by African American women at the end of the nineteenth century, Angel David Nieves underscores the difficulty in determining from our current historical distance the symbolic resonances of the architectural choices made at these schools. Nevertheless, he "maintain[s] that the use of the so-called 'elegant Ionic portico' has always held a deeper meaning and is symbolic of Black attempts to express political, social, and economic advances in the New South."[95] Similarly, in her examination of architect Robert R. Taylor's work at Tuskegee Normal and Industrial Institute in the opening decades of the twentieth century, Ellen Weiss posits that "Tuskegee insiders might have been silent about architectural equality, but that does not mean that they did not understand their porticos as just that [representations of architectural equality] when safe among family and friends or in the quiet of their own thoughts."[96] Undoubtedly, no one at the GEB, let alone Meharry's president or the architects at Gordon and Kaelber, intended to create an exterior that subverted prevailing norms by using Meharry's Gothic revival style to place the Black medical college within the European-American cultural tradition. Weiss reminds us that "a classical portico could also be best practice for any ambitious institution," regardless of the race of its occupants.[97] The same could be said of a Gothic revival exterior.

African American architect Albert Cassell's 1927 colonial revival building for Howard University's medical school may have been read as contesting racial hierarchies, however. W. Montague Cobb was a medical student at Howard when the building opened, and he recalled the condemnation of the structure's portico by individuals he does not name (see fig. 3.8): "The general attitude of the times . . . was not one to regard either Howard or Meharry as being important for national research potential, but as significant merely to train the largest number of general practitioners who would serve as shock troops, as it were, in an area of enormous need. *As a consequence*, the 1927 Howard medical building represented almost the ultimate in economy. . . . Even so, the architect was severely criticized as wasteful, because a simple portico employing four columns and steps was used to break the monotony of a vast expanse of red brick wall and windows."[98] Cobb implies an expectation that, because they were not elite research schools, Black colleges would construct unadorned buildings in keeping with their position within the medical profession. When Cassell refused to adhere to this expectation, he crossed a racial boundary within the profession. Underscoring the role of race in this critique, no historical evidence suggests that Woman's Medical College, with its predominantly white student body and from which research was not expected, received similar criticism of the portico on its 1930 medical school–hospital.

From one hundred years' historical distance, intent and reception in the 1920s and 1930s can be challenging to distill. At the least, however, in constructing buildings in the same styles typically chosen by the faculties at schools with predominantly white and male student bodies, the leadership at Meharry, Howard, and Woman's Medical College positioned these schools alongside the white and male institutions as part of the esteemed medical profession. In so doing, they expanded the profession's demographics. But the example of Howard's medical school makes clear that claiming professional space could come at a price, particularly for African Americans.

"Momentous" Activities to Engage the Public

Architectural style mattered, but medical school administrators had long sought additional ways to communicate with the public. In 1812, Colonel John Eager Howard laid the cornerstone during ceremonies marking the beginning of construction for the College of Medicine of Maryland (see fig. I.3).[99] A century later, medical faculty and others continued to celebrate the various stages of construction, from groundbreaking to dedication, with at times elaborate exercises.

The year before Vanderbilt University School of Medicine's 1925 facility was to open, Abraham Flexner wrote passionately about the importance of such events for connecting with the public. Vanderbilt occupied a critical position in Flexner's plan to bring reformed medical education to all parts of the country. Flexner explained, "South of Washington [DC] and East of the Mississippi there has been up to now no such thing as a modern medical school." He had high hopes for the 1925 building in Nashville and called for a dedication ceremony commensurate with the impact of the school: "the significance of this new departure ought to be impressed upon the South at the dramatic moment when the new institution is thrown open for the reception of students." Flexner suggested inviting internationally renowned American and European medical leaders and noted that the Europeans in particular "will signalize to the country and to the South that something momentous is happening."[100] Flexner's hopes were fulfilled; a dedication ceremony coupled with academic proceedings took place the following fall. Flexner's vision for Vanderbilt's dedication was unusual only in its scale. During the early twentieth century, medical schools around the country collectively hosted an almost constant parade of construction-related events, with multiple points during the building process often recognized for each structure.

Columbia-Presbyterian Medical Center hosted its groundbreaking on a sunny day in January 1925. A commemorative booklet provides a detailed description of the event. To help attendees envision the future building, stakes—standing out against the snow and connected with tape—traced the outline of the medical school–hospital. During the ceremonies, six hundred people listened to a series of speakers before witnessing a dramatic and triumphant finale. Edward Harkness, a major donor and the driving force behind the medical center, turned the first scoop of dirt using a silver spade engraved for the occasion, and "immediately there came a shrill blast from the excavator near by, and the automatic shovel dropped to gather up a load of earth and rock." The chairperson of the board of Columbia University then declared, "Ladies and gentlemen, work on the Medical Center has begun." The program ended with a benediction given by the bishop of the Episcopal Church's Diocese of New York.[101]

When the groundbreaking began to fade from memory, the laying of the cornerstone provided an opportunity to involve the local and sometimes also the broader community in heralding the construction efforts.

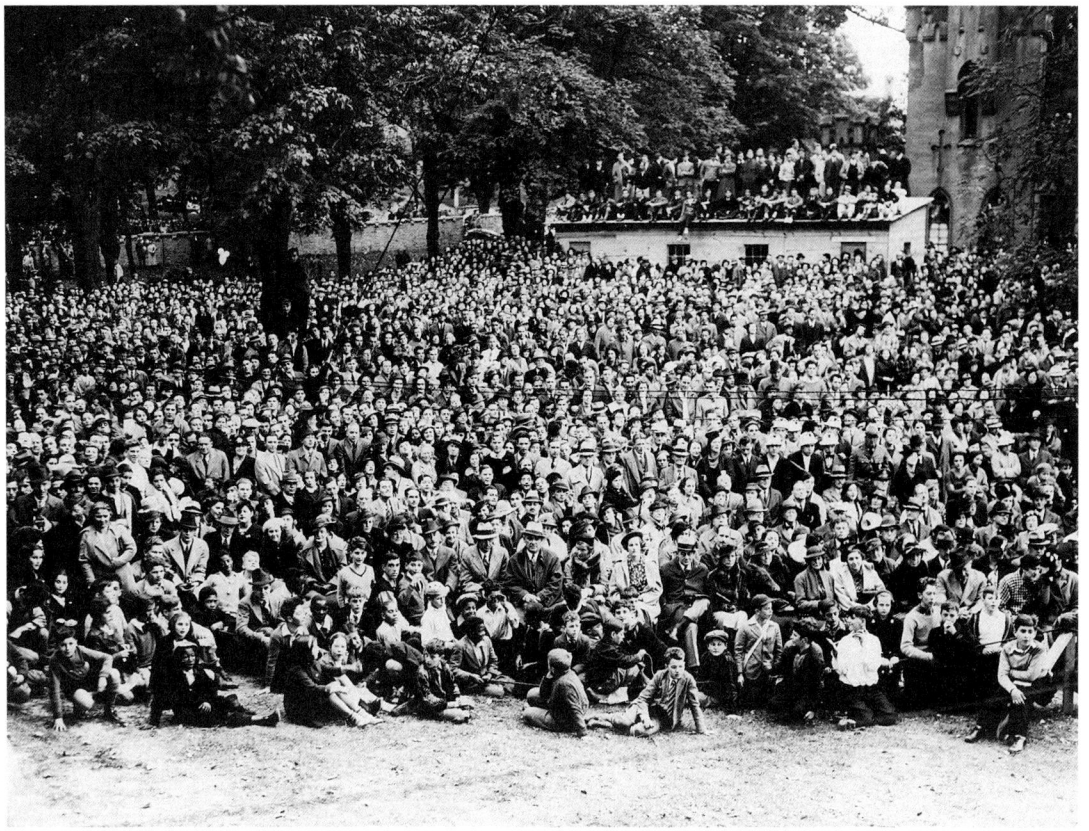

4.10.   Spectators watching medical school cornerstone ceremony at Syracuse University, September 1936.

In Syracuse enthusiasm ran particularly high in September 1936, when President Franklin D. Roosevelt participated in the ceremony for the laying of the medical school cornerstone ahead of the New York State Democratic Convention later in the evening. More than twenty-five thousand spectators gathered to watch his motorcade move through the city ahead of the 4:00 p.m. cornerstone ceremonies. In addition to being broadcast on the radio, the proceedings were open to the public, but most of the approximately four thousand people who crowded the university grounds were students, faculty, and their families (fig. 4.10).[102]

Not every school held such elaborate programs. Meharry promised its cornerstone "exercises will be comparatively informal and simple, in keeping with the general spirit and atmosphere of Meharry Medical College," although its guest list included "representatives from all the Negro organizations."[103] No doubt President Mullowney thought carefully about his audience at the ceremony when he affirmed in his speech, later published with emphasis in the original, "In this new and greater educational center that will arise in Northwest Nashville, Meharry will try to mind her own business and *live at peace with her neighbors.*"[104] Courting the public involved both inspiring the local community and improving community relationships.

Like Flexner, medical educators tended to place particular emphasis on events surrounding the completion of the building, and the public often responded with high attendance numbers. In the fall of 1913, to coincide with the annual alumni clinical week, the University of Nebraska College of Medicine held a reception to show off its school, which was not quite finished but already occupied. The structure was cleaned and decorated especially for the evening occasion, musicians played, a group of women served refreshments, students acted as tour guides, and faculty answered questions about the various departments. The efforts were rewarded when more than eight hundred people attended the event.[105]

Duke University planned a staggered opening for its medical school–hospital, with the hospital and outpatient department commencing activity on 21 July 1930, the medical school on 1 October 1930, and the nursing school on 2 January 1931. The day before the clinical facilities began accepting patients, the medical school's dean, Wilburt C. Davison, welcomed the public to the complex, an experience he remembered vividly three decades later: "It was the hottest day I have ever encountered. I lost six pounds and ruined a white linen suit showing visitors through the building and repairing overloaded elevators. The suit shrank so much that I gave it to a friend half my size. Approximately fifteen thousand visitors from the Carolinas and Virginia accepted the invitation to this 'Open House' which had been announced in the newspapers."[106]

Davison may have invited the populations of three states, but other schools' leaders took a more targeted approach to their audience. In September 1930, Woman's Medical College of Pennsylvania held a typical dedication day, with public tours of the building as well as more formal exercises.[107] A few months later, however, the administration focused its attention on representatives of college women: the members of 28 college alumnae groups with Philadelphia branches, deans of women at coeducational colleges, and deans and presidents of women's colleges, mostly from the greater Philadelphia area. The guests toured the facility and discussed ways to forge closer relationships between Woman's Medical College and the female students of the visiting institutions. The leadership at Woman's Medical College had its eye on recruitment and hoped to raise its enrollment from 120 medical students to 200. As part of this effort, Woman's Medical College dean Martha Tracy positioned the structure as an emblem of the school's progress. She pointed out that many in academic circles continued to equate the medical college with its antiquated 1875 building, but "we want to convince them that we have kept abreast of the times by acquainting them with our new building, its facilities and equipment. We are up-to-date and modern."[108] Guests appear to have understood Tracy's point. In a comment described as characteristic of the visitors' responses, the dean of Bryn Mawr College declared, "I think it is a perfectly splendid institution. Both Dr. Park [president of Bryn Mawr] and I are delighted with it. It is so completely and thoroughly equipped."[109]

To broaden the impact of the buildings, medical school leaders also strove to reach people outside of the region and unable to visit the facilities. They generated books and pamphlets about the structures so that the material could be personally distributed or mailed to donors and other concerned parties. Harvard printed one thousand copies of the book published in conjunction with the completion of the 1906 quadrangle. Recipients of the volume included donors to the complex, faculty, special guests present at the dedication, and leading medical schools and libraries.[110] George Eastman, a contributor to Meharry Medical College's 1931 building, received a copy of the richly illustrated commemorative publication created to celebrate the opening of that medical college.[111] School leadership also sought and received exposure in the popular press, sometimes far from their campuses. Faculty shared materials with the press, including architectural plans, information about public events, and announcements of major donations, and these efforts could produce results. Sketches of Duke University's medical campus-in-progress appeared in the *New York Times* and further piqued the interest of Duke's inaugural medical college dean, who hoped to lead the school under development in Durham.[112] J. P. Morgan's gift to Harvard Medical School received extensive news coverage, which included a drawing of the planned quadrangle, in both Boston and New York newspapers. This publicity refocused John D. Rockefeller's attention on the project, and he ultimately gave substantially to the undertaking.[113] Profiles in national medical journals further expanded awareness of the medical facilities. For example, the *Journal of the National Medical Association*, the publication of the country's professional organization for Black physicians, who were often excluded from the American Medical Association in this period, closely followed news of Meharry Medical College and Howard University College of Medicine.

Offering tours through the buildings or publishing plans and photographs of the structures provided medical faculty with the opportunity to educate the public in the foundations of modern medicine through the site where it was taught, and the expanding laboratory spaces represented a critical component of the transformed educational environment. Historian James Hopkins has investigated the late nineteenth-century facilities for Owens College Medical School in Manchester, England. According to Hopkins, because laboratories had become symbolic of scientific knowledge and authority, the medical profession allied itself with science's rising prestige when it adopted the laboratory for teaching and research.[114] At the same time, as the reputation of physicians grew, medical educators' promotion of the laboratory simultaneously elevated the status of science.

Community engagement did not stop once the building's paint began to fade. Although Harvard Medical School did not have a lecture hall designed for public use, in 1911 more than seven thousand individuals attended eighteen lectures on a broad spectrum of topics, with at least fifteen hundred people unable to gain admittance even if they were willing to stand. Faculty member Harold C. Ernst affirmed, "These Public Lectures are unquestionably a valuable part of the activity of the School. The interest of the public in them appears to be increasing, and the prediction that this interest would diminish has not as yet been verified."[115] In his president's address to the American Medical Association in 1908, Harvard professor of surgery Herbert L. Burrell argued that, with the development of scientific medicine, the profession had an obligation to share its expanding knowledge with the nonmedical community. Among his many ideas for this transfer of information, he lauded the lecture series given at the University of Chicago and at Harvard. An education in scientific medicine would benefit an individual's health, and such "judicious publicity" would result in multiple advantages for the profession, not least of which was "the recognition by the world that the medical profession is a great public benefactor."[116] Beyond improving attendees' well-being, lectures for laypersons had the potential to strengthen the community's appreciation for scientific medicine, as well as for the men and women who practiced it.

Shaping Public Opinion on Animal Experimentation

In their efforts to promote scientific medicine, the faculty also responded to the negative opinions some members of the public held about certain types of laboratory work. One troubling laboratory practice was animal experimentation, or vivisection, as it was often called at the time.[117] Antivivisectionists denounced the practice. Medical scientists feared that public condemnation of animal experimentation could lead to legislation that would significantly curb or prohibit using animals in the laboratory. They worried as well that criticisms of animal experimentation could diminish the local community's enthusiasm for the medical school, a situation with a cascade of consequences for an organization that depended on its home city for patients, students, and donations. In his 1908 address to the American Medical Association, Harvard Medical School's Herbert L. Burrell suggested animal experimentation as a potential topic for contributions to magazines and other publications: "Let a series of articles be published in order that the public may know the truth as to the inestimable benefits that have come from animal experimentation. . . . Let circulars of information . . . be placed in the hands of every legislator . . . [and] of every citizen who is misinformed as to the truth."[118] The year before Burrell gave this address, the American Medical Association had created the Council for the Defense of Medical Research. Led by Burrell's colleague at Harvard Medical School, Walter Cannon, the council disputed antivivisectionists' charges. In addition, it developed a code of conduct for animal laboratories that reduced public support for the antivivisectionists but did not end the antivivisectionists' calls for abandonment, or at the least further reform, of animal experimentation.[119] As the leader of organized medicine's reaction to the antivivisection movement, Cannon also wrote articles for laypersons that highlighted the role experimentation on dogs played in advances in medical science and clinical practice.[120]

Troublingly for the medical scientists, their critics could literally enter the medical school. In 1926, the University of Rochester Medical School fired Calvin Simmonds from his position in the animal house after learning he had falsified his background during the hiring process. The dean reported, "We are convinced that this individual was sent here by these officers of the Dog Protective Association to make trouble for us."[121]

Despite the efforts of proponents of animal experimentation, they faced a renewed antivivisection movement in the 1920s, the same decade that saw an increase in the construction of medical colleges.[122] The anxiety of medical faculty about condemnation from the antivivisectionists and the arousal of public anger permeated discussions of animal facilities. In 1921 the faculty at Western Reserve University School of Medicine outlined the school's need for a new home, and they described the subpar conditions for animals in blunt terms:

> The use of animals is essential to modern teaching and research in very nearly all divisions of the preclinical years. Common humanity directs that they should be properly cared for and this is not possible where roofs, basements, tin

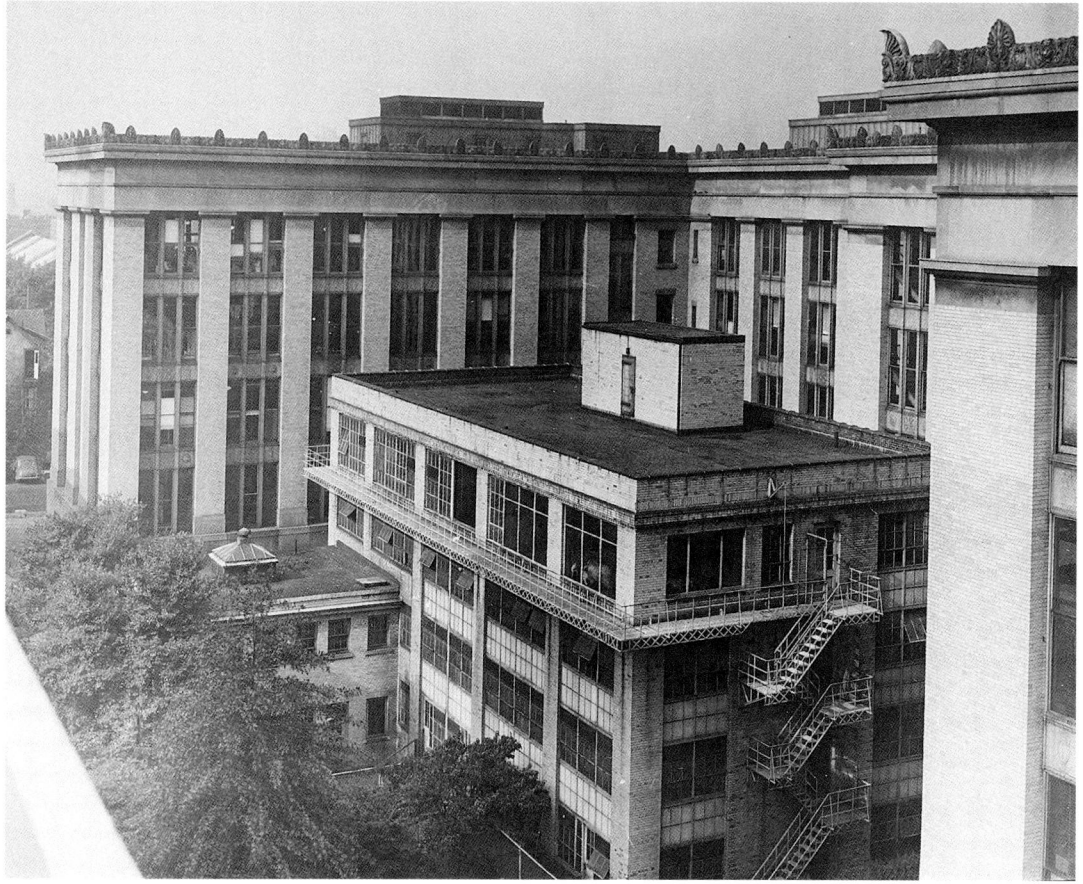

4.11.   Animal House (*center*), Western Reserve University School of Medicine, 1930, Garfield, Stanley-Brown, Harris, and Robinson, architects. Photograph 1943. Note remaining section of two-story 1924 animal house (*left, partly obscured*) designed by architects Coolidge and Shattuck.

garages and similar quarters are provided. Proper quarters would avoid deaths from fighting, deaths from invasion by rats and even death from freezing. The future of this School depends in large part upon maintaining a position before the public such that our care of animals cannot be criticized. Under present conditions any improvement is impossible. The efforts of all members of the staff are directed toward humane treatment of animals but they are sadly handicapped at present.[123]

In 1924, Western Reserve University School of Medicine occupied a new facility. Between the wings of the U-shaped building stood a separate animal house composed of two stories in addition to the basement. Within six years, however, much of the original animal house was demolished and a four-story structure that dramatically expanded the animal facilities was attached to the remaining portion of the 1924 building (fig. 4.11).[124] The many windows on both edifices, particularly the 1930 animal house, suggest the faculty's determination not to repeat the "over heated [*sic*], dark, ill-ventilated and entirely unsanitary" conditions of the pre-1924 accommodations for animals.[125]

The University of Rochester also constructed a separate animal house as part of its 1925 medical school–hospital complex. George Hoyt Whipple, dean and professor of pathology, detailed the two-story structure for *Methods and Problems of Medical Education*. The article included the building's architectural plans along with photographs of the cages for rabbits, guinea pigs, and dogs. Whipple asserted confidently, "In planning this house the object in mind was to provide quarters for animals which would be in every way comparable to those supplied to patients in a modern hospital." He reviewed the cutting-edge ventilation and heating systems, the design elements that aided in cleaning the facility, the management of distemper among the dogs, and even the dogs' typical diet: "carefully selected table scraps from the hospital and a standard dog-biscuit." He went so far as to offer descriptions of the special cages for unusual animals, such as monkeys, to "any interested person who may wish to write for this information."[126] Editors, scientists, and educators knew that antivivisectionists read research reports in medical and scientific journals for anything that could be considered evidence of animal abuse, so they strove to eliminate statements that could be taken out of context as evidence of cruelty.[127] Whipple may have anticipated that antivivisectionists might read his article, and he went out of his way to emphasize the school's humane management of its animals and to suggest a level of transparency about their care. Facilities carefully designed to promote humane treatment of animals became part of medical educators' defense of animal experimentation.

Likely in an attempt to stave off criticism, educators and architects also housed the animals discreetly.[128] Animal quarters tended to sit on the less public edges of campus. At the University of Rochester, the designers located the animal house directly behind the medical school–hospital, far from the main entrance and backing up to an open field. At Western Reserve University, the animal house occupied the space between the wings of the U-shaped medical school, itself placed at one end of the group of medical buildings. At Harvard Medical School, a cluster of trees shielded the animal house, sited behind Building D and close to the front of the quadrangle, so that it was not visible from the nearby road (see fig. 1.17 and fig. 4.3). Rather than building separate animal facilities, some colleges cared for the animals in the medical school, probably to

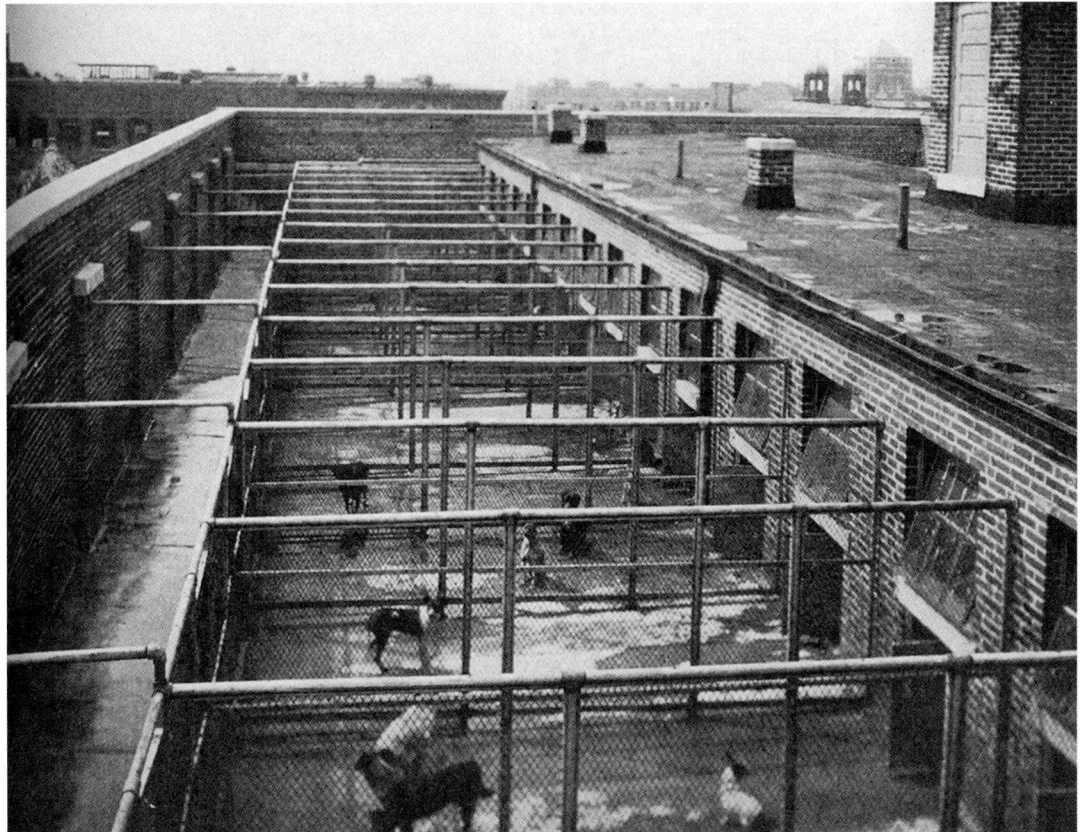

4.12.   University of Michigan physiology department dog runs and kennels, ca. 1930.

reduce construction costs, and basements and roofs proved popular as
relatively inconspicuous sites for the animals. It was fairly easy not to see
animals in basements and on roofs, but they made their presence known
in other ways. Although well-designed ventilation could diminish the
unpleasant smells wafting into adjacent departments, noise was harder
to manage. In the University of Nebraska's 1913 medical college, the dogs
barking in the basement irritated at least one person attempting to work
upstairs.[129]

Housing animals in the medical school may have been less pleasant
for the building's human occupants, but medical educators promised
that the facilities offered humane accommodations in terms similar to
those applied to separate structures. The physiology department at the
University of Michigan's medical school cared for its animals on a top
floor where it had rooms for rats, birds, and rabbits, with dog runs on
the adjacent roof (fig. 4.12). For dog noise, the roof seems to have worked
better than the basement, although the professor of physiology's review

of the situation's acoustics was somewhat tepid: "There is relatively little noise and this is reflected skyward fairly well by the high encircling parapet." The professor emphasized the provisions for dogs, which occupied most of the space. Dogs received particular attention from the antivivisectionists, which may also account for the physiologist's affirmation of the department's respect for the canine: "Mindful of the fine traits of this animal and his sensitive nature we have attempted to make him as comfortable as our means would permit." He described the dog runs, indoor rooms, heating, and ventilation. He reported no deaths from dogfights but enough communication between animals to relieve the dogs' monotony. Despite the author's intentions, however, the text hints at the harsh realities of animal experimentation.[130]

Housing Anatomy and "Much That Is Grim and Unpleasant"

Unlike the members of other esteemed professions, such as law or theology, physicians in training engaged in activities that some in the public found objectionable. Not just animal experimentation but human dissection as well could fuel the disapproval of the nonmedical community. Awareness of the discomfort with dissection impacted a building's circulation, as well as the location and glazing of the gross anatomy laboratory.

Historian Michael Sappol has examined the complicated history of anatomy in the United States in the nineteenth century. Sappol contends that medicine's identification with anatomy allowed the profession to adopt the prestige of the most developed of the European medical sciences and to separate itself from its competitors, including clergy, midwives, and lay healers. Outrage over body snatching plagued the profession, however, especially as the number of medical schools burgeoned between 1865 and 1890 and the demand for cadavers grew rapidly. Bolstered by the rising cultural authority of scientific medicine, anatomists in this period rededicated themselves to gaining support from the public and political leaders for anatomy legislation. By 1913, all but four states with medical schools had laws that enabled medical colleges to obtain the corpses of the indigent. According to Sappol, "Body-snatching scandals disappeared from the front pages. Anatomical dissection, so fiercely contested for much of the eighteenth and nineteenth centuries, was made invisible, regularized. And so it remains today." And yet this narrative of professional authority and public opposition is challenged by the proliferation of "popular anatomy," which included the instruction of anatomy in public schools, anatomical books, lectures, and museums that targeted a nonmedical audience, as well as the sensationalist material of the penny press, dime novels, magazines, and minstrel shows. In fact, the boundaries between professional and popular anatomy were fluid. Medical faculty themselves offered anatomical lectures for the public that frequently even involved the dissection of animals and humans. In the end, both the privileged practice of anatomy within the medical college and the public experience of anatomy promoted the cultural authority of the medical profession and the physician's position within the hierarchy of medical knowledge. The many physicians of the mid-nineteenth century who decorated their offices with skeletons, memento mori, or anatomy charts and books implicitly made this claim.[131]

In the early twentieth century, the faculty of reformed medical schools understood both the public's fascination with and its aversion to anatomy, but the facilities they helped to design strove to minimize anatomy's visibility. In an exception that proves the rule about discretion regarding anatomical instruction in the modern medical college, Harvard Medical School's Warren Anatomical Museum, magnificently housed in Building A at the head of the 1906 quadrangle, did welcome members of the public (see fig. 1.24). A 1908 description of the museum explains, "As the Museum is open all day, it is visited by people of all classes as well as our own students, and, although not generally advertised, it is surprising to find how many from outside visit it."[132] Despite its academic focus, the museum catered in part to its lay clientele: "While the primary use is for the student, large guide labels enable the casual visitor to readily find his way about and understand the general arrangement."[133] Moreover, the visitor could reach the museum fairly easily by ascending the central stairway from the building's entrance hall to the third floor.

Harvard's unusual museum likely stemmed from several causes. These factors included the prestige of the medical school's holdings; the collection's connection to John Collins Warren (1778–1857), a member of a venerable Boston medical family; the museum's established position within the medical school (by 1906 it enjoyed an endowment for maintenance of the collection and an endowed curatorship); and the interest at the time of the quadrangle's construction in using the museum for public education, although it is not clear that this goal was realized beyond admitting the community to the museum.[134] Only rarely, however, did schools include massive exhibition spaces for their teaching collections or accommodate laypersons by providing relatively direct access from the entrance to the museum.

In contrast, virtually every medical college building rendered dissection nearly invisible to the visitor or passerby, continuing an element of medical school construction from before medical education reform.

Johns Hopkins Medical School professor Franklin P. Mall reported that medical colleges in the nineteenth century often used the top floor for anatomy, and he maintained this practice in the 1894 Women's Fund Memorial Building. The skylights made possible by this location allowed for brighter rooms.[135] In addition, diffuse overhead light better illuminated the cadaver than windows along the wall. Anatomy laboratories on the top floor also likely enjoyed better access to prevailing breezes via the windows that punctuated the walls than laboratories on lower floors, a benefit for the famously malodorous practice of dissection. Even more, the top floor offered privacy from members of the public who might look through the windows, and it provided distance from possible mobs on the streets below.

Almost all medical schools in the late eighteenth and early nineteenth century experienced some form of anatomy-related violence incited by anger over the grave robbery used to procure bodies for dissection. In 1852, the final major riot against an American medical college, in this case a homeopathic school, occurred.[136] However, relatively small acts of violence continued to take place. J. Collins Warren, Harvard Medical School class of 1866, described the attack he experienced as a student and reveals the danger of a first-floor anatomy room:

> The class in dissecting was often held in the evening in the little one-story dissecting room at the foot of the western wall of the building on North Grove Street. In the daytime it was lighted by a skylight. The character of this wing was well known to the hoodlum element of the neighborhood, and at night, when work was going on there, the light always shone brightly through the roof. One evening while we were absorbed in class work, a brickbat crashed through the glass. [Demonstrator of anatomy] Dr. Cheever's equanimity did not forsake him, but calmly looking upwards and then down at us he said, 'Up, guards, and at them!' We needed no further urging and sallied forth *en masse* to drive off the intruders.[137]

Not surprisingly, Harvard Medical School's next home, the 1883 facility on Boylston Street, housed anatomy on the building's top floor. Increasingly, though, for members of reformed medical schools, violent attacks by the public persisted only as memories from a bygone era, and some faculty involved in constructing modern buildings chose to move the gross anatomy laboratory down from the rafters.

Improvements in artificial lighting and ventilation undoubtedly contributed to this change. Shortly before the completion of Howard University's 1927 medical school, architect Albert Cassell described the

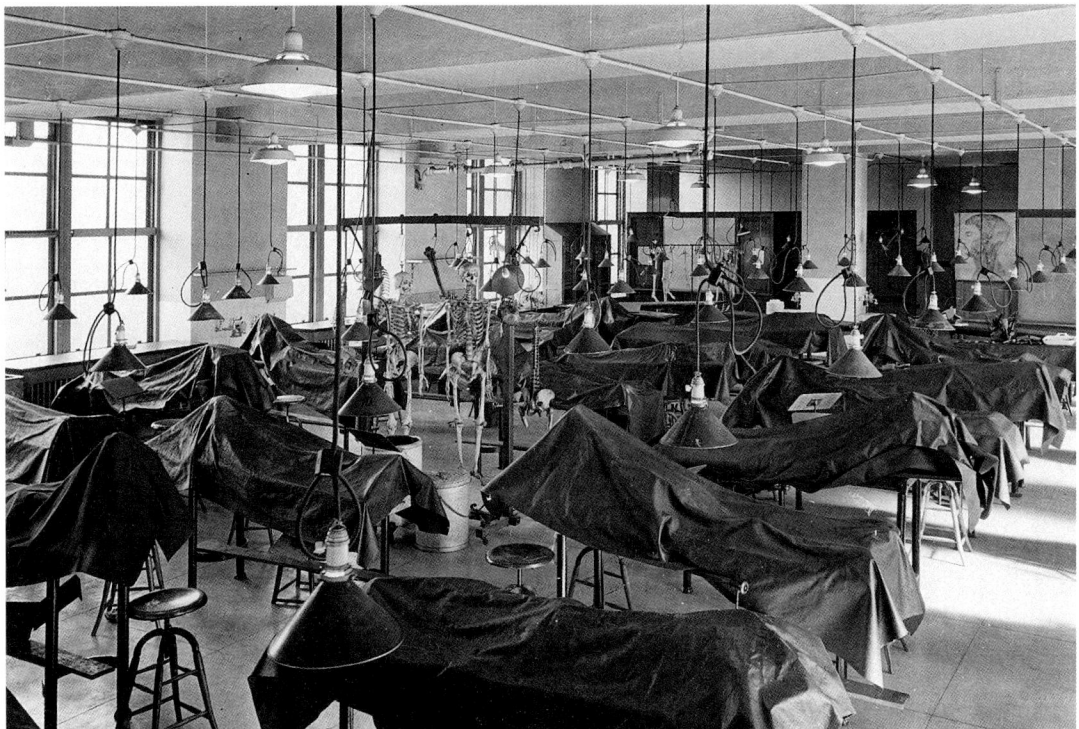

4.13.   New York Hospital–Cornell Medical College, 1932, Coolidge, Shepley, Bulfinch, and Abbott,
         architects, gross anatomy laboratory with overhead lamps hanging just above most of the dissecting
         tables. Photograph ca. 1932–1939.

system that would provide each dissecting table in a ground-floor laboratory with multiple forms of overhead light. The room was to be wired
such that "goose-neck table lamps . . . [could] be attached to the edge of
the table by a thumb screw clamp." Additionally, above each table seven
and a half feet from the floor would hang "two nitrogen lamps with
x-ray shades" (fig. 4.13). As for ventilation, the laboratory's "floor [will
be] spotted with mushroom ventilators of sufficient exhaust capacity
to remove all odors at the source of their origin and it will be possible
to effect a total change of the air in this area once during every eight
minutes."[138] A floor system of ventilation may have functioned particularly well since formaldehyde had replaced heavy metal salts and become
the preferred chemical for embalming human cadavers by approximately
1906–1910.[139] At room temperature, formaldehyde is a gas that weighs
slightly more than air. With formaldehyde accumulating near the floor,
venting the room from this location would have been efficient and likely
also more effective.

        If requirements of light, ventilation, and safety no longer necessitated

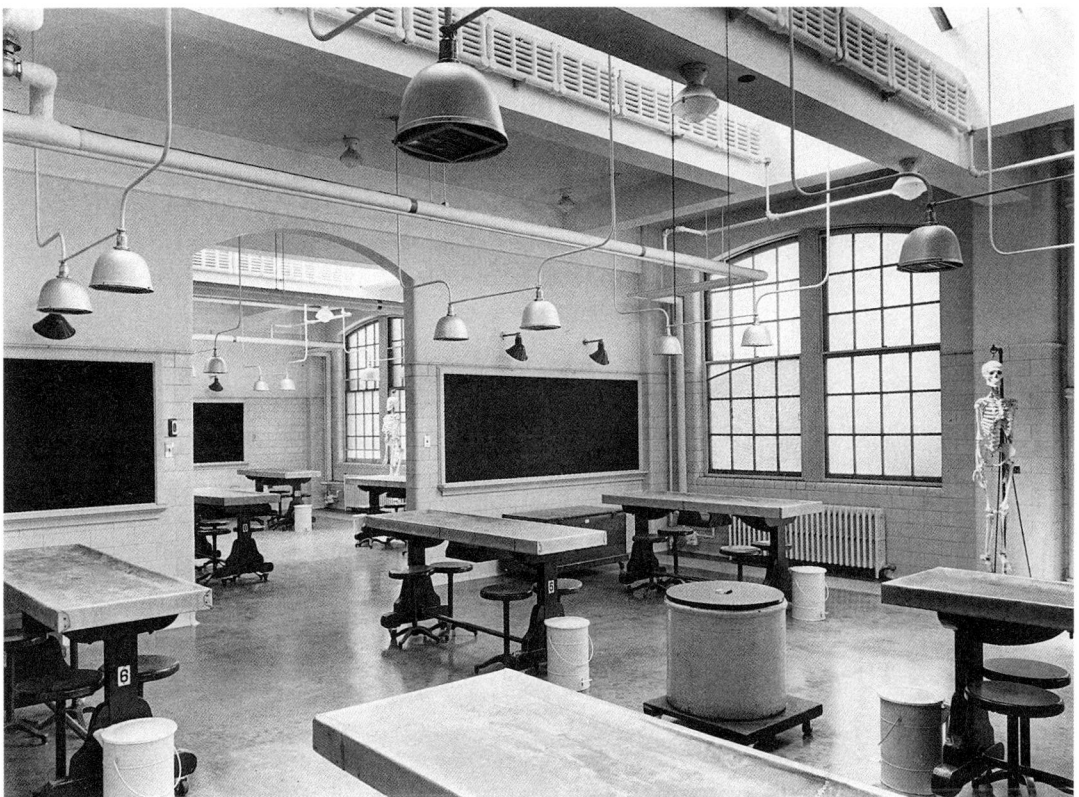

4.14.   Syracuse University College of Medicine, 1937, Baum and Pope, architects, gross anatomy laboratory.

placing the laboratory for dissection directly under the roof, then a logical place for it was the ground floor, where cadavers were not only received but also typically embalmed and stored. Syracuse University College of Medicine made this choice, although it managed to achieve the best of both the top- and ground-floor locations. The dissecting rooms occupied a single-story extension off of the main building, which enabled the anatomy laboratories to have skylights while sitting near the cadaver receiving, embalming, and storage sites on the ground floor (fig. 4.14).

As the Syracuse example suggests, artificial illumination did not eliminate anatomists' dedication to natural light. At Columbia-Presbyterian Medical Center, the faculty decided not to locate the anatomy department on the top floor but to keep it higher rather than lower in the tall building to improve access to light for dissection.[140] Similarly, at Woman's Medical College of Pennsylvania, dissection took place on the fourth of the building's five stories.

Grave robbery may have substantially decreased by 1913 and all but ended by 1930, but even as the public's outrage over body snatching

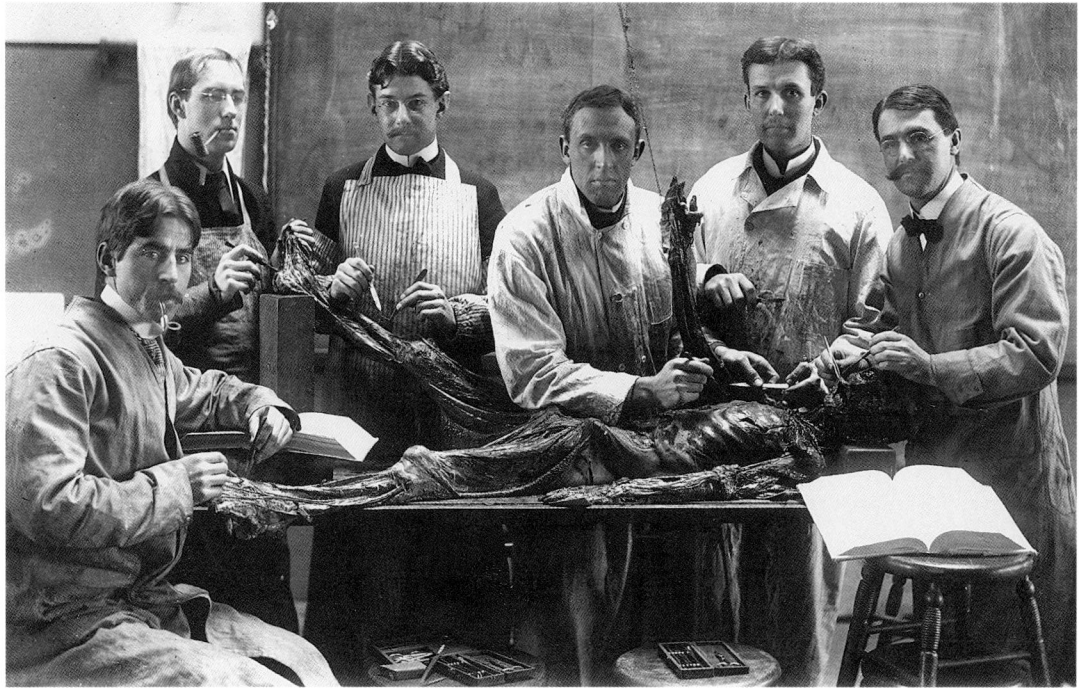

4.15.   Students at dissecting table, Yale University School of Medicine, ca. 1910.

diminished, some laypersons remained uncomfortable with dissection.[141]
This ongoing uneasiness likely stemmed from the engagement with
death represented by the cadaver and the failure of dissection to respect
the body of the deceased in accordance with long-standing customs of
the nonmedical community.[142] Historian John Harley Warner explains
that a "culture of secrecy" encircled dissection in the nineteenth and early
twentieth centuries, a reality that makes the proliferation of dissecting
room photographs beginning in the 1880s all the more surprising. In
addition, although the study of anatomy, the oldest of the basic medical
sciences, was fading from prominence by the late nineteenth century in
the face of recently established laboratory fields, the dissecting room
portrait became probably the most typical group photographic depiction
of medical students at work. The portraits showcased students of every
demographic and remained commonplace into the 1920s. In a photograph taken around 1910 at Yale University School of Medicine, six men
surround a cadaver; open instrument cases and anatomy books, objects
that mark the undertaking as one of science rather than butchery, appear prominently in the scene (fig. 4.15; see also fig. 1.12 and dissection
image on cover). Warner demonstrates that, although a more complete
reading of the photographs requires careful attention to race, gender,

class, power, and violence, the portraits primarily recorded the dissectors' transition from laypersons to physicians. Posed in environments that the nonmedical community might consider shocking and gruesome, the dissectors frequently seem determined not to convey emotion and instead to present the detachment expected by the 1880s in laboratories in general. The photographs themselves fail to reveal whether this demeanor was, according to Warner, "deliberate self-restraint or the outward signs of a hard-won inner transformation in character," but students' diaries and letters suggest the accuracy of both assessments. While these images did have some circulation outside the medical community, Warner argues that they were "not the public face of modern medicine."[143]

If students and physicians did not widely distribute dissection room photographs among laypersons, neither did educators and architects want dissection to be easily visible at the medical school. The discomfort some members of the public felt about dissection inflected assessments of school buildings. When an osteopathic medical school opened in 1895, a reporter sensationally referred to the attic dissecting room as the "chamber of horrors," even as he lauded the structure overall and noted that "within and without, [it] gives the impression of beauty, convenience, and stability."[144]

Not surprisingly, when the anatomy department had space on the ground floor, shielding dissection from passersby who might look through the windows remained a concern. The anatomy department at Vanderbilt University School of Medicine did occupy the first (ground) floor of one side of the medical school court (see fig. 2.14). Opaque glass concealed the activities within the laboratories, and when dissectors wanted ventilation, they lowered an upper section of the window rather than opening the bottom portion, thus maintaining the visual barrier. Similarly, opaque glass in the windows along the walls of Syracuse University College of Medicine's dissecting area ensured that no one outside inadvertently viewed the cadavers (see fig. 4.14).

The desire for discretion further required that the arrival of anatomical material remain a private affair, so medical schools included a separate entrance for cadavers. Some architects also found ways to screen the entrance area. At Vanderbilt's medical school–hospital, a porch shielded the movement of anatomical material from vehicle to door (see fig. 2.14). The Women's Fund Memorial Building at Johns Hopkins Medical School had an internal driveway that brought anatomical material directly into the building (see fig. 1.13). Similarly, at Washington University School of Medicine, a vehicle could enter the small L-shaped structure in the courtyard behind the building housing the anatomy department (see fig. 2.8). From here, an elevator took the body down to

a tunnel that connected with the embalming rooms in the basement of
the anatomy building.[145] Other schools devised simpler arrangements;
a University of Nebraska College of Medicine student reported that "a
row of trees was discretely [sic] placed on the street side of the driveway
to hide the transfer of the bodies from the neighbors."[146]

Within buildings, faculty and their assistants also worked to move
anatomical material as unobtrusively as possible. The design of Vanderbilt University's medical school–hospital ensured that the cadavers
remained in one wing, where they were received, embalmed, stored,
and dissected. A passage immediately adjacent to the cadaver entrance
provided access to the embalming and storage areas without the use of
the main hallway (see fig. 2.14). Not all designs resulted in the same
level of inconspicuousness for cadavers, however. At Syracuse University
College of Medicine, the cadavers never left the basement, but to reach
the cadaver storage area from the receiving, embalming, and dissecting
wing required transfer past the locker rooms for male and female help,
the lounge and locker room for women students, the locker room for men
students, a classroom, and an office.

Schools with dissection on an upper floor faced the challenge of
transporting cadavers to the top of the building. W. Montague Cobb,
Howard University medical class of 1929, described the situation at Howard before its new medical school opened in 1927: "Each one [cadaver]
had to be hauled up the five floors by hand pulley through the stairwell.
This work was done by the janitor and whoever he could get to help
him. Naturally, there were few eager volunteers."[147] In contrast, modern
buildings at the very least had elevators, and they sometimes included
an extra elevator in the anatomy wing that allowed cadavers to be moved
with greater privacy. At Woman's Medical College of Pennsylvania, a
freight elevator connected the receiving, embalming, and storage space
in the basement directly with the anatomy department on the fourth
floor.[148] The University of Colorado School of Medicine reserved one elevator for the unobtrusive transfer of two potentially distressing laboratory
requirements: animals and cadavers.[149] Circumspection thus dominated
progressive medical school design in an attempt to ensure that no one
accidentally viewed a cadaver in transit or during dissection.

Medical schools promoted not only the accomplishments and aspirations of medical education but also the uncomfortable elements. In
his 1906 article about the Harvard Medical School, journalist Ralph
Bergengren expressed a sentiment that, if not directly from the medical
educators, certainly would have been endorsed by them: "The anatomy
and histology building must necessarily provide much that is grim and

unpleasant to the general reader except as he realizes that it is only by the path of dissection that the physician or surgeon can reach the knowledge that has made his profession noble and supremely necessary to human existence; the study of disease in living animals, leading as it already has, to medical discoveries that have ameliorated the condition of thousands of human beings, is another necessity of medical instruction that must here be given the best, and therefore the most humane, environment."[150] Educators and architects knew that the animal quarters and dissecting rooms would attract particular attention. They worked to create facilities that encouraged humane and unobtrusive housing of animals and discreet dissection in order to soothe the anxieties some members of the public felt about medical training and the laboratory practices it involved.

The Success of School Buildings as Marketing Agents

As donors, large numbers of laypersons, state legislatures, and later the federal government embraced modern medical education, it developed into an entrenched and well-funded enterprise. Buildings participated in this shift and proved to be a good investment. Not only did they make possible the schools' redesigned curriculum, but they also represented a primarily positive force in the marketing of reformed medical training.

As medical leaders no doubt hoped they would, newspapers celebrated the facilities and the scientific medicine and education they represented. In his investigation of images of medical achievements in the mass media, Bert Hansen has described the coverage of the first structure for the Rockefeller Institute for Medical Research (RIMR) (see fig. 3.25): "A photograph of the RIMR's new building opened a general article in the *American Review of Reviews* about the institute's activity. As with the [New York] Pasteur Institute building erected in the prior decade, the substantial and expensive edifice was an important symbol of the magnitude and permanence of the investment in the experimental laboratories housed therein. But what the public saw was not limited to exteriors. In some magazines, readers were invited to look inside the laboratories and view technicians at work."[151] Similarly, newspaper coverage of medical schools often included an image of the building's exterior, itself a commanding visual statement about the medical community's, donors', and state legislatures' commitment to the transformed training. In some cases, the articles took readers inside the structure as well. The Sunday before the November 1937 dedication of Syracuse University's medical college, readers of the *Syracuse Herald* encountered several photographs of the facility. In addition to the building's exterior, readers observed the library (the same image as fig. 2.5); the technician's room, where "members of the faculty and graduate students are given expert assistance in their research problems"; and a scene of students "busy on experiments in physiology."[152] Medical schools capitalized on and encouraged the media's attention.

Donors also enjoyed the recognition that came with the press's coverage of the buildings. The *New York Times* lauded the Columbia-Presbyterian Medical Center as the "largest and most modern in the world" and a "great scientific project," and it listed the undertaking's major patrons.[153] For the General Education Board, the complementary associations between the buildings and its gifts may have been particularly welcome. Critics questioned the intentions of the Rockefeller foundations and argued that the GEB wielded too much control over medical education.[154] But the GEB's contributions to medical school construction were applauded.

As we know, beyond the media reports the construction of a medical school itself stimulated regional interest, and visitors came in droves to mark the progress on the building. Mary S. Hoffschwelle has discussed how cornerstone and dedication ceremonies for Rosenwald schools (schools for African American children paid for by Julius Rosenwald Fund grants, local donations, and state money) showcased community pride and enthusiasm for the projects.[155] Similarly, positive descriptions in the hometown newspaper and the turnout at medical school construction events underscored the neighboring population's identification with and excitement for the medical colleges.

Medical school leadership recognized that buildings also helped to recruit faculty and students. Prominent medical educator G. Canby Robinson affirmed that research space in particular appealed to potential faculty: "The best teachers demand facilities, time and assistants in order that they may constantly pursue scientific investigations."[156] The faculty at Western Reserve University School of Medicine feared that other schools in the region with more up to date buildings would lure prospective students away from their college: "Students and the profession at large should judge a school by the personnel of the teaching staff[,] but they all too often base opinions upon physical equipment. One of our near competitors, the University of Pittsburgh[,] has more modern buildings. Another, the University of Cincinnati, has buildings of international fame. The recent endowment of the University of Rochester, N.Y., will provide modern buildings and staff which may well attract students from our field."[157]

The concerns of the Western Reserve medical faculty were justified. By students' own accounts, buildings did shape their decisions to attend a school. Walter F. Riker Jr. described his first time seeing New York Hospital–Cornell Medical College: "In 1934, while driving into Manhattan with my father, he suddenly detoured from his usual midtown route, saying 'I want to show you a beautiful new hospital that is associated with Cornell. This is where you ought to think about going to medical school.' As we approached, I was struck by the sight of the spectacular gleaming white buildings rising skyward. The magnificence of its neo-gothic architecture not only enhanced its beauty but endowed it with a façade that made the overall structure unique. One would hardly think it a hospital but more suggestive of a cathedral."[158] Riker graduated from Cornell Medical College nine years later.

Students did not have to see the schools in person to feel awestruck. Images of medical colleges could have a similar effect. Alice Baker, a student at Louisiana State University School of Medicine, wrote in 1937 to her future husband, Joe Holoubek, at the University of Nebraska College of Medicine on paper that included a view of her medical school. He responded with admiration: "I cannot match stationery with you—and what a medical center you must have. I hope to see it someday. What a grand building."[159] From the image of the school, Holoubek extrapolated that the medical center—the conglomerate of school and teaching hospital(s)—must also be exceptional.

In the opening decades of the twentieth century, postcards were ubiquitous. Postcards of medical colleges distributed images of the schools and likely impressed recipients. Architectural historian Paula Lupkin has examined YMCA postcards. She explains that the 1893 World's Columbian Exposition in Chicago popularized postcards in the United States, and more than 770 million postcards were sold in 1906 alone. Local promoters, news groups, national companies, and even the YMCA published postcards. Often generated in series, postcards exhaustively documented the institutions, houses, streets, parks, and special events of a city or town. More than a record of travels, postcards provided a rapid, inexpensive, and easy form of correspondence employed by many types of people. In addition, collectors would save postcards in scrapbooks and mail cards depicting their hometown to numerous pen pals. Drawing on the work of Alison Isenberg, Lupkin notes that postcards offered the opportunity to encourage the ideal representation of a community. Lupkin also asserts that postcards influenced widespread ideas about the YMCA and promoted the institution.[160]

The growing appetite for postcards in the years following 1893 coincided with the reform of medical education and the rebuilding of medical schools. Publishers frequently made postcards of the recently constructed medical colleges, which represented significant additions to the urban fabric. In fact, medical schools of all reputations, from Harvard Medical School and Columbia-Presbyterian Medical Center to Meharry Medical College and the University of Nebraska College of Medicine, appeared on postcards (see fig. 3.9). The creation of postcards of nearly every medical college suggests that the public's enthusiasm for these schools—at least as it was perceived by postcard publishers—had little, if anything, to do with the institution's standing among medical colleges.

Some people with the interest and means, predominantly physicians and medical educators, were not content with a postcard of a medical school; they traveled to see it. After the opening of Western Reserve University School of Medicine's 1924 facility, the dean proudly reported, "Numerous visitors from various parts of the United States and from foreign countries have expressed a high appreciation and admiration of the New Buildings."[161] Carl J. Wiggers, professor of physiology, concurred: "The sincere remarks of visitors leave no doubt that we are making an impression in medical circles."[162] Wiggers detailed the widespread enthusiasm for the structure among the medical community: "The interest shown by the Rockefeller Foundation in inviting 'write-ups' of various departments [for *Methods and Problems of Medical Education*], the fact that this school has lately been the subject of discussion for a considerable part of an evening at a Council Meeting of the Society for Experimental Biology and Medicine in New York, the remarks of scientists at meetings, 'Well, I hear wonderful stories of your new laboratory building and the work being done there'—all are evidence that the Medical School has suddenly risen in the esteem of medical and scientific men."[163] An up-to-date edifice could improve the reputation of a medical college.

In many senses, medical school buildings successfully endorsed reformed medical education, but a closer look reveals the limits of architecture to change a medical school's trajectory. The 1937 facility for Syracuse University College of Medicine and the 1930 structure for Woman's Medical College of Pennsylvania provided the enlarged and upgraded buildings the schools desperately needed to remain abreast of the growing requirements for medical education. But both also left the colleges, which had long struggled to find donors of significant means, saddled with debt. In the case of Syracuse's medical college, the loan undertaken during the construction of its 1937 structure likely contributed to the university's desire in the late 1940s to shed its expensive medical school with its outstanding debts. In 1950, Syracuse University transferred the medical college to the State University of New York (SUNY).[164]

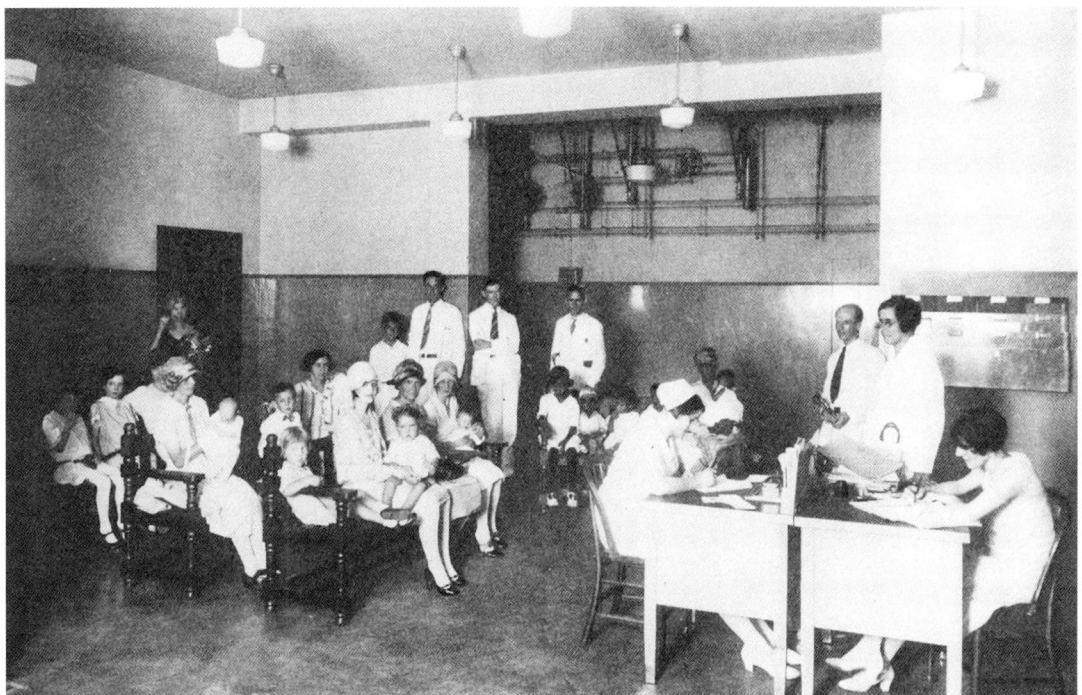

4.16.   Vanderbilt University School of Medicine and Hospital, 1925, Coolidge and Shattuck, architects,
          pediatrics waiting room. Photograph ca. 1929. White women and children sit in the center of the room
          while a Black woman and children sit in the alcove of a terminal for the Lamson carrier system, a
          noisy and temperamental belt and pulley apparatus for transporting patient records.

    Similarly, Meharry Medical College's modern educational and clini-
cal facility in North Nashville could not itself fuel sufficient trust among
the Black community to fill the school's wards and clinics. Historian
Darlene Clark Hine describes African American residents' assessment
of Meharry before 1921, when Meharry's Hubbard Hospital, still located
in South Nashville, closed each summer due to inadequate funds: "Perhaps its limited operating period was a blessing in disguise; such a cloud
of incompetence, suspicion, and lack of confidence hung over Meharry
and Hubbard that blacks in Nashville suffered the indignities accompanying requests for medical treatment at the segregated white hospitals
rather than risk their . . . lives . . . at Hubbard 'for the colored.'"[165] As
time passed, African American Nashvillians saw little reason to change
their opinion of Meharry, and they continued seeking medical care at
the hospitals serving white residents despite the degrading experience
(fig. 4.16). During his constant fundraising efforts, John J. Mullowney,
Meharry's president from 1921 to 1938, expressed publicly his racist views
of African Americans. After the school's 1931 move to North Nashville,

Mullowney's prejudice further diminished Meharry in the eyes of its African American neighbors, many of whom remained frustrated by the institution's displacement of numerous Black homeowners. African American Nashvillians so frequently chose the facilities for white residents, at City Hospital and Vanderbilt University Hospital, for their medical care that Meharry's recently completed hospital functioned at just an estimated 50 percent capacity.[166] In 1937, six years after Meharry moved to its in North Nashville location, Edward L. Turner, who would become Meharry's president the following year, commented, "It is going to be a very long pull to build up confidence in the Negro public as well as in the Negro practitioner here," and he noted that he "was not surprised that Negroes prefer the white hospitals when I watch some of our clinical staff."[167] Meharry's 1931 facility may have been a definite improvement over its previous home, but many other factors kept significant numbers of Black Nashvillians from choosing Meharry's hospital and outpatient department.

———————

By the 1930s, educators, architects, donors, and laypersons generally expected medical education to take place in noteworthy facilities. In 1939, Augusta Tucker published her novel *Miss Susie Slagle's*, about a Baltimore boardinghouse and the group of Johns Hopkins medical students who lived there between 1912 and 1916. The carefully researched work that became a best-seller describes the students' surprise when they encounter for the first time the relatively unadorned and aging structures of the renowned Johns Hopkins Medical School, whose buildings ranged from seven to eighteen years old in 1912 (see fig. 1.6): "In the sharp features of Elbert Riggs there was a sudden flicker of disappointment. Were these boxy old buildings the famous Johns Hopkins Medical School? These old red brick piles! They couldn't touch the University of Pennsylvania. Clay Abernathy had a similar reaction. The State University in West Virginia still smelled of new paint, had a view, looked the part."[168] Clearly medical colleges did not need marble exteriors or Gothic revival exuberance to be a top-tier institution, but most medical faculty wanted a building that would distinguish itself among medical schools and within the urban landscape. Faculty leaders strove to have the grandest buildings possible given constraints of money and sometimes donors; Eastman's and Flexner's aversion to ornament comes to mind. Educators and many benefactors, however, desired medical schools that would architecturally impress so that they might reflect with particular favor on the transformed medical profession and its financial backers.

Although the number of medical schools decreased in the reform era, the size of the buildings and their visibility increased. Not only were modern medical schools much larger than their proprietary counterparts, but they also functioned as cornerstones of prominent new campuses—sometimes part of and sometimes separate from the university—composed of medical college and teaching hospital(s) and encapsulated in the phrase "medical center" that came into use at the end of the 1920s. Other types of practitioners, including traditional healers such as midwives and members of medical sects such as osteopaths and homeopaths, may have felt the expanded physical presence of "regular" medicine particularly strongly.

The buildings of reformed medical colleges both grew out of and encouraged the rising cultural authority of physicians. Faculties responded to the urban environment when planning their campuses, but they also shaped the city, an action that itself marked the power of the profession's authority. Educators, however, did not assume that laypersons would support the redesigned medical training, the science upon which it was based, or the individuals who championed it, and they recognized that the public encapsulated a diversity of opinions and perspectives. Some observers protested animal experimentation, while others remained concerned about dissection. Some welcomed a medical school to their neighborhood, while others resisted its presence. In the end, educators used the buildings to court the nonmedical community with its varied factions, and when laypersons experienced the structures in person or in print, they encountered facilities designed to celebrate medical education, the laboratory science that underpinned it, and the physicians who embraced it.

5

CONSTRUCTING
A PROFESSION

Cohesion and Hierarchy in the Medical School

MEDICAL EDUCATION ONE HUNDRED YEARS AGO, LIKE MEDICAL training in the early twenty-first century, developed professional character in addition to laboratory and clinical knowledge. Medical school leaders in the opening decades of the twentieth century strove to inculcate in their students the identity of a respected modern medical doctor, and they utilized the schools' buildings in advancing this goal. The buildings, however, reveal a dual reality for the students and faculty. At the same time that the structures encouraged a unified, privileged professional consciousness, they also advanced hierarchies among physicians.

In its examination of foundation support for medical schools, chapter 3 argued that paucity of funding coupled with expectations about race and gender resulted in Howard University College of Medicine, Meharry Medical College, and Woman's Medical College of Pennsylvania having little in the way of research facilities. As research became an increasingly influential barometer of medical school prestige, the coeducational Black medical colleges and the women's school enrolling mostly white students fell behind the elite schools predominantly composed of white men and reinforced the differentiation of physicians based on race and sex. This chapter expands the discussion of disparities within the profession and introduces external hierarchies between physicians and other medical fields, specifically nurses, dentists, and pharmacists. Medical school buildings contributed to the creation of this complex professional identity.

Uniting Physicians around a Privileged Professional Consciousness

Medical schools, like other educational and laboratory spaces, fostered collective identity.[1] Even if experiences were mixed, the time spent in training with classmates, friends, professors, and mentors generated powerful associations and a sense of communal history. As the literal stage for these interactions and an agent constantly molding daily life, the buildings themselves and their features—from a leaky laboratory roof to open porches used for smoking breaks—often held a prominent place in students' descriptions and, later, their memories of medical school.[2] When recounting their student years, alumni to this day continue to share anecdotes about the buildings and their physical experiences within them, recalling the frustration of slow elevators, the odor of the anatomy laboratory (despite all attempts at adequate ventilation), and the fixed-arm desks too small to accommodate pregnant students' bodies. Experiences like these that were specific to a particular time and place connected students to alma mater more than to profession.

In other ways, however, the buildings and campuses cultivated students' commitment to the profession in addition to the school. The facilities were the local manifestation of a relatively standardized national educational program. Regardless of where one studied, for example, all physicians experienced the rite of passage of gross anatomy. Medical historian Michael Sappol singles out dissection as "*the* ritual that inducted young men into the cult of medical knowledge."[3] When students entered the anatomy laboratory in the first half of the twentieth century, not only did they increasingly conform to elevated standards of professional behavior, but they also participated in a type of training reserved for physicians and few others. Dissection could not take place under modern conditions without a specially designed and maintained laboratory, and this space became inseparable from students' initiation into the ranks of medical doctors. When the University of Nebraska's medical college opened in 1913, a student reporter for the school newspaper provided a firsthand account of the anatomy laboratory and particularly its improved smell, albeit with tongue firmly in cheek:

> The anatomy laboratory has always been the piece de resistance for trembling curious visitors. But alas this is no more. The old atmosphere of ghoulish mystery has given place to one of culture and refinement. The very smell

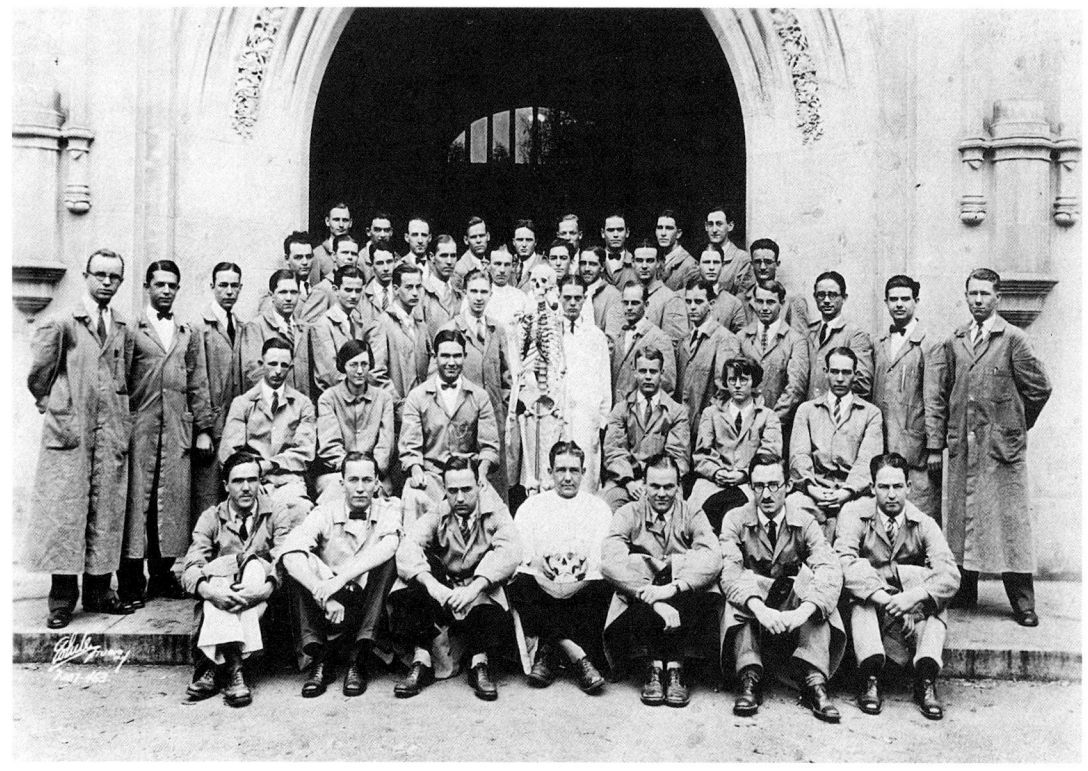

5.1.   First-year medical students, Vanderbilt University, 1925.

has changed, and where we formerly breathed the pestilential odor of formaldehyde and carbolic acid the place is now heavy with the incense of rare
and costly perfumes. In an interview with the Pulse reporter[,] Dr. Poynter
[professor of anatomy] stated that an immense quantity of attar of roses had
just been received and would be used on the next group of subjects, by way of
giving variety to the incense.[4]

If the portraits of medical students at the dissecting table underscored the significance of gross anatomy in transforming laypersons
into physicians, perhaps nowhere was the identification of student with
facility clearer than in the many class photographs taken on the stairs
of North American medical schools. Architectural historian Annmarie
Adams has described this trend. She notes that the tiered stairs allowed
each person's face to be visible. In the case of McGill University's 1911
Strathcona Building, the Asclepius symbol—the snake encircling a staff
associated with the Greek god of healing—adorned the railings and affirmed the students' place within the medical profession.[5] When included
in the composition of the photograph, the inscriptions frequently carved

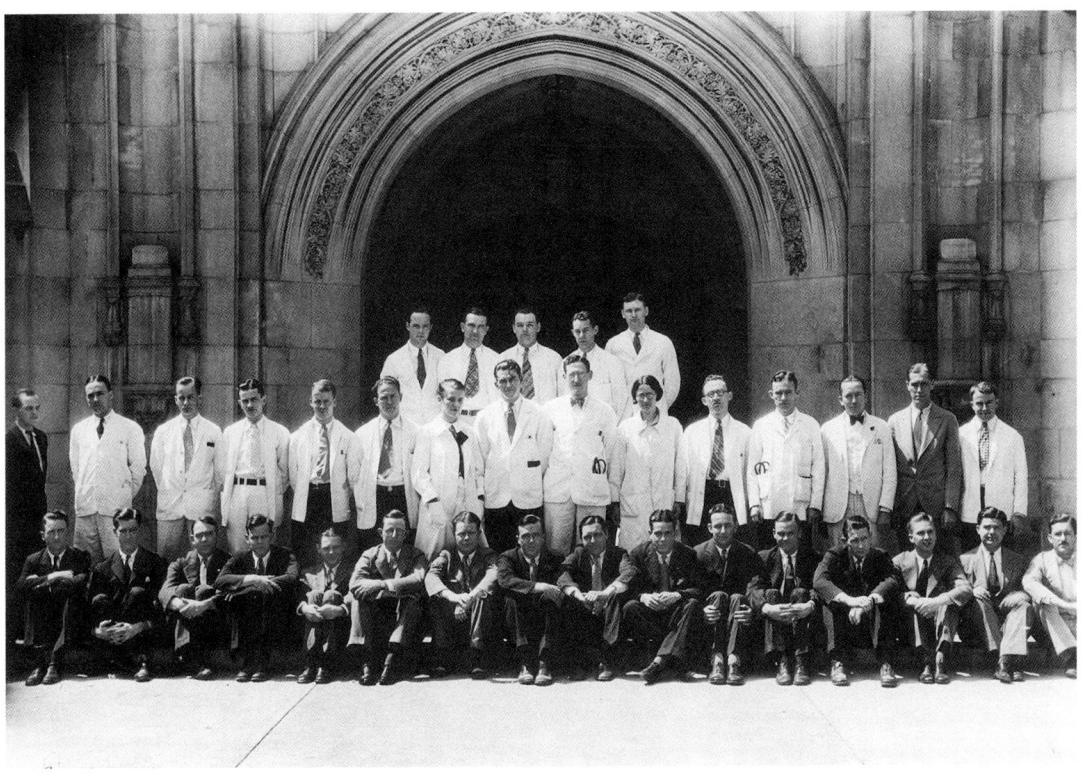

5.2.   Fourth-year medical students, Vanderbilt University, 1929.

above the schools' doorways would have similarly confirmed the group's
professional identity. At Vanderbilt University, the medical school entrance was a favored spot for photographing faculty, house staff, and
medical students (see fig. 2.18).[6] A photograph of Vanderbilt's incoming
medical class of 1925, the year the medical school–hospital opened, shows
forty-four men and two women—the college's first female medical students—on the school's steps (fig. 5.1). Here the young people continue
the student tradition of taking their photograph with skeleton and skull
and lacing the composition with a dose of dark humor: the skeleton
smokes a pipe and is posed in a standing position, as if it is just another
medical student.[7] The skeleton, skull, and gray laboratory coats worn in
the dissecting room clearly mark the men and women as physicians in
training. Four years later, the students returned to the steps for another
photograph on the eve of their graduation (fig. 5.2). With anatomy long
past, half now wear the white apparel of clinical clerks, and stethoscopes
protrude from some pockets. Ready to embark on their medical careers,
they present a serious face to the camera.[8] Although a seemingly passive backdrop and identifier in these photographs, the buildings were

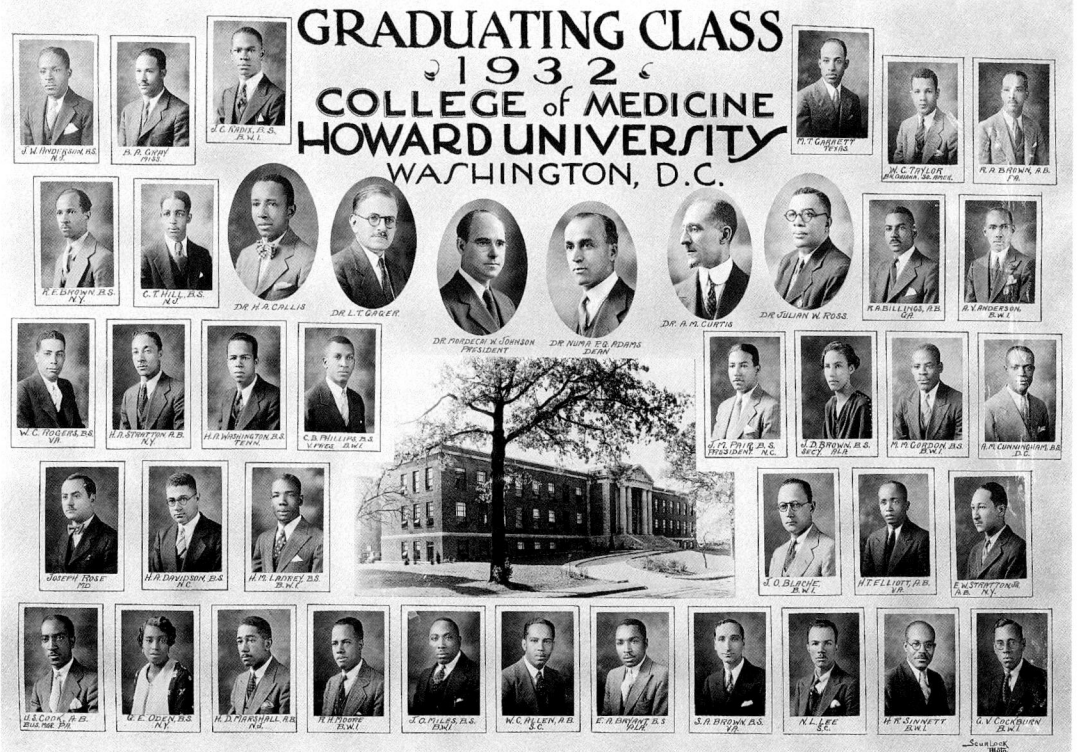

5.3.   Medical class photograph, Howard University, 1932.

synonymous with alma mater and medical training for the students. Even in class pictures in which students appeared individually rather than collectively, the building featured prominently at some schools (fig. 5.3).

Medical school gathering areas also connected students to alma mater and profession. Alumni rooms, boardrooms, libraries, and sitting rooms often contained portraits of previous generations of physicians. When Columbia-Presbyterian Medical Center opened, Frederick van Beuren, a medical school associate dean who was also an alumnus, oversaw the furnishing of an alumni visitors' "lounging room" that included "a large number of oil portraits of prominent graduates" (fig. 5.4).[9] Portraits of two former faculty members hung in the library of Vanderbilt University's medical school–hospital, while three portraits of alumnae who were also outstanding faculty members lined the boardroom at Woman's Medical College of Pennsylvania.[10] These portraits typically commemorated someone who had an association with the medical college, but some of these people, especially the alumni, presumably earned their recognition for work done elsewhere. These portraits celebrated the history of both the college and the profession. Portraits of prominent physicians

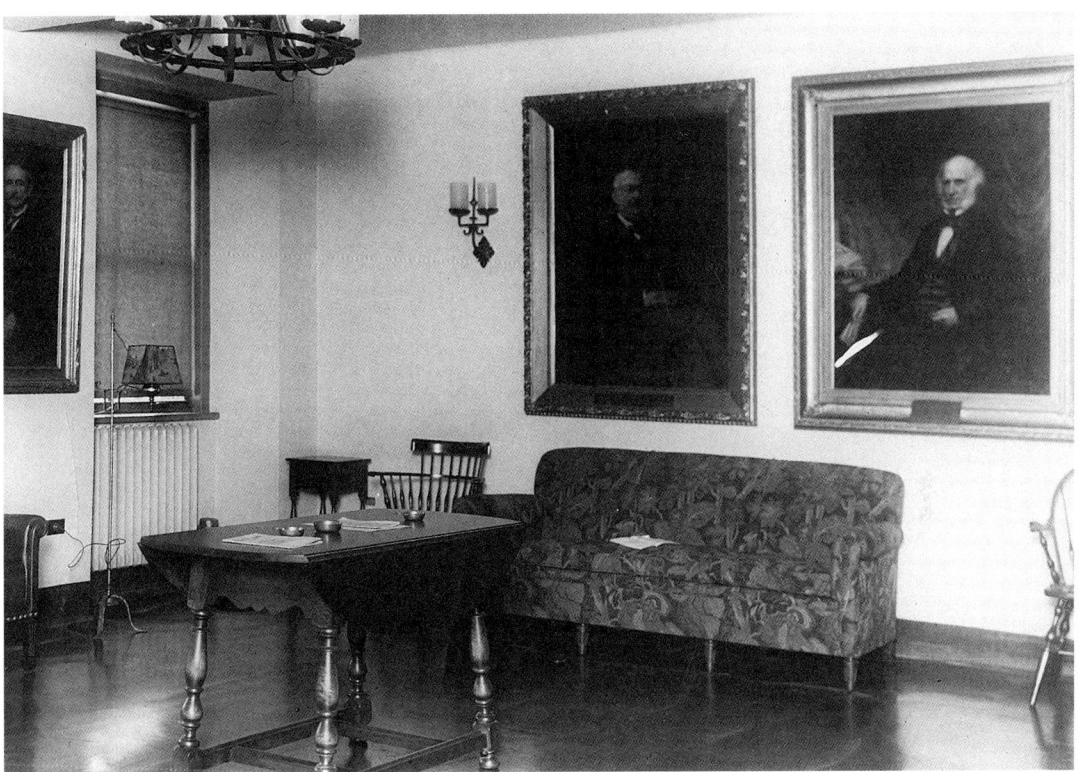

5.4.   College of Physicians and Surgeons, Columbia-Presbyterian Medical Center, 1928, James Gamble
Rogers, architect, alumni room. Photograph ca. 1928.

had hung in medical schools before the era of education reform, but
by continuing this practice, physicians maintained a connection with
their forebears even as they created a new form of education that bore
little resemblance to the training of previous generations. This ongoing
interaction with prestigious physicians of the past helped to facilitate an
elite, communal identity among students, faculty, and alumni.

Faculty and students articulated the feeling of connection generated
for them by the portraits. In 1947, Charles W. Johnson Sr. joined the
faculty at Meharry Medical College, where he would remain for more
than four decades. He later described the significance for him when he
first came to Meharry of the portraits hanging in the hallway that led
to the Public Health Lecture Room:

> In a sense, this corridor was a sort of pantheon. On its walls were class grad-
> uation photographs of Meharrians I had known, who had gone before my
> arrival. I saw the photographs of Dr. Rogers (my family physician) and my
> Uncle Son (James Arthur Johnson, D.D.S., 1933) . . . and others. In my mind's

eye I could see each of them as I knew them before and as I saw them at the point of transformation to professionals. I stood in awe as I recognized that I was now, somehow, on the verge of being a part of the process through which they had achieved their dreams.[11]

In May 1938, Joe Holoubek, a senior medical student at the University of Nebraska, wrote to Alice Baker, a student at Louisiana State University School of Medicine, New Orleans, from the card room of his fraternity house. Looking at the photographs of Nu Sigma Nu alumni, he affirmed, "Gee, they are a grand group of physicians—every one of them. I hope that someday my students & patients, if any, will think one-tenth as much of me as we think of them. Therefore we must try to follow the standards that they set up."[12] For faculty and students alike, portraits cultivated the sense of a shared, privileged identity.

Medical school events generated professional cohesiveness as well. A dedication ceremony typically marked the conclusion of the construction effort and the school's opening. The proceedings not only invited the public to explore the buildings but also gathered the leaders of medical colleges from across the nation. In October 1926, the University of Rochester dedicated its medical school and hospital, and guests at the event represented seventy American and Canadian medical schools and hospitals.[13] These programs became national and sometimes international celebrations of a medical college's achievement—and by extension the country's advance in medical training. They also provided participants with time for informal and formal investigations of modern buildings and progressive pedagogical ideas.

In October 1925, Vanderbilt University dedicated its medical school–hospital as part of the observation of the fiftieth anniversary of the university's founding. Events related to the medical complex received prime billing and took place during the first afternoon and evening of the four day celebration. The medical proceedings began with talks related to medical education and delivered by two nationally recognized physicians. After the panel, which took place in a nearby auditorium, guests then visited the medical facilities. They took tea in the nurses' home, another part of the recent construction effort, and toured the medical school–hospital. Later the medical school hosted dinner on site for the guests.[14] Over the course of half a day, delegates reflected together on broad issues in medical education and examined one school's system for training physicians and caring for patients.

Dedication programs often involved some combination of formal ceremonies, speeches, medical conferences, social gatherings, and tours, like the one at Vanderbilt, but the delegates in Nashville also had an extra opportunity to become acquainted with one another and the buildings. More than twenty-five delegates, representing a number of the elite schools as well as a handful of the struggling medical colleges, stayed in the medical facilities, as did architect Charles Coolidge. The honored guests occupied the suites for the hospital's resident physicians, while the others resided in the hospital's rooms for private patients and in the fourth floor of the nurses' home.[15] The time spent together away from formal duties likely provided the delegates with additional opportunities to renew old friendships and meet more members of the medical education leadership. In this era of widespread medical school construction, dedication events occurred relatively frequently; they encouraged the growing solidarity within medical education and among physicians and underscored for members of the medical community, as they did for laypersons, the ongoing transformation in medical training.

Medical schools also developed the profession's collective identity and sense of accomplishment when they hosted major professional conferences. Harvard Medical School rushed construction of its 1906 quadrangle in order to make it available to the American Medical Association three months before the school began offering classes at the site. In June 1906, thousands of physicians from around the world arrived in Boston for the American Medical Association meeting. In addition to hosting some of the academic proceedings, the Harvard Medical School quadrangle provided space for social activities and scientific exhibitions (see fig. 4.9).[16] Harvard's immense medical campus stood on full display, with its institute design and the pedagogy and science it promoted open to discussion, debate, and frequently celebration by the conference's many participants.

Hierarchies among Physicians and the Limits of Professional Cohesion

Although medical schools supported the development of an elite professional identity in the early twentieth century, not everyone shared equally in this group consciousness. White men dominated the profession, a reality highlighted by the individuals honored in the buildings. In most schools, the portraits lining the walls displayed images of white men. Despite Syracuse University's long and storied history of coeducation—the first woman to earn the MD degree graduated from its predecessor institution—the portraits hanging in the library, men's study, and women's study of its 1896 building appear only to have commemorated

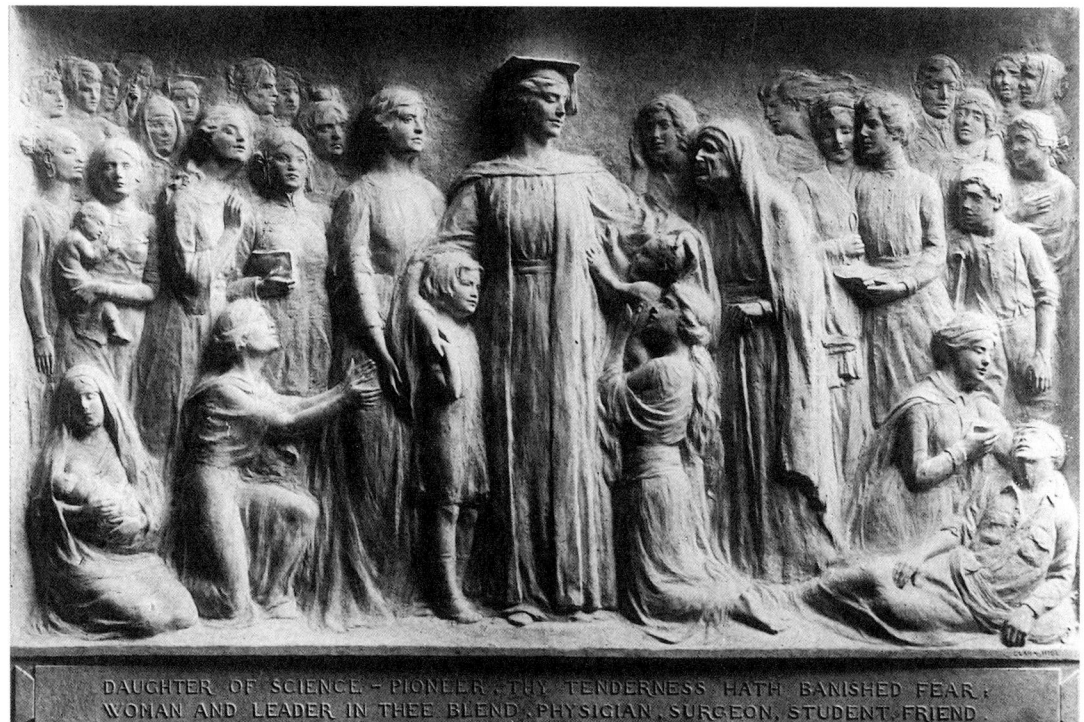

DAUGHTER OF SCIENCE ~ PIONEER : THY TENDERNESS HATH BANISHED FEAR :
WOMAN AND LEADER IN THEE BLEND . PHYSICIAN . SURGEON . STUDENT . FRIEND

5.5.   Clara Hill, *The Woman Physician*, 1916. Relief sculpture, 52 by 96 inches. The inscription reads,
          "Daughter of Science—Pioneer. Thy tenderness hath banished fear: woman and leader in thee blend.
          Physician, surgeon, student, friend."

men.[17] When Duke University opened its medical school in 1930, the
wards and clinics, as the founding dean later explained, bore the names
of "physicians and surgeons to remind the staff and students of what has
been accomplished in medicine" and to encourage the study of prominent
historical figures.[18] Even with Duke University School of Medicine's
coeducational student body, only men received this distinction. In this
segregated university, all were also white.

No doubt the commitment to educating women at Woman's Medical
College of Pennsylvania resulted in the display of images of women
physicians in the college's 1930 medical school–hospital. In 1916, Woman's Medical College alumna Rosalie Slaughter Morton had given the
school a bas-relief, *The Woman Physician*, of her own conception and
executed by sculptor Clara Hill (fig. 5.5). The sizable relief, measuring
fifty-two by ninety-six inches, contains a female physician in academic
attire at the center of a group of people. The editors of the *Woman's
Medical Journal* published a detailed description of the work shortly
after its presentation to the school. Although a fuller analysis of the

sculpture requires examination of the specialties it promotes for women and the relationships between the figures, it celebrates women physicians by displaying the individuals, nearly all female, who turn to them for help. It also includes nurses (exclusively women in this period), a female intern, and women medical students. The medical students are clustered in the very back left corner, with one exception. Far more visible than her counterparts, this student stands near the front of the crowd on the left side of the composition and has a book tucked under her right arm. The *Woman's Medical Journal* identifies the woman as "a Chinese student, representative of the foreigners who come to this country for medical training," a rare, perhaps unique, depiction of a medical student or physician of color in a predominantly white medical school in the early twentieth century.[19] When Woman's Medical College relocated in 1930, the bas-relief moved, too, and ultimately received prominent placement in the main entrance of the building.[20] The sculpture's acknowledgment of the diversity of students within the college, where small numbers of international students and African American women enrolled, does not appear to have occurred in other parts of the 1930 facility, however.[21] The portraits of physicians that hung in the school's boardroom all seem to have commemorated white women.[22]

For marginalized members of the profession, portraits of predecessors who looked like them offered particular inspiration. Camilla Graham graduated from Medical College of Pennsylvania in 1994, nearly twenty-five years after Woman's Medical College of Pennsylvania became coeducational and changed its name. Despite the addition of men to the student body, the college's origin as a women's medical school remained visible. Graham explained, "It was when I walked down the hallway that I knew I was in the right place. I passed large beautiful portraits of commanding appearing women—*all* women."[23] Although the collection did include a few men, women dominated both the hallway and Graham's recollection.[24]

Outside of Meharry Medical College, Howard University College of Medicine, and Woman's Medical College of Pennsylvania, however, medical campuses emphasized the profession's most powerful members: white, Protestant men. Women, African Americans, Jews, Catholics, and immigrants and various combinations thereof became physicians in this period, but they endured discrimination from the profession.[25] White women and Jewish individuals, for instance, faced stringent medical school admissions quotas, and the majority of African American men and women trained at Meharry and Howard. Black women, marginalized by their sex and their race, composed small percentages of the primarily male student bodies at Howard University College of Medicine and Meharry Medical College and of the predominantly white student body of Woman's Medical College. By 1923, American medical colleges had graduated only approximately ninety Black women, with thirty-nine receiving their degrees from Meharry, twenty-five from Howard, and sixteen from Woman's Medical College. The remaining Black women who had completed their degrees by 1923 studied at various northern coeducational schools.[26]

Students' experiences of the medical colleges perpetuated these hierarchies. Vanderbilt University, located in the segregated South, constructed separate facilities for white and Black patients and for white and Black personnel who staffed the building. With only white students enrolled in the medical college, however, the educational section of the medical school–hospital did not include duplicate facilities for Black students. At racially integrated schools, the architectural plans did not contain additional spaces designed to segregate African Americans, or their Jewish classmates, from their white, Christian counterparts, but occupants could—and did—use the buildings in discriminatory ways. African American students, for example, sometimes had to dine in separate rooms from their white colleagues when on call and, like their Jewish classmates, struggled to obtain university housing.[27] After the integration of the University of Pennsylvania's medical school, Black and white students dissected in separate teams.[28] These behaviors, although not formally built into the architecture, powerfully shaped students' lives.

Occupants also could use the structures to separate men and women in coeducational schools. In the late nineteenth century, the University of Michigan was the largest of the nation's state universities and had the strongest reputation. When it started enrolling women in its medical school in 1870, coeducational medical training began in earnest in the United States. Admitting women, however, required a compromise between the regents of the university and the medical school faculty. The faculty insisted that women and men take all courses separately and that the faculty's compensation be increased for duplicating their classes. In 1881, with women composing more than 20 percent of the first-year class, the medical faculty requested a change in policy to allow each instructor to decide personally how to handle coeducation. Faculty took a variety of approaches: some hung a curtain that allowed women to listen to the lectures without being seen by their male classmates, others marked a red line on the classroom floor to divide the sexes (men would drive back women who crossed the line by chanting, "red line, red line"), and still others continued to teach women and men entirely separately.[29] A

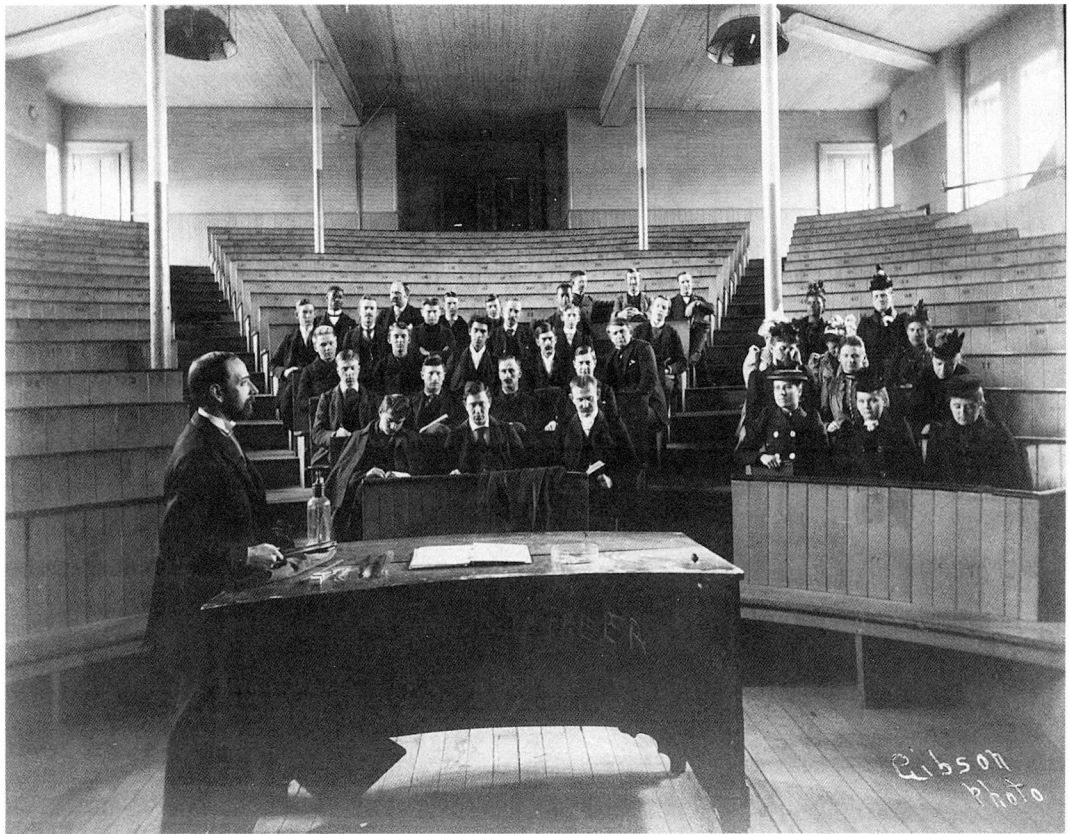

5.6.   Medical students attending a lecture in physics, University of Michigan, ca. 1893.

photograph of medical students at the University of Michigan attending a lecture in physics circa 1893 reveals men and women grouped by sex (fig. 5.6). In this case, the aisle demarcates the male and female spaces. In her examination of this image, urban historian Dolores Hayden asks whether the students may also be separated by race, with African American students sitting at the back, behind their white classmates.[30]

As Sappol has explained, eighteenth- and nineteenth-century dissecting room hijinks, smoking, and drinking, along with body snatching, made dissection a cornerstone of the fraternal medical school culture, and coeducation posed a challenge to this masculine environment.[31] Anatomy faculty at the University of Michigan continued to instruct women and men separately. When a new building for anatomy opened in 1889, the women dissected on the ground floor and the men on the second floor.[32] Moreover, Johns Hopkins Medical School's acclaimed anatomist, Franklin P. Mall, advocated replacing the single large anatomy laboratory with a number of small dissecting rooms. At schools that adopted Mall's design, women could easily have studied anatomy in a different room from the men due either to institutional requirements, faculty insistence, or personal choice. Pauline Stitt described her experience at the University of Michigan's medical school in 1929. By this point, women and men at Michigan dissected together, but male and female students typically self-segregated. As Stitt explained, "I was one of the only girls—I guess I might have been the only girl—that landed with the men at the dissection table."[33]

In educational spaces, the occupants themselves rather than the architecture divided students by sex. In contrast, the extracurricular areas of the medical school were themselves designed to segregate students by sex. For portions of each day, medical students abandoned laboratory, lecture hall, and library for extracurricular facilities. For example, students used locker rooms for changing clothes before and after the notoriously odorous and messy anatomy lab, and they might eat in a dining room while on the medical campus. Ludmerer has mentioned the inequality built into the medical campuses and the barrier these designs created between groups of students. Women sometimes ate in separate dining rooms when on call, and some medical colleges failed to provide an adequate number of toilets for women.[34] A more comprehensive examination of these extracurricular areas reveals that they not only separated students by sex and inculcated occupants in a sex-based hierarchy, but they also promoted gendered behavioral expectations.

Cultural norms dictated that men and women have separate locker rooms and bathrooms, but these facilities did not provide equivalent experiences for men and women. At Columbia University's College of Physicians and Surgeons, part of Columbia-Presbyterian Medical Center, the men occupied a 450-person locker room with a large internal bathroom on the first floor. The women used a much smaller locker room with adjoining lounge and bathroom on the second floor. Dissection, however, occurred on the ninth floor, a significant distance away from the changing facilities for both men and women. Nevertheless, only one locker room connected with the gross anatomy laboratory. Built to support roughly the same number of students as the men's locker room on the first floor, the ninth-floor locker room presumably accommodated the male students. Women appear to have traveled seven floors to change for dissection. Architectural design contributed to the lack of parity for women in early twentieth-century medical education.

If the absence of space in these buildings encouraged a male-dominant gender hierarchy, so too did the addition of space. The 1894 Women's Fund Memorial Building at Johns Hopkins Medical School offered the women a "dressing room" with lockers, sinks, and toilets on the second floor, but no parallel facility existed for the men, who had lockers along the hallways of the third floor and male-designated bathrooms on the third floor and in the basement. (Presumably either sex used the buildings' private toilets.)[35] Women and men enjoyed the same physical amenities—lockers and toilets—but those for the women were well removed from the corridors and completely private. This design encouraged women to retreat from the school's main thoroughfares when not in class. Similarly, the placement of the women's rooms on the second floor at Columbia University's College of Physicians and Surgeons pulled the women away from the busier first floor with its entrance to the street, men's locker area and toilet facilities, reception and cloak rooms, alumni room, and combined lounge, reading, and smoking room. This last space, prominently located near the school's main entrance and across from the alumni room, apparently provided the male students with a place to relax. Unlike the women students, the men did not have a rest area attached to their locker and toilet facilities. Instead, they would have taken their leisure time in the lounge, where they could read and smoke. The room's designation as a place for smoking, not to mention its shared vestibule with a men's toilet, further reinforced that this space did not welcome women. Cultural norms discouraged women not only from smoking but also from entering the locations where men smoked.[36] Including a "dressing room" for women at Johns Hopkins and removing women to the second floor at Columbia also adhered to contemporary conventions of affording women greater privacy than men. It is possible that the spaces for women at Johns Hopkins and Columbia provided the female students with a welcome escape from the male-dominated medical school. Nevertheless, by separating the women from their male classmates and discouraging their presence in the schools' more public areas, the designs at Johns Hopkins and Columbia diminished the visibility and participation of women in the masculine medical school environment and discouraged casual, noneducational contact between the sexes.

In fact, women's spaces typically provided female students with more privacy than the facilities for their male counterparts. Schools often included a locker room, rest area, and bathroom for both men and women. In the women's case, however, one entrance would lead to all three rooms, with interior doorways connecting one room to the next. In contrast, the men's area would have multiple doors, to allow male students to enter directly into the lounge, locker room, or bathroom from the hallway. This difference in design appears in Howard University's

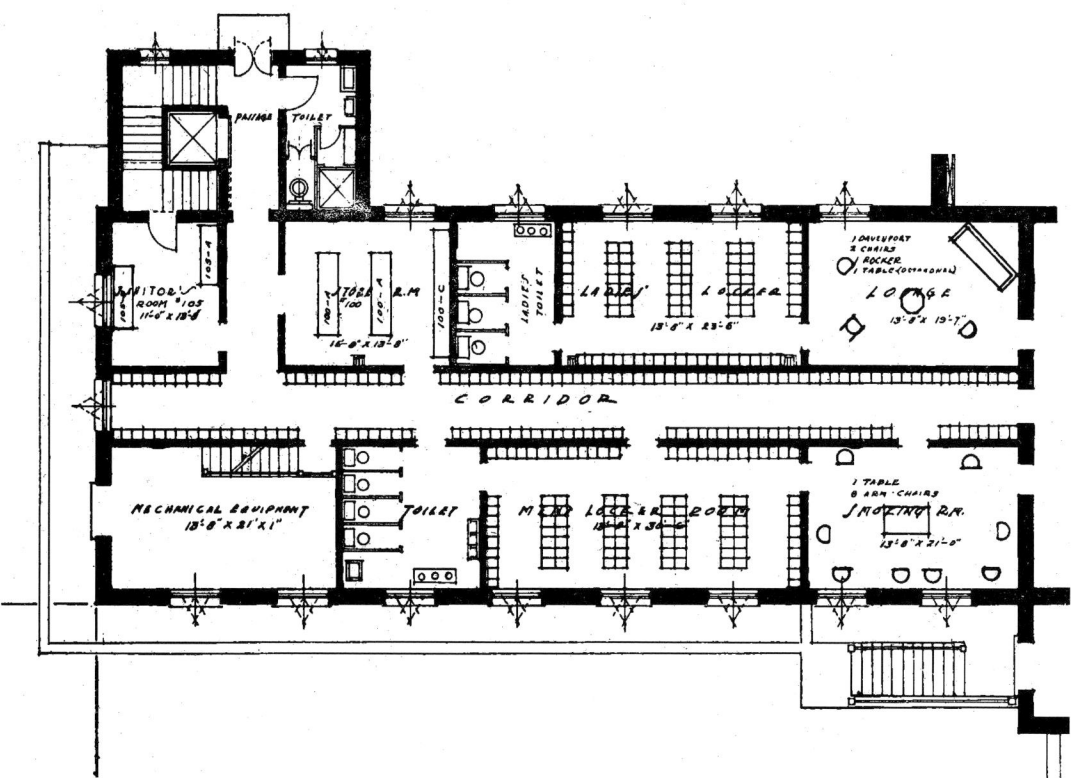

5.7.   Howard University College of Medicine, 1927, Albert I. Cassell, architect, plan with equipment, ground floor, wing with extracurricular areas for male students (lower side of hallway) and female students (upper side of hallway).

1927 medical school building (fig. 5.7). In the women's rooms, a single entrance led to a "lounge," followed by a locker room and then a toilet room. In the men's section, multiple entrances led to a "smoking room," locker room, and toilet room.

Beyond the design, the furnishings for the men's and women's extracurricular areas at Howard University's medical school also varied by the sex of the occupant. The women's "lounge" contained one davenport, one rocker, two chairs, and an octagonal table, while the men's "smoking room" offered its occupants eight chairs and a rectangular table. In giving women the opportunity to recline or rock, the architect and medical educators presented the women with ways to rest more completely than was possible in the men's "smoking room." Furthermore, the davenport and rocking chair have close associations with domestic spaces. The furnishings both reflected and encouraged the connection between women and the domestic (private) sphere and the expectation that women needed to lie down on occasion.

The labels assigned to these spaces on the architectural plans, and possibly adopted by the students and faculty, underscored gendered behavioral expectations as well. At Howard, women had a space to "lounge," a more passive descriptor than the one applied to their male colleagues' "smoking room," itself a reference to a culturally male activity. At the University of Nebraska College of Medicine, women used spaces with domestic titles: the "dressing room" attached to the "parlor." The men, however, occupied the "locker room" connected to a "lounging room." No consistency existed between schools for the naming of these rooms, but when the men's and women's spaces did not have the same titles, the names given to the women's areas tended to suggest docility and home life more than the titles affixed to the men's rooms. In design and function, the extracurricular facilities privileged men over women by encouraging women to retreat into more private spaces and to conform to traditional notions of passivity and domesticity. Even as women pushed their way into medical coeducation, barriers continued to limit their full inclusion in medical training.

No architectural barrier curbed women's participation in medical education more than the total absence of facilities for women. When the leadership at Yale University considered including women in its medical school in 1916, the decision to accept women was conditioned on acquiring funds to alter the building; the school needed to construct women's bathrooms. The father of a young woman who wanted to attend the medical school came forward with the money.[37]

When areas for women—bathrooms, lounges, and locker rooms—did exist, they generally remained smaller than the parallel facilities for male students. These spaces codified architecturally the expectation that fewer women would attend medical school than men. Paucity of space for women could then easily shift from a response to admissions decisions to a justification for continuing admissions quotas. In other words, these rooms literally set in stone the expectation that medical schools would predominantly enroll men.

Scholars have documented the discrimination against women in coeducational medical schools in the early twentieth century. According to historian Regina Morantz-Sanchez, this hostility explains in part why the spread of coeducation in the early twentieth century, a shift simultaneous to the closure of all but one of the women's medical colleges, did not immediately increase the number of female students relative to male students. In fact, the proportion of women medical students declined significantly in the early twentieth century, from 5 percent of students in 1899 to just 2.9 percent of students in 1910. Morantz-Sanchez notes that coeducational schools often "grudgingly allowed [women] a few places each year in the freshman class—just enough, so the old joke went, to form a dissecting team."[38] Investigating architecture broadens our understanding of how hierarchical educational environments are created and expands the discussion of medical education's "hidden curriculum."

Medical training encompasses more than formal scientific knowledge. It also includes the acquisition of an appropriate demeanor, accepted values, and professional identity. Every experience teaches students, in the words of Ludmerer, "what it mean[s] to be a physician." Although not overt, this "hidden curriculum" also is not random. Scholars first focused on the "hidden curriculum" of primary schools but came to recognize it in the context of medical training as well. According to Ludmerer, the "hidden curriculum" in medical education encompasses "the implicit messages continually conveyed, the education that occurred by example rather than word, and the imprinting of attitudes and values that regularly" were demonstrated. Ludmerer called for greater study into this mode of learning in order not only to understand better the medical education of the past but also to create positive change in medical education today.[39] Ludmerer made this call at the very end of the twentieth century, but the architectural component of medical education's "hidden curriculum" has remained largely unstudied. As the example of the bathrooms and rest areas indicates, architecture contributes significantly to the "hidden curriculum" and in particular to the development of professional identities that can remain long after medical training ends. Perhaps nowhere is this clearer than in medical student dormitories.

Dormitories and the Creation of Elite White Male Physicians

As medical colleges grew in complexity in the early twentieth century, they became in a functional sense universities in microcosm. Like the universities of which they usually formed a part, medical colleges provided their students with laboratories, lecture halls, libraries, museums, and administrative suites. This parallel with the university only expanded when, as occasionally happened, the medical school constructed a dormitory.

Medical students, like college undergraduates, required places to live, eat, and socialize, but unlike for college undergraduates, in the opening decades of the twentieth century dormitories for medical students remained rare. Poor housing contributed to the physical toll that medical training took on some students. Many medical students spent their educational years in rundown, inexpensive boardinghouses in the neighborhood around the medical school; in some cases these accommodations did not even offer consistent heat or running water.[40] Mary Bruins Allison, Woman's Medical College of Pennsylvania class of 1932, recalled, "Our rooms were cold. We took our meals at cheap restaurants. There were seven of us students in one house."[41]

With little financial aid in this period, students of limited means struggled. Frequently they paid for their food and lodging by taking on outside work, a reality that made eight- or nine-hour academic days that much lengthier. Blood donations also helped cover necessary expenses.[42] After graduating from Woman's Medical College, Allison took an unpaid internship, during which, as she explained, "I wanted some new clothes so I gave 500 cc of blood and received $25.00."[43]

Inadequate diet, repeated blood donations for cash, and exposure to illness in the clinic and hospital compounded the physical effects of long days and subpar housing and resulted in significant health risks for students. Tuberculosis, for which antibiotic treatment did not exist until the mid-1940s, represented the most notorious threat and took the lives of a few students each year at many medical colleges.[44] Joe Holoubek, who graduated from medical school at the University of Nebraska in 1938, wrote vividly in his memoir of students' fear of this disease: "I remember the service in Douglas County Tuberculosis Hospital. . . . I hated to go there. I did the bare essentials for my patients because I was dreadfully frightened of tuberculosis. One of the medical students obtained an extra long tube for his stethoscope so he wouldn't have to even come near the patients when he examined them. He had the patient place the bell of the scope on places on the chest while he listened." It was not until his future wife, Alice Baker, contracted the dreaded disease during her medical training that Holoubek "suddenly got over [his] mortal fear of tuberculosis."[45]

Students did have other options outside of boardinghouses, however. Some lived at home, while others resided with their classmates in fraternities. Marginalized groups, such as Jewish people and women, traditionally excluded from fraternities, formed their own fraternities and sororities.[46] Students could also live in a hospital, where they presumably worked as well.[47] Beyond these typical options, individual schools might provide unique solutions to housing students.

Although unusual, medical college dormitories did exist.[48] Washington University in St. Louis opened a dormitory for medical students in 1917. At Johns Hopkins Medical School, the Women's Medical Association, created to help women students locate a suitable place to eat, rented a house in 1918 to provide the women with a dining room along with seven bedrooms to rent. In 1920, the Women's Medical Association officially incorporated and purchased a home, which the male students dubbed the "Hen House."[49] "Hen House" played on the phrase "hen medics," a common moniker for female medical students and physicians in this period. In the early 1930s, Howard University set aside part of a campus dormitory for men pursuing professional and graduate training.[50] Before its 1930 relocation, some students at the Woman's Medical College of Pennsylvania, which enrolled white, African American, and racially diverse international students, lived in area houses owned and run by the college or in the school's branch of the Young Women's Christian Association, which also assisted students looking for room and board.[51] Many of these medical schools and related organizations made arrangements for white women, Black women, other women of color, and Black men, a response perhaps to the particular challenges faced by these students in obtaining housing and, at least in the case of the women, possibly also an outgrowth of patriarchal attitudes and societal expectations that encouraged institutions to offer housing for women.

It may seem surprising, then, that two leading medical schools predominantly composed of white men spent decades working to construct dormitories. These dormitories require investigation not because they were typical but because they highlight the desire to indoctrinate students in an elite professional identity during medical training. Harvard Medical School and Columbia University's College of Physicians and Surgeons, two wealthy schools with established and deep donor pools, found patrons to build up (literally) this powerful element of the "hidden curriculum." The medical school leadership at Harvard and Columbia understood the dormitories as tools for improving enrollment, expanding the curriculum, and—most importantly—inculcating in young white men the demeanor and behavior befitting a prestigious physician.

In both cases, realizing the dormitories took decades. At Harvard, the call for a medical student dormitory began as early as 1895.[52] After a number of attempts to get the project off the ground, Harvard Medical School alumni undertook raising the necessary funds in 1923. The alumni canvassed Harvard Medical School graduates from around the world and collected donations from more than thirteen hundred alumni before expanding the campaign. Harold S. Vanderbilt, who had graduated from Harvard College in 1907 and Harvard Law School in 1910, gave $700,000 to complete the fundraising effort, and the school named the building in his honor (fig. 5.8).[53] Coolidge, Shepley, Bulfinch, and Abbott (a Shepley, Rutan, and Coolidge successor firm) designed Vanderbilt Hall. The dormitory sits directly across the street from the base of the Harvard Medical School quadrangle at the head of Avenue Louis Pasteur and to

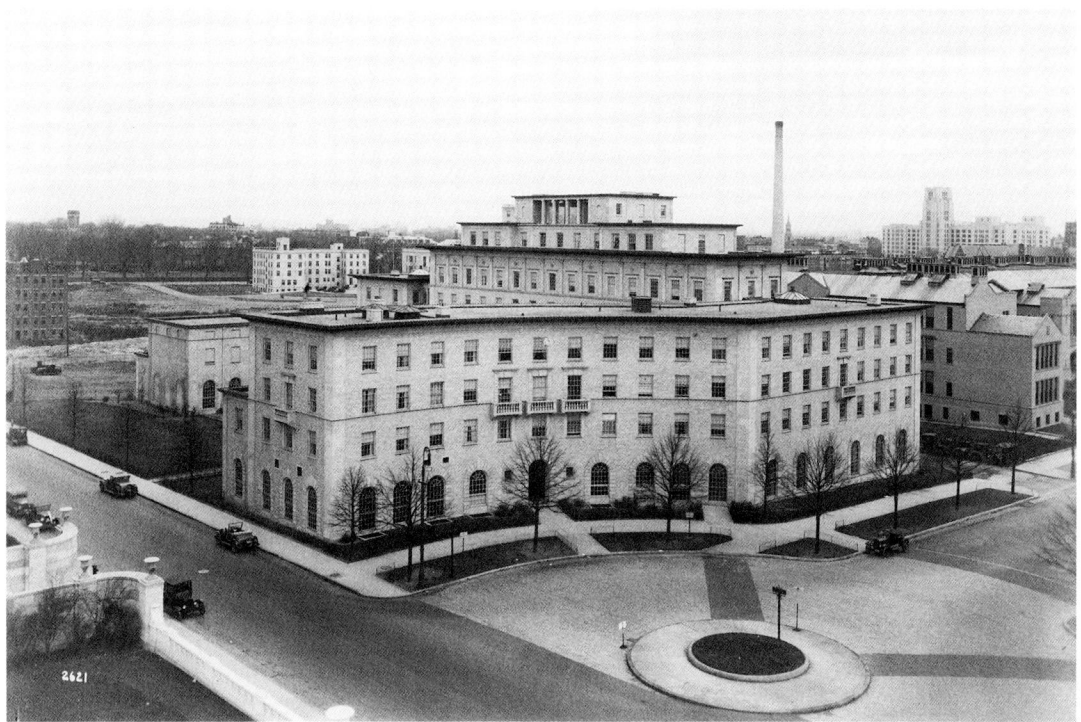

5.8.   Vanderbilt Hall, Harvard Medical School, 1927, Coolidge, Shepley, Bulfinch, and Abbott, architects.
Photograph ca. 1928. A 1930 addition connected the wings at the far left and enclosed the courtyard.

this day contains living, dining, and recreational facilities for Harvard
medical students.

At Columbia, the call for a dormitory began at least two decades
before Bard Hall received its first occupants.[54] In early 1927, Columbia's
medical school dean, William Darrach, requested information about
the nearly complete Harvard Medical School dormitory, and a Harvard
Medical School faculty member wrote to an administrator at Columbia-Presbyterian Medical Center with an overview of the project as well
as a sketch of the building.[55] After the Columbia-Presbyterian Medical
Center opened in October 1928, Darrach persuaded Edward S. Harkness,
his friend, his Yale classmate, and the principal benefactor of Columbia-Presbyterian Medical Center, to donate the $2 million needed to
purchase the land for and to build and equip Bard Hall (fig. 5.9).[56] James
Gamble Rogers, the primary architect of the Columbia-Presbyterian
Medical Center group, a fellow Yalie, and Harkness's personal architect
and friend, designed the dormitory located a short walk from the medical
college.[57] Like Vanderbilt Hall, Bard Hall combined living, dining, and
recreation, and it, too, remains in use today.

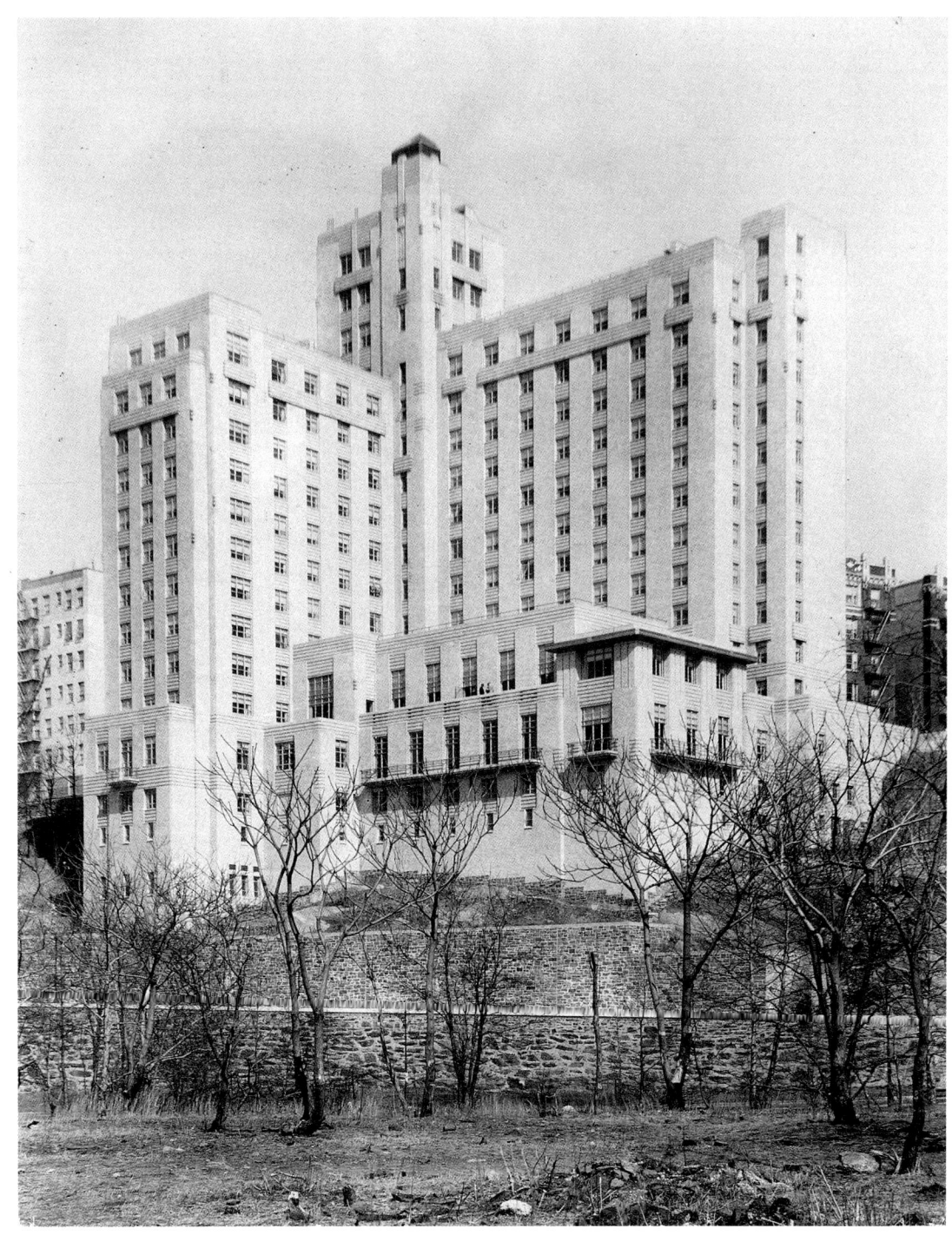

5.9.   Bard Hall, Columbia-Presbyterian Medical Center, 1931, James Gamble Rogers, architect. Photograph 1941.

The extended call for the dormitory at Harvard Medical School, followed by the long fundraising campaign, required proponents of the dormitory to articulate time and again their ambitions for the facility. Together they presented a layered series of arguments in support of the building. Most basically, they affirmed that the dormitory would provide much-needed housing and dining facilities. Harvard's medical school sat too far from the university for its students to access the housing, dining, recreation, and social opportunities available closer to the main campus. In addition, young men increasingly traveled significant distances to attend the school, which made living at home less practicable. Moreover, once clinical sites began to be constructed near the school in 1913, the demand for area housing increased as third- and fourth-year students undergoing their clinical training wanted to live in the neighborhood as well. Replacing the existing inadequate and unnecessarily expensive options with quality, affordable housing and dining in the neighborhood of the medical school would fill a pressing need and improve the health of the students. Better student health would benefit academic performance.[58]

The emphasis on health went beyond providing more hygienic living quarters. The gymnasium—although not added to the building program until Harold Vanderbilt offered to donate one—came to play a prominent role in the dormitory's mission.[59] Undoubtedly the gymnasium served as an athletic and social resource for the students, but in a letter to the *New York Times* Francis M. Rackemann, the general secretary of the fundraising campaign, highlighted several additional functions for the space. Rackemann noted that the gymnasium aligned with the teaching of Hippocrates, who "wrote that medical students should be taught how to take care of themselves in order that they could better take care of others." He also quoted Harold Vanderbilt, who had asserted that, "from . . . personal experience . . . the students would learn the benefit which would accrue to their future patients and mankind, by prescribing and encouraging exercises of a similar nature." Moreover, the gymnasium would correlate with the students' academic courses. It would show students personally the significance of preventive medicine and function, according to Rackemann, as "a sort of laboratory" for the physiology class by enabling students to experience for themselves the mental and physical effects of exercise.[60]

Supporters of the dormitory also expressed more pragmatic concerns. They argued that the building would help Harvard Medical School remain competitive among its peer institutions, such as the University of Pennsylvania, where the medical students had the opportunity to live in that university's dormitories.[61] Furthermore, as Ludmerer has observed, "faculties knew that contented students were more likely to become loyal alumni—a crucial source of financial and political support for a school."[62] Although Ludmerer refers to a later generation of faculty, the medical leadership pushing for dormitories in the early twentieth century believed that the dormitory would shape students' current and future relationship with the medical school by fostering a sense of community. As they explained it, the dormitory would provide young men new to the area with organized social opportunities, it would bring together "rich and poor alike," and it would give men from different medical school classes the chance to interact, a point of particular concern since the concentration system of teaching limited interactions between the various classes during the academic day.[63] In addition, the faculty would eat and possibly live in the dormitory, and this "throwing together of students . . . and their instructors will foster good-fellowship [sic] and loyalty to the School."[64] The camaraderie and networking of the school years would produce a band of brothers willing to support one another in their future careers and would ensure that the schools' coffers remained full as the decades passed.

At the same time, dormitory proponents asserted that the medical profession would also benefit from the stronger community spirit. In 1912, Harvard Medical School student Lewis Wendell Hackett wrote to prominent faculty member and dormitory supporter J. Collins Warren about the need for a dormitory. Hackett asserted that "a humanizing amount of social activity will be good not only for the student, but for the School and the profession."[65] In this line of thinking, fraternization went hand in hand with personal growth, dedication to alma mater and fellow graduates, and development of the profession.

As Hackett's words also suggest, the final argument for the dormitory focused on enriching students' minds and characters. In a letter to potential donors, Rackemann quoted Harvard University president A. Lawrence Lowell, who affirmed, "A large part of the training comes from the students themselves discussing the matters they have been studying, and by that process greatly clarifying one another's ideas and fixing the essentials in the memory." Beyond academics, such an environment would, according to Rackemann, "develop the personality of the students." Rackemann explained that "when medical students live together, eat together, and meet their young instructors outside of the classroom, interest in the School and in the School work will be stimulated and the ability to meet and deal with men will be developed."[66] The strengthening of students' character and their ability to interact well with

others spoke to an ongoing concern in medical education. According to
Warren, the medical classes no longer included the "rough and uneducat-
ed" men found in the school in the past, but room for improvement still
existed. In addition to scientific training, the medical student required
social development that would make each future doctor into "a friend
who would be acceptable and welcome in any household."[67] In other
words, the dormitory would help ensure that students excelled academ-
ically and came to behave in ways befitting members of the professional
class. More than creating a healthy living and dining environment, the
dormitory would cultivate bodies, minds, and characters. Molded into
refined members of society, the young men would embody the privileged
identity of modern physicians.

The discussion of a dormitory for Columbia University's College of
Physicians and Surgeons revealed similar circumstances and ambitions.
As at Harvard Medical School, Columbia's medical school sat at some
distance from the main university campus and its resources for students.
Columbia University's president, Nicholas Murray Butler, promised that
the dormitory would provide "comfortable, commodious and hygienic
living rooms and good food" in proximity to the medical school as well
as serve as a social center.[68] Moreover, Butler explained, in addition to
helping recruit talented students, the dormitory would begin "a new era
in the history of the Medical School, for it will mean building up in the
students and junior teachers of the future a new spirit of association,
inter-dependence, and personal as well as scholarly devotion to the great
profession in which they are engaged, and to the Medical Center at
which they have found their training."[69] In bringing young faculty and
students together outside of class, the dormitory would promote a unified
(elite white Protestant male) culture that would help to generate a strong
profession and loyalty to alma mater—loyalty that administrators no
doubt hoped would cause alumni to become future donors.

Observers of undergraduate life in this period would have found
many familiar themes in the calls for medical school dormitories. By
1910, the German university's emphasis on research and specialized
graduate study had become prominent at many leading American institutions. This shift did not go uncontested, however, and dissidents,
including Lowell, Harvard's president, worried about the impact on
undergraduates of the growing research orientation and the expanding
size of the university. They felt that the German-trained researchers
failed to develop the close student-teacher relationships that they believed had existed in the past, a change they perceived as detrimental to
undergraduates' personal development. To rectify this situation, some

university leaders championed the model of Oxford and Cambridge. Adopting some form of the English universities' collegiate structure, which included students and teachers living together in enclosed quadrangles, would enable American universities to retain their research focus while increasing student-faculty contact. The dormitory had lost favor in American universities at the end of the nineteenth century, but it regained popularity at the beginning of the twentieth. Not only did it offer a university-controlled alternative to fraternities and boardinghouses, but it also created an opportunity to shape students' character in line with some aspects of the Oxford and Cambridge system.[70]

One outgrowth of this movement was the residential colleges constructed at Harvard and Yale, both of which had close ties to the medical school dormitories at Harvard and Columbia. Lowell, who was quoted in fundraising material for Harvard's medical student dormitory, had transformed the undergraduate experience at Harvard with the construction of four freshman dormitories between 1914 and 1926 and the requirement that most freshmen live in university housing. Like Lowell, Edward S. Harkness greatly admired the English collegiate system.[71] In 1928, he provided Lowell with the funds to create Harvard's House Plan, whereby sophomores, juniors, and seniors, along with tutors and faculty, lived, ate, studied, and socialized together in one of seven houses. At the end of that same year, Harkness pledged to fund Columbia's medical school dormitory. Shortly thereafter, Harkness returned to his alma mater, Yale University, to fund its College Plan, an undergraduate residential system similar to Harvard's House Plan, and the first College Plan buildings opened in 1933. Further connecting these collegiate experiments with the medical school dormitories, architects Coolidge, Shepley, Bulfinch, and Abbott designed both Harvard's medical school dormitory and Harvard's residential colleges, while James Gamble Rogers designed eight of the original ten colleges at Yale after completing the plan for Columbia's medical school dormitory. The leadership at the Harvard and Columbia medical schools were familiar with the changes taking place in undergraduate housing. In 1929, during preparations for the expansion of Vanderbilt Hall, Harvard Medical School's dean referenced a handful of models, including Harvard's House Plan, Oxford, and Cambridge, for the inclusion of a Master's House in the larger dormitory.[72]

Despite the boom in collegiate dormitories in this period, dormitories for medical students remained relatively few in number. The medical school faculties at Harvard and Columbia understood that the dormitories represented, in the words of Columbia University's medical school dean, "a new departure in medical education."[73] The dean's description

of the proposed dormitory as an *educational* rather than a *residential* innovation reveals again that proponents of these facilities saw them as
much more than living quarters.

Steeped in expectation, Vanderbilt Hall opened at Harvard Medical School in 1927 and Bard Hall at Columbia University's College
of Physicians and Surgeons in 1931. Vanderbilt Hall housed about 250
students, or approximately half of the student body. It offered areas for
dining, recreation, socializing, and study.[74] Two years after the dormitory
opened, Harold S. Vanderbilt donated an additional $450,000 in order
to expand the facility by nearly 90 student rooms.[75] At Columbia-Presbyterian Medical Center, Bard Hall contained accommodations for 10
tutors and around 250 students, or about 60 percent of the student body.
The building included multiple dining areas, rooms where students could
gather, facilities for the students' Young Men's Christian Association,
and recreational amenities.[76] While Vanderbilt Hall was enlarged almost
immediately, Bard Hall received no major alterations until the 1970s.[77]

The men responsible for both buildings believed that environment
shaped behavior, a conviction expressed by Harvard Medical School
faculty member J. Collins Warren when he called for a student dormitory
in 1922. Warren quoted the late George Hodges, erstwhile dean of the
Episcopal Theological School in Cambridge, Massachusetts, who said,
"So long as the dormitory is a tenement, the men will live in the street.
. . . But, when the dormitory takes on the aspect of cultivated life, with
lawn about it and flowering shrubs . . . these influences summon men
with pipes and books to sit in the shade, to talk and read and dream."[78]
While perhaps not as verdant or utopian a setting as this vision imagined,
Vanderbilt Hall, and to a lesser extent Bard Hall, existed as a separate
enclave from the rest of the medical center. Once expanded, Vanderbilt
Hall formed a relatively low, enclosed quadrangle—two or four stories
along its street-facing sides and six stories at the back—in keeping with
many of the new undergraduate dormitories that drew on the tradition
of Oxford and Cambridge.[79] In her discussion of undergraduate dormitories that utilized the quadrangle plan, Carla Yanni writes, "The
importance of the enclosed outdoor room cannot be overemphasized, as
it was intended to create community by forcing the residents into a shared
space."[80] Although a twelve-story skyscraper rather than a quadrangle
with private interior courtyard, Bard Hall sat at the northernmost edge
of the medical center, a location that removed it from the area's main
thoroughfares. Within these retreats, young men would sleep, eat, socialize, and exercise in a carefully crafted environment designed to mold
the character of a privileged group of professionals.

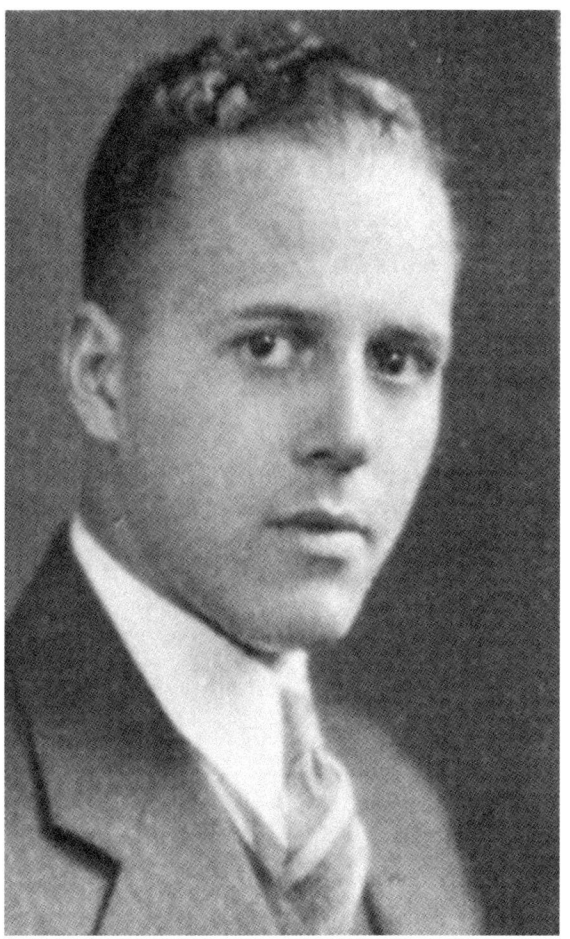

5.10.   Frederick Douglass Stubbs, ca. 1931.

Medical school dormitories mirrored undergraduate residences in cultivating a circumscribed leadership class. As historian of education Alex Duke explains, "Lowell [Harvard's president] saw the residential colleges as vehicles for the creation of an intellectual and a social elite among those whom he considered to be assimilable into the American common culture." Although the administrations at Harvard and Yale strove to populate the colleges with cross sections of the all-male undergraduates, mixing students of varied academic interests and economic and religious backgrounds, this goal did not extend to every student. Jewish pupils faced informal quotas, and African American undergraduates at Harvard were not welcome in the residential colleges.[81]

Vanderbilt and Bard Halls also celebrated a culture that was white, male, and Protestant. Harvard Medical School accepted no women students in this period, and—as we will see shortly—women students at Columbia University's College of Physicians and Surgeons occupied a marginalized position within the medical school dormitory. In Harvard's Vanderbilt Hall, room sizes and special amenities—such as semiprivate studies and bathrooms—varied in order to provide rooms at different rates and house together students of diverse financial means.[82] Despite this nod toward economic inclusivity, extant documents do not reveal whether Jewish medical students actually lived in Vanderbilt Hall, although the dean of Harvard Medical School appears to have considered housing Jewish students in the dormitory at least on an individual basis.[83]

African American medical students did reside in Vanderbilt Hall, but the experience was not congenial. Historian Nora Nercessian investigated the history of Black students at Harvard Medical School, which in the early twentieth century admitted small numbers of African Americans;

thirty-six Black students matriculated between 1900 and 1927. In 1927, the year Vanderbilt Hall opened, three Black students enrolled at Harvard Medical School, and then fourteen years ensued when no African American students entered the school. One of the three 1927 enrollees, Frederick Douglass Stubbs, became the first Black student to reside in the dormitory when he occupied room 211 (fig. 5.10). Nercessian described Stubbs's experience: "According to his close friend, Dr. Wilbur Strickland, . . . no one at Vanderbilt Hall would speak to him. Stubbs himself would discuss, in later years, his race-related problems, and incidents involving discrimination while at Harvard Medical School."[84] Hildrus A. Poindexter, another of the African American students who matriculated in 1927, lived off campus with his wife. He later contrasted his generally favorable academic experience during his two years at Harvard Medical School (he entered the school as a third-year student) with the social isolation imposed on him by many of his fellow students: "Harvard as an academic institution is wonderful. It is fair to students without regard to race and is generous to those in financial need. However, it has no control over the extra-curricular activities of its students and the majority of the class of 1929 was affluent and conservative to the point of excluding the poor and the black from their social life outside of the classroom and ward assignments."[85] Vanderbilt Hall's design did not explicitly segregate or exclude, but the occupants created a discriminatory environment that underscored the racial hierarchy endemic to medicine and American culture more generally.

In Bard Hall, the suite of rooms set aside for the medical student chapter of the Young Men's Christian Association (YMCA) signaled the school's commitment to Protestantism. Religious studies scholar Paul Kemeny has argued, "Despite the 'second disestablishment' of old-stock Protestant hegemony over the national culture in the 1920s, mainstream Protestantism remained firmly entrenched" at a number of elite, officially nondenominational institutions. Even as these universities widened their civic missions in the early twentieth century, they remained dedicated to furthering the nation's supposed Christian character. The YMCA played a significant role in maintaining many schools' long-standing adherence to Protestantism in this period.[86] When Bard Hall opened, the medical school's branch of the YMCA—the P&S Club—received a suite of rooms on the eleventh floor that included a comfortable lounge with large windows, fireplace, and built-in bookshelves; a pantry for storing and preparing food; and a sitting room, bedroom, and bathroom for the club's secretary.[87] The secretary also functioned as Bard Hall's athletic director, a role believed to "surely help his [Young Men's Christian] Association Service."[88]

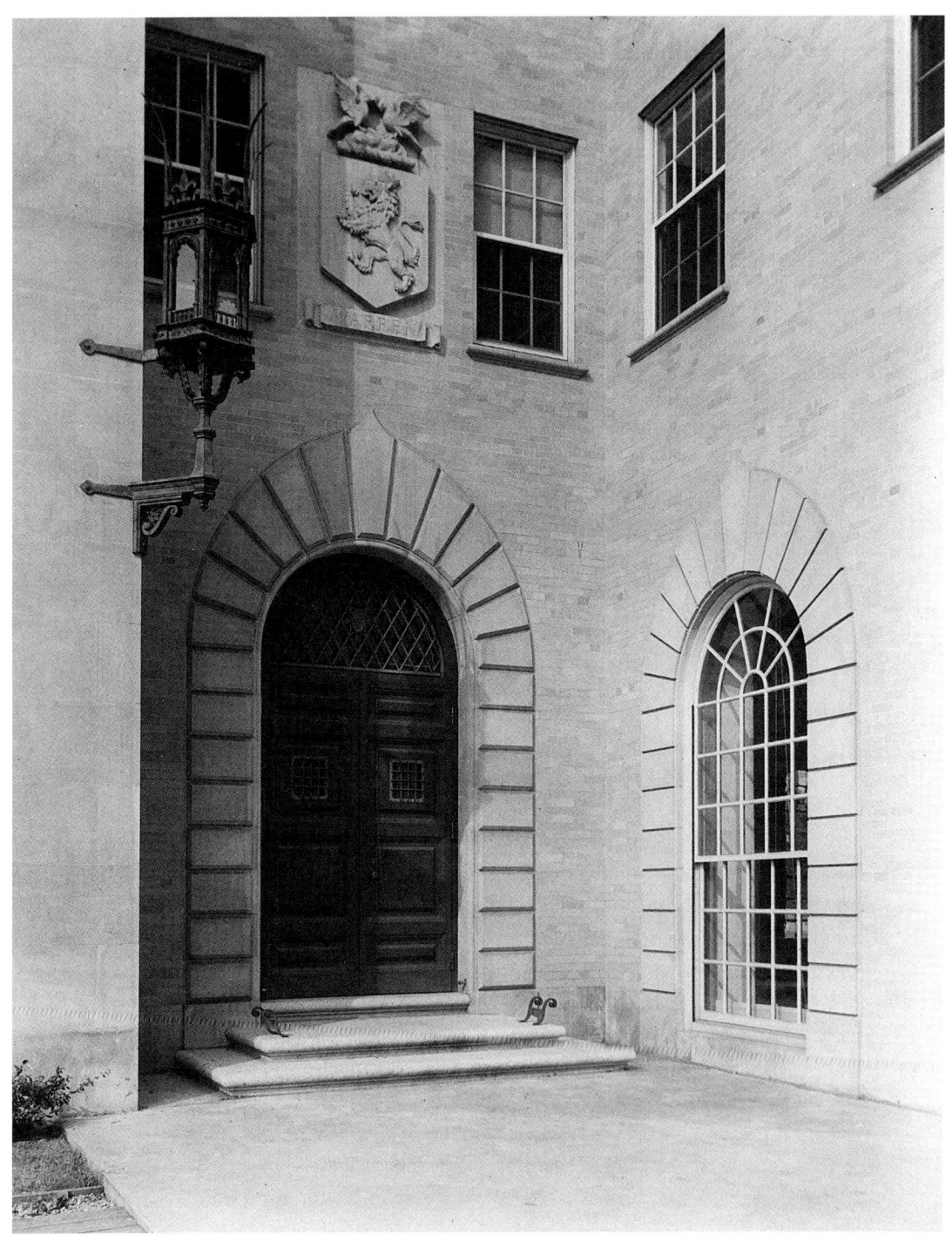

5.11.   Vanderbilt Hall, Harvard Medical School, 1927, Coolidge, Shepley, Bulfinch, and Abbott, architects, courtyard entrance with Warren family crest. Photograph ca. 1928.

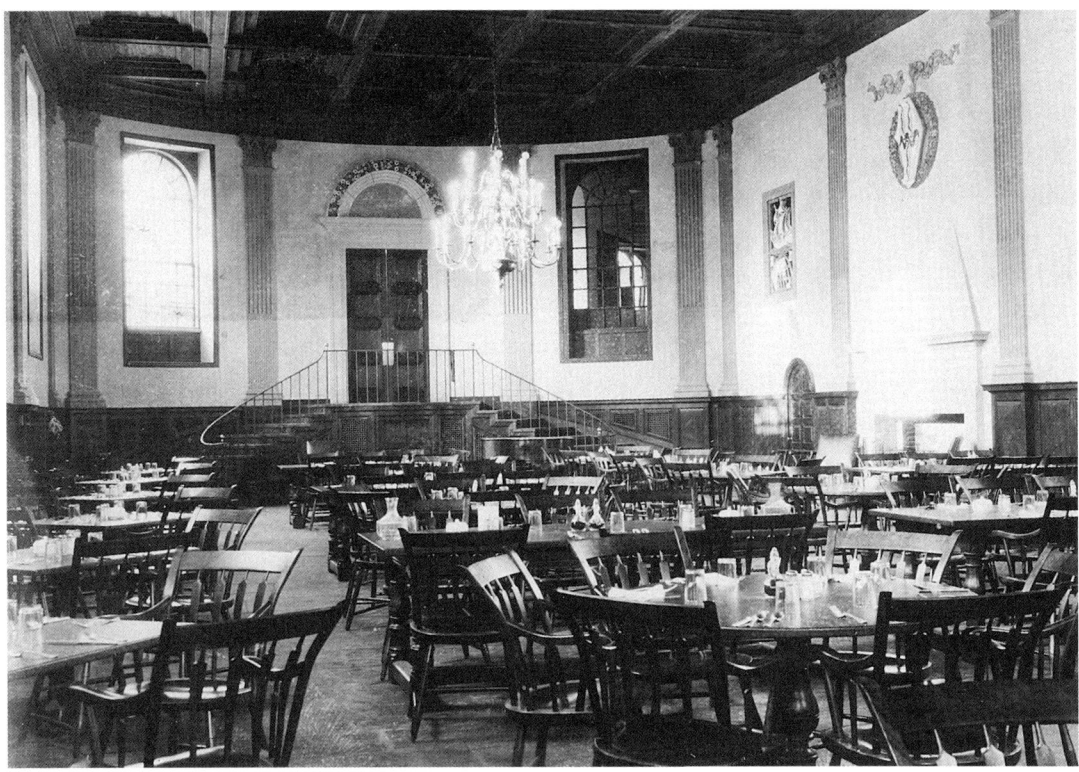

5.12.   Vanderbilt Hall, Harvard Medical School, 1927, Coolidge, Shepley, Bulfinch, and Abbott, architects, Henry Pickering Bowditch Dining Hall. Photograph ca. 1929.

The design and decoration of Vanderbilt and Bard Halls also encouraged an elite professional identity for their occupants. In Vanderbilt Hall, several memorial rooms honored prominent physicians. Although conceived as an incentive for donors, these rooms formed a connection between students and faculty and various medical luminaries.[89] They inculcated in residents and visitors an ethos of medical achievement and contributed to an environment of cultural sophistication. In keeping with undergraduate colleges, including the buildings designed by Rogers for Yale, Vanderbilt Hall contained heraldic shields.[90] These aristocratic symbols heightened the sense of history and privilege and suggested that the medical students—or at least the white, Protestant ones—were adopted sons of prestigious families. For example, the crest of the Warren family, an esteemed Boston family connected for generations with Harvard Medical School, marked one courtyard doorway (fig. 5.11). In addition, the Bowditch coat of arms enlivened one wall of the Henry Pickering Bowditch Dining Hall, named for a former professor and dean at Harvard Medical School (fig. 5.12). The dining hall's chandelier

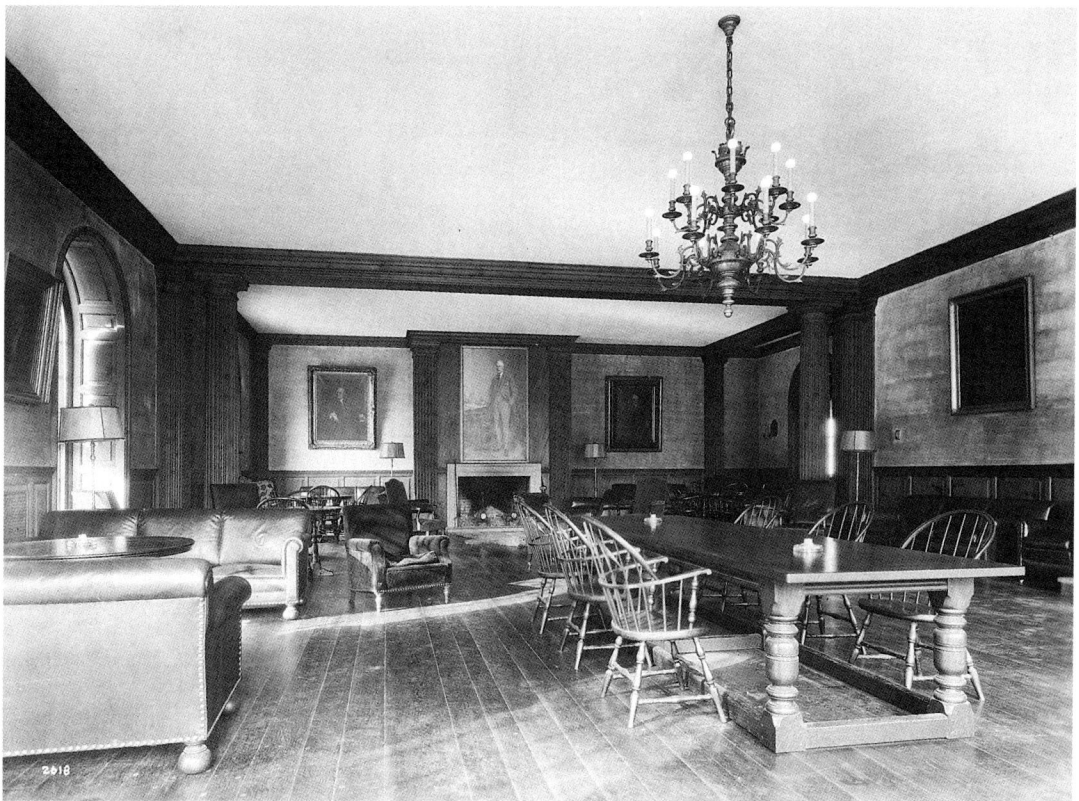

5.13.   Vanderbilt Hall, Harvard Medical School, 1927, Coolidge, Shepley, Bulfinch, and Abbott, architects,
           Charles H. Best Room. Photograph ca. 1928.

contributed to the creation of a genteel environment, and dormitory supporters hoped the chairs by the fireplace would induce faculty and students to linger "before and after meals [so that] all men may congregate
to promote sociability and to exchange ideas."[91] The dramatic entrance
balcony and stairway made stepping into the room an opportunity to see
and be seen as students and faculty declared themselves members of an
exclusive physician class.

Organized activities within the dormitories made it clear that the
faculties expected (or at least hoped) students' behavior would match
the buildings' refinement. At Vanderbilt Hall, faculty wives took turns
hosting tea each Sunday afternoon. The teas took place in the Charles
H. Best Room, named for one of the men responsible for discovering
insulin, and gave students the opportunity for socially choreographed
interactions with faculty and their families (fig. 5.13).[92] Moreover, in providing squash courts, Vanderbilt and Bard Halls offered their students
opportunities to participate in a sport closely connected with the nation's

white male elite through members-only clubs, fancy tournaments, and select private high schools and universities, where the sport's popularity took off in the 1920s and 1930s. Harvard University's program stood out in these decades under the leadership of famed coach Harry Cowles, whose "Hints for Those Wishing to Become Champions" culminated with "always be a gentleman." Squash was so popular among Harvard undergraduates in the early 1920s that each week some five hundred students played the game, and in 1923 they resorted to breaking into the squash courts on Sundays, the one day each week that the university closed the facility.[93] The squash courts in Vanderbilt and Bard Halls undoubtedly responded to student demand and enabled those students who had developed a passion for the game at prestigious high schools or universities to continue playing it in medical school. At the same time, those students who had not been exposed to squash could learn this gentlemen's sport from their peers. Student enthusiasm for squash at Harvard Medical School proved so great that the school constructed more courts in the 1931 addition to Vanderbilt Hall.[94] The leadership at Columbia and Harvard hoped that in these carefully designed dormitories students would leave behind any lingering habits associated with the undereducated and unrefined doctor of the previous century and instead come to embody a respected professional.

Reality, however, did not always match expectations. In the winter of 1931, in the midst of the national prohibition against alcohol, students in Vanderbilt Hall reportedly brewed beer and exhibited intoxicated behavior.[95] Later that spring, a concerned alumnus reported that occupants of the maternity hospital across the street found immense entertainment in watching the events at Vanderbilt Hall between midnight and 3:00 a.m., specifically the large number of young women exiting the residence.[96] As Francis D. Moore, class of 1939, recalled, "a widespread tendency to uproarious alcoholic parties was certainly notable in our medical school years. While these parties sometimes bothered the neighbors, they seemed to be a generally harmless way of blowing off steam and getting out from under the intense pressures of medical school."[97] Henry A. Christian, prominent faculty member and former dean, did not agree with Moore's sanguine assessment of the parties. In 1939, he contacted current dean C. Sidney Burwell about poor behavior among Harvard's medical students. He singled out Moore's class for their actions, which were "cause for a very considerable criticism of the medical profession." Christian believed that Harvard faculty and alumni implicitly condoned the medical students' behavior by not condemning it and were in large part responsible for the students' misconduct.[98] Medical leaders could not dismiss students' transgressive actions as youthful rowdiness; they reflected on the school and on the profession. Educators worked hard to shape students' behavior, but the task remained a challenge.

Molding students' character required careful management of the people interacting with the aspiring physicians, and each group on the medical campus received careful examination to determine its appropriateness for the dormitory environment. From the beginning, Harvard Medical School leadership intentionally housed some international students, whether graduate students in medicine or in the School of Public Health, in Vanderbilt Hall, noting that they "constitute an exceptionally valuable type of men for our medical students to meet intimately and freely; and . . . they provide a very cosmopolitan and intellectually interesting group." Similarly, lodging unmarried faculty in the dormitory benefited medical students "socially and intellectually."[99] When the dining hall repeatedly ran a deficit, however, Harvard Medical School set up a system whereby ten dollars secured membership in the "Vanderbilt Club." Club membership provided access to the dining hall, common room, and library, but only those club members who were also Harvard Medical School students and faculty had access to the athletic facilities as well. In addition to students, faculty, and alumni of Harvard Medical School, faculty and students affiliated with the School of Public Health and the graduate courses could join the club, but only Harvard Dental School faculty—not the dental students—could become club members.[100] Such a system created a hierarchy that privileged medical students over those training in public health, graduate programs, and dentistry and also prioritized public health and graduate students over dental students. Harvard Medical School did not enroll women until 1945, but female secretaries, technicians, and graduate students could obtain guest passes at Vanderbilt Hall during lunchtime.[101]

As at Harvard Medical School, use of Columbia University's medical student dormitory reinforced the power structure within the medical center. In particular, dormitory access marginalized Columbia's dental students. Bard Hall housed male medical students and a small number of unmarried medical faculty but no students from the dental school. As Columbia's medical school dean explained, "one of the great needs of the Medical School is to improve the character of the student body. This is also true of the Dental School and even to a greater degree, but we have reached a higher point than they have."[102] Thus, dental students would degrade the refined environment of the dormitory. Moreover, the presence of dental students would discourage medical students from living in Bard Hall. The dean felt sure that with dental students in Bard

Hall the building would become a recruitment liability for the medical school rather than an impetus for enrollment.[103] In the end, the administration hoped that the dormitory would help bring the top collegians to the medical school at Columbia. Once lodged at Bard Hall, the medical students—surrounded only by others like themselves—would be elevated socially and intellectually by contact with the young faculty.

When the dormitory opened in the fall of 1931, however, it failed to fill, a particularly problematic turn of events for Columbia, where the leadership—unlike at Harvard—hoped that rentals in the dormitory would generate income for the university.[104] The medical school dean explored a number of options to remedy this problem. He considered setting aside floors for married medical students and women medical students, renting rooms to the medical fraternities, and reserving space for dental students.[105] Ultimately the administration invited the forty women medical students (who made up 10 percent of the medical school's students), women graduate students, and women faculty and research staff to live on the second floor at Bard Hall.[106] While the dean's perception that dental students lived at home or lacked the financial resources to afford residence in Bard Hall may have influenced this decision, professional hierarchies did as well, with dental students considered a less desirable addition to the dormitory than female medical students.[107] After the change in policy, women immediately filled the second floor and required additional rooms on the first floor.[108]

The decision to allow women to live in Bard Hall underscores complex dialogues about the economic bottom line, gender, and professional identity. Columbia University expected Bard Hall to generate revenue for the school, and filling the dormitory became a critical goal. Early twentieth-century Americans considered separate housing for male and female students standard practice.[109] In choosing to buck cultural norms and admit medical women to the dormitory rather than male dental students, Columbia's leadership demonstrated the power of professional hierarchies. Even deeply entrenched gender expectations could not eclipse a desire to keep physicians and dentists separate.

Included out of necessity, however, the women received a lukewarm reception at Bard Hall. Most basically, they were restricted to the first and second floors rather than interspersed among their male classmates on all eleven residential floors. The first floor included the front office, entrance hall, foyer, lounge, and grill. The second floor contained a gallery that opened onto the lounge and a corridor with a row of large windows overlooking the foyer, which, although glazed with "obscure wire glass," may have allowed some visibility from the space below and particularly the front office.[110] Women usually received greater levels of privacy than their male peers, but the choice to place women on the more public first and second floors likely stemmed from a desire to supervise their behavior in this unconventional living situation.

In addition, from the opening of the dormitory, women could not become members of the Bard Hall Club. Modeled on the Vanderbilt Club at Harvard, the Bard Hall Club offered dues-paying members access to the building's dining and athletic facilities. Only men who were medical students, medical school alumni, medical or dental faculty and administrators, special students and graduate students with recommendation, and residents and interns at the medical center could join. Women in these positions could obtain guest privileges in order to enter the reception room, lounge, dining room, and cafeteria during certain hours. Bard Hall remained entirely closed to dental students.[111] Women appear not to have received expanded access to the dining or athletic areas once they began living in the dormitory. Designed only for men, the athletic facilities at Bard Hall did not have locker rooms or toilets for women, which no doubt discouraged a change in policy. Even before Bard Hall opened, the nursing students had invited the women medical students to use the pool in the nurses' home.[112] Presumably this arrangement continued once the women moved into Bard Hall.

As places to congregate and dine with male members of the same (or soon-to-be same) socioeconomic circle, Vanderbilt Hall and Bard Hall paralleled upper-class urban men's clubs. It is no coincidence that both dormitories called their dining and recreational organizations a *club*. Architectural historian Annmarie Adams has shown how elite urban men's clubs expressed masculinity and class architecturally. Adams demonstrates the ways in which elements of the aristocratic home, the control of movement through the building, and an emphasis on male-only leisure activities generated a message of manliness and power.[113]

Versions of all of these architectural features existed at Vanderbilt and Bard Halls. Adams highlights rooms that are "dark and cozy, an ambience traditionally associated with men's residential spaces, such as libraries, dens, and dining rooms, which in the nineteenth century frequently showcased dark paneling, fine wooden furniture, leather upholstery, and books."[114] These decorative motifs appear at Vanderbilt and Bard Halls, as indicated by Vanderbilt Hall's Charles H. Best Room (see fig. 5.13), where the ashtrays on every table further demarcate this room as a masculine preserve. Indeed, smoking rooms and heraldic emblems further aligned the dormitory—and some medical schools' educational buildings—with private men's clubs.[115]

At the same time, both dormitories carefully controlled how visitors moved through the space. At Bard Hall, a visitor to the building immediately encountered a two-story foyer under the direct surveillance of a front office. A reception room to the left of the entrance with adjoining women's toilet indicated where female guests should wait for their male hosts. Across the foyer from the entrance, the visitor faced three pairs of glass doors that restricted access to the lounge and demarcated the limits of the visitor's progression into the building. Whereas a central entrance organized circulation at Bard Hall, Vanderbilt Hall combined a staircase (entry) plan with a main entrance. In dormitory architecture, staircase plans allowed for less control over the occupants because a series of staircases with external doors gave students direct admittance to the residential quarters.[116] At Vanderbilt Hall, the building's residential section had a staircase plan, while the more public section open also to members of the Vanderbilt Club had a single entrance that gave guests admission only to the main dining room, living room, and library. From the more public section of the building one had either to leave the main floor or exit the building to enter the dormitory area.

Once inside the medical student dormitories, as in the men's clubs, occupants conversed, ate together, and engaged in leisure activities, with some—such as squash—clearly associated with men. The bonds produced by these communal activities were reinforced in spatial terms. Like the men's clubs, the designs of the dormitories ensured that occupants constantly saw one another, validating visually their shared membership in an exclusive group.[117] At Bard Hall, a gallery on the second floor opened onto the lounge. At Vanderbilt Hall, a dramatic corridor window connected arriving guests with diners before the dining room door opened (fig. 5.14).

It was no coincidence that the medical school dormitories created an environment that paralleled in many ways prominent urban men's clubs. Both strove to envelop their members in a prestigious, white male world separated from the rest of the city.[118] In her work on undergraduate dormitories, Yanni explains that "women *were* second-class citizens in the educational landscape of the late nineteenth and early twentieth centuries. . . . Coeds were women. Students were men."[119] Similarly, men were "medics" or "medicos," while women were "medico-eds."[120] The most elite young men could move fluidly from select male preparatory school to exclusive, all-male or predominantly male college, and then urban men's club. As members-only masculine preserves, the medical dormitories at Harvard and Columbia inserted male medical students into this extended indoctrination in class and power. In this way, the dormitories proclaim

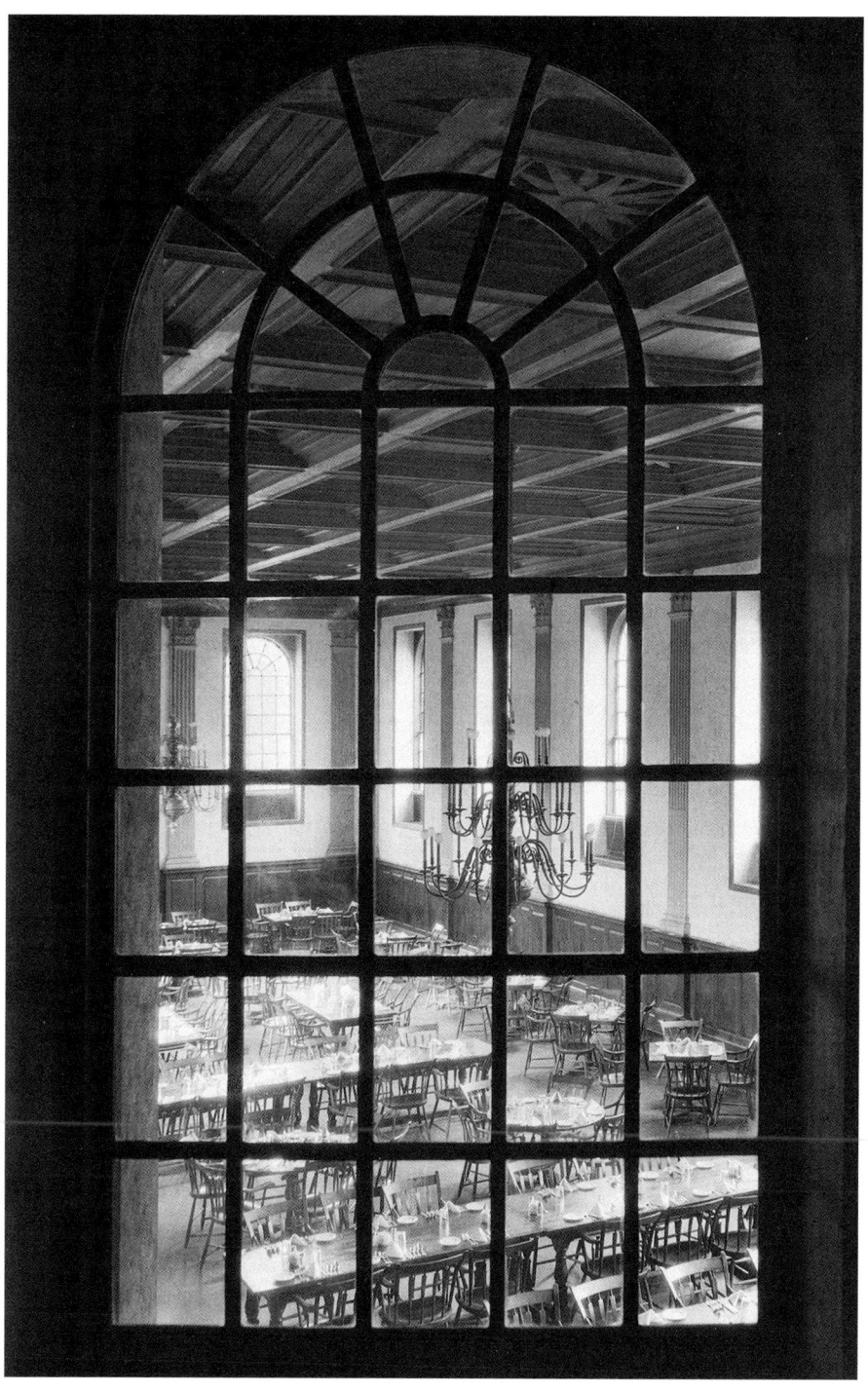

5.14.   Vanderbilt Hall, Harvard Medical School, 1927, Coolidge, Shepley, Bulfinch, and
         Abbott, architects, view through window between dining room and hallway.
         Photograph ca. 1928.

boldly what the medical schools' educational buildings reveal more mutedly: these facilities steeped students in a privileged, white, Protestant, masculine professional identity.

Given this environment, the women's enthusiasm for living in Bard Hall may seem surprising. Likely the lack of housing near the medical center disproportionately affected women students.[121] Women students may also have had a greater need than their male classmates for the community of colleagues and faculty mentors established by their relatively separate living quarters within Bard Hall. During Alice Baker's senior year at Louisiana State University School of Medicine in 1938, she wrote of the comfort provided by the presence of other women students (fig. 5.15): "Gretchen is on OB

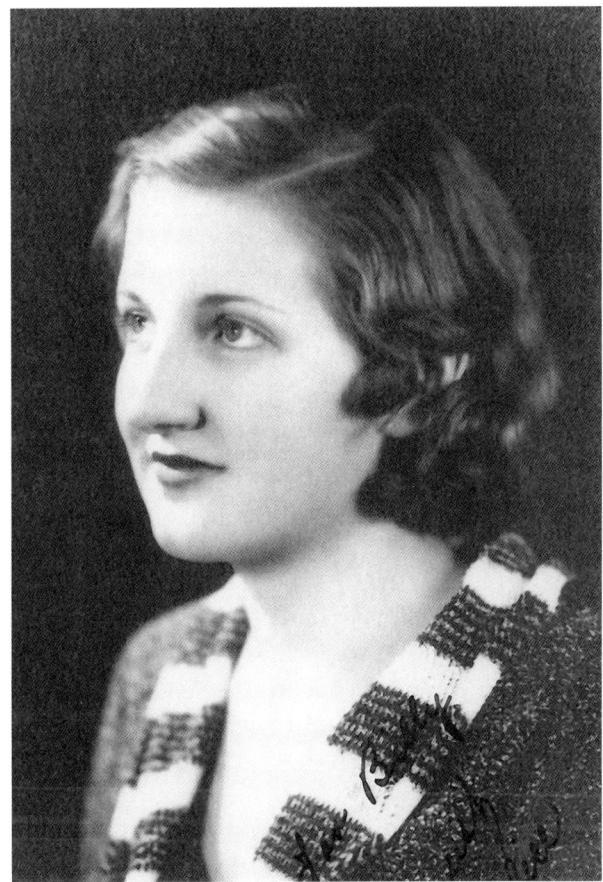

5.15.   Alice Baker, ca. 1934.

duty this week, so with Dot away and Alice Tisdale in California . . . I'm trying to hold up the feminine side of the class. It's quite a job to withstand all the teasing and jibes without someone to share it with, but I believe I can take it by now!"[122] Indeed, Baker had plenty of experience with verbal attacks, sometimes from the highest quarters of the profession. When Morris Fishbein, the long-standing and powerful editor of the *Journal of the American Medical Association*, spoke at her medical school the previous year, Baker had reported that "he picked out the female sex to insult and—well, he made every girl who listened to him furious. Not content with belittling our mental capacity, he informed the group that one only had to look around even in a medical class to see how women wasted money on cosmetics."[123] Historian Regina Morantz-Sanchez has described the psychological toll of even subtle and frequently unperceived discrimination against women in coeducational medical schools, and she notes in particular the shortage of female faculty to act as role models and offer support.[124] Although living in the dormitory opened women to possible surveillance by the office staff and others in Bard Hall, the clustering of rooms at Bard Hall for women students and faculty may have created a temporary retreat from the male-dominated environment of the rest of Bard Hall and the medical center. The construction of Bard Hall stemmed in part from a desire to strengthen male medical students' professional consciousness, but it may have been the marginalized women medical students whose professional identity gained the most from the dormitory. Moreover, even with their second-class status, women in Bard Hall affirmed their place within the ranks of current and future physicians when they moved into the dormitory.

Significant disparities in students' experiences based on race and sex notwithstanding, medical schools and dormitories inculcated in medical students an elite identity and promoted the elevated socioeconomic status of the modern American physician. Establishing the profession, however, required more than cultivating doctors' privileged cultural position. As has already been hinted, creating modern physicians also meant defining the profession in relation to other medical fields. American medical schools reflected and encouraged a hierarchy among medical personnel.

Physicians, Nurses, Dentists, and Pharmacists in the Medical Hierarchy

More types of medical personnel than physicians trained in medical schools and their affiliated hospitals. By the early twentieth century, many American hospitals had opened schools for nurses. By 1923, one in four hospitals across the nation included a nursing school, but the ratio could be much higher. In 1910, nearly twice as many hospitals in Massachusetts housed a nursing school as did not. Although billed as educational programs, the nursing schools in reality provided inexpensive labor for the hospital, and most of the student nurses' time in the wards involved working rather than learning.[125] In contrast, education represented the primary focus of physicians' student years. Difference in professional status compounded this educational divide, with nurses subordinated to physicians.[126] Gender conventions further reinforced this unequal relationship between female nurses and doctors, most of whom were men. The buildings promoted this hierarchy. They emphasized the primacy of medical education over nursing education and codified greater levels of autonomy and independence for the physicians-in-training than for their nursing counterparts.

The first fully fledged nursing schools opened in the United States in 1873 in Boston, New York, and New Haven. The schools' leadership envisioned their students replacing untrained nurses in the hospital wards by providing patient care while they learned the practical and theoretical components of nursing, but the hospitals' need for cheap labor and the nursing schools' fiscal reliance on the hospitals—nursing schools had no endowments—resulted in more work than education. The practical training intended to move pupils through increasingly technical tasks dissolved in the face of emergencies and staffing shortages. Physicians offered lectures to supplement pupils' time on the ward, but these sessions typically took place in the evening after ten- or twelve-hour shifts had already left students exhausted.[127] Moreover, because physicians taught these courses, the nursing leadership had little control over the material covered, not to mention the physicians' enthusiasm or commitment. Even with these hurdles, however, nursing students did become proficient in the new scientific language and skilled techniques, and they used this knowledge to distinguish themselves from untrained nurses. Trained nurses enjoyed the authority to act as physicians' able assistants at the same time that they had to accept their inferior position within a hierarchical, and gendered, medical structure.[128] Despite her expanded knowledge and discipline, the student nurse undertook much of the same work as her earlier counterparts. By 1900, phrases such as "hospital machine" and "industrial slave" had come into use for the student nurse, and popular culture underscored the drudgery of her work, her lack of individuality, and her subordination within the hospital hierarchy (fig. 5.16). After completing either two or three years of training, graduates usually became private nurses who offered personal care to those who could afford it. A handful of women filled leadership positions in hospitals. Not until the 1930s did most nurses obtain employment on hospital staffs.[129]

As the educational rhetoric, knowledge, and discipline, if not much of the day-to-day work, changed with the rise of nursing schools, so too did the architecture. Before the advent of nursing schools, untrained nurses typically lived with the hospital service staff in attics, basements, or empty wards—locations that connoted low status and subservience.[130] Architectural historian Karen Kingsley has shown that student nurses in the early training schools endured similarly makeshift accommodations, including at Massachusetts General Hospital. Its first nursing students lodged two to a bed in small rooms between wards that frequently functioned as clinical spaces during the day. Nursing and hospital leadership, however, quickly called for separate homes for student nurses. These autonomous

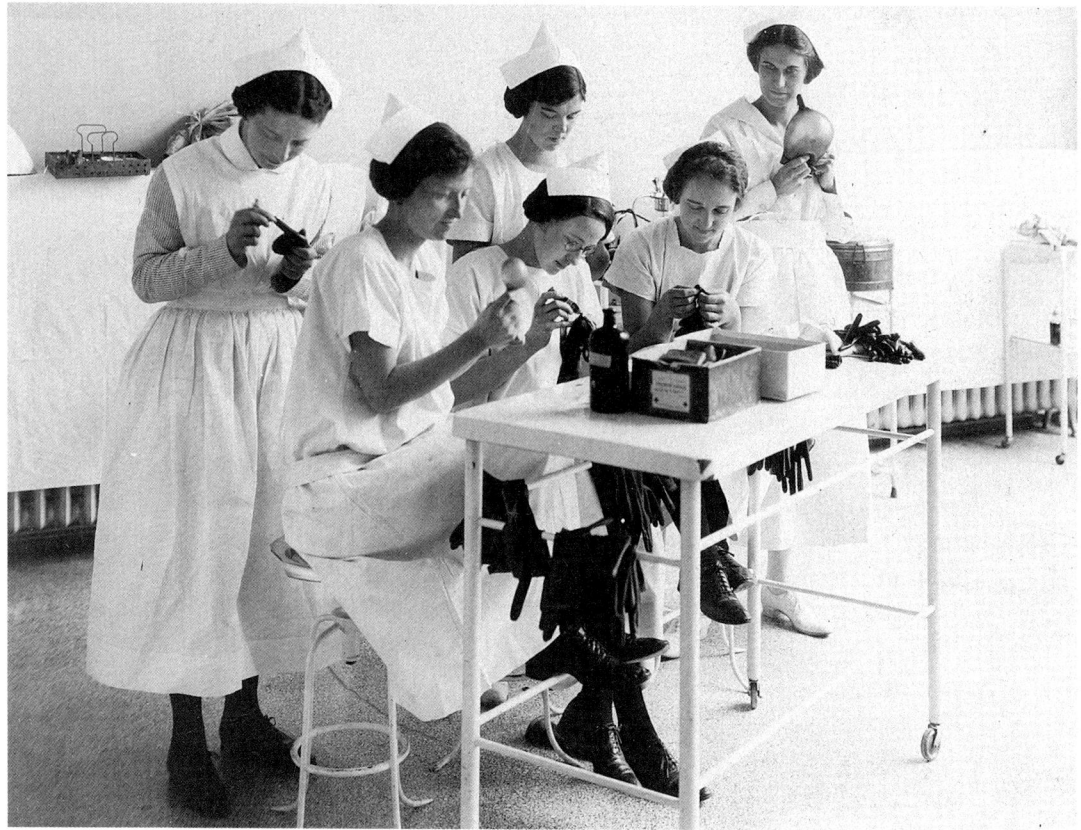

5.16.   Nursing students, all dressed for the operating room except for one (*far left*), patch gloves under the supervision of a faculty member (*far right*), University of Nebraska School of Nursing, 1922.

buildings affirmed for the public, student and graduated nurses, and the broader medical community the professional image of the trained nurse. Much like modern medical schools, "the architecture [of the nurses' home] had to erase the old image of the nurse from the mind of the public and establish a new one." The nurses' residences also appealed to nursing school leaders and donors because the structures attracted stronger applicants and helped the young women maintain their physical and mental strength once they enrolled. Healthy and happy student nurses, so the thinking went, provided better patient care.[131] But not every hospital had the land or financial resources to construct a separate building for its student nurses; instead, they continued to carve out space for the nursing students within the hospital or rented or bought nearby houses.[132] Presbyterian Hospital had the good fortune to have both the land and the money to construct a model nurses' residence; Maxwell Hall opened as part of the larger Columbia-Presbyterian Medical Center in 1928 (fig. 5.17).

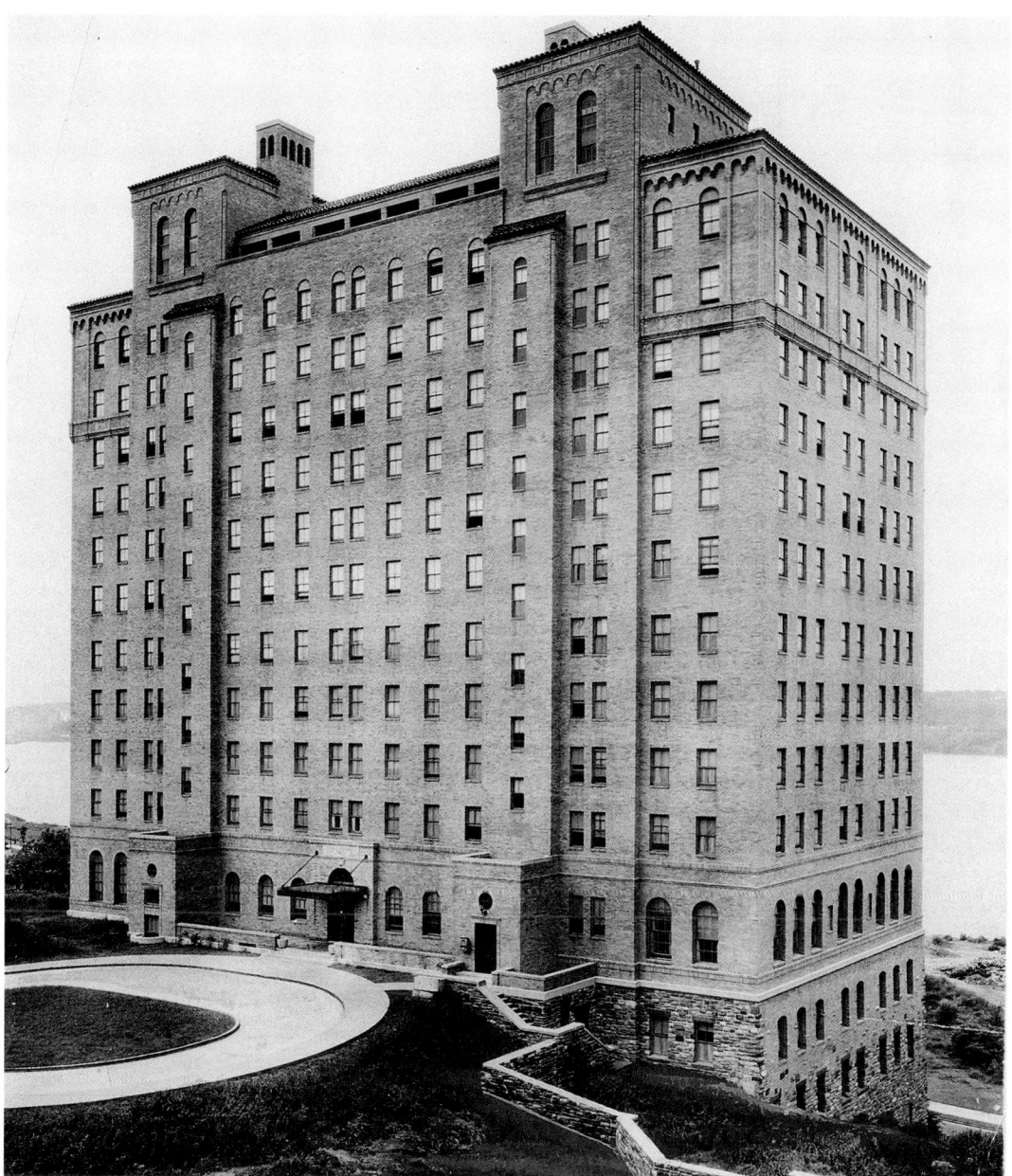

5.17.   Maxwell Hall, Columbia-Presbyterian Medical Center, 1928, James Gamble Rogers, architect.

  The Presbyterian Hospital School of Nursing, like Columbia University's College of Physicians and Surgeons, grew out of the highest pedagogical standards. From its founding in 1892, the nursing school had taught the medical sciences alongside compassionate care, cleanliness, and discipline. When the school relocated to Columbia-Presbyterian

Medical Center, it continued to provide exceptional educational opportunities. Nursing students at Columbia-Presbyterian trained in a
massive, modern medical complex. The medical center provided the
students access to a wide variety of specialty wards, outpatient clinics,
cutting-edge equipment, and renowned physicians. Presbyterian Hospital School of Nursing also augmented the extensive ward experience
with classroom instruction and took academic learning seriously. At
Presbyterian, for example, the schedule received careful organization to
eliminate, among other potential problems, students on the night shift
attending daytime classes.[133] In contrast, at Vanderbilt University's School
of Nursing the students' ward duties left them unable to prepare properly
for lectures and laboratory courses.[134] To house its educational program,
the Presbyterian Hospital School of Nursing enjoyed its own practice
rooms and small amphitheater within the main medical school–hospital
building. In addition, the nursing students could use the medical school's
library, and they took their classes in anatomy and physiology, chemistry,
pathology, and bacteriology in the medical school.[135]

Nursing students' time within the medical school may have been
carefully monitored, however. Nancy Caroline King Cost, who earned
her bachelor of science in nursing from Vanderbilt University in 1939, recalled that "the nursing faculty chaperoned us when we attended classes
in the medical school."[136] Nursing students could not forget that they
were invited guests rather than the medical school's primary occupants.

The planning for the medical complexes also differentiated between
the medical fields and privileged medical students over nursing students,
even in the case of progressive nursing programs with extensive facilities.
At Columbia-Presbyterian and Vanderbilt, the nursing schools utilized
the medical school laboratories, and the leadership of the Nashville
nursing school expressed frustration at having to organize its program
around that of the medical school.[137] Not surprisingly, none of the documents related to the design of the medical student laboratories at Columbia-Presbyterian or at Vanderbilt mentions the unique needs of the
student nurses. The facilities at Columbia-Presbyterian and Vanderbilt
promoted the idea that scientific education remained less important
for nursing students than for medical students. Although exposed to
laboratory training, student nurses primarily remained ward workers,
while medical students became men of science. Underscoring this point,
physicians earned the title "doctor" upon graduation, but nurses received
the title "nurse" when they arrived on the wards as students. In essence
then, during their student years, doctors trained, while nurses showed
up and worked.[138]

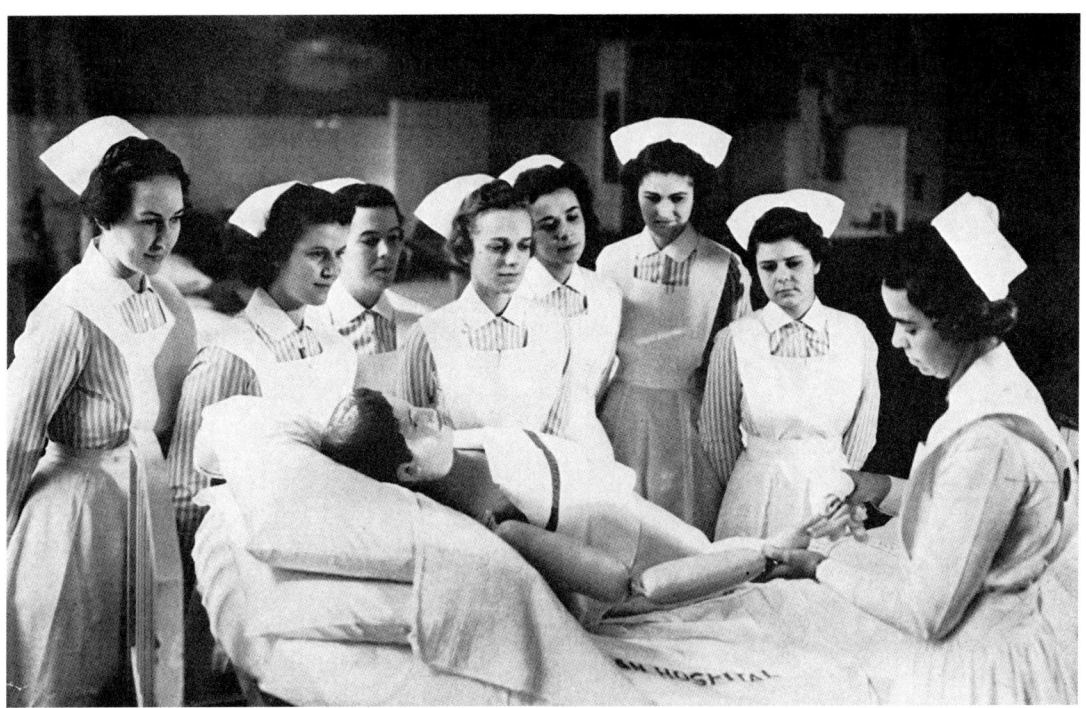

5.18.   Members of the Presbyterian Hospital School of Nursing class of 1940 receive instruction with a
patient manikin.

The nursing students' experience on the wards at Presbyterian Hospital School of Nursing further reinforced that their education remained
less of a priority than the medical students' education. An internal study
of the student nurses' ward and clinical experience in 1930–1931 catego-
rized only 58 percent of a student nurse's time as educationally significant, and only 13 percent of this time involved organized instruction and
classroom study. A student nurse, therefore, dedicated 42 percent of her
day to service in the hospital. Student nurses at Presbyterian Hospital
enjoyed many advantages, including the latest hospital equipment and a
state-of-the-art patient manikin in the practice rooms (fig. 5.18).[139] Nevertheless, a significant proportion of their days provided cheap labor for the
hospital. By contrast, although medical students' clinical years involved
patient care and inevitably redundancies of procedures, service to the
hospital was not as dominant an element of their four years of training.
    Divided between education and service, work and care, the student
nurses at the medical center experienced the same ambiguity as the
members of their profession more generally. The field's diverse con-
stituents responded to these dichotomies differently, but nursing school
leaders attempted a pluralistic approach. They strove to celebrate service

to patients and womanly virtues while simultaneously insisting on control over their work life. The patriarchal system under which this female workforce functioned compounded the situation. Physicians and hospital administrators, most of whom were men, opposed nurses' attempts at professionalization out of reluctance to allow women to act autonomously and from fear both of competition and of losing the inexpensive hospital labor supplied by student nurses.[140] As physicians solidified their professional status in the early twentieth century, nurses struggled to do the same. Maxwell and Bard Halls, the dormitories for nursing students and medical students, respectively, at Columbia-Presbyterian Medical Center further underscored the distinct professional identities of these two groups.

In February 1928, the student nurses' residence, Maxwell Hall, welcomed its first occupants. The nursing school's alumnae association had worked tirelessly to raise the necessary $1 million for the edifice. Current and former students contributed more than $225,000. The sale of the previous nurses' home provided an additional $500,000, and the campaign benefited from several friends of the school who made substantial gifts, including Anna M. Harkness and Mary Stillman Harkness, who together donated $275,000. The fifteen-story building designed by James Gamble Rogers included single rooms for 360 students, a small ward for infirm students, accommodations for 15 faculty members, a roof designed for sleeping and sunbathing, dining facilities, lounge, swimming pool, room equipped for exercise and dancing, 300-seat auditorium, large classroom, and library, all of which eventually pushed the project over budget by $400,000.[141]

Ultimately, however, the school's 1928 announcement could promise that Maxwell Hall offered "every facility for study, recreation, and hygienic living."[142] In fact, the former director of the school of nursing, Anna Maxwell, chose the hall's site not only for its spectacular view of the Hudson River and the New Jersey Palisades but also for its access to light and air.[143] Understandably, the students appreciated the new structure. One alumna affirmed, "In the 'good old days' when the P.H. [Presbyterian Hospital] Training School inhabited the upper floors of the Hospital Buildings and nurses were pigeonholed in small cubicles, the conception of a residence like Maxwell Hall would have been merely another air-castle."[144]

The grand edifice generally followed national trends of the 1920s, when concerns about recruitment and retention prompted some hospitals to construct expensive, large, and lavish nurses' homes.[145] Nursing educators and hospital architects in this decade called for a building

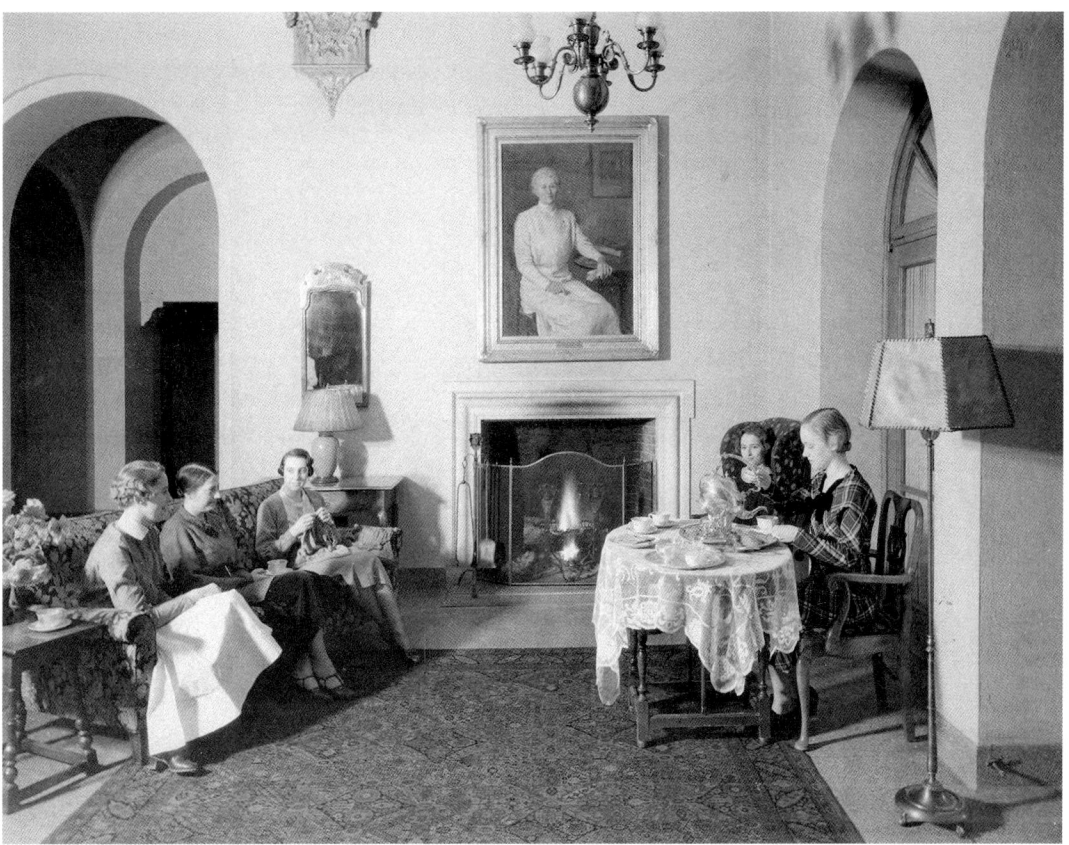

5.19.   Maxwell Hall, Columbia-Presbyterian Medical Center, 1928, James Gamble Rogers, architect, lounge.

detached from the hospital and providing single bedrooms, spaces for socialization, and opportunities for recreation. Despite the fact that these sizable homes were inherently institutional, carefully decorated parlors, lobbies, and sitting areas, in addition to outdoor patios and roof gardens, were linked to a home-like atmosphere intended to offer students a retreat from the institutional environment of the hospital.[146] In addition, architectural historian Annmarie Adams argues that the emphasis on refined, domestic residences was likely intended to ease the adjustment to the workplace for middle-class women, to calm the fears of concerned parents, and to recruit wealthier—and presumably more dignified—women to the profession.[147]

The annual announcements for the nursing school at Presbyterian Hospital underscored these points for potential applicants. One image published in the 1935–1936 announcement presented a staged scene within the lounge on the hall's first floor (fig. 5.19). Consistent with other nurses' residences in this period, mass-produced furniture reflective of

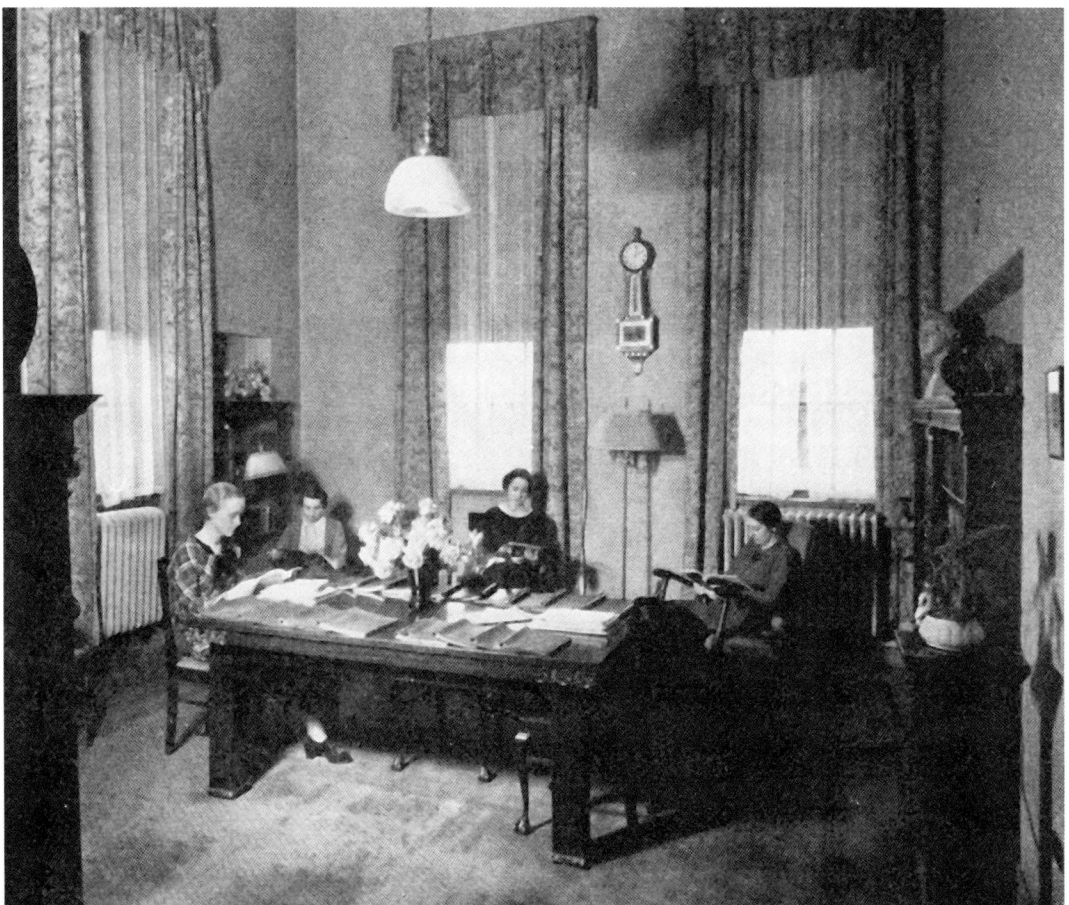

5.20.   Maxwell Hall, Columbia-Presbyterian Medical Center, 1928, James Gamble Rogers, architect, library.

middle-class homes and casually arranged around the fireplace suggested
a cozy middle-class interior. Although the prominent portrait of Anna
Maxwell—founder of the Presbyterian Hospital nursing school, national
leader in nursing education reform, and the person whose name the
structure bore—left no doubt about the work these women performed,
the scene highlighted their domestic qualities rather than their nursing
skills, with the women shown taking tea and making handicrafts.[148]
Moreover, although the 1935–1936 announcement for the nursing school
at Presbyterian Hospital asserted that Maxwell Hall's "reference library"
contained "the latest editions of approved reference books," the accompanying image displayed an intimate, home-like setting suggestive of casual review rather than serious academic work (fig. 5.20). Those students
"desiring advanced professional study," the announcement explained,
could find the necessary resources at the medical school library.[149] The

domestic, middle-class interiors of the nurses' home may also have inculcated in working-class women the middle-class values desired by the
field's academic leadership.[150]

If a domestic atmosphere infused the building, so too did competing
experiences of autonomy and control. The movement of student nurses out of hospital attics and into purpose-built structures undoubtedly
increased the field's visibility and granted women some freedom from
the hospital. At the same time, however, in a recognition of students'
dedication to nursing and their demanding schedules on the wards, close
physical ties remained between the hospital and the nearby residence.[151]
In the case of Columbia-Presbyterian, an underground tunnel connected
the nurses' home with the hospital across the street. Furthermore, although likely an unintentional reminder of the hospital's influence over
the students' lives, the roof of Maxwell Hall, used for both recreation
and sleep, fell within the sight lines of the upper stories of the hospital,
a reality the students lamented in their 1936 yearbook.[152]

Rules and regulations augmented the architectural controls.[153]
When students or visitors used the main entrance to Maxwell Hall,
they passed in front of an open office, which maintained a direct view of
the doorway. School historian Gary Goldenberg notes that arrivals and
departures were closely monitored, particularly after curfew at 10:30 p.m.
In addition, the school recorded both students' hours of sleep and their
recreation. Physical appearance also received scrutiny. A 1930 graduate
recalled the review of students by the school's director before they entered the hospital: "On our way down to the tunnel to the hospital, Miss
Young inspected us, especially to check for hairnets. No hairnet—back
you went."[154]

The nursing students' apparel itself further underscored the paradoxes of their position in the medical center. With the development of
nurses' training schools came nurses' uniforms. Nursing pioneers needed
to make the vocation acceptable for young women, and with the field's
historical associations with religious orders and the military, nursing
leaders knew well the symbolic value of a uniform. The elaborate early
uniforms ensured that no one would confuse the nurses with scrub-
women in the hospital or domestic servants in the home. After Bellevue
Hospital's nursing school adopted a uniform, other American schools
followed suit. Each school designed its own uniform, and graduates typically wore the uniform of their alma mater for life, regardless of whether
they worked in hospitals, on private duty, or even internationally. As
Goldenberg explains, "the uniform . . . became a wearable [résumé],"
and nurses took pride in this marker of their training.[155]

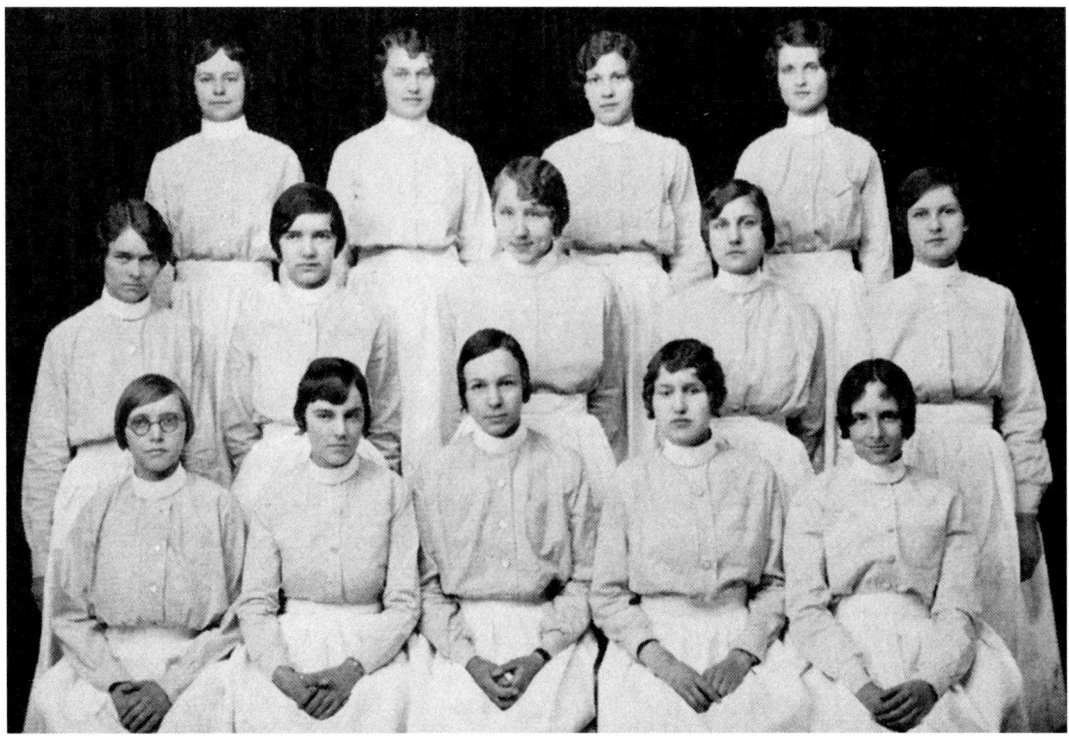

5.21.   Nursing students wearing the probationer uniform required during the early part of their training, University of Nebraska School of Nursing, 1930.

Within nursing schools, the uniform also conveyed one's educational level. Students wore a different uniform during the first phase of training, the probationary period, and a 1936 Presbyterian Hospital graduate recalled that this uniform "protected the students while they were working in the clinical area . . . and it protected the patients."[156] Students obtained the full school uniform, including the cap, upon completion of the probationary session (figs. 5.21 and 5.22). The "capping" ceremony at the University of Nebraska School of Nursing marked the conclusion of the probationary period and underscored the personal, institutional, and professional significance of both this accomplishment and the new uniform. Attended by students' friends and family, the ceremony took place either on campus or in a church. During the ceremony, the student nurse knelt while the director of the school affixed the cap to her head and her "big sister" gave her a lighted "Nightingale lamp." Music by the school's choir, an inspirational message, and a tea given by the School of Nursing Alumnae Association and usually held in the lounge of the nurses' residence rounded out the day. Many nurses described the capping ceremony as the most significant event of their school years.[157]

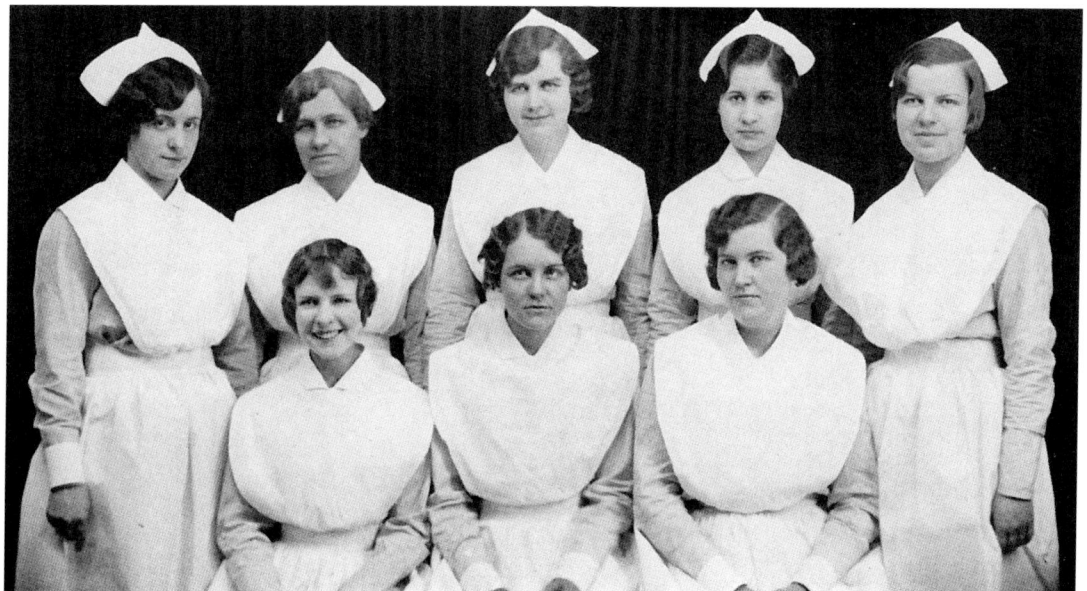

5.22.   Big Sister Organization, University of Nebraska School of Nursing, 1930. These nursing students have completed the probationary period and no longer wear the probationer uniform. In the senior year, the students added white cuffs to their sleeves (compare student on far left with student on far right). The nursing students in the front row presumably removed their caps for the photograph in order not to block the women behind them.

Finer variations in dress also existed. At Nebraska, students added white cuffs to their uniform in their senior year.[158] At Presbyterian Hospital, although the student nurse received her distinctive striped outfit and her cap upon completion of the probationary period, she did not exchange her black stockings and shoes for white ones until graduation.[159]

If student nurses found their uniforms prescribed to the smallest detail, no parallel clothing requirements existed for medical students. Underscoring that profession and not sex determined one's dress, the female medical students of Woman's Medical College of Pennsylvania, like their male counterparts elsewhere, did not wear matching uniforms (fig. 5.23). By the 1920s, the white coat increasingly represented the modern physician, both within the medical community and in popular culture. For medical students, the designation as a physician-in-training was marked by longer laboratory coats, often white, in the preclinical years and shorter white coats donned for clinical training in the second two years.[160] But medical students, like physicians, wore clothes of their own choosing underneath the coats (see figs. 5.1 and 5.2). Even the nearly entirely white outfits expected of interns and residents still allowed for some individual variation (fig. 5.24). Nevertheless, medical

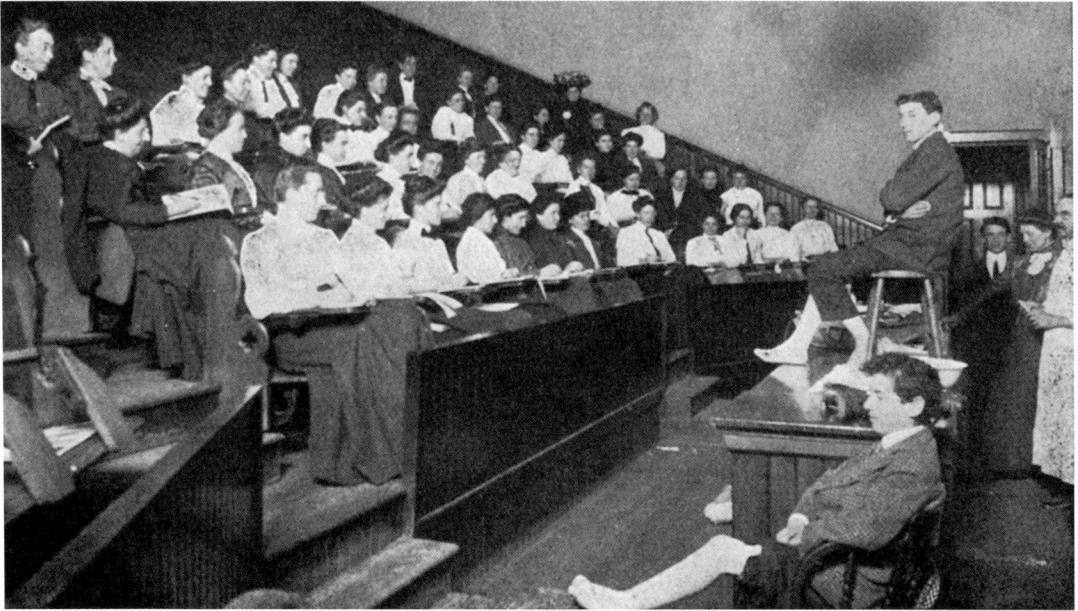

5.23.   Woman's Medical College of Pennsylvania students attending an orthopedics clinic, ca. 1911.

students' clothing did receive scrutiny. Joe Holoubek recalled the words the dean spoke to his class on his first day of medical school in 1934: "You are now members of a respected profession and I want you to act accordingly. I don't ever want to see or hear of any one of you appearing in public without a coat and a tie, unless you are going to or coming from an athletic event in which you are taking part."[161] While administrators may have expected medical students to look professional, particularly once they had contact with patients in their third and fourth years, they did not have to dress identically.

In contrast, student nurses dressed with complete uniformity and found their individuality erased as a result. Those trained in Presbyterian Hospital's nursing school, which became part of Columbia University in 1937, wore a uniform whose cloth had a distinctive blue stripe. A 1960 graduate warned, "A seeming loss of individuality may be one of the clouds which you will experience as you see yourself mirrored in the sea of blue uniforms."[162] If student nurses felt their personal identity dissolved by the uniform, so too did others cease to distinguish them as individuals. In a 1913 novel, *The White Linen Nurse*, a surgeon fails to identify the main character despite a long exchange and apologizes, "Excuse me for not recognizing you, but you girls all look so much alike!" The student nurse's response includes, "I tell you, sir, I'm sick to death of being nothing but a type. I want to look like *myself*!"[163] The uniform became a

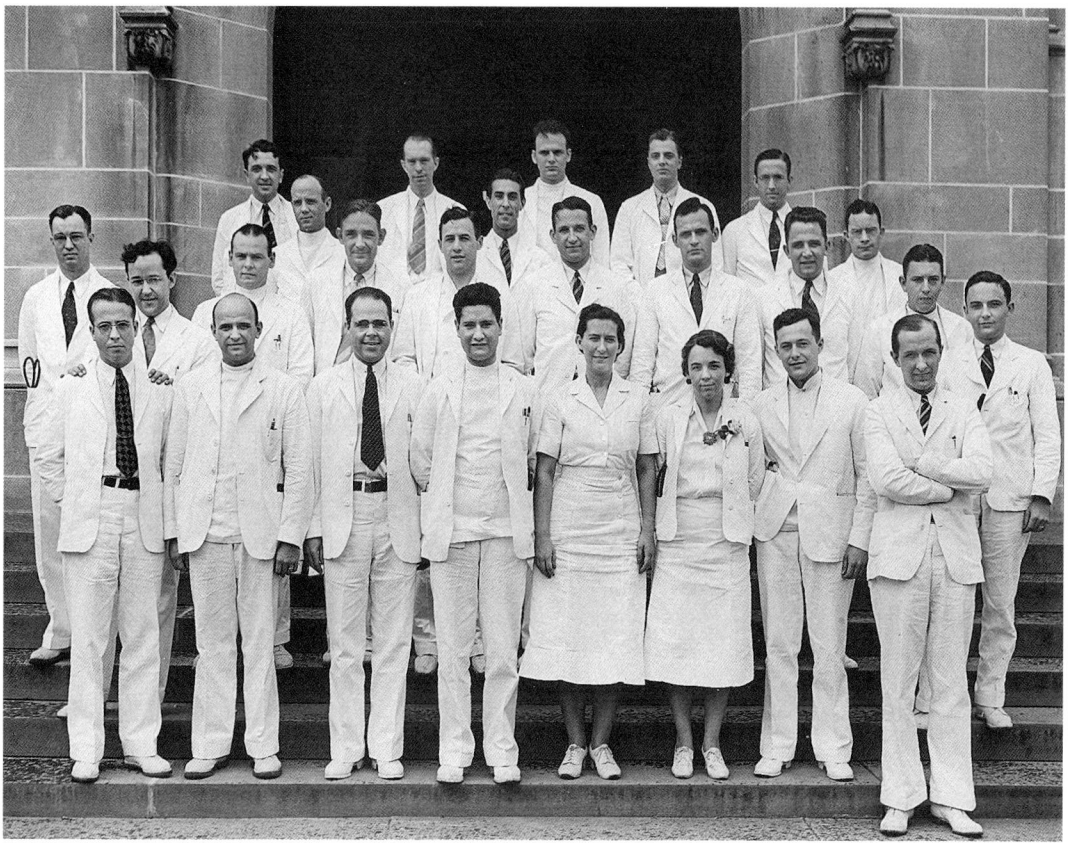

5.24.   Vanderbilt University Hospital House Staff, 1938–1939.

symbol of nurses' education and the creation of a new profession, but at
the same time it rendered individuals nearly invisible.

Fraught with contradictions between autonomy and service, innovation and traditional values, the design and experience of nurses' educational and residential facilities made manifest the field's professional
paradoxes and inculcated in the young women their incongruities. Conversely, the residential space for male medical students formulated a less
conflicted professional identity. Their dormitory, Bard Hall, positioned
these students as independent young people and future members of a
powerful profession, all capable of making their own decisions.

Compared to Maxwell Hall, Bard Hall offered its inhabitants greater freedom of choice. Maxwell Hall provided only single rooms, but students at Bard could reside in single rooms or small suites.[164] With regard
to dining, all of the nursing students in Maxwell Hall ate in one dining
area, but in Bard Hall medical students had two eating options: a large
dining room or a more intimate grill. Furthermore, Bard Hall's location

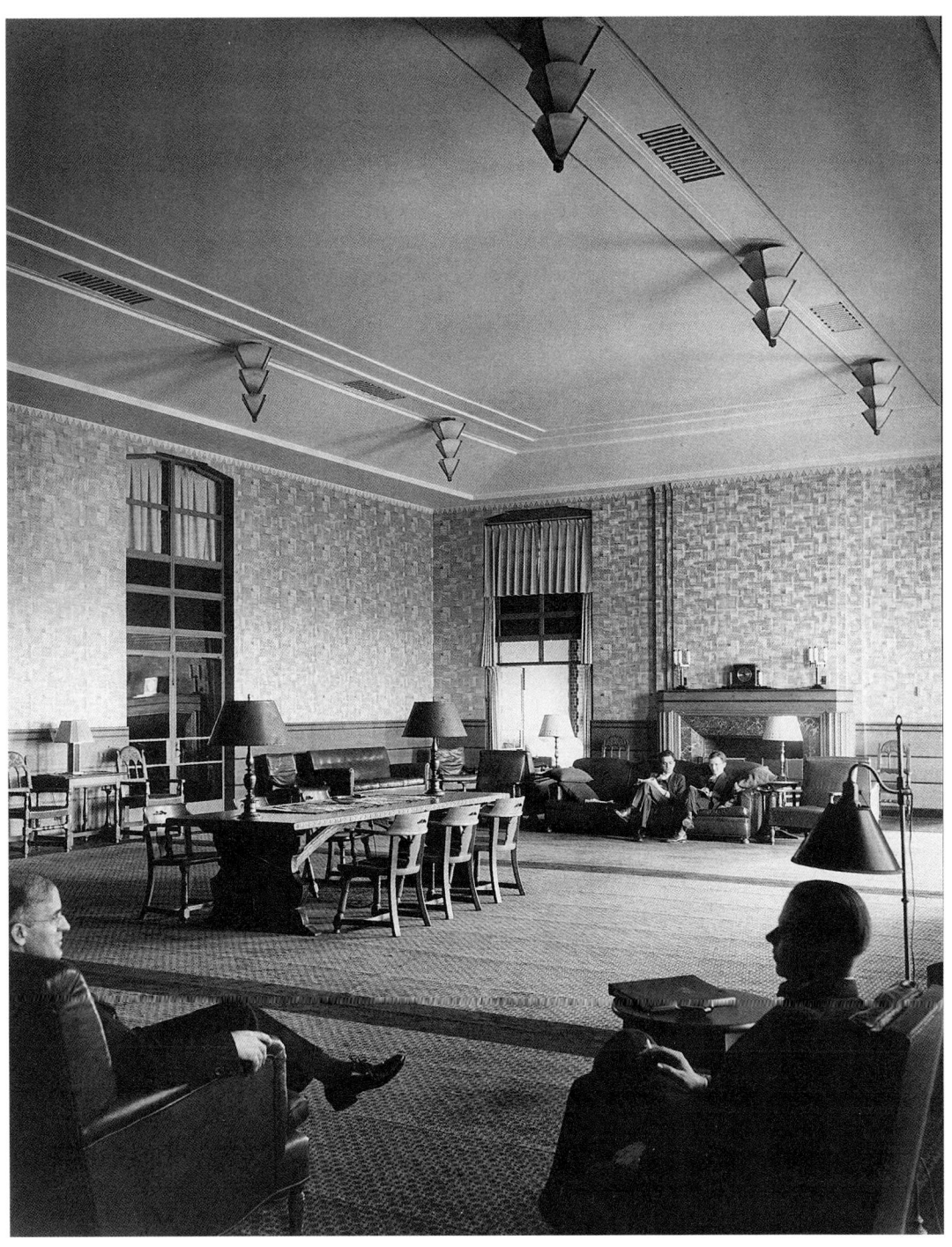

5.25.   Bard Hall, Columbia-Presbyterian Medical Center, 1931, James Gamble Rogers, architect, living room.

on the periphery of campus, with no direct tunnel to the medical school and hospital complex, gave its inhabitants a larger degree of separation from their academic work. An open office in the entrance hall did allow for direct surveillance of Bard's main doorway, but far fewer regulations structured life in Bard Hall. Unlike at Maxwell Hall, no curfew existed, and the only detailed rules explained when women could visit and where they could venture within Bard.[165] Designed originally for male medical students, Bard Hall codified gender and professional expectations by encouraging male medical students to act autonomously. Of course, the most basic option afforded medical students was the decision to live in Bard Hall at all. Unlike the nursing students, medical students could opt out of dormitory life.

The role of faculty in Maxwell and Bard Halls also communicated different behavioral standards to nursing students and medical students. In Maxwell Hall, where fifteen faculty members, including the school's director, lived, the faculty closely monitored students within the residence, as the hairnet inspections revealed.[166] Underscoring the differentiation between students and faculty, Maxwell Hall's design separated the faculty from the students by creating distinct spaces in which the faculty would live and eat within the dormitory. The relatively private south hallway on the first floor, for instance, housed the school's director and a pair of graduated nurses but no students. Moreover, although the walls enclosing the staff dining room in the original plan ultimately were not built, the nursing faculty still ate in a separate alcove, apart from their pupils.[167] This division of faculty and students reinforced that their relationship was hierarchical. In many ways, the obedience demanded of student nurses on the wards continued when they entered the dormitory.

Conversely, life in Bard Hall fostered collegial engagement between students and faculty. Accordingly, no separate dining space existed for faculty at Bard. In addition, a staged photograph highlighted in the foreground a conversation between an older and a younger man, with the junior member casually smoking a cigarette. The image suggests friendly faculty-student interaction, a contrast with the seemingly student-only domestic scene promoted at Maxwell Hall (fig. 5.25; see also fig. 5.19). Furthermore, the tutors—members of the medical faculty who resided in Bard Hall—lived in continuous contact with the students. The tutors' suites occupied one end of each floor and opened directly onto the main dormitory corridor. Early projections imagined that the tutors would have some controlling influence on the behavior of Bard Hall occupants.[168] But when associate dean Frederick T. van Beuren Jr. wrote to a prospective tutor in 1931, he mentioned no regulatory role. Instead, he envisioned that "the work will be to act in effect as older brothers or friends of the students and help to inspire them by example rather than by precept and to arouse their enthusiasm for medical study and practice or research."[169] If nursing students learned deference to their faculty at Maxwell Hall, medical students may have found some relief in their dormitory from the faculty-student hierarchy typically associated with the medical school and hospital. Bard Hall encouraged medical students to see themselves as fledgling members of a professional community that valued independence and autonomy.

Within this environment, women medical students occupied a complex position that underlined their convoluted place in the medical hierarchy. Elevated by professional status but restricted by gender expectations, they navigated competing identities. Overall, however, women medical students' identity as physicians-in-training outstripped their identity as women.[170] Women medical students at Columbia-Presbyterian may have had to swim in the nursing students' pool, but they received an invitation to live in Bard Hall, unlike male dental students. Similarly, when Woman's Medical College of Pennsylvania relocated in 1930, it provided housing, initially on the top floor of the medical school–hospital building, for its nursing students but not for its medical students (all women).[171] Moreover, women medical students may have had to retreat to their more private lounges within the coeducational medical schools, but their individualized clothing and white coats clearly marked them as medical students.

Professional identity can begin to form in the educational environment before one enters the workplace. Hospitals, as sites of both work and education, may provide particularly intensive immersion in expected professional behavior. Due to its emphasis on the education obtained during the four years of medical school, this study does not consider the hospital employees that sometimes lived in the medical center. For example, when Columbia-Presbyterian opened, it housed in its main medical school–hospital building five floors of personnel, including kitchen workers, cleaners, general duty nurses, dietitians, and interns, the last being recently graduated physicians who worked and lived in the hospital while they expanded their training. Not surprisingly, the male intern's experience paralleled in many ways that of the male medical student. Underscoring the continuity of professional indoctrination, Adams's examination of the residence for male interns at the Royal Victoria Hospital in Montreal reveals an emphasis on autonomy, power, masculinity, and individuality.[172] In contrast, the relatively small number of female interns in this period may have found themselves removed from the main circulation routes of the hospital, an experience that would have felt very similar to the women's experiences during medical school. According to Vanderbilt faculty member Rudolph H. Kampmeier, the Nashville medical school–hospital had "a segregated suite of rooms for the few women house officers [interns], reached by the more private stairwell."[173]

Besides medicine and nursing, medical centers trained people for other work. As health care burgeoned, medical centers came to include smaller, ancillary educational programs. Duke University, for example, launched the country's first program in hospital administration when its medical school–hospital opened in 1930.[174] Some medical centers also educated those studying to enter more established professions such as dentistry and pharmacy. As they did with nurses and physicians, the medical campuses reinforced these groups' positions within the hierarchy of medical personnel.

Not all medical centers included dental schools and schools of pharmacy, but when they did, the architecture clearly articulated the primacy of medical education. Both Harvard Medical School and Columbia University's College of Physicians and Surgeons restricted dental students' access to the medical school dormitories, and the academic buildings privileged medicine over dentistry as well. When Harvard Medical School relocated in 1883, it gave its former home on North Grove Street to Harvard Dental School (fig. 5.26). Although presumably an improvement in space for the dental school, the move into the vacated medical school created a contradictory message. The transfer of the structure generated a positive association between dentistry and the more elite profession of medicine, but it also suggested that what was obsolete for medicine was appropriate for dentistry.

Not an isolated event, medical colleges often received updated facilities more swiftly than dental schools. Prior to the construction of the 1925 medical school–hospital on the main campus of Vanderbilt University, Vanderbilt's medical and dental schools shared the South Campus.[175] Emphasizing the divide between the medical and dental professions, dental education drew almost no support from philanthropic foundations in the early twentieth century. Neither Vanderbilt University nor the organizations that supported its medical school allocated money for the simultaneous relocation of the dental school when the medical school–hospital opened in 1925. The dental school remained by itself on the South Campus for a year after the medical school moved, and it suspended operations in 1926.[176] Similarly, Howard University's College of Medicine, College of Dentistry, and College of Pharmacy occupied

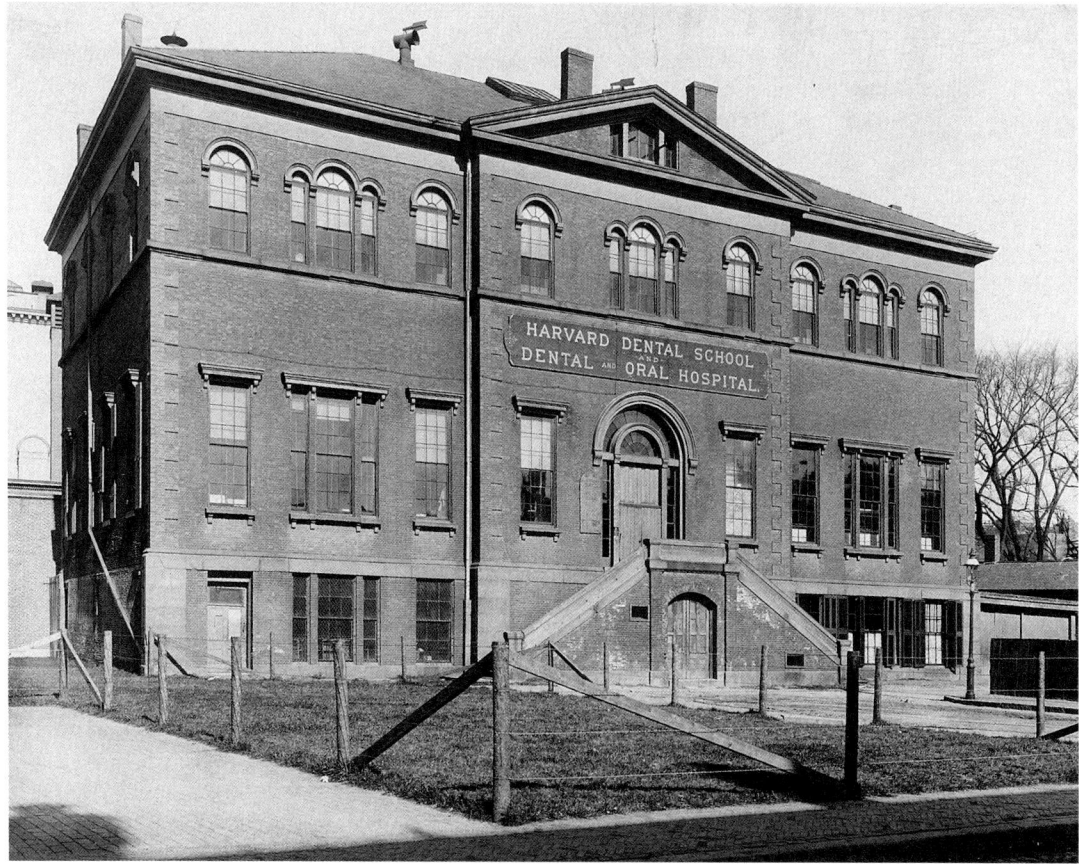

5.26.   Harvard Medical School North Grove Street building, rebranded for use by Harvard Dental School.

a single educational building, first constructed in 1869 and expanded in 1892, until Howard's new medical school structure opened in 1927 (see fig. 3.8). The 1927 building housed the College of Medicine, which shared the facility's laboratory space with the College of Dentistry and the College of Pharmacy. The College of Dentistry and College of Pharmacy remained in the remodeled 1869 building (fig. 5.27). They would have to wait until 1955 for their own new facilities.[177]

Even when modern medical centers did provide space for dentistry, the facilities highlighted the relative professional status of dentistry and medicine. Three years after Harvard Medical School's 1906 facilities opened, the dental school moved into a building next to the quadrangle (fig. 5.28). Designed by the architects of the medical college, the dental school, with its modestly ornamented brick exterior, was overshadowed by the far larger and more elaborate marble-clad medical school. The dental school building contained that school's clinical facilities, while all

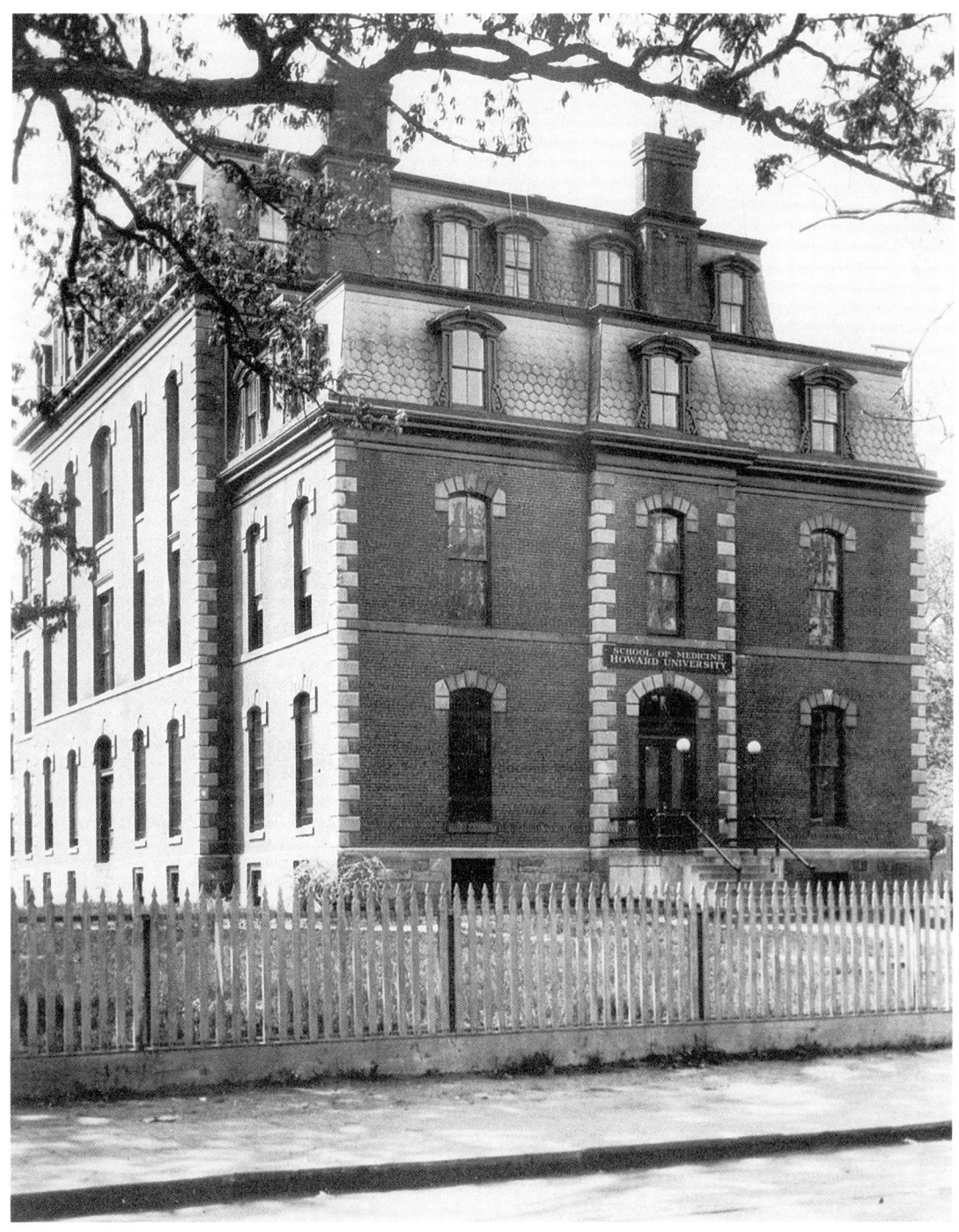

5.27.   Medical building, Howard University, constructed in 1869 and expanded in 1892. Photograph ca. 1920.

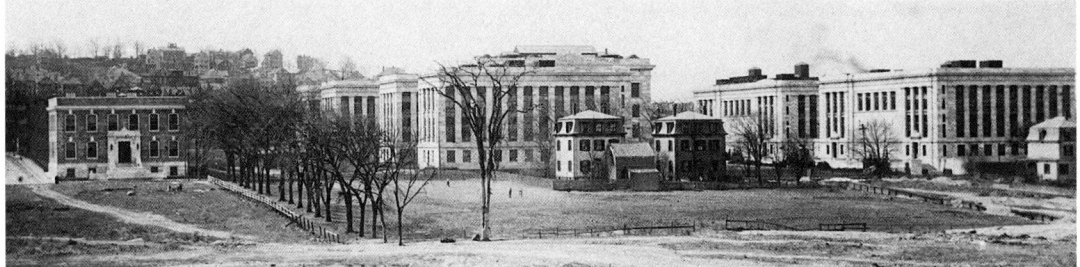

5.28.   Harvard Dental School (*far left*), 1909, Shepley, Rutan, and Coolidge, architects. At right is the
Harvard Medical School quadrangle. Photograph ca. 1911.

nonclinical instruction took place in the adjacent medical school, which
was easily accessible by tunnel.[178]

A similar relationship between medical school and dental school existed at Columbia University. The 1928 Columbia-Presbyterian Medical
Center housed Columbia's School of Dental and Oral Surgery on three
floors over the outpatient clinic. The dental students followed a schedule
almost identical to that of the medical students during the first two years
of their program.[179] They depended on the facilities of the medical school
for this training, and the specific needs of the dental school received
consideration during the design of the medical school.[180] Constructing
laboratory departments for use by all students—medical, nursing, dental,
and others—increased efficiency and reduced costs when compared with
building unique departments for each school, as one planning document
explained. Nevertheless, the same document affirmed, "The main and
most important function of the School [of Medicine] naturally is the
teaching of students who are expecting to receive the MD degree at the
termination of their course."[181] Ultimately, the move provided the dental
school with more laboratory space, but it left behind a two-building
campus that had been separate from the medical school and hospital.[182]

Not only did the dental school give up its autonomous physical identity for inclusion within Columbia-Presbyterian Medical Center, but
the dental program also found itself reduced to near invisibility at the
medical center. When Columbia-Presbyterian Medical Center opened,
an entrance with the medical school's name inscribed over the doorway
broadcast the existence of the medical college (fig. 5.29). Similarly, the
nursing school had Maxwell Hall to declare its presence. The dental
school, however, had no public marker. Dental students used the medical school entrance, after which they embarked on a trek through the
building wherein they could "take the elevators to the sixth floor and
walk across to their quarters in the northeast wing of the main group

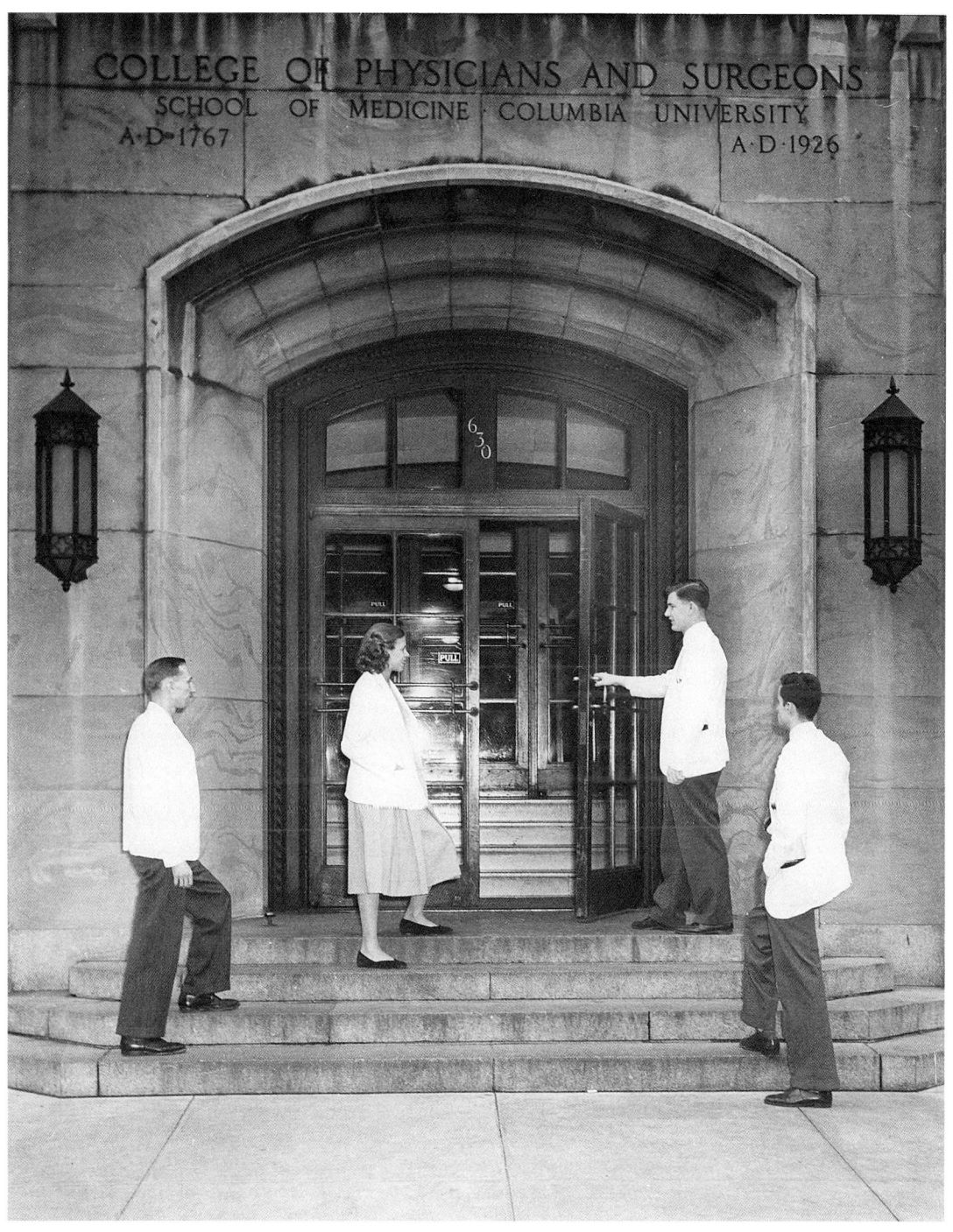

5.29.   College of Physicians and Surgeons, Columbia-Presbyterian Medical Center, 1928, James Gamble
         Rogers, architect, entrance. Photograph ca. 1949.

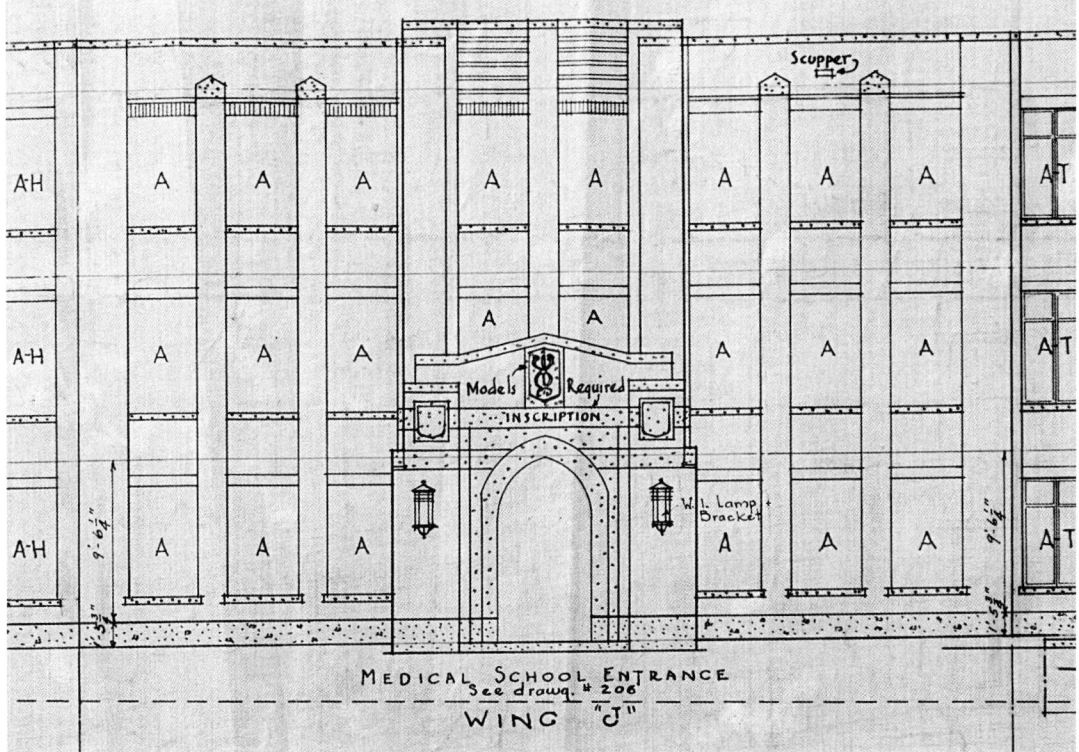

5.30.   Meharry Medical College, 1931, Gordon and Kaelber, architects, elevation of medical school entrance.

of buildings."[183] Although one dental school publication promoted the shared doorway as "illustrating the integration of the School of Dental and Oral Surgery with the Medical Center institution," the dental school not only lacked its own school entrance but also a dedicated clinical entrance.[184] For dental care, patients entered through the Vanderbilt Clinic, the medical center's outpatient department, and then proceeded to one of the wing's top three floors. As university-based dental programs at top institutions, the dental schools at Harvard and Columbia represented the upper echelon of dental education in the early twentieth century. Nevertheless, neither university understood dental and medical education as equals, and students could hardly have misinterpreted the architectural codification of this hierarchy.

As the Howard University example hinted, the architectural articulation of professional status also extended to pharmacists. The 1930 medical school–hospital at Meharry Medical College included facilities for training pharmacists in addition to physicians and dentists. Medicine, the most elite profession, enjoyed the central entrance on the educational side of the building. A series of architectural features highlighted the

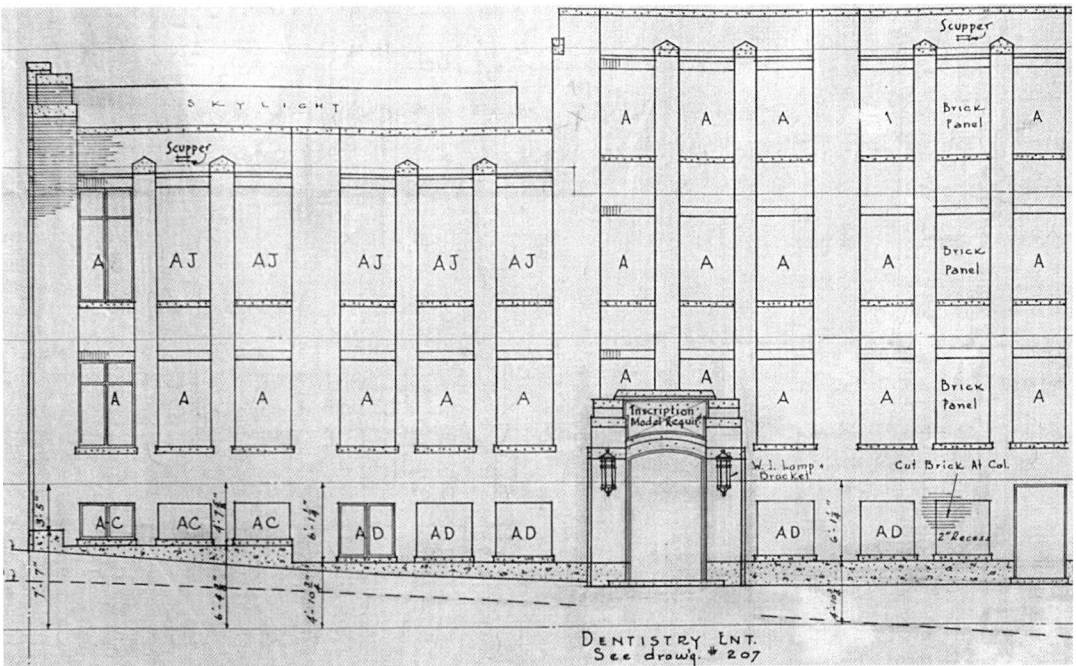

5.31. Meharry Medical College, 1931, Gordon and Kaelber, architects, elevation of dental school and dental clinic entrance.

doorway, including a small porch, a projection in the façade, and a change in the roofline. The entrance also contained relatively ornate decorative elements (fig. 5.30; see also fig. 3.12). Dental students and faculty used a more modest entrance closer to the hospital's main clinical entrance. Unlike their counterparts in medicine, they shared this doorway with their patients (fig. 5.31). Underscoring the lack of separation from their patients, dental students heading to their locker room had to pass in front of the open alcove that demarcated the dental waiting room. Such a merging of public and private space was unusual, as typically medical facilities were designed to ensure a certain "professional" distance between patient and practitioner. Last, and in this case also least, the pharmacy school doorway stood at the back of the building down a half story from the floor that contained the medical and dental entrances (fig. 5.32). Pharmacy represented in this period a less established and respected profession than either dentistry or medicine, and the pharmacy school entrance contained almost no ornament. These physical features paralleled other barometers of professional recognition, specifically the amount of overall floor space in the new building reserved for medicine,

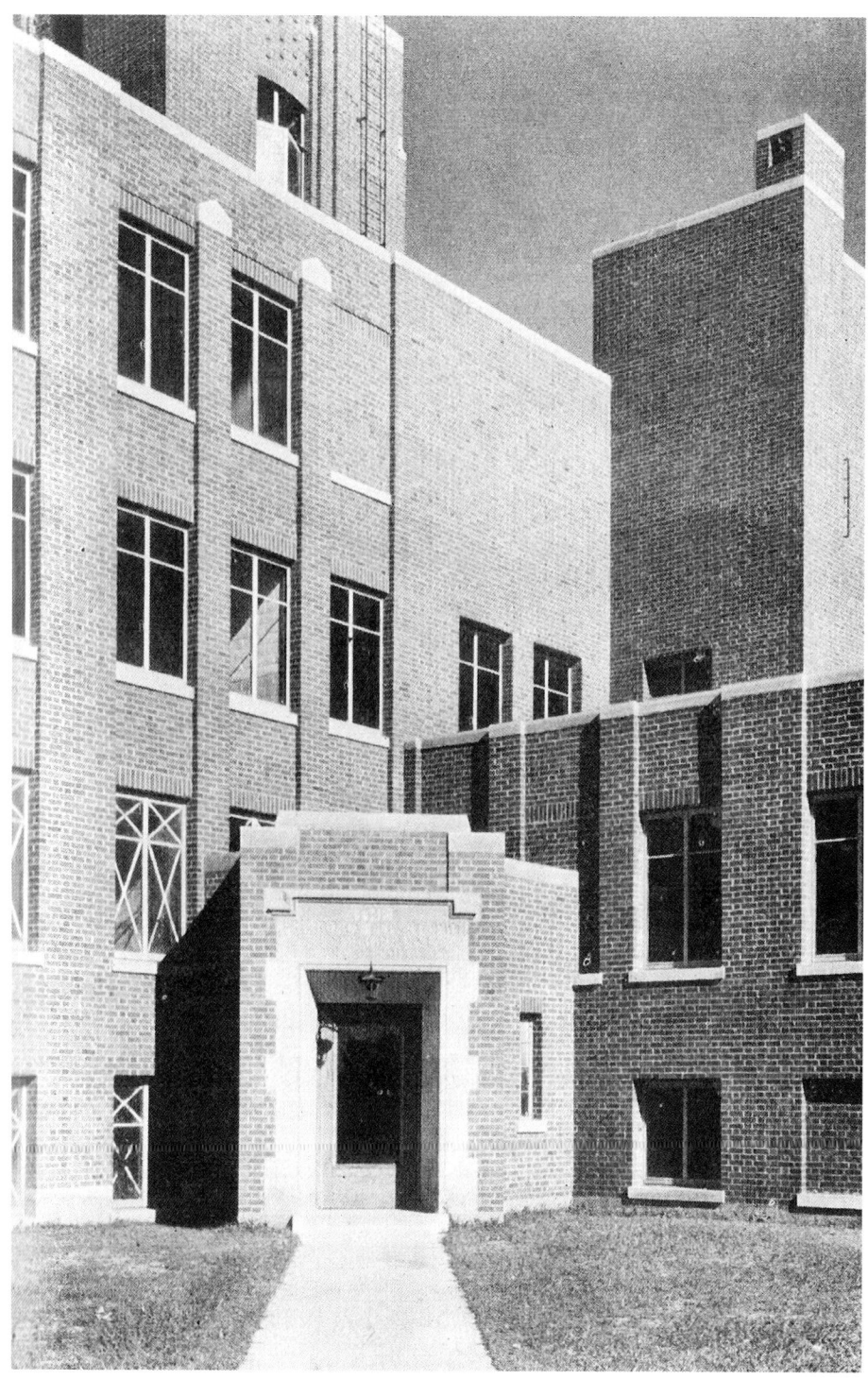

5.32.   Meharry Medical College, 1931, Gordon and Kaelber, architects, pharmacy
         school entrance.

dentistry, and pharmacy, respectively, and the budget allocated to each school.[185] Together they laid bare the hierarchies between the medical fields.

———————————

As the physical embodiment of the reformed, standardized curriculum, medical schools celebrated the modern medical profession, a function reinforced by walls of historical portraits and elaborate dedication ceremonies. Simultaneously, however, medical centers privileged white, male medical students and promoted disparities between medical fields. With most of these buildings in use today and many of these hierarchies still present, this form of analysis remains deeply relevant.

EPILOGUE

THE REVOLUTION IN MEDICAL EDUCATION THAT TOOK PLACE during the end of the nineteenth century and beginning of the twentieth famously reduced the number of American medical schools. Concurrently, however, nearly all of the medical colleges that survived the transformation in training rebuilt, generating a massive nationwide construction effort largely unrecognized by scholars. The educators, architects, and donors who participated in this building boom conceived of medical schools as pedagogical tools that would shape how students learned and how they conceptualized and practiced medicine. At the same time, they utilized the buildings to expand physicians' cultural authority and to define for the public and members of this hierarchical profession what it meant to be a modern American physician. Since 1940, the end date of this study, no widespread, from-the-ground-up rebuilding of American medical schools has occurred. Instead, schools have generally remodeled and expanded their existing facilities. Most reform-era medical colleges continue as medical schools today, and in recent decades buildings on medical campuses across the country have passed the one-hundred-year mark. Simultaneously, nearly three dozen medical schools have been founded since 2001, an undertaking that engages many of the conversations and ambitions held by educators, architects, and donors a century ago.

Modern Medical Schools at One Hundred

Unlike nurses' homes, mental hospitals, and tuberculosis sanitariums, the majority of medical schools constructed during the reconceptualization of medical education still serve their original purpose a century after they opened. Exceptions most often concern the structures from early in the redesign of medical training. These facilities generally lacked the space necessary to meet the growing demands of the modern educational program. Some of these schools were replaced relatively quickly, as happened at Harvard Medical School (completed 1883; vacated by medical school 1906; demolished 1967) and Syracuse University College of Medicine (completed 1896; vacated by medical school 1937; extant). Although the first Johns Hopkins Medical School campus, constructed between 1893 and 1899, retained its usefulness well into the next century, none of the structures exists today. In 1920, the pathology laboratory burned; in 1959, the Physiological Building was demolished; and in 1979, the Women's Fund Memorial Building was razed.

Among the schools constructed later in the transformative period, almost all continue as parts of medical colleges. The case studies in this book include only one facility constructed after 1900 that no longer supports medical instruction: Woman's Medical College of Pennsylvania (1930). Woman's Medical College admitted men among its students for the first time in 1970 and dropped the word *Woman's* from its name. A series of acquisitions and mergers between 1987 and 2002 resulted in the formation of Drexel University College of Medicine, the legacy institution of both Medical College of Pennsylvania and Hahnemann University (previously Hahnemann Medical College and Hospital). Drexel continued to use the former Woman's Medical College campus until 2005. The following year, Iron Stone Real Estate Partners purchased the complex and undertook a mixed-use redevelopment project. The property was listed on the National Register of Historic Places in 2008. The original medical school–hospital is now the Preston Apartments at Falls Center, named after prominent Woman's Medical College alumna and dean Ann Preston.

More typically, however, reform-era structures retain their initial function, thanks to ongoing renovations to meet the evolving requirements of medical education, science, and research. For administrators, fitting out a new laboratory was one thing, but their work became more difficult when fundamental components of the building's original design ceased to align with current pedagogical and scientific ideas. In his investigation of scientific research laboratories, Stuart W. Leslie writes that "laboratory architecture, however flexible in theory, necessarily stabilizes scientific practice, since a philosophy of research is embedded in the very structure of the building and persists far longer than the initial vision and mission that gave it life."[1] Leslie draws on the work of Thomas Gieryn and notes that, although buildings preserve scientific practice, neither the architecture nor the science it contains are fixed; both change continuously through modification and reinterpretation.[2] The leadership of Harvard Medical School faced these very scenarios.

In 1945, the dean of Stanford University School of Medicine wrote the dean of Harvard Medical School, C. Sidney Burwell, to request information on the Massachusetts school and its nearby hospitals in advance of the California school's renovation and expansion.[3] The deans' correspondence occurred two decades after unified designs had replaced the institute plan as the preferred medical school building types, and Burwell felt he could provide little guidance to his West Coast counterpart. "This is a curiously decentralized School," he declared, before explaining, "The actual Medical School buildings were begun in 1904 and represent in their outward plan the educational philosophy which ruled the roost at that time. The philosophy of today is quite different and we have had to cut the inside of the buildings about, *to build bridges both material and psychological*, and otherwise bring matters up to date."[4] Although designed with a focus on flexibility and expandability, Harvard Medical School's institute plan still codified a segmented conception of medical education and science. In time, the buildings failed to support current educational tenets, and the once progressive campus had to be altered.

Despite these changes, Harvard Medical School's open quadrangle remains, with the famous columned administration building, Building A, still immediately visible from Avenue Louis Pasteur (see fig. I.1), but at a number of medical colleges the reform-era buildings are now surrounded by later construction. If Harvard Medical School's distinctive exterior serves as a continual acknowledgment of the school's past, other structures from the same period have been nearly erased from the campus landscape. At Howard University, the Seeley G. Mudd Building, completed in 1979, sits directly in front of the 1927 building, now known as the Numa P. G. Adams Building, with the original portico the point of connection between the two structures (fig. E.1). Similarly, at Vanderbilt University the Learned Labs, opened in the early 1950s, closed off the medical school courtyard that initially faced the university, and the cherished—and much photographed—medical school entrance no longer functioned as a prominent entryway for the medical college (see figs. 2.18, 5.1, and 5.2). The medical school entrance, however, fared better than the hospital entrance, which in the early 1970s was demolished in the construction of the Joe and Howard Werthan Building.

Although later buildings all but envelope Vanderbilt's 1925 medical school–hospital, some of the ideas that informed the early structure

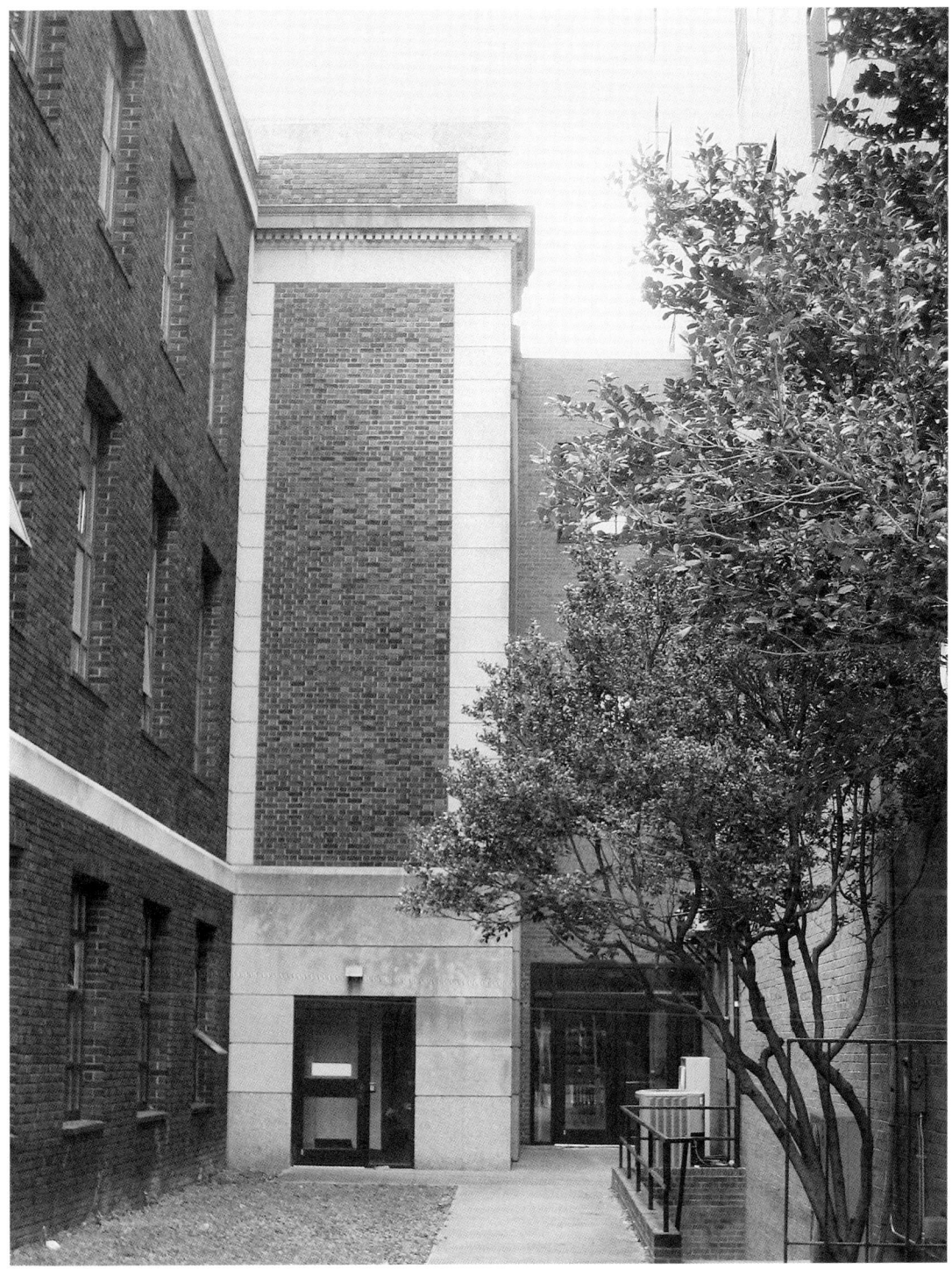

E.1.   Howard University College of Medicine, connection between Numa P. G. Adams Building (1927) on
left and Seeley G. Mudd Building (1979) on right. Photograph 2008.

remain. In 1994, longtime faculty member Robert Collins reflected on the tremendous growth in the medical center facilities since 1981, writing, "Our new library, the Annette and Irwin Eskind Biomedical Library, has just been completed and located properly in the center of the medical complex, as was the original library in 1925."[5] This shift may have felt particularly gratifying because in 1964 the library had moved to the northeast corner of the medical center. In 2006, Cyril Stewart, director of facility planning at Vanderbilt University Medical Center, explained that the faculty continued to prefer a program of proximity, wherein a person can easily redirect between tasks to see a clinic patient, return to the lab, check on an inpatient, go teach a class, and so forth. Proximity was part of the culture at Vanderbilt; physicians set up their day to move between activities and asked for the physical integration of the various facilities. Stewart described how the medical center maintained zones for teaching, research, and patient care, with the various clusters in close physical connection to one another, similar in concept to the 1925 medical school–hospital.[6]

At the one-hundred-year anniversary of the medical college reform period, medical campuses also reveal these institutions' legacies in other ways. The buildings of Meharry Medical College and Howard University College of Medicine, the two historically Black medical schools that survived the transformation of medical education, tell a story of achievement despite tremendous challenges. Howard University College of Medicine's first African American dean, Numa P. G. Adams, assumed his position in 1929. Among his many accomplishments over the next eleven years, he recruited and nurtured young African American faculty members in the preclinical and clinical departments.[7] In 1990, the 1927 medical school and a 1957 addition were named for Adams. At Meharry, Gordon and Kaelber designed a nurses' home adjacent to the 1931 medical school–hospital. Placed on the National Register of Historic Places in 1998, it reopened after a major renovation in 2013, one part of a $25 million campus-wide construction effort. Support from the National Park Service and President Barack Obama's American Recovery and Reinvestment Act stimulus grant for HBCUs (historically Black colleges and universities) contributed to the building's renovation. Although the nursing school closed in 1962, the structure retains the name given it in 1946: Hulda Margaret Lyttle Hall. Lyttle graduated from Meharry in 1913 and returned in 1916 to lead its nursing program. In time she became director of nurse training and superintendent of the hospital and then dean of the nursing school, an appointment that made her the first Black woman to lead an academic division at Meharry. Lyttle's portrait hangs prominently over the fireplace in the building's former living room (fig. E.2).

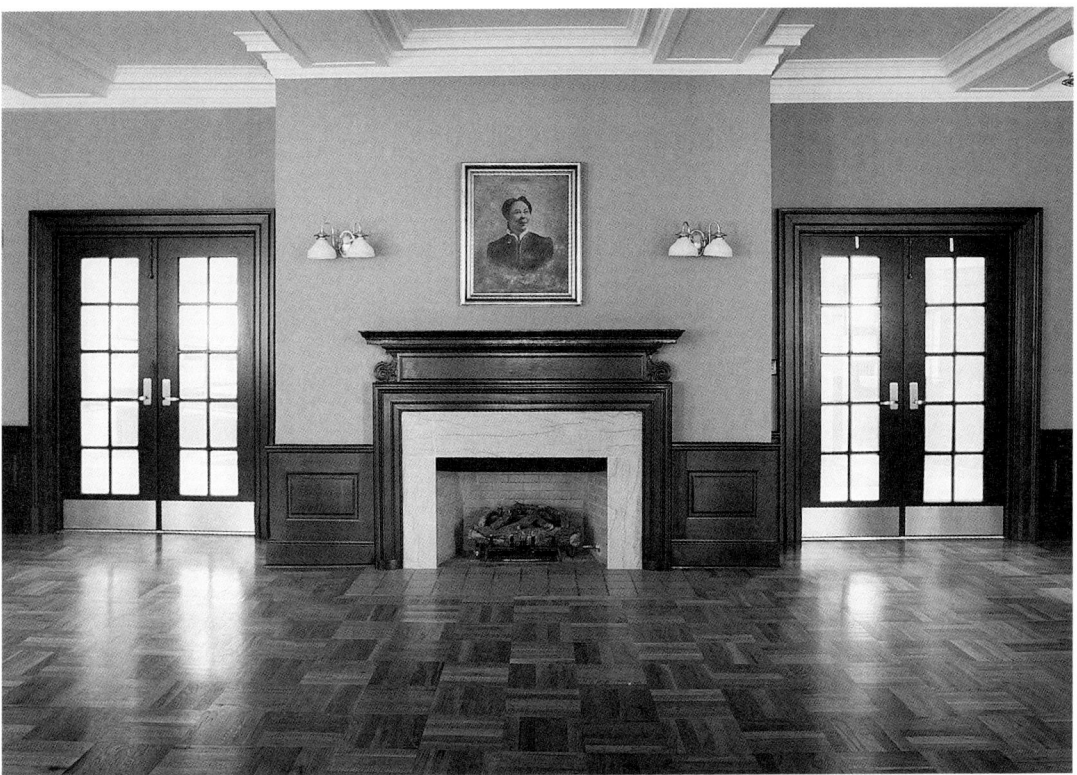

E.2.   Nurses' Home (now Hulda Margaret Lyttle Hall), Meharry Medical College, 1931, Gordon and
         Kaelber, architects, former living room transitioned to use as event space with portrait of Hulda
         Margaret Lyttle (artist unknown).

Howard University and Meharry Medical College continue to play
critical roles in training African American physicians and other medical
professionals. As of 1991, more than 80 percent of all African American
physicians and dentists had earned their medical or dental degree at
Howard or Meharry.[8] In the 2017–2018 academic year, Meharry Medical College, Howard University College of Medicine, and Morehouse
School of Medicine, accredited in 1985 to award medical degrees, enrolled 350, 304, and 247 Black students, respectively, or 14.6 percent of all
Black medical students nationwide. The same year, Indiana University
enrolled 128 Black students, the largest number of Black students at a
predominantly white medical college.[9] Howard and Meharry, like historically Black colleges and universities generally, struggle with lack of
funding, a reality that has impacted critical areas, including facilities.[10]
As Wayne Frederick, a surgeon who trained at the Washington, DC,
school and who became president of Howard University in 2014, put it,
"Out-punching your weight class is really the hallmark of HBCUs."[11]

Nationally, African American men and women represent a far smaller percentage of medical students than the percentage of African Americans in the population, and much remains to be done to create an inclusive educational environment. In the 2018–2019 academic year, only 7.1 percent of accepted applicants to US medical schools identified as Black or African American.[12] Between 1980 and 2012, Harvard Medical School ranked eighth among all American medical schools for its total number of Black graduates, but during the search for a new dean in 2016 its students highlighted the ongoing inequalities at the institution. In a petition to the university's president, students observed that Black, Hispanic, and American Indian academics together represented only 5.9 percent of Harvard Medical School's full-time faculty. Across the country, similar numbers existed, with just 5.3 percent of faculty identified as underrepresented minorities in medicine. Individuals who identified as Asian or Pacific Islander composed 18.9 percent of the faculty at Harvard Medical School, and the Association of American Medical Colleges does not consider these groups "underrepresented" in medicine, although this lack of designation does not mean that people who identify as Asian or Pacific Islander fail to experience race-based discrimination. Far more diverse than its instructors, the student body at Harvard Medical School was 21.7 percent Black, Hispanic, or American Indian in 2016, but only 6.6 percent of the 2015–2016 first-year class was African American.[13]

Medical education marked a major milestone in 2017, when more women than men enrolled in American medical colleges for the first time, but other statistics provide a fuller perspective on women in medicine. Only 34 percent of physicians nationwide are women, and far fewer women hold leadership roles, with women making up just 16 percent of medical school deans and department chairs.[14] For African American women, the numbers are even lower. In 2016, male and female Black academics accounted for only 3 percent of all medical faculty. While women outstripped men in numbers of Black faculty overall, men held more full and associate professorships.[15]

As students and faculty examine the disparities in medical education, they recognize the impact of the physical environment. In keeping with Abraham Flexner's approach of publishing medical schools' accomplishments and deficits, White Coats for Black Lives, a national, medical student–run advocacy organization, released in 2018 its *Racial Justice Report Card*, a report that graded ten medical schools on fifteen metrics. One metric focused on the recognition of underrepresented minorities in medicine, specifically whether "the physical space of the medical school acknowledges the contributions of alumni and other physicians of color (through plaques, statues, portraits, and building names) and does not celebrate racist or white supremacist individuals."[16] Sixty percent of the schools, including Harvard Medical School, received a C, the lowest rating, in this category. With regard to Harvard, the reviewers noted that one of the school's academic societies was named for Oliver Wendell Holmes Sr., who as dean in 1850 expelled the school's first three Black students after white students protested their enrollment. In addition, the writers of the *Racial Justice Report Card* explained, "the overwhelming majority of individuals whose likenesses are present in Harvard Medical School public spaces are white men." But the report also mentioned the creation of the Dean's Standing Committee on Artwork and Cultural Representation.[17] In the 2019 *Racial Justice Report Card*, Harvard Medical School retained its C grade in the metric on the recognition of underrepresented minorities in medicine. The report's compilers, however, documented instances where the school had commemorated diverse faculty, and they described the efforts of the Dean's Standing Committee, which resulted in the exhibition of medical student Pamela Chen's self-portraits in the dean's offices and the display of a bust of Alice Hamilton, the first woman appointed to the Harvard Medical School faculty.[18] In 2019, a painting of William Augustus Hinton was unveiled at the school as part of larger efforts to display more portraits of diverse alumni and faculty at the university, and the following year, the medical school's Oliver Wendell Holmes academic society became the William Augustus Hinton Society (fig. E.3). Hinton, a graduate of Harvard College (1905) and Harvard Medical School (1912) and a Harvard Medical School faculty member, achieved international distinction for his research on infectious diseases and was the first Black full professor at Harvard Medical School and Harvard University.[19]

The actions at Harvard Medical School reflect the ongoing work at a number of medical schools to diversify portraits and reconsider who is commemorated, an initiative also under way at many colleges and universities across the country.[20] In 2019, researchers at Yale School of Medicine documented the negative impact on some students of the portraits in the Sterling Hall of Medicine (Yale School of Medicine's main building), where the individuals celebrated in art included three white women and fifty-two white men.[21] Yale medical student Max Jordan Nguemeni Tiako described his experience of the portraits: "There are times when you're having a really bad day—someone says something racist to you, or you're struggling with feeling like you belong in the space—and then you see all those photos and it kind of reinforces whatever you might have been feeling at the time."[22] Yale has commissioned additional portraits, including

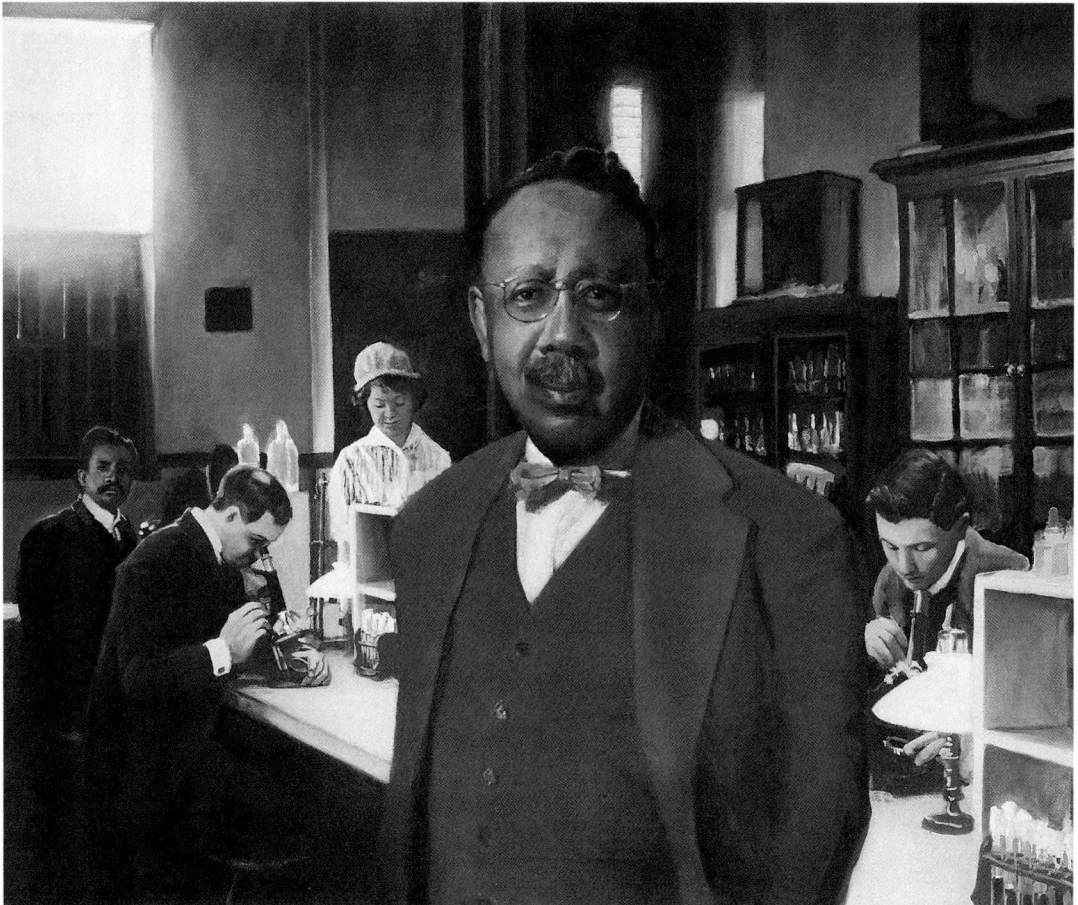

E.3.   Stephen Coit, *Dr. William A. Hinton*, 2019. Oil on canvas, 34.5 by 42 inches. The painting depicts
        Hinton in a microbiology laboratory that the artist based on a 1920s photograph of a laboratory at
        Howard University. A woman features prominently in the background in recognition of Hinton's
        dedication to women's education, including establishing a school, the first of its type in the country, to
        train women as laboratory technicians.

one of Beatrix Hamburg, an innovator in developmental psychiatry and
the medical school's first Black female graduate. In 2018, Betsy Nabel,
president of Brigham and Women's Hospital and the first woman to
lead a major Harvard teaching hospital, decided to remove the portraits
of former department chairs—all men, of whom thirty were white and
one was Asian—from the Louis Bornstein Family Amphitheater and
disperse them throughout the hospital as part of wider diversity efforts
(fig. E.4). Harvard's medical students attend events in the auditorium,
and Titilayo Afolabi, a member of the first-year medical class, supported
the decision to redistribute the portraits but remained "very wary of the

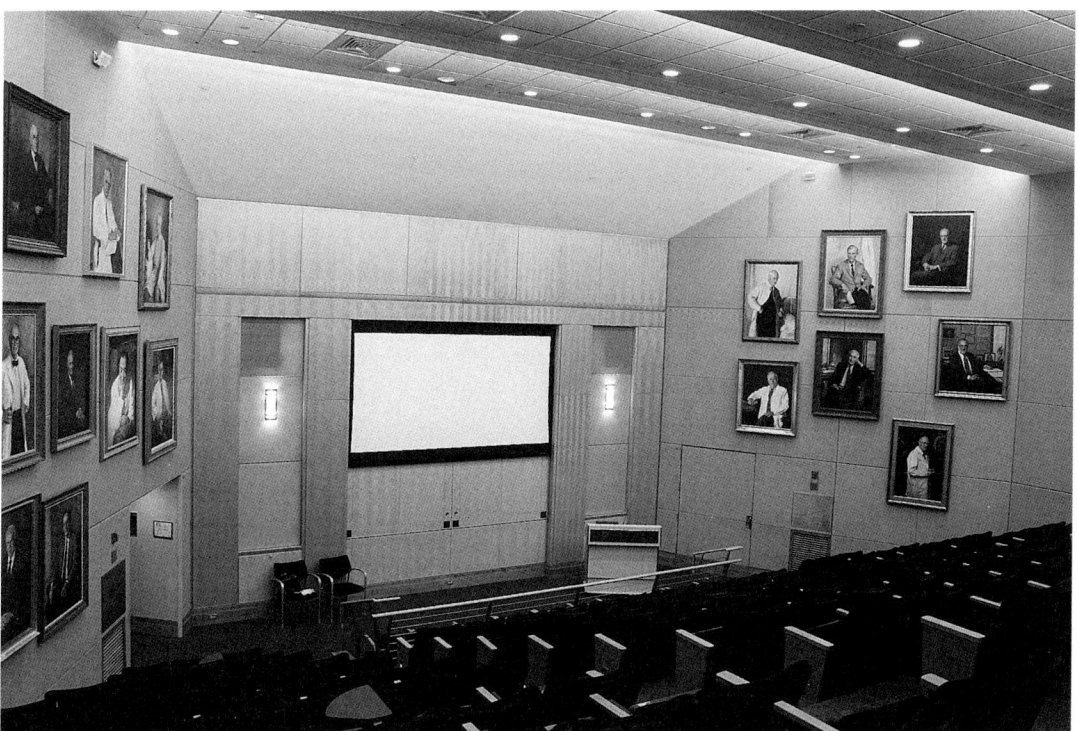

E.4.   Portraits in the Louis Bornstein Family Amphitheater at Brigham and Women's Hospital in Boston
        before their removal in 2018.

image of change rather than actual change. It's easy to remove people
from the wall. It's more difficult putting people of color in power."[23]
As reform-era medical schools mark their centennials, educators and
students continue to grapple with the legacies these spaces communicate
with regard not only to pedagogy and science but also to professional
identity.

Constructing a New Era in Medical Education

In 1940, 77 medical colleges existed in the United States. In 2019, the
country was home to 154 medical schools, with more in development.
The growth in medical colleges primarily occurred in two waves.

    The first wave took place in the late 1960s and 1970s. Between 1965
and 1980, the number of US medical colleges increased from 88 to 126,
with the number of graduates doubling in the same period. Calls for
more physicians had begun in the late 1940s. Most critically, the growing
conception of medical care as a basic right had resulted in an increase in
demand for medical treatment and physicians. At the same time, rural

and other underserved communities pressed for more doctors. Medical educators also found themselves rather embarrassed by their inability to admit many qualified applicants in the face of expanded college enrollments. The simmering concerns about physician supply had come to a head in 1959, when a report was published by the Surgeon General's Consultant Group on Medical Education; it stunned the public with its projection of a deficit of almost 40,000 physicians across the country by 1975. Congress responded with the Health Professions Educational Assistance Act of 1963, the provisions of which included federal funds for the expansion and creation of medical schools. After a series of renewals, the last Health Professions Educational Assistance Act lapsed in 1980. Even with federal aid, private universities rarely had the resources to build and run a medical college, and thus it was state institutions that developed most of the medical schools.[24]

Between 1980 and 2005 the number of medical schools, as well as the number of students they enrolled, plateaued amid concerns of an impending physician surplus, but as the twenty-first century began predictions again suggested that a physician shortfall was looming. In 2006, the Association of American Medical Colleges called for a 30 percent increase in first-year medical school enrollment over 2002 figures. In 2019, the Association of American Medical Colleges announced that the 2006 target had been reached. Since 2002, medical school enrollment had expanded by 31 percent, and in roughly the same period, between 2001 and 2019, a staggering twenty-nine medical colleges had opened. In addition, many of the schools founded in earlier eras had enlarged their enrollment, some through the creation of branch campuses.[25]

Unlike at the start of the twentieth century, in the twenty-first century having more medical school graduates does not itself create more practicing physicians. In the early 1900s, few internships existed to provide hospital-based clinical education after medical school graduation. By the 1930s, the internship had become standard; nearly every medical graduate completed an internship, typically one year in length, although Black men and women faced racially discriminatory policies that significantly curtailed the number of internships available to them. After 1942, the Advisory Board for Medical Specialties required physicians seeking specialty certification to have finished a residency lasting at least three years.[26] As of 2021, physicians in most states become eligible for licensure after finishing one year of an accredited residency, but nearly all physicians complete residency training. The US Congress has mostly frozen federal support for residency training for more than twenty years, however, and residency positions have expanded at a rate of only 1 percent per year, or less swiftly than medical school enrollment growth. For the United States to produce significantly more practicing doctors, more residency positions are needed. Medical advocacy groups are calling for additional residency spots. In 2017, the Texas legislature passed a bill designed to increase residency positions in that state. As of winter 2020, the US House and the US Senate had referred the Resident Physician Shortage Reduction bill to committees.[27]

The expansion in medical school enrollment has occurred amid simultaneous efforts to reimagine medical training. The medical school model inaugurated more than a hundred years ago has long felt restrictive, obsolete, and unresponsive to students' needs. Since 2005, three-quarters of medical colleges have begun to restructure their curricula. Dominant themes include introducing clinical training earlier; arranging the curriculum around systems, such as respiratory or cardiovascular, instead of subjects or disciplines, such as anatomy and pathology; and reducing the amount of time spent on lectures in favor of learning in small groups, frequently with case-based instruction.[28] In addition, medical educators and organizations have made recommendations for change; for example, the Carnegie Foundation for the Advancement of Teaching commissioned a report on medical education in 2010, the centennial of the Flexner Report.[29] As in the past, regulation also impacts medical training. The Liaison Committee on Medical Education, the accrediting agency for medical schools, is encouraging curricular modifications, specifically the implementation of new types of instruction and more clinical training in the first two years of medical school.[30]

Medical educators and architects today, no less than their counterparts one hundred years ago, view the buildings under construction—at both established and recently founded medical colleges—as participants in the transformation of medical education. A century ago medical educators succeeded in reforming medical training. In the 1960s and 1970s, however, medical educators learned that the process of opening and building schools grounded in progressive ideas does not necessarily result in lasting change; over time, inventive educational programs may return to conventional modes of instruction.[31] As for the current wave of construction and innovation still in progress, the long-term outcome cannot yet be determined.

The medical schools created in the last two decades utilize a variety of spaces. Some start out in temporary or existing facilities, others occupy buildings that have been renovated or expanded, and still others welcome their first classes in purpose-built structures. Dell Medical School at the University of Texas at Austin, which opened in 2016, falls into the last of these categories.

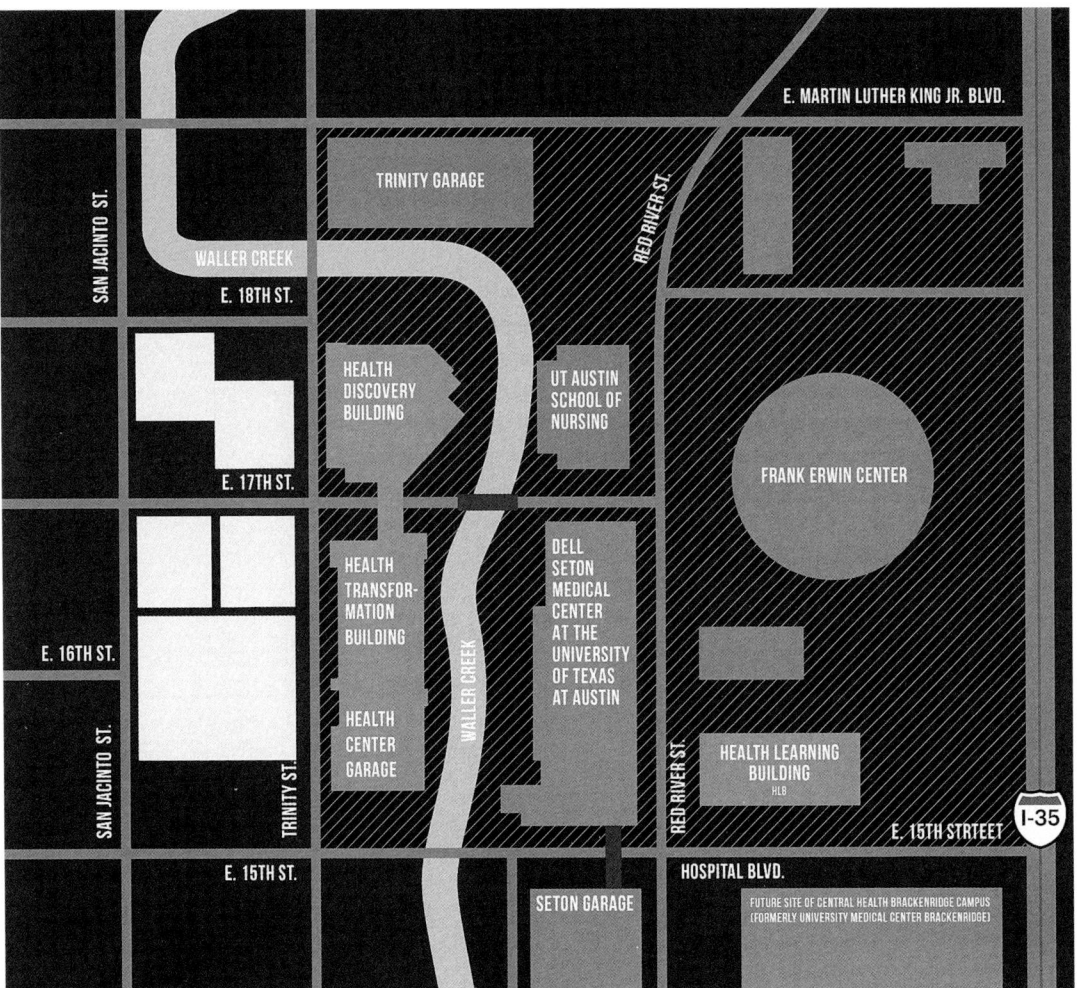

E.5. Health District, the University of Texas at Austin, ca. 2019. The hatched lines demarcate the university's growing health district. To enable expansion of the medical school, the Frank Erwin Center, the university's multipurpose events arena, was scheduled for demolition.

If medical education in the early twentieth century was big business, in the early twenty-first century it is enormous business. Primary funding for Dell Medical School included $65 million from the University of Texas Board of Regents; a $50 million naming gift from the Michael and Susan Dell Foundation; and $35 million annually from Travis County, where voters approved an increase in property taxes to support the school's operations. Located on the campus of the University of Texas at Austin, the medical school currently includes the Health Learning Building, for educational and administrative space; the Health Discovery Building, a research facility; and the Health Transformation Building, a

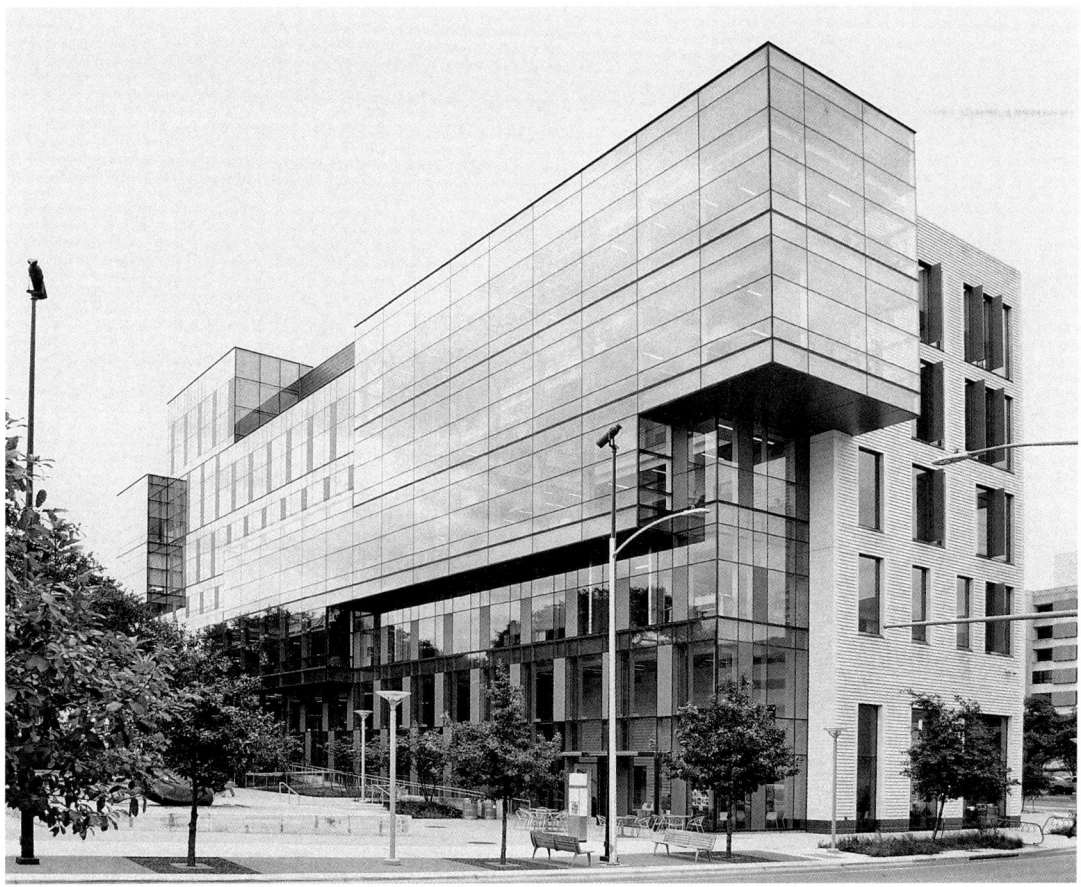

E.6.   Health Learning Building, Dell Medical School at the University of Texas at Austin, 2016, Page with
        the S/L/A/M Collaborative, architects.

site for clinical services. Steps away are the Dell Seton Medical Center, a $295 million, 211-bed hospital and Level I trauma center that opened in 2017 as the medical college's primary teaching hospital, and the School of Nursing, which predated the medical school (fig. E.5).

   In the Health Learning Building, where preclinical training takes place at Dell Medical School, few of the features that distinguished medical school design a century ago remain (fig. E.6). Gone are the museum; the central library; the suite for receiving, embalming, and storing cadavers; separate wings for each department; and numerous large teaching laboratories. Like museums, libraries have become obsolete—at least in the traditional sense of housing books. In the Health Learning Building, a section of the third floor contains an information commons with individual study carrels, group tables, and a librarian but no stacks. Dell Medical School obtains cadavers as needed from other medical schools, so no embalming or cadaver storage facilities exist in the Health Learning Building. Further, Dell Medical School's preclinical curriculum is not divided by subject, and neither is the building. As for the disappearance of teaching laboratories, this shift relates directly to the movement away from laboratory instruction in the second half of the twentieth century, a change Kenneth Ludmerer has described. Simply put, lectures were more efficient for faculty, for whom—like their colleagues in other parts of the university—promotions depended mainly on research output rather than distinction in teaching. In 1982, one study of full-time medical faculty estimated that 60 percent of instructors dedicated less than five hours per week, inclusive of preparation and assessment, to teaching.[32] With this shift, medical school administrators reallocated teaching laboratories for faculty research.[33]

Students responded to the focus on lectures and memorization by skipping class and studying independently.[34] This trend continues, especially with the option to watch or listen to lectures remotely and the pressure to forgo lectures entirely in order to study for the licensing exam undertaken at the end of the second year of medical school—the United States Medical Licensing Examination Step 1, the score from which becomes a critical component of residency applications.[35] As one student reported, "there were times that I didn't go to a single class, and then I'd get to the actual exam and it would be my first time seeing the professor. Especially, when Step [the licensing exam] was coming up, I pretty much completely focused on studying outside materials."[36]

Although the issue of memorizing massive amounts of information for the high-stakes medical licensing exam remains (at least for the time being; the Step 1 will become pass/fail no earlier than January 2022), medical schools are moving away from the preclinical lecture, an agenda similar to the call for experiential learning a century ago.[37] At Dell Medical School, the shift away from lectures is built into the curriculum and the Health Learning Building. As Susan Cox, executive vice dean of academics, chair of the medical education department, and principal designer of Dell Medical School's curriculum, explained, "We were able to design the building that would serve the curriculum needs and student needs best."[38] According to Cox, half of the training at Dell Medical School involves case-based learning. With case-based learning, groups of students work together to solve a medical problem, a process intended to encourage asking questions and examining different approaches. The students, Cox explains, are "not just going to do things because we've always done them that way. They're going to challenge."[39] The first floor of the Health Learning Building contains the school's one lecture hall,

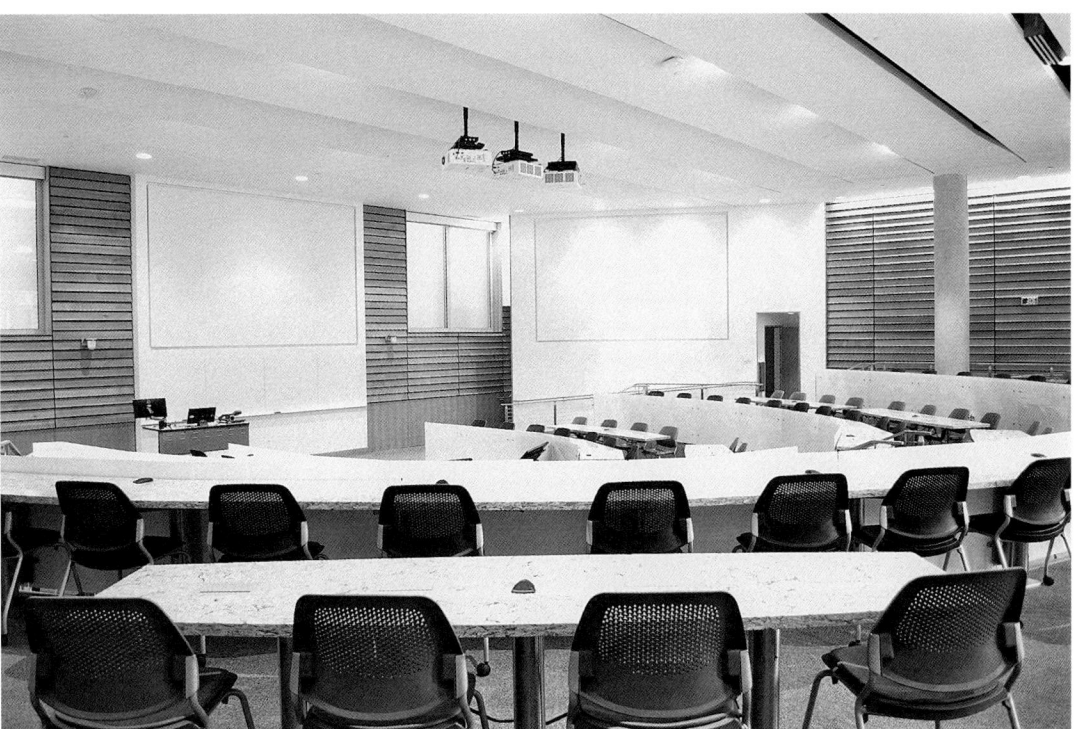

E.7.   Health Learning Building, Dell Medical School at the University of Texas at Austin, 2016, Page with
        the S/L/A/M Collaborative, architects, lecture hall.

but the faculty tries not to lecture (fig. E.7). In the "large-group inter-
actives" faculty present cases and students work together to formulate
solutions. Student Anatoli Berezovsky describes the experience: "It's not
just one person talking at you. It's thinking through problems with people around you. It's a structured way to learn as a group."[40] To promote
this type of learning, the auditorium contains flexible seating and panels
of whiteboards behind most rows of chairs, along with wiring for sound
and internet throughout the room.

    Similar to other recently constructed spaces for medical education,
the design of the Health Learning Building supports active learning,
collaboration, interaction, and technology beyond just the lecture hall.[41]
On the third floor, ten small rooms line one wall of the building, with
half available as student study spaces and half reserved for instruction.
On the fourth floor, students receive hands-on training. In the large
anatomy laboratory students access audiovisual technology and the
internet at each workstation in addition to traditional cadavers. The
design team had first planned to forgo cadavers in favor of digitized
anatomy tables, but students requested cadavers. Page architectural firm's

principal and design lead, Josh Coleman, explained, "We were told over and over again how integral it is—essentially a medical school rite of passage."[42] The fourth floor also contains the multipurpose teaching laboratory, where students use mannequins, and a mock clinic, where students begin to develop their clinical skills through engagement with standardized patients—individuals trained to present a simulated patient experience. Moving through the Health Learning Building generally involves climbing the structure's dramatic five-story open staircase, its so-called social edge. One reviewer of the building, Canan Yetmen, put this feature in context: "The notion of encouraging social function in the academic realm through architecture has taken a firm hold in the interdisciplinary sciences, fostering cross-pollination among scientists who previously might have preferred to shut themselves away in their offices."[43] In the Health Learning Building, numerous lounges, seating areas, and the café further promote interaction among students, faculty, and staff.

Dell Medical School also joins other medical colleges exploring ways to break down the now traditional format of two years of preclinical training and two years of clinical training, specifically by moving clinical training to an earlier point in the program. Referred to as the Leading EDGE (essentials, delivery, growth, and exploration), the Dell Medical School curriculum begins with the essentials year, when the material typically covered in two years of preclinical instruction is completed in twelve months. Next comes the delivery year, dedicated to clerkships, followed by the growth year, when students follow their individual interests and either earn a dual master's degree or undertake a project in a distinction area. In the exploration year, students complete additional clinical rotations with time reserved for electives and applying and interviewing for residency. Three courses focus on relationship building—understood at Dell Medical School as a critical tool for future physician leaders—and continue throughout all four years: Developing Outstanding Clinical Skills, Leadership, and Interprofessional Education.[44] In the early twentieth century, nursing students used medical school laboratories when medical students were not in class, but at Dell Medical School, the Interprofessional Education course is designed to bring students of medicine, nursing, social work, pharmacy, and other fields together with the goal of "producing physicians who are prepared for interprofessional collaborative practice."[45] At the beginning of the last century, progressive medical educators and Flexner hoped that their ideas would spread across the nation, and the leadership at Dell Medical School had similar aspirations. As Cox affirmed, "We have a unique

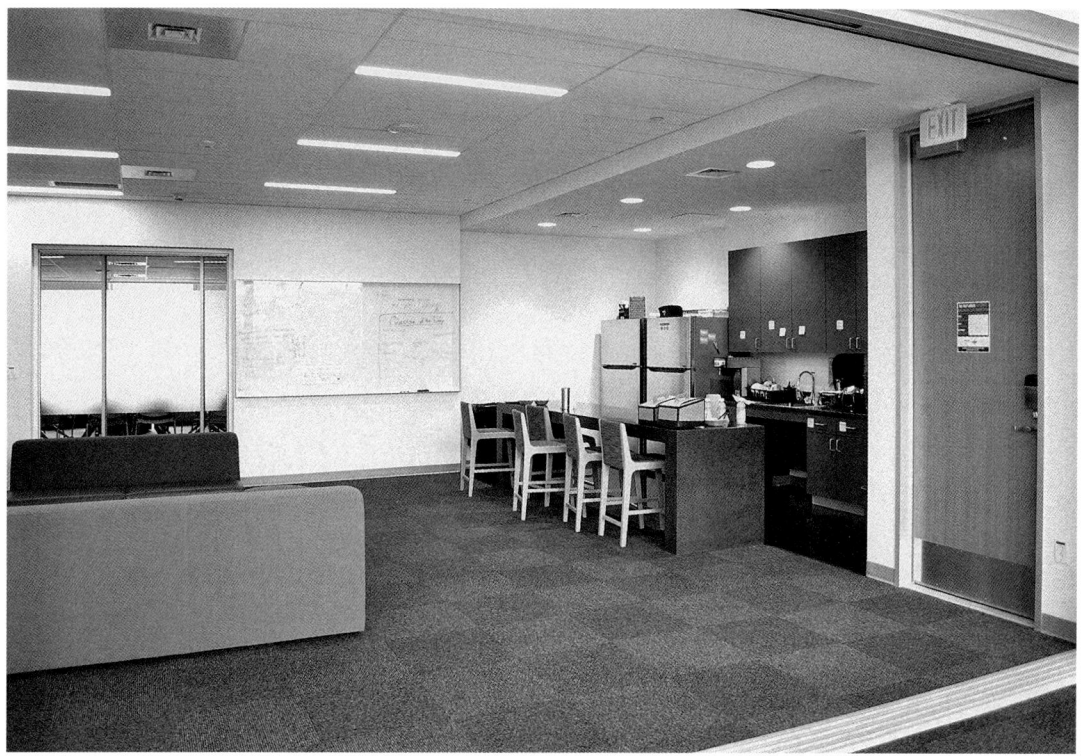

E.8.   Health Learning Building, Dell Medical School at the University of Texas at Austin, 2016, Page with
        the S/L/A/M Collaborative, architects, student society lounge.

opportunity to design a medical education program entirely from scratch.
. . . That's a luxury that existing medical schools don't have. But as we
and other schools demonstrate the effectiveness of new practices and
procedures, other schools will start to embrace changes, if only to remain
competitive."[46]

Medical educators today, like their counterparts a century ago, remain concerned with students' experiences away from their academic
work. At Dell Medical School, the leadership strives to promote camaraderie among students and to encourage advanced students to mentor
their schoolmates. To this end, all students are placed in one of two societies. On the third floor of the Health Learning Building, each society
has a dedicated lounge, which includes a kitchen and casual furniture
(fig. E.8). The building also reflects and supports the increased diversity
among students, faculty, staff, and visitors, with gender-inclusive bathrooms and a lactation room.

With many student features concentrated on the third and fourth
floors, students serve as the conceptual and physical center of the five-story

Health Learning Building. The first floor is home to the most communal and public spaces—the café and lecture hall; the second floor is administrative, with recruitment, admissions, counseling, and faculty offices; the third floor includes lounges for the student societies, small group rooms, and the information commons; the fourth floor contains instructional facilities; and the fifth floor houses the school's leadership. Cox explains, "Putting the students in the middle [on the third floor] meant they could go up easily to [the fourth floor to] anatomy and the multipurpose room for training around mannequins and other kinds of trainings, and down to student affairs on the second floor. Students are the hub."[47]

The Health Learning Building emphasizes the experience of students and, in sharp contrast to medical schools a century ago, contains no research facilities. Instead, research takes place a short walk away on the other side of Waller Creek, in the Health Discovery Building. Medical campuses in the early twentieth century sometimes divided their schools into separate buildings based on discipline, but they did not typically create autonomous structures for research. One hundred years ago, research and instruction were far less distinct activities than they are today. Until World War II, Ludmerer explains, it was a "relatively short distance from the standard student courses to the forefront of medical research. . . . A congruence existed between the required teaching of the medical school courses and the specific research problems faculty were pursuing when not teaching." In the decades following the war, a growing wedge between teaching and research developed, especially after 1970, when biomedical research became more and more molecular in its focus. In the early twenty-first century, particularly in the basic sciences, the research undertaken by most faculty bears little direct relationship to the topics covered in medical school classes.[48] The campus at Dell Medical School reinforces the split between medical research and instruction.

Early promotional material for the Health Discovery Building highlighted its commitment to bringing together "seemingly unrelated disciplines" in the hope of sparking innovation, and its design encourages this objective.[49] Of the recent medical structures, the Health Discovery Building is sited closest to the heart of the university campus, a location that underscores the desire to create joint research appointments between the medical school and other sectors of the university. The Health Discovery Building contains wet and dry labs and a cutting-edge imaging center—all intended to serve the needs of a diverse group of scientists. Adding to the spectrum of uses within the facility, one floor was reserved for a biotech accelerator that would support startups—partnerships that presumably would generate revenue for the medical school.

The Health Discovery Building connects directly to the Health Transformation Building for clinical services through a multistory bridge. This bridge speaks to the emphasis on translational research, what Chris Webb, chief research officer and associate dean for research, describes as "projects that promise to move new knowledge from the laboratory to the bedside quickly and efficiently."[50] This is a sentiment G. Canby Robinson and others would have appreciated. One of the occupants of the bridge between the two buildings is the Design Institute for Health. Reportedly the nation's first institute to grow out of a collaboration between a medical school and a college of fine arts, it seeks to use human-centered design to improve health systems.[51]

Many medical colleges constructed since 2001 have not maintained the early twentieth-century ideal of locating the medical school adjacent to the university and the primary teaching hospital.[52] But Dell Medical College has continued this ideal, a choice that also places the school in the heart of Austin, Texas. The medical school and its teaching hospital are intended to anchor a multipartner innovation district, currently under development, that would transform a section of downtown Austin with high-density and mixed-use construction. Planned to expand on Austin's strengths, particularly in software, information technology, and semiconductors, the nascent district offers a unique opportunity, according to Dell Medical School dean Clay Johnson, "to make advances in the whole digital health arena, so where technology meets health."[53] Innovation districts, however, have had uneven success nationwide.[54] The outcome of this one cannot be predicted, but in summer 2021 construction was under way and the alteration of the city's landscape assured.

In 2012, when Travis County voters agreed to use property tax revenue in support of the proposed medical school, the intended return on investment included physicians, students, pioneering initiatives, and related economic growth that together would improve the health of the community.[55] A decade later, the community remained engaged with the young medical school. Although the hospital, the clinics in the Health Transformation Building, the economic impact of the medical school, and the fledgling innovation district may draw the greatest attention, the Health Learning Building does more than provide mute testimony of the presence of medical students in Austin. In keeping with the guidelines of the Liaison Committee on Medical Education, which require medical schools to work on improving the "pipeline" of applicants who are underrepresented minorities in medicine, Dell Medical School hosts health science summer camps on its campus each summer to introduce middle and high school students from traditionally underrepresented groups to careers in the health sciences.[56] When people of all ages experience the Health Learning Building by attending camps, taking a tour, or learning about the school in the news, they see an articulation of progressive medical training and receive an introduction to the professionals who strive to improve American health care.

———————————

Dell Medical School, like a number of recently founded and long-standing medical colleges, hopes to reinvent medical education and to produce innovative leaders prepared to address broader health systems challenges. Whether or not the current era in medical education turns out to be the desired revolution, medical campuses across the country promote the aspirations of this generation of medical educators. Despite the effort to create flexible buildings, the present pedagogy will continue to shape medical training, research, and patient care for the foreseeable future. In many ways, medical schools today are far different from medical colleges one hundred years ago, but medical school buildings remain tools for pedagogical and professional development and expressions of scientific ideas and physician identity.

ABBREVIATIONS
FOR ARCHIVES

Albany Medical College
Albany Medical College Archives, Albany, New York

Case
Case Western Reserve University Archives, Cleveland, Ohio

Chesney Medical Archives
Alan Mason Chesney Medical Archives of the Johns Hopkins Medical
Institutions, Baltimore, Maryland

Columbia Health Sciences
Archives and Special Collections, Columbia University Health Sciences
Library, New York, New York

Columbia University
University Archives, Rare Book and Manuscript Library, Columbia
University Libraries, New York, New York

Countway
Center for the History of Medicine, Francis A. Countway Library of
Medicine, Boston, Massachusetts

Drexel
Legacy Center, Drexel University College of Medicine, Philadelphia,
Pennsylvania

Eastman Museum
George Eastman Museum, Rochester, New York

Eskind
History of Medicine Collections, Eskind Biomedical Library, Vanderbilt
University, Nashville, Tennessee

Hamburger University Archives
Ferdinand Hamburger University Archives, Johns Hopkins University,
Baltimore, Maryland

Harvard University Archives
Harvard University Archives, Cambridge, Massachusetts

Howard University Archives
University Archives, Moorland-Spingarn Research Center, Howard University, Washington, DC

Howard University Library Division
Library Division, Moorland-Spingarn Research Center, Howard University, Washington, DC

Howard University Manuscript Division
Manuscript Division, Moorland-Spingarn Research Center, Howard University, Washington, DC

LC
Library of Congress, Washington, DC

Meharry Medical College
Meharry Medical College Archives, Meharry Medical College, Nashville, Tennessee

MHS
Massachusetts Historical Society, Boston, Massachusetts

NLM
National Library of Medicine, National Institutes of Health, Bethesda, Maryland

RAC
Rockefeller Archive Center, Sleepy Hollow, New York

Shepley Bulfinch
Archives of Shepley Bulfinch Richardson and Abbott, Shepley Bulfinch Richardson and Abbott, Boston, Massachusetts

SUNY Upstate
Archives and Special Collections at the SUNY Upstate Health Sciences Library, Syracuse, New York

Syracuse University
University Archives, Special Collections Research Center, Syracuse University Libraries, Syracuse, New York

University of Nebraska
Archives and Special Collections, University of Nebraska–Lincoln Libraries, Lincoln, Nebraska

University of Nebraska Medical Center
McGoogan Health Sciences Library, Special Collections and Archives, University of Nebraska Medical Center, Omaha, Nebraska

Vanderbilt University
Vanderbilt University Archives, Nashville, Tennessee

NOTES

Introduction

1. G. Robinson, "Relation of Medical Education to the Medical Plant," 321.

2. Rothstein, *American Medical Schools*, 151.

3. William P. Few to J. L. Jackson, 16 November 1925, quoted in Gifford, *Evolution of a Medical Center*, 42 (also quoted in Ludmerer, *Learning to Heal*, 205).

4. Ludmerer, *Learning to Heal*, 205.

5. Davison, *Duke University Medical Center*, 17.

6. Two articles are the exceptions that prove the rule. Medical historian Steven Peitzman's "Style and Space" examines the 1875 building for the Woman's Medical College of Pennsylvania. Although working on a British rather than American topic, historian James Hopkins's "(Dis)assembling of Form" investigates the 1874 building for the Owens College Medical School in Manchester, England, and its 1894 extension.

7. Adams, *Medicine by Design*; Kisacky, *Rise of the Modern Hospital*; Yanni, *Architecture of Madness*. The handful of chapters and articles by architectural historians of nonclinical medical spaces include Gournay, "L'architecture hospitalo-universitaire"; Adams, "Designing the Medical Museum"; and Kingsley, "Architecture of Nursing."

8. I am not alone in emphasizing the usefulness of architecture for understanding the history of medicine. For example, see Adams, "Designing the Medical Museum," 185; and Strickland, "Passive and Active," 233.

9. See, for example, Leslie, "'Different Kind of Beauty'"; Gieryn, "What Buildings Do"; and Schlich, "Surgery, Science and Modernity."

10. Horowitz, *Alma Mater*; P. Turner, *Campus*.

11. Yanni, *Living on Campus*; Grubiak, *White Elephants on Campus*; C. Robinson, "Architecture in Support of Citizenry."

12. See, for example, Adams, *Medicine by Design*; and Yanni, *Living on Campus*.

13. Examples of this perspective include Ludmerer, *Learning to Heal*, 231; Jacobson, *Making Medical Doctors*, 121–26; and Peitzman, "Style and Space."

14. Kisacky, *Rise of the Modern Hospital*, 8.

15. Ludmerer, *Learning to Heal*, 11–15.

16. Ludmerer, *Learning to Heal*, 11–15.

17. Kisacky, *Rise of the Modern Hospital*, 58–60, 138.

18. Kisacky, *Rise of the Modern Hospital*, 214.

19. D. Riesman, "Clinical Teaching in America with Some Remarks on Early Medical Schools," *Transactions and Studies of the College of Physicians of Philadelphia*,

4th ser., 7 (1939): 109, quoted in Hudson, "Abraham Flexner in Perspective," 550 (also quoted in Kisacky, *Rise of the Modern Hospital*, 214).

20. On the amphitheater, see Johns, "*The Gross Clinic*," 259n11, 259n12.

21. On the identity of the woman, see Burns, *Painting the Dark Side*, 283n33.

22. M. Smith, "*The Agnew Clinic*," 169–71. See also Long, "Medical World of *The Agnew Clinic*," 192–94.

23. Ludmerer, *Learning to Heal*, 3.

24. J. Howard Ferguson, "A Chronological Calendar of Events of the College of Medicine at Syracuse, 1872–1968, with Some Later Additions," 1968, vol. 1 (PDF), SUNY Upstate.

25. Dyson, *Founding the School of Medicine of Howard University*, 6; Dyson, *Howard University*, 44–45.

26. Lavoie, "Davidge Hall"; John G. Waite Associates, "College of Medicine of Maryland (Davidge Hall)," National Historic Landmark Nomination, 1997, https://np gallery.nps.gov/NRHP/GetAsset/NHLS/97001275_text; *Davidge Hall*, 4–7; Cordell, *Historical Sketch of the University of Maryland School of Medicine*, 22. On the connection between anatomical and operating theaters, see Adams, *Medicine by Design*, 14.

27. Billings, "Ideals of Medical Education," 2.

28. Ludmerer, *Learning to Heal*, 16–19, 29–38; Bonner, *American Doctors and German Universities*, 3–5, 41–42, 79–81.

29. Ludmerer, *Learning to Heal*, 38–63; Bonner, *Becoming a Physician*, 264–68, 291–92.

30. Eliot, "Exercises in Huntington Hall," 38.

31. "Description of the New Building Erected for the Medical School of Harvard University," 339–43.

32. "Description of the New Building Erected for the Medical School of Harvard University," 340; Douglass Shand-Tucci, "City-State," Back Bay Historical, accessed 10 October 2011, http://www.backbayhistorical.org/blog/archives/781 (site discontinued); Warren, *To Work in the Vineyard of Surgery*, 187; Morgan, *Buildings of Massachusetts*, 95, 146.

33. Examples of various forms of press coverage include: "Dedication of the New Harvard Medical Building and Celebration of the Centennial Anniversary of the School," *Boston Daily Globe*, 18 October 1883; and "Description of the New Building Erected for the Medical School of Harvard University," 339–43.

34. Ludmerer, *Learning to Heal*, 69; Bonner, *Becoming a Physician*, 267, 292–94.

35. C. M. Jackson, "On the Improvement of Medical Teaching," in *Medical Education and Research*, ed. J. McKeen Cattell (New York: Science Press, 1913), 371, quoted in Bonner, *Becoming a Physician*, 293.

36. Franklin P. Mall, "The Value of Research in the Medical School," *Michigan Alumnus* 8 (1904): 396, quoted in Ludmerer, *Learning to Heal*, 69–70.

37. Bonner, *Becoming a Physician*, 293.

38. Ludmerer, *Time to Heal*, xxii–xxiii.

39. See especially Kisacky, *Rise of the Modern Hospital*.

Chapter 1. An Alternative to Unification

Parts of chapters 1 and 2 appeared in Carroll, "Creating the Modern Physician," 48–73.

1. Ludmerer, *Learning to Heal*, 11–12.

2. Ludmerer, *Time to Heal*, 66. For more on reformed preclinical training, see Bonner, *Becoming a Physician*, 329.

3. On the architecture of surgical spaces, see Kisacky, *Rise of the Modern Hospital*, 62, 138–44, 214–18; on clinical medical education, see Ludmerer, *Learning to Heal*, 152–60, 219–33. See also Adams, *Medicine by Design*, 14–15, 126.

4. On the parallels between Dewey's ideas and modern medical education, see Ludmerer, *Time to Heal*, 6, 10; and Ludmerer, *Learning to Heal*, 64, 67–68. For more on Dewey's ideas, see Gyure, "Creating Friendly School Environments," 71.

5. Boster and Howell, *Medicine at Michigan*, 53.

6. Ludmerer, *Time to Heal*, 10 (quote), 66, 68–70.

7. Ludmerer, *Time to Heal*, 66–68.

8. Ludmerer, *Time to Heal*, 72.

9. Moore, *Miracle and a Privilege*, 18.

10. Ludmerer, *Time to Heal*, 72, 75.

11. Ludmerer, *Time to Heal*, 66.

12. Charles W. Eliot, "President's Report for 1898–99," in *Annual Reports of the President and the Treasurer of Harvard College, 1898–99* (Cambridge, MA: Harvard University, 1900), 25–26.

13. Gifford, *Evolution of a Medical Center*, 106–8.

14. Joe E. Holoubek, "Memories of My Medical School Years and Internship at the University of Nebraska College of Medicine, 1934–1939," [2001?], n.p., University of Nebraska Medical Center.

15. J. Holoubek, "Memories of My Medical School Years."

16. Mall, "Anatomical Course and Laboratory of the Johns Hopkins University," 85.

17. Moore, *Miracle and a Privilege*, 16–17.

18. J. Holoubek, "Memories of My Medical School Years."

19. See Ludmerer, *Learning to Heal*, 57–58; Bonner, *Becoming a Physician*, 292; and P. Starr, *Social Transformation of American Medicine*, 115–16.

20. On Hopkins's request, see Chesney, *Johns Hopkins Hospital and the Johns Hopkins University School of Medicine*, 1:16–17.

21. Chesney, *Johns Hopkins Hospital and the Johns Hopkins University School of Medicine*, 1:68–69, 95–97; Harvey et al., *Model of Its Kind*, 1:16–17; Sander, *Mary Elizabeth Garrett*, 155–57.

22. For the conditions of Garrett's gift, see Chesney, *Johns Hopkins Hospital and the Johns Hopkins University School of Medicine*, 2:42.

23. For the slow expansion of the student body, see the school's annual announcements, including Johns Hopkins Medical School, *The Johns Hopkins Medical School Announcement for 1893–1894* (Baltimore: Johns Hopkins Press, 1893), 10.

24. Henry Mills Hurd, *Fourth Report of the Superintendent of the Johns Hopkins Hospital* (Baltimore: Johns Hopkins Press, 1893), 15.

25. For the conditions of the gift, see Chesney, *Johns Hopkins Hospital and the Johns Hopkins University School of Medicine*, 2:42.

26. Johns Hopkins Medical School, *The Johns Hopkins Medical School Announcement for 1895–1896* (Baltimore: Johns Hopkins Press, 1895), 12–13.

27. Henry Mills Hurd, *Seventh Report of the Superintendent of the Johns Hopkins Hospital* (Baltimore: Johns Hopkins Press, 1896), 7.

28. Henry Mills Hurd, *Eighth Report of the Superintendent of the Johns Hopkins Hospital* (Baltimore: Johns Hopkins Press, 1897), 7.

29. Chesney, *Johns Hopkins Hospital and the Johns Hopkins University School of Medicine*, 2:208–9.

30. Osler, "On the Library of a Medical School," 111.

31. "Woman's Fund Building [*sic*]: The First of the Johns Hopkins Medical School Group," *Baltimore Sun*, 16 April 1894. For another mention of the proposed group, see George Archer to Daniel Coit Gilman, 12 November 1894, Ms. 1, Folder 31, Box 1.2, Series 1, Hamburger University Archives.

32. Osler, "On the Library of a Medical School," 111.

33. Weed, "William H. Welch Medical Library," 8.

34. William H. Welch, "Regarding Medical Instruction in the Johns Hopkins University," March 1891, Folder "Regarding Medical Instruction in the JHU, by Welch. Prefaced by Henry Hurd letter, March 1891," Box 2, Series A, RG 1, Chesney Medical Archives.

35. Billings, "Ideals of Medical Education," 2.

36. W. Coleman and Holmes, "Introduction," 6.

37. W. Coleman and Holmes, "Introduction," 8.

38. McClelland, *State, Society, and University in Germany*, 280–81.

39. W. Coleman and Holmes, "Introduction," 9.

40. P. Turner, *Campus*, 6.

41. Chesney, *Johns Hopkins Hospital and the Johns Hopkins University School of Medicine*, 1:12–17 (quote, 16).

42. Cameron, "Early Contributions to the Johns Hopkins Hospital by the 'Other' Surgeon," 270–72.

43. Cox, "Johns Hopkins Hospital, Baltimore, Maryland," 26.

44. "Building the Hospital," 15.

45. On the medical school site and hospital block plan, see Chesney, *Johns Hopkins Hospital and the Johns Hopkins University School of Medicine*, 1:44, 61–62; and for a reproduction of the block plan, see vol. 1 of that work, following p. 312.

46. Chesney, *Johns Hopkins Hospital and the Johns Hopkins University School of Medicine*, 1:65.

47. Chesney, *Johns Hopkins Hospital and the Johns Hopkins University School of Medicine*, 1:65.

48. Ingleby, "Department of Pathology," 13.

49. Ingleby, "Department of Pathology," 11.

50. Ingleby, "Department of Pathology," 13.

51. Flexner, *Medical Education in the United States and Canada*, 235.

52. For Archer's involvement in the pathology addition, see Minutes, 4 April 1893, 2 May 1893, Minutes of the Executive Committee of the Johns Hopkins Hospital, Chesney Medical Archives. On Archer's involvement in the Physiological Building, see "Action of the Trustees," Folder "'New' Medical Laboratory, 1897," Box 2, Series A, RG 1, Chesney Medical Archives. For biographical information on Archer, see Irma Walker and James T. Wollon Jr., "George Archer," Baltimore Architecture Foundation, accessed 5 September 2019, http://baltimorearchitecture.org/biographies/george-archer/.

53. "Woman's Fund Building [*sic*]," *Baltimore Sun*.

54. William H. Welch to Daniel Coit Gilman, 27 June 1894, reprinted in Chesney, *Johns Hopkins Hospital and the Johns Hopkins University School of Medicine*, 2:45 (see also 2:42–43).

55. Tilton, "William H. Welch Medical Library," 21.

56. Mall, "Anatomical Course and Laboratory of the Johns Hopkins University," 85.

57. Mall, "Anatomical Course and Laboratory of the Johns Hopkins University," 86.

58. Mall, "Anatomical Course and Laboratory of the Johns Hopkins University," 93.

59. Mall, "Anatomical Course and Laboratory of the Johns Hopkins University," 94.

60. Mall, "Anatomical Course and Laboratory of the Johns Hopkins University," 85.

61. Mall, "Anatomical Course and Laboratory of the Johns Hopkins University," 96. On concerns associated with large laboratories, see Minot, "Further Study of the Unit System of Laboratory Construction," 410.

62. Flexner, *Medical Education in the United States and Canada*, 88 (also quoted in Barzansky, "Growth and Divergence of the Basic Sciences," 23).

63. Mall, "Anatomical Course and Laboratory of the Johns Hopkins University," 96.

64. Chesney, *Johns Hopkins Hospital and the Johns Hopkins University School of Medicine*, 2:43.

65. "College of Medicine," *The Hilltop*, 10 October 1924, 5. *The Hilltop* is the student newspaper of Howard University.

66. G. Robinson, *Adventures in Medical Education*, 42.

67. Hertzler, *Horse and Buggy Doctor*, 43 (also partially quoted in Sappol, *Traffic of Dead Bodies*, 81). For Mall's smoking prohibition, see Mall, "Anatomical Course and Laboratory of the Johns Hopkins University," 96.

68. Mall, "Anatomical Course and Laboratory of the Johns Hopkins University," 88.

69. Mall, "Anatomical Course and Laboratory of the Johns Hopkins University," 89.

70. Cox, "Johns Hopkins Hospital, Baltimore, Maryland," 26. See also Fair, "'Laboratory of Heating and Ventilation,'" 357–81; and Billings, "Plans and Purposes of the Johns Hopkins Hospital," 506–7.

71. Mall, "Anatomical Course and Laboratory of the Johns Hopkins University," 89–90 (quote, 89).

72. Mall, "Anatomical Course and Laboratory of the Johns Hopkins University," 90.

73. Mall, "Anatomical Course and Laboratory of the Johns Hopkins University," 90–93 (quote, 93). See also Chesney, *Johns Hopkins Hospital and the Johns Hopkins University School of Medicine*, 2:43–44.

74. Hertzler, *Horse and Buggy Doctor*, 43. On the role of janitors, see Warner, "Witnessing Dissection," 20.

75. Ludmerer, *Learning to Heal*, 63.

76. Bluestone, "From Pasture to Pasteur," 1–2, 17.

77. Mall, "Anatomical Course and Laboratory of the Johns Hopkins University," 85–87 (quote, 85).

78. Mall, "Anatomical Course and Laboratory of the Johns Hopkins University," 85, 94–95 (quote, 95). For more on the histology course, see Barker and Bardeen, "Outline of the Course in Normal Histology and Microscopic Anatomy," 100–109.

79. Hopkins, "(Dis)assembling of Form," 39–40, 44, 46–48, 53.

80. Howard A. Kelly, "Address Delivered by Howard A. Kelley [*sic*] of Johns Hopkins University, at Dedication of New Building," in *Schedule of Clinics, Conferences and Entertainments: Fourth Annual Alumni Clinical Week of the University*

of Nebraska, College of Medicine ([Omaha?]: [University of Nebraska College of Medicine?], [1913?]), 141, University of Nebraska Medical Center.

81. J. Collins Warren and Henry Pickering Bowditch to Andrew Carnegie, 2 March 1901, Folder "J. C. Warren Mar. 1902," Box 19, John Collins Warren Papers, MHS.

82. On the cost of the Harvard Medical School buildings, see Charles W. Eliot, "President's Report for 1906–07," in *Reports of the President and the Treasurer of Harvard College, 1906–07* (Cambridge, MA: Harvard University, 1908), 38. On the cost of the Johns Hopkins Medical School buildings, see Chesney, *Johns Hopkins Hospital*, 2:47, 209.

83. Warren, *To Work in the Vineyard of Surgery*, 204.

84. Bluestone, "From Pasture to Pasteur," 8 (visual supplement), 16–18.

85. For a ground plan showing future additions, see Shepley, Rutan, and Coolidge, "New Harvard Medical School Buildings," 203.

86. For a description of the buildings, see "New Harvard Medical School," *Harvard Graduates' Magazine*, 616–17.

87. Mallory, "Medical School," 670.

88. Harvard Medical School, *Harvard Medical School, 1782–1906*, 177. See also Warren, *To Work in the Vineyard of Surgery*, 203.

89. Bowditch, letter to the editor, 305. Jack Eckert introduced me to this letter.

90. Fye, "Carl Ludwig and the Leipzig Physiological Institute," 920; W. Coleman and Holmes, "Introduction," 5. For a critical discussion of the formation of this institute, see Lenoir, "Science for the Clinic."

91. Kremer, "Building Institutes for Physiology in Prussia," 73.

92. Bowditch, letter to the editor, 306.

93. For a description of the building, see Bowditch, letter to the editor, 306.

94. For the plans for this institute, see Pistor, *Anstalten und Einrichtungen des öffentlichen Gesundheitswesens*, 95.

95. Shepley, Rutan, and Coolidge, "New Harvard Medical School Buildings," 204.

96. On the linear plan, see Yanni, *Architecture of Madness*, chap. 2.

97. J. Collins Warren, "Memoir #4," 217 (emphasis added), Folder "Memoir #4," Box untitled, John Collins Warren Additions, 1849–1929, MHS.

98. For Coolidge's comments, see "Triennial Dinner," 620.

99. On housing in German medical institutes, see Carroll, "Creating the Modern Physician," 70n38.

100. On the schedule and methods of instruction, see Harvard University, *Official Register of Harvard University* 3, no. 39 (1906–7): 17–30.

101. Bergengren, "New Harvard Medical School," 54.

102. For the schedule and the courses for the first and second years, see Harvard University, *Official Register of Harvard University* 3, no. 39 (1906–7), 17–36. For more on Harvard's block system, see Henry A. Christian, "The Concentration Plan of Teaching Medicine," paper presented at a meeting of the Association of American Medical Colleges, 21 and 22 [Mar.?] 1910, 1–4, Folder "Harvard University, 1904–1910," Box 20, Abraham Flexner Papers, Manuscript Division, LC. For the assignment of space within the buildings, see Harvard Medical School, *Harvard Medical School, 1782–1906*, 189–91.

103. For this criticism, see Christian, "Concentration Plan of Teaching Medicine," 8.

104. Councilman, "Ideals and Methods of the New Harvard Medical School," 586.

105. For the curriculum at Syracuse University College of Medicine, see *Syracuse University Bulletin: College of Medicine, 1938–1939* (Syracuse: [Syracuse University?], [1938?]), 25–26.

106. Christian, "Concentration Plan of Teaching Medicine," 7–8.

107. Coburn, "Mechanical Plant of the Harvard Medical School," 62–66 (quotes, 62, 65, 66). For more on the mechanical plant, see Densmore and LeClear, "Mechanical Plant"; and Densmore and LeClear, "Report to the President and Fellows of Harvard College upon the Mechanical Plant of the New Harvard University Medical School," no. 1, 15 June 1903, Folder "Densmore and LeClear, 1899–1903," Box 36, General Correspondence Group 2, Records of the President of Harvard University, Charles W. Eliot, UAI 5.150, Harvard University Archives. See also Carroll, "Modernizing the American Medical School," 62–64.

108. McClelland, *State, Society, and University in Germany*, 279.

109. Adams, "Designing the Medical Museum," 171.

110. McLeary, "Science in a Bottle," 36–41, 230–31.

111. McIsaac, "Rise and the Fall of the University of Michigan's Medical Museums," 68.

112. Harvard Medical School, *Harvard Medical School, 1782–1906*, 66.

113. McLeary, "Science in a Bottle," 160.

114. Adams, "Designing the Medical Museum," 172, 182–83. On the design of natural history museums, see Yanni, *Nature's Museums*.

115. John Shaw Billings, quoted in Rose Lincoln, "Hidden Spaces: Where Time Stands Still," *Harvard Gazette*, 10 March 2015, https://news.harvard.edu/gazette/story/2015/03/hidden-spaces-where-time-stands-still/.

116. For a description and history of the Warren Anatomical Museum, see Nercessian, *Legacy So Enduring*, 26–29.

117. Dominic Hall, quoted in Lincoln, "Hidden Spaces."

118. "Dedication of the New Medical School," 238.

119. Terry, "Washington University School of Medicine," 1–20 (quote, 15–16).

120. Mall, "Anatomical Course and Laboratory of the Johns Hopkins University," 96, 98–99 (quote, 96).

121. Mall, "Anatomical Course and Laboratory of the Johns Hopkins University," 98.

122. McLeary, "Science in a Bottle," 194–96, 195n69.

123. McLeary, "Science in a Bottle," 16, 160, 208–10, 225.

124. McIsaac, "Rise and the Fall of the University of Michigan's Medical Museums," 68.

125. Reinarz, "Age of Museum Medicine," 435.

126. For examples, see Reinarz, "Age of Museum Medicine," 435; and Nercessian, *Legacy So Enduring*, 44–54.

127. See Minot, "Unit System of Laboratory Construction," 390–91; and Minot, "Further Study of the Unit System," 409–15. On Porter's role, see Harrington, *Harvard Medical School*, 1441–42.

128. Minot, "Unit System of Laboratory Construction," 390; Biscoe, "University of Colorado School of Medicine and Hospital at Denver," 323.

129. Minot, "Unit System of Laboratory Construction," 390–91. On Minot's role in planning the 1883 building, see Lewis, "Charles Sedgwick Minot," 149.

130. Minot, "Further Study of the Unit System," 409–13 (quotes, 410, 409,

respectively). For mention of Minot's furniture, see Terry, "Washington University School of Medicine," 13.

131. Minot, "Unit System of Laboratory Construction," 391.

132. Minot, "Further Study of the Unit System," 409–10, 413–15.

133. Minot, "Further Study of the Unit System," 409–10, 413–15 (quotes, 409, 413).

134. Charles Coolidge, "Random Jottings," n.d., 3, Charles A. Coolidge Personal Files, Shepley Bulfinch.

135. Harvard Medical School, *Harvard Medical School, 1782–1906*, 178–79.

136. Harvard Medical School, *Harvard Medical School, 1782–1906*, 179.

137. Harrington, *Harvard Medical School*, 1204–5.

138. Charles S. Minot to Charles W. Eliot, 9 April 1902, Folder "Charles S. Minot, 1893–1903," Box 54, General Correspondence Group 2, Records of the President of Harvard University, Charles W. Eliot, UAI 5.150, Harvard University Archives (also quoted in Bluestone, "From Pasture to Pasteur," 67).

139. Bluestone, "From Pasture to Pasteur," 69.

140. Bluestone, "From Pasture to Pasteur," 69.

141. Charles S. Minot to Charles W. Eliot, 12 August 1903, Folder "Charles S. Minot, 1893–1903," Box 54, General Correspondence Group 2, Records of the President of Harvard University, Charles W. Eliot, UAI 5.150, Harvard University Archives (also cited in Bluestone, "From Pasture to Pasteur," 141n126).

142. Charles S. Minot to Charles W. Eliot, 26 February 1907, Folder "Medical School 1904–09," Box 103, General Correspondence Group 3, Records of the President of Harvard University, Charles W. Eliot, UAI 5.150, Harvard University Archives.

143. Corner, "Foundation and Earliest Years," 46–47.

144. Munby, "Design of Science Buildings," 76.

145. For a summary of these ideas, see Adams and Schlich, "Design for Control," 305.

146. Starr, *Social Transformation of American Medicine*, 134–38.

147. Howell, *Technology in the Hospital*, 2, 19–21, 89–91, 126–27, 178–79, 185–86, 232, 234–36 (quote, 91).

148. On the slow clinical adoption of x-rays, see Howell, *Technology in the Hospital*, chap. 4.

149. J. Holoubek, "Memories of My Medical School Years."

150. See Hopkins, "(Dis)assembling of Form," 48.

151. See, for example, Kisacky, *Rise of the Modern Hospital*; Schlich, "Surgery, Science and Modernity"; and Adams, *Medicine by Design*.

152. The exceptions are Peitzman, "Style and Space"; and Hopkins, "(Dis)assembling of Form."

153. H.H.L., "New Medical Buildings at Yale University," 390.

154. Bergengren, "New Harvard Medical School," 56.

155. Reinarz, "Age of Museum Medicine," 437.

156. See also Adams, "Designing the Medical Museum," 173.

157. Herman G. Weiskotten, "Problems in the Establishment of a New Medical School," address, 7 February 1949, 12–13, Folder untitled, Box 1, Papers of Herman G. Weiskotten, SUNY Upstate.

158. Harvard Medical School, *Harvard Medical School, 1782–1906*, 185–86.

159. Charles S. Minot to Charles W. Eliot, 24 September 1902, Folder "Charles S. Minot, 1893–1903," Box 54, General Correspondence Group 2, Records of the President of Harvard University, Charles W. Eliot, UAI 5.150, Harvard University Archives.

160. Ludmerer, *Learning to Heal*, 32. For more on this migration, see Bonner, *American Doctors and German Universities*.

161. For example, see G. Robinson, *Adventures in Medical Education*, 166–70.

162. On the autonomy of German institutes, see McClelland, *State, Society, and University in Germany*, 279.

Chapter 2. Unification Triumphs

1. Ludmerer, *Learning to Heal*, 235.

2. Rothstein, *American Medical Schools*, 144, 146.

3. Ludmerer, *Learning to Heal*, 235–36.

4. See, for instance, John J. Mullowney to Trevor Arnett, 27 May 1930, Folder 1234, Box 134, Subseries 1, Series 1, General Education Board Archives, RAC; and G. Robinson, "Relation of Medical Education," 323.

5. Ludmerer, *Learning to Heal*, 113–17.

6. Blake, "Laboratories, Hospitals, Libraries and Museums," 335.

7. Corner, "University of Rochester School of Medicine and Dentistry: Department of Anatomy," 22.

8. Adolph, "Perspectives of the First Faculty," 62.

9. "Editorial," *Bulletin of the Woman's Medical College of Pennsylvania* 79, no. 4 (December 1929), 2; "Educators Praise $1,000,000 College," *Public Ledger*, 25 January 1931, clipping, p. 882aaj, Clippings Scrapbook #14, July 1926–May 1936, ACC 133, Drexel.

10. Starr, *Social Transformation of American Medicine*, 143.

11. Rothstein, *American Medical Schools*, 151; Weiskotten et al., *Medical Education in the United States*, foreword by Ray Lyman Wilbur (quote, unpaginated) (also quoted in Rothstein, *American Medical Schools*, 151). For statistics, see chart in Rothstein, *American Medical Schools*, 143.

12. For statistics, see chart in Rothstein, *American Medical Schools*, 143 (see also 149).

13. Ludmerer, *Learning to Heal*, 170, 173.

14. Ludmerer, *Learning to Heal,* 171–72.

15. For a thorough discussion of the Flexner Report, see Ludmerer, *Learning to Heal*, chap. 9, and 235–37, 240, 245.

16. Ludmerer, *Learning to Heal*, 241.

17. Ludmerer, *Learning to Heal*, 241.

18. N. P. Colwell, "Inspection Made by Dr N. P. Colwell, Secretary of Council on Medical Education and Hospitals of the American Medical Association," 29 November 1921, Folder "Mullowney, John J.—Meharry Medical College—President—Inspection Made November 29, 1921. Inspection Made by Dr. N. P. Cornwell [*sic*] Secretary of Council on Medical Education and Hospitals of the American Medical Association," Box 1, John J. Mullowney Papers, Meharry Medical College.

19. Hine, "Pursuit of Professional Equality," 180–81.

20. J. Stanley Durkee, *Annual Report of President J. Stanley Durkee to the Board of Trustees: Howard University, Washington, D.C., 1922–23* (Washington, DC: Howard University Press, [1923?]), 4.

21. "To Accompany Budget for 1931–1933," 22 September 1930, Folder 14, Box 2, ACC 42, Drexel.

22. Council on Medical Education of the American Medical Association, "An Outline of the Essentials of a Satisfactory Medical College," 1 January 1910, 3, 5, 6, Folder "Cornell University 1909–1910," Box 19, Abraham Flexner Papers, Manuscript Division, LC.

23. Galpin, *Syracuse University*, 2:73–74; Wright, *Foundations Well and Truly Laid*, 26. For architectural plans, see Luft, *SUNY Upstate Medical University*, 73.

24. Flexner, *Medical Education in the United States and Canada*, 272–73, 276.

25. On fundraising for the 1896 building, see Luft, *SUNY Upstate Medical University*, 72.

26. Wright, *Foundations Well and Truly Laid*, 53–54, 58–59, 113.

27. Mould, "Dr. Ward L. Mould Remembers," 12.

28. [Herman G. Weiskotten?], "Syracuse University College of Medicine; Copy of Outline to Mr. Straus," 19 September 1936, 3, Folder "Historical—College of Medicine," Box 13, Papers of Herman G. Weiskotten, SUNY Upstate. See also F. Gordon Smith to William P. Graham and the Executive Committee of the Board of Trustees, 10 October 1940, 2, Folder "Smith, F. Gordon, 1937–41," Box 13626, Chancellors Charles Flint and William Graham Papers, RG 01/Flint and Graham, Syracuse University.

29. Ludmerer, *Learning to Heal*, 257.

30. [Weiskotten?], "Syracuse University College of Medicine," 2–3.

31. *Syracuse University Bulletin: College of Medicine, 1938–1939* (Syracuse: [Syracuse University?], [1938?]), 22.

32. For an outline of Syracuse's medical curriculum, see *Syracuse University Bulletin: College of Medicine, 1938–1939*, 23–30. The final architectural plans do not label the various departments in the medical college, but the earlier plans dated 10 October 1935 do. By correlating the physical needs (e.g., types of laboratories) in the two plans, I determined which departments occupied which spaces on the later plans. The plans dated 10 October 1935, along with a set of the final plans, are available at University Archives, Special Collections Research Center, Syracuse University Libraries. I also depended on the partial description of the building provided in J. Howard Ferguson, "A Chronological Calendar of Events of the College of Medicine at Syracuse, 1872–1968, with Some Later Additions," 1968, vol. 2, physiology section, and vol. 3, pathology section (PDFs), SUNY Upstate.

33. Waite, *Western Reserve University Centennial History of the School of Medicine*, 428.

34. For statistics on the prevalence and location of the central library in 1940, see Weiskotten et al., *Medical Education in the United States*, 89.

35. For the new schedule, see *Syracuse University Bulletin: College of Medicine, 1939–1940* (Syracuse: [Syracuse University?], [1939?]), 23–26.

36. Davison, *Duke University Medical Center*, 17.

37. On university and medical school fundraising efforts, see Ludmerer, *Learning to Heal*, 203. On the boom in hospital construction between the end of World War I and the Great Depression, see Kisacky, *Rise of the Modern Hospital*, 239, 296.

38. For descriptions of the campus, see Kampmeier, *Vanderbilt University School of Medicine*, 26–28; and James H. Kirkland to Abraham Flexner, 27 June 1921, Folder 1408, Box 152, Subseries 1, Series 1, General Education Board Archives, RAC.

39. For the earlier sketch, see unsigned sketch attached to James H. Kirkland to Wallace Buttrick, 13 October 1919, Folder 1406, Box 152, Subseries 1, Series 1, General Education Board Archives, RAC.

40. G. Robinson, *Adventures in Medical Education*, 155.

41. G. Canby Robinson, "Plan for the Proposed Reorganization of the Vanderbilt University Medical School," received 25 September 1920, 1–2, Folder 1407, Box 152, Subseries 1, Series 1, General Education Board Archives, RAC.

42. G. Robinson, "Plan for the Proposed Reorganization," 2.

43. G. Robinson, "Plan for the Proposed Reorganization," 3.

44. On Robinson's travels, see G. Robinson, *Adventures in Medical Education*, 160–61; and G. Canby Robinson to James H. Kirkland, 14 August 1920, Folder 22, Box 100, RG 300, Vanderbilt University.

45. G. Robinson, *Adventures in Medical Education*, 157.

46. Washington University School of Medicine, *Dedication of the New Buildings*, 180 (emphasis added).

47. G. Robinson, "Vanderbilt University School of Medicine," 1, 8. Timothy C. Jacobson provides a thorough description of the funding and final design for Vanderbilt University's 1925 medical school and hospital facility. See Jacobson, *Making Medical Doctors*, esp. 79–140. Jacobson recognizes the landmark nature of the facility's combination of preclinical and clinical teaching and research (121). See also Heskel, *Shepley Bulfinch Richardson and Abbott*, 47–49.

48. Robinson's other sketches are located in Folder 2, G. Canby Robinson Biographical File, Eskind.

49. G. Robinson, "Relation of Medical Education," 321–23.

50. G. Robinson, "Relation of Medical Education," 321; G. Robinson, "Vanderbilt University School of Medicine," 8. See also Jacobson, *Making Medical Doctors*, 123–24.

51. G. Robinson, "Vanderbilt University School of Medicine," 8.

52. Davison, *Duke University Medical Center*, 17.

53. On Robinson's work in the 1930s related to the concept of the patient as a whole, see T. Brown, "George Canby Robinson and 'The Patient as a Person,'" 137, 145–51. Brown briefly considers the design of the Vanderbilt plant (139, 141).

54. Warner, "Art of Medicine in an Age of Science," 58, 61–63, 69. For Warner's discussion of Robinson, see 68–69.

55. Davison, *Duke University Medical Center*, 17.

56. John J. Mullowney, "Training for Medicine and Dentistry," reprinted in *Opportunity: Journal for Negro Life* (December 1936), n.p., in Folder 1251, Box 136, Subseries 1, Series 1, General Education Board Archives, RAC.

57. Kampmeier, *Recollections*, 179–80.

58. G. Robinson, "Vanderbilt University School of Medicine," 11.

59. For the schedule before the move, see *Bulletin of Vanderbilt University, School of Medicine of Vanderbilt University, 1924–1925* (Nashville: [Vanderbilt University?], 1924), 57–59.

60. G. Robinson, "Relation of Medical Education," 321. See also Davison, *Duke University Medical Center*, 17.

61. Lemkau, "Crossroads," 147, 156–57.

62. Flexner, *Medical Education in the United States and Canada*, 82.

63. Howell, "Changing Structure of Medical Education," 17–18.

64. Holt, "Library of the Harvard Medical School," 32–35, 38; "Description of the New Building," 341.

65. Mallory, "Medical School," 670–71 (quotes, 670).

66. Robert, "Libraries at P. and S.," 214–15 (quotes, 214, 215). See also Lemkau, "Crossroads," 146–47.

67. Robert, "Libraries at P. and S.," 214–15 (quote, 215).

68. Holt, "Library of the Harvard Medical School," 38–39.

69. H. Shepley, "Considerations in Planning a Teaching Hospital," 94.

70. Weiskotten et al., *Medical Education in the United States*, 89–90.

71. Weiskotten et al., *Medical Education in the United States*, 90.

72. Sollmann, "Departmental Libraries of the School of Medicine of Western Reserve University," 177–81 (quotes, 177, 178).

73. Holt, "Library of the Harvard Medical School," 38.

74. Holt, "Library of the Harvard Medical School," 38–40; Nercessian, *Legacy So Enduring*, 33–35.

75. See "Wood Building," Case Western Reserve University Archives, accessed 13 November 2019, https://case.edu/its/archives/Buildings/woobui.htm.

76. Weed, "William H. Welch Medical Library," 3–9.

77. Weiskotten et al., *Medical Education in the United States*, 89.

78. Abbott, "Library Research Infrastructure for Humanistic and Social Scientific Scholarship in the Twentieth Century," 64. On the monumentality and frequently prime locations of these university libraries, see Gyure, "Heart of the University," 118–23.

79. Abbott, "Library Research Infrastructure for Humanistic and Social Scientific Scholarship in the Twentieth Century," 64–65.

80. Sollmann, "Departmental Libraries of the School of Medicine of Western Reserve University," 177.

81. Lemkau, "Crossroads," 145–46. Lemkau outlines these changes but does not directly link them to the development of medical librarianship.

82. See Stefanacci, Wood, and Huff, "Departmental Libraries," 433–37; Kasses, Taylor, and Jones, "Departmental Libraries," 177–84; Moran, "Role of the Medical Departmental Library," 25–31.

83. Cushing, "Binding Influence of a Library on a Subdividing Profession," 35.

84. Cushing, "Binding Influence of a Library on a Subdividing Profession," 35.

85. Cushing, "Binding Influence of a Library on a Subdividing Profession," 41–42 (quote, 41). On the understanding of medical history as a stimulus for cohesion and humanization and a counterbalance for specialization in this period, by Cushing in particular, see Warner, "Aesthetic Grounding of Modern Medicine," 18–31, esp. 26–27.

86. *Presbyterian Hospital and the Medical Center*, pamphlet, Folder "Columbia-Presbyterian Medical Center: Construction of CPMC and Early Years, 1920s–1930s; [Folder] 1/2, Development/Promotional," Development/Promotional Literature A–N, Columbia Health Sciences.

87. G. Canby Robinson to James H. Kirkland, 25 May 1926, annual report, 4, Folder 10, Box 109, RG 300, Vanderbilt University.

88. Rappleye, "Survey of Medical Education," 844 (also quoted in Rothstein, *American Medical Schools*, 155).

89. Weiskotten et al., *Medical Education in the United States*, 85 (also quoted in Rothstein, *American Medical Schools*, 155).

90. Weiskotten et al., *Medical Education in the United States*, 85.

91. Souers and Parnall, "New Medical Unit," 73–75.

92. Souers and Parnall, "New Medical Unit," 75.

93. G. Robinson, "Relation of Medical Education," 321.

94. Conversation with the author during tours of the building, 29 August 2006 and 14 October 2008.

95. Cullen, "Vanderbilt University School of Medicine," 38.

96. Conversation with the author during tour of the building, 30 July 2009.

97. *Woman's Medical College of Pennsylvania: Freshman Handbook, 1945–1946* (Philadelphia: [Woman's Medical College of Pennsylvania?], [1945?]), "Clothes" section, n.p., Folder "Student Handbook, 1945," ACC 72, Drexel.

98. G. Canby Robinson, "Discussion of the Address of Dr. Thomas Ordway on Four Years in Medicine: The Hospital Medical School," 1, in Thomas Ordway, "Four Years in Medicine: The Hospital Medical School," publication of address read before the Association of American Medical Colleges, 2 March 1923, Item 21, Box 2, Thomas Ordway Papers, Albany Medical College.

99. Gieryn, "Two Faces on Science," 448.

100. Robinson to Kirkland, 25 May 1926, annual report, 4.

101. Ordway, "Four Years in Medicine," 5.

102. G. Robinson, "Influence of Environment in Medical Education," 11.

103. Adolph, "Perspectives of the First Faculty," 64–65.

104. Whipple, "Autobiographical Sketch," 283.

105. Adolph, "Perspectives of the First Faculty," 65.

106. Rothstein, *American Medical Schools*, 159, 173–74.

107. Henry H. Donaldson to Frederick [*sic*] S. Lee, 28 October 1912, Folder 8, Box 5, Frederic Schiller Lee Papers, Columbia Health Sciences. See also [Frederic S. Lee?] to Franz Boas, T. H. Morgan, E. B. Wilson, J. McK. Cattell, and R. S. Woodworth, 25 October 1912, Folder 8, Box 5, Frederic Schiller Lee Papers, Columbia Health Sciences. I assume that Donaldson is responding to an inquiry from Lee similar to that dated 25 October 1912.

108. Harvard Medical School, *Harvard Medical School, 1782–1906*, 177.

109. G. Robinson, "Vanderbilt University School of Medicine," 11.

110. Harrison quoted in Kampmeier, *Recollections*, 38.

111. Kampmeier, *Recollections*, 38–39; R. Collins, *Ernest William Goodpasture*, 140.

112. Kampmeier, *Recollections*, 43.

113. Adolph, "Perspectives of the First Faculty," 66.

114. Adolph, "Perspectives of the First Faculty," 66; G. Robinson, "Vanderbilt University School of Medicine," 11.

115. R. Collins, *Ernest William Goodpasture*, 140.

116. R. Collins, "Dr William DeMonbreun," 459, 461–62, 464 (quote, 464). Collins introduced me to a number of his and others' publications related to Vanderbilt University School of Medicine, including this article.

117. John B. Youmans, "Vanderbilt–Yesterday, Today and Tomorrow," address to the medical alumni reunion, 5 June 1965, reprinted in *Journal of the Tennessee Medical Association* 59, no. 1 (1966): 41, quoted in R. Collins, *Ernest William Goodpasture*, 138.

118. Souers and Parnall, "New Medical Unit," 75.

119. Ludmerer, *Learning to Heal*, chap. 12. On the proximity of medical schools and hospitals, see Rothstein, *American Medical Schools*, 113.

120. Kisacky, *Rise of the Modern Hospital*, 99.

121. For a discussion of these events at Woman's Medical College of Pennsylvania, see Peitzman, *New and Untried Course*, 21–25, 39–40, 125–28. For students' difficulty obtaining access to hospitals, see [Woman's Medical College of Pennsylvania?], *Natural Guardians of the Race* (Philadelphia: Woman's Medical College of Pennsylvania and Holmes Press, 1926), 13, Butler Scrapbook, ACC 123, Drexel. On the 1875 medical school, see Peitzman, "Style and Space," 28–43.

122. "Inspection of the Woman's Medical College of Pennsylvania," William Pepper and Samuel W. Lambert to W. S. Carter, Association of American Medical Colleges, 28 February 1919, Folder 7, Box 1, ACC 290, Drexel (emphasis added).

123. Kisacky, *Rise of the Modern Hospital*, esp. 91–95, 168, 253–57 (quote, 240). A passing comment from Kisacky encouraged me to reconsider the similarities between the two building types.

124. On these trends in hospitals, see Kisacky, *Rise of the Modern Hospital*, 135, 167, 198–204, 239–40, 250–51 (quote, 198).

125. Samuel W. Lambert, "Memorandum on the Ideal Development of Hospital and Medical School Addressed to the Trustees of Columbia University and the Managers of the Presbyterian Hospital," March 1912, 2, Folder "545 Medical Center Development, 1910–1918," Box 631, Office of the Vice President for Health Sciences Central Records, Columbia Health Sciences.

126. Stevens, *American Hospital of the Twentieth Century*, 2nd ed., 396–399.

127. Stevens, *American Hospital of the Twentieth Century*, 2nd ed., 399–402.

128. Kisacky, *Rise of the Modern Hospital*, 255–57.

129. Stevens, *American Hospital of the Twentieth Century*, 2nd ed., 399.

130. Leroy, "Columbia-Presbyterian Medical Center," 186.

131. Ludmerer, *Learning to Heal*, 230–33 (quotes, 230, 232). In his analysis of Columbia-Presbyterian, Ludmerer quotes *A Medical Center for New York* (New York: Presbyterian Hospital, 1924), 23, Folder "Columbia-Presbyterian Medical Center: Construction and Early Years, 1920s–1930s; Folder 2/2; Development/Promotional Material," Development/Promotional Literature A–N, Columbia Health Sciences.

132. On modern medical centers, see Ludmerer, *Time to Heal*, 114. On the earlier use of the term, see Kisacky, *Rise of the Modern Hospital*, 115.

133. Minutes, 23 November 1926, 22 March 1927, Minutes of the Joint Administrative Board, Columbia Health Sciences.

134. *A Medical Center for New York: The Alliance between Columbia University and Presbyterian Hospital* ([New York?]: Columbia University, May 1915), Folder "545 Medical Center Development, 1910–1918," Box 631, Office of the Vice President for Health Sciences Central Records, Columbia Health Sciences.

135. *A Medical Center for New York* (New York: Presbyterian Hospital, 1924).

136. Minutes, 23 November 1926, Minutes of the Joint Administrative Board.

137. Minutes, 22 March 1927, 9 February 1928, 27 March 1928, 24 April 1928, Minutes of the Joint Administrative Board, Columbia Health Sciences.

138. *Build New York a Medical Center: Handbook of Information; Presbyterian Hospital Building Fund*, 4–5 (see also 6–7), Folder "Columbia-Presbyterian Med-

ical Center: Construction of CPMC and Early Years, 1920s–1930s; [Folder] 1/2, Development/Promotional," Development/Promotional Literature A–N, Columbia Health Sciences. On the fundraising campaign, see Lamb, "Story of the Founding of the Columbia-Presbyterian Medical Center," 760.

139. Edward S. Van Duyn, "Dr. Van Duyn Tells Aims of Medic Center," *Syracuse Herald*, 21 November 1937, 4-C.

140. Brandt and Sloane, "Of Beds and Benches," 294.

141. Brandt and Sloane, "Of Beds and Benches," 294–95.

142. See Kisacky, *Rise of the Modern Hospital*, 208–10.

143. Stevens, *American Hospital of the Twentieth Century*, 2nd ed., chap. 15. For the original text, see Stevens, *American Hospital of the Twentieth Century* (1918). For the intermediate edition, see Stevens, *American Hospital of the Twentieth Century*, rev. ed. (1921). Citing Stevens, Ludmerer recognizes that by the late 1920s texts on hospital architecture had begun to explore the physical relationship between hospitals and medical schools. See Ludmerer, *Learning to Heal*, 231. See also Shepley, "Considerations in Planning a Teaching Hospital," 91–96.

144. Charles Coolidge to James H. Kirkland, 30 October 1922, Folder 13, Box 100, RG 300, Vanderbilt University.

145. See Coolidge and Shattuck et al., "New Plant of the Vanderbilt University Medical School and Hospital"; and Biscoe, "University of Colorado School of Medicine and Hospital at Denver."

146. On the time line for the Colorado facility, see Meader, "University of Colorado School of Medicine and Hospital," 287.

147. Robinson, "Vanderbilt University School of Medicine," 8.

148. On the time line for the Rochester facility, see Whipple, *Planning and Construction Period of the School and Hospitals*, 5, 7.

149. Whipple, "University of Rochester School of Medicine and Dentistry: School and Hospital Plans," 8; Whipple, "Autobiographical Sketch," 272.

150. G. Robinson, "Vanderbilt University School of Medicine," 8.

151. On this competitiveness, see Ludmerer, *Learning to Heal*, 84–85.

152. Davison, *Duke University Medical Center*, 17.

153. [Woman's Medical College of Pennsylvania?], *Natural Guardians of the Race*, 14–15, 20, 24 25. See also "National Plans of Campaign Are Discussed," *Bulletin of the Woman's Medical College of Pennsylvania* 77, no. 3 (1926): 8.

154. On the shortfall, see Peitzman, *New and Untried Course*, 158.

155. Sarah Logan Wister Starr, "Talk by Mrs. Star [sic]," *Transactions of the Fifty-Third Annual Meeting of the Alumnae Association of the Woman's Medical College of Pennsylvania, June 7 and 8, 1928* (Philadelphia: Alumnae Association of the Woman's Medical College of Pennsylvania, 1928), 21

156. Martha Tracy, "Report to the Alumnae Association of the Woman's Medical College of Pennsylvania–June, 1929," *Transactions of the Fifty-Fourth Annual Meeting of the [Alumnae Association of the] Woman's Medical College of Pennsylvania, June 13 and 14, 1929* (Philadelphia: Alumnae Association of the Woman's Medical College of Pennsylvania, 1929), 26. George Thomas also notes the pioneering nature of the unified medical school–hospital facility at Woman's Medical College. See George E. Thomas, nomination, Woman's Medical College of Pennsylvania, National Register of Historic Places, sec. 8: 14, accessed 24 June 2019, https://www

.dot7.state.pa.us/CRGIS_Attachments/SiteResource/H054170_54076_10.pdf (site discontinued).

157. Stevens, *American Hospital of the Twentieth Century*, 2nd ed., 399.

158. Harrison quoted in Kampmeier, *Recollections*, 38.

159. Spock and Morgan, *Spock on Spock*, 99.

160. Davison, *Duke University Medical Center*, 17.

161. Kisacky, *Rise of the Modern Hospital*, 248 (see also 293).

162. Flexner quotes his report under preparation in Abraham Flexner, "Confidential Comments on the Memorandum Prepared by Messrs. MacCallum, Howland, and Weed," 24 February 1923, 7, Folder 6277, Box 590, Subseries 4, Series 1, General Education Board Archives, RAC.

163. Davison, *Duke University Medical Center*, 17. See also Robinson, "Vanderbilt University School of Medicine," 11.

164. Stevens, *American Hospital of the Twentieth Century*, 2nd ed., chap. 15.

165. Ray Lyman Wilbur, foreword to Weiskotten et al., *Medical Education in the United States*, n.p.

166. Herman G. Weiskotten, "Problems in the Establishment of a New Medical School," address, 7 February 1949, 13, Folder untitled, Box 1, Papers of Herman G. Weiskotten, SUNY Upstate.

Chapter 3. Donors, Architects, and Medical School Design

Parts of chapter 3 were previously published in Carroll, "Incorporated Philanthropy," 77–95.

1. Ludmerer, *Learning to Heal*, 139–46.

2. Ludmerer, *Learning to Heal*, 146.

3. Ludmerer, *Learning to Heal*, 147; Rothstein, *American Medical Schools*, 111.

4. Pusey, "Importance of Being Historically Minded," 2080 (also quoted in Rothstein, *American Medical Schools*, 111). On 29 October 1884 *Puck* ran a cartoon similar to the one described by Pusey, or Pusey may have been misremembering the 29 October 1884 cover. See Hansen, *Picturing Medical Progress from Pasteur to Polio*, 35–36.

5. Ludmerer, *Learning to Heal*, 151, 167, 191–92, 202–4.

6. Ludmerer, *Learning to Heal*, 192, 198–99.

7. Abraham Flexner, "Medical Education, 1909–1924," *Educational Record*, April 1924, 15, reprint, located in Folder "Articles and Lectures: Printed, 1917–1925," Box 33, Abraham Flexner Papers, Manuscript Division, LC.

8. For a fuller list, see Ludmerer, *Learning to Heal*, 198.

9. Sander, *Mary Elizabeth Garrett*, 159–82, 268–69; Jarrett, "Raising the Bar," 22–24.

10. Sander, *Mary Elizabeth Garrett*, 182–86. On coercive philanthropy, see Jarrett, "Raising the Bar," 26.

11. Sander, *Mary Elizabeth Garrett*, 194–95.

12. On the Harvard Medical School campaign for its 1906 quadrangle, see Ludmerer, *Learning to Heal*, 148.

13. For a complete reprint of Murphy's report, including original sections later left unpublished, see "Harvard University: Papers Concerning the Proposed New Buildings and Endowment for the Medical School," 19–41, Folder "Farrar Cobb,

1893–1901, folder 2 of 2," Box 32, General Correspondence Group 2, Records of the President of Harvard University, Charles W. Eliot, UAI 5.150, Harvard University Archives.

14. Harvard Medical School, *Harvard Medical School, 1782–1906*, 181.

15. Warren, *To Work in the Vineyard of Surgery*, 216.

16. See Harrington, *Harvard Medical School*, 1197; and Bluestone, "From Pasture to Pasteur," 60.

17. Ludmerer, *Learning to Heal*, 200–203.

18. Bethell, *Harvard Observed*, 34.

19. Hertzler, *Horse and Buggy Doctor*, 59.

20. Ludmerer, *Learning to Heal*, 192–93; Wheatley, *Politics of Philanthropy*, 84–85, 112–13. Neither of these two authors mentions construction.

21. Zunz, *Philanthropy in America*, chap. 1 (quote, 22). On Rockefeller's youthful charitable giving, see Brown, *Rockefeller Medicine Men*, 32–33.

22. On the development of the professions, see Wiebe, *Search for Order*, chap. 5.

23. Fosdick, *Adventure in Giving*, 8–9 (quote, 8).

24. Chernow, *Titan*, 491.

25. Ludmerer, *Learning to Heal*, 200–202.

26. Bonner, *Iconoclast*, 100–107, 112–13.

27. Fosdick, *Adventure in Giving*, 161, 172–73, 336, 339.

28. Wheatley, *Politics of Philanthropy*, 112, 159–62, 168.

29. Fosdick, *Adventure in Giving*, 172.

30. Ludmerer, *Learning to Heal*, 193–94, 197.

31. Ludmerer, *Learning to Heal*, 172–73, 178, 193–94. For the rise and fall of Flexner's system of philanthropic management, see Wheatley, *Politics of Philanthropy*, esp. chaps. 3–5.

32. Collins, *Ahmic Lake Connections*, 53–70.

33. Wheatley, *Politics of Philanthropy*, 99–106.

34. Ludmerer, *Learning to Heal*, 172–73, 204–5.

35. Ludmerer, *Learning to Heal*, 205, 210–13; Wheatley, *Politics of Philanthropy*, 62, 69–82, 86, 153.

36. See also Rothstein, *American Medical Schools*, 145.

37. Flexner, *Medical Education in the United States and Canada*, 256.

38. Flexner, *Medical Education in the United States and Canada*, 243.

39. Flexner, *Medical Education in the United States and Canada*, 119.

40. "Progress of the College," 65–66 (quote, 66).

41. Flexner, *Medical Education in the United States and Canada*, 261.

42. Wheatley and Ludmerer recognize an architectural component to Flexner's ideal medical school. See Wheatley, *Politics of Philanthropy*, 86; and Ludmerer, *Learning to Heal*, 177.

43. John L. Heffron to James R. Day, 6 May 1914, Folder "Correspondence: Heffron, John L.," Box 31349, Chancellor James Roscoe Day Papers, RG 01/Day, Syracuse University.

44. "Great Medical Plant Planned at University," newspaper clipping, 10 June 1922, Folder 33, Box 3, Papers of Dr. John L. Heffron (1851–1924), SUNY Upstate.

45. Carroll, "Modernizing the American Medical School," 202–6.

46. Abraham Flexner to James H. Kirkland, 20 June 1919, Folder 1406, Box 152,

Subseries 1, Series 1, General Education Board Archives, RAC. See also Brown, *Rockefeller Medicine Men*, 173–74.

47. See, for example, James H. Kirkland to Abraham Flexner, 10 February 1921, and attached outline, Folder 29, Box 98, RG 300, Vanderbilt University.

48. Since publication of my essay "Incorporated Philanthropy" in 2019, I have removed Washington University in St. Louis from this list; the GEB made its endowment gift to that school as the new buildings for the medical college neared completion, and the gift was intended to support full-time clinical faculty. I have also added the 1929 Institute of Pathology at Western Reserve University to this list. The institute supported the work of the medical school, dental school, nursing school, and the University Hospitals of Cleveland.

49. See Flexner, *Medical Education in the United States and Canada*, 240.

50. Abraham Flexner, "Confidential Comments on the Memorandum Prepared by Messrs. MacCallum, Howland, and Weed," 24 February 1923, 7–8 (quote, 7); "Memorandum by Howland, MacCallum, and Weed," February 1923, both in Folder 6277, Box 590, Subseries 4, Series 1, General Education Board Archives, RAC.

51. James H. Kirkland to Abraham Flexner, 10 February 1921, Folder 29, Box 98, RG 300, Vanderbilt University.

52. Robert H. Bremner describes Flexner's understanding of GEB gifts as "hardheaded investments." See Bremner, *American Philanthropy*, 130.

53. Abraham Flexner, "Memorandum Regarding Southern Trip: December 1–10, 1924," Folder 1410, Box 152, Subseries 1, Series 1, General Education Board Archives, RAC.

54. Abraham Flexner to G. Canby Robinson, 30 December 1924, Folder 1410, Box 152, Subseries 1, Series 1, General Education Board Archives, RAC.

55. Flexner, *Medical Education in the United States and Canada*, 71.

56. Flexner, *Medical Education in the United States and Canada*, 59. See also Kisacky, *Rise of the Modern Hospital*, 209; and George E. Thomas, nomination, Woman's Medical College of Pennsylvania, National Register of Historic Places, sec. 8: 14, accessed 24 June 2019, https://www.dot7.state.pa.us/CRGIS_Attachments/SiteResource/H054170_54076_10.pdf (site discontinued).

57. Jacobson, *Making Medical Doctors*, 110.

58. James H. Kirkland to Abraham Flexner, 4 November 1919, Folder 1406, Box 152, Subseries 1, Series 1, General Education Board Archives, RAC. See also unsigned and undated sketch attached to James H. Kirkland to Wallace Buttrick, 13 October 1919; and, for announcement of GEB gift, "Memorandum," 7 November 1919, both in Folder 1406, Box 152, Subseries 1, Series 1, General Education Board Archives, RAC.

59. Abraham Flexner to James H. Kirkland, 7 November 1919, Folder 1406, Box 152, Subseries 1, Series 1, General Education Board Archives, RAC.

60. James H. Kirkland to Abraham Flexner, 4 November 1920, Folder 1407, Box 152, Subseries 1, Series 1, General Education Board Archives, RAC.

61. James H. Kirkland to Charles Coolidge, 30 January 1922, Folder 12, Box 100, RG 300, Vanderbilt University.

62. For the relationship between the two plants, see G. Robinson, "Vanderbilt University School of Medicine," 8.

63. Rush Rhees to Abraham Flexner, 6 November 1926, Folder 1231, Box 133, Subseries 1, Series 1, General Education Board Archives, RAC.

64. On the coordination between philanthropic foundations, see Wheatley, *Politics of Philanthropy*, 84–85, 112–13.

65. Pearce, "Prefatory Note," 3.

66. George E. Vincent, "President's Review," in *The Rockefeller Foundation: Annual Report, 1926* (New York: Rockefeller Foundation, [1927?]), 52, accessed 25 June 2021, https://www.rockefellerfoundation.org/wp-content/uploads/Annual-Report-1926-1.pdf.

67. George E. Vincent, "President's Review," in *The Rockefeller Foundation: Annual Report, 1925* (New York: Rockefeller Foundation, [1926?]), 61, accessed 25 June 2021, https://www.rockefellerfoundation.org/wp-content/uploads/Annual-Report-1925-1.pdf.

68. Minutes, 4 November 1927, Rockefeller Foundation Minutes, Folder 10, Box 1, Series 906, RG 3.1, Rockefeller Foundation Archives, RAC. Tom Rosenbaum at the RAC provided valuable assistance in locating documents related to *Methods and Problems of Medical Education*.

69. See, for example, unsigned review of *Methods and Problems of Medical Education*, 13th ser. (1929), in *Journal of the American Medical Association* 93, no. 15 (12 October 1929): 1172; and unsigned review of *Methods and Problems of Medical Education*, 3rd ser. (1925), in *Journal of the American Medical Association* 86, no. 2 (9 January 1926): 141. See also unsigned review of *Methods and Problems of Medical Education*, 9th ser. (1928), in *New England Journal of Medicine* 199, no. 10 (6 September 1928): 502; and unsigned review of *Methods and Problems of Medical Education*, 18th ser. (1930), in *New England Journal of Medicine* 204, no. 5 (29 January 1931): 242. Note that each issue of *Methods and Problems of Medical Education* was called a series. Each series (issue) received a unique number.

70. For an example of authors using illustrations from *Methods and Problems of Medical Education* in their own article, see Munby, "Design of Science Buildings," 75, 77. The images published by Munby appeared four years earlier in *Methods and Problems of Medical Education*; see Wiggers, "Western Reserve University School of Medicine: Department of Physiology," 47, 52.

71. Offices of Dwight James Baum and John Russell Pope to Robert A. Lambert, 14 November 1935, Folder "Medical College," Box 15410, RG 44, Syracuse University.

72. Rockefeller Foundation Inter-Office Correspondence, 11 September 1931, Folder 10, Box 1, Series 906, RG 3.1, Rockefeller Foundation Archives, RAC; and Minutes, 4 November 1927, Rockefeller Foundation Minutes (quote).

73. [Alan Gregg?], "The Medical Sciences," in *The Rockefeller Foundation: Annual Report, 1932* (New York: [Rockefeller Foundation?], [1933?]), 210, accessed 25 June 2021, https://docuri.com/download/rockerfeller-foundation_59a8d-692f581719e12adaaf6_pdf.

74. See *Methods and Problems of Medical Education*, 7th series (1927) on Rochester; 13th series (1929) on Vanderbilt; 15th series (1929) on Albany; and 19th series (1931) on Chicago.

75. For the foundation's affirmation of neutrality, see George E. Vincent, "President's Review," in *The Rockefeller Foundation: Annual Report, 1924* (New York: Rockefeller Foundation, [1925?]), 15–16, accessed 25 June 2021, https://www.rockefellerfoundation.org/wp-content/uploads/Annual-Report-1924-1.pdf.

76. P. Starr, *Social Transformation of American Medicine*, 121.

77. Bailey, "Flexner Report," 219.

78. On the medical training of Black women, see Ward, *Black Physicians in the Jim Crow South*, 52–53.

79. The scholarship on Black women physicians is growing. See, for example, Gamble, "'Sisters of a Darker Race.'"

80. Flexner, *Medical Education in the United States and Canada*, 178–79 (quote, 179).

81. For the medical schools supported by the GEB and their respective appropriations, see Fosdick, *Adventure in Giving*, 328.

82. Peitzman, *New and Untried Course*, 1–2, 77.

83. Bonner, *To the Ends of the Earth*, 154.

84. Peitzman, *New and Untried Course*, 130.

85. S. Starr, "To the Alumnae of the Woman's Medical College of Pennsylvania," 1. Starr confused the Rockefeller Foundation with the GEB.

86. S. Starr, "To the Alumnae of the Woman's Medical College of Pennsylvania," 2–3.

87. See also Sarah Logan Wister Starr, "Statement Prepared for Corporators' Meeting," 15 May 1922, Folder untitled, Box 1, ACC 268, Drexel. Starr again confused the Rockefeller Foundation with the GEB.

88. Peitzman, *New and Untried Course*, 122–23.

89. See Jacob Billikopf to Sarah Logan Wister Starr, 14 December 1927, Folder untitled, Box 1, ACC 293, Drexel; and Ellen Culver Potter to Walter Lee Sheppard, 25 January 1936, Folder 16, Box 1, ACC 42, Drexel.

90. Potter to Sheppard, 25 January 1936.

91. "Our Proudest Possessions," 3–4.

92. Minutes, 23 April 1930, Minutes of the Special Meeting of the Corporation of the Woman's Medical College of Pennsylvania, Drexel.

93. Peitzman, *New and Untried Course*, 167–72, 176–81.

94. Carroll, "Modernizing the American Medical School," 202–7.

95. On the Woman's Medical College building's teaching emphasis, see Kuhlenbeck, "Department of Anatomy and Histology," 14. On the long-term, and largely unfulfilled, faculty interest in research before 1935, see Peitzman, *New and Untried Course*, 174.

96. For the written description and plan, see Bunzell, "Chemistry at the Woman's Medical College of Pennsylvania," 5–7.

97. Bickings-Thornton, "Department of Anatomy," 16; Bunzell, "Chemistry at the Woman's Medical College of Pennsylvania," 9; Rose, "Department of Bacteriology and Immunology," 17.

98. Peitzman, *New and Untried Course*, 167–76.

99. Kuhlenbeck, "Department of Anatomy and Histology," 14.

100. On the addition to the building, see Peitzman, *New and Untried Course*, 189–90. On the ensuing growth in research, see Medical College of Pennsylvania, *Pioneer-Pacesetter-Innovator*, 23.

101. Joe E. Holoubek, "Memories of My Medical School Years and Internship at the University of Nebraska College of Medicine, 1934–1939," [2001?], n.p., University of Nebraska Medical Center.

102. J. Holoubek, "Memories of My Medical School Years."

103. J. Holoubek, "Memories of My Medical School Years."

104. Peitzman, *New and Untried Course*, 174–76 (quote, 175; emphasis added).

105. G. Thomas, nomination, Woman's Medical College of Pennsylvania, National Register of Historic Places, sec. 8: 9.

106. Gamble, "'Sisters of a Darker Race,'" 169–73, 181–88, 197.

107. On women and these specialties, see Morantz-Sanchez, *Sympathy and Science*, 61–62.

108. Martha Tracy, "Report of the Woman's Medical College of Pennsylvania," in *Transactions of the Fifty-First Annual Meeting of the Alumnae Association of the Woman's Medical College of Pennsylvania, June 10 and 11, 1926* (Philadelphia: Alumnae Association of the Woman's Medical College of Pennsylvania, 1926), 28–29.

109. Tracy, "Report of the Woman's Medical College of Pennsylvania," 29–31.

110. Morantz-Sanchez, *Sympathy and Science*, 261.

111. Peitzman, *New and Untried Course*, 2, 136.

112. Morantz-Sanchez, *Sympathy and Science*, 281–83, 314–15. See also Fee and Greene, "Science and Social Reform," 164–70.

113. Peitzman, *New and Untried Course*, 81–82, 135–39.

114. On women's frustration with the expectation that they practice particular specialties, see Marion Spencer Fay, interview by Regina Markell Morantz-Sanchez, 11 July 1977, transcript, 34–35, Oral History Project on Women in Medicine, ACC 31, Drexel.

115. Morantz-Sanchez, *Sympathy and Science*, 271–73; Blustein, *Educating for Health and Prevention*, 21. See also *The Woman's Medical College of Pennsylvania*, pamphlet, August 1926, Butler Scrapbook, ACC 123, Drexel.

116. Peitzman, *New and Untried Course*, 157. For the pamphlet, see *Twenty-One Reasons for Giving the Woman's Medical College of Pennsylvania Your Support*, pamphlet, ca. 1926, Butler Scrapbook, ACC 123, Drexel.

117. Peitzman, *New and Untried Course*, 139, 190. See also G. Thomas, nomination, Woman's Medical College of Pennsylvania, National Register of Historic Places, sec. 8: 9, 12.

118. Anne H. Thomas, "Report of the Hospital of the Woman's Medical College of Pennsylvania, June 1, 1926–May 31, 1927," in *Transactions of the Fifty-Second Annual Meeting of the Alumnae Association of the Woman's Medical College of Pennsylvania, June 9 and 10, 1927* (Philadelphia: Alumnae Association of the Woman's Medical College of Pennsylvania, 1927), 31.

119. "Vanderbilt University was selected by the General Education Board . . . ," 25 March 1935, Rockefeller Foundation Inter-Office Correspondence, Folder 1416; "Gifts Improve V.U. Med School," *Morning Tennessean*, 31 July 1938, clipping, Folder 1419; G. Canby Robinson to Raymond B. Fosdick, 13 March 1930, Folder 1414, all in Box 153, Subseries 1, Series 1, General Education Board Archives, RAC.

120. Moore, *Miracle and a Privilege*, 12–13.

121. J. Holoubek, "Memories of My Medical School Years."

122. Moore, *Miracle and a Privilege*, 13.

123. Moore, *Miracle and a Privilege*, 13; J. Holoubek, "Memories of My Medical School Years."

124. Allison, *Doctor Mary in Arabia*, 16.

125. On the ward's location, see G. Thomas, nomination, Woman's Medical College of Pennsylvania, National Register of Historic Places, sec. 7: 3.

126. On the increasing emphasis on research, see Ludmerer, *Time to Heal*, 49–51.

127. G. Thomas, nomination, Woman's Medical College of Pennsylvania, National Register of Historic Places, sec. 8: 3–4. See also Peitzman, *New and Untried Course*, 140–42.

128. Gamble, "'Sisters of a Darker Race,'" 178–82.

129. Peitzman, *New and Untried Course*, 65–67, 160–62, 174–75, 293n47; Gamble, "'Sisters of a Darker Race,'" 191.

130. See also Bailey, "Flexner Report," 213–14.

131. Flexner, *Medical Education in the United States and Canada*, 180–81 (quote, 180).

132. K. Thomas, *Deluxe Jim Crow*, 16–19; Gamble, *Making a Place for Ourselves*, 109–10; Goldberg and Shubinski, "Black Education and Rockefeller Philanthropy from the Jim Crow South to the Civil Rights Era," n.p. For more on the work of northern philanthropies in the South, see Zunz, *Philanthropy in American*, 30–40.

133. Baker et al., "Creating a Segregated Medical Profession," 501, 508–10.

134. Gamble, *Making a Place for Ourselves*, 125.

135. Ward, *Black Physicians in the Jim Crow South*, 26.

136. Ward, *Black Physicians in the Jim Crow South*, 25–26; Hine, "Pursuit of Professional Equality," 173–92; Gamble, *Making a Place for Ourselves*, 123.

137. K. Thomas, *Deluxe Jim Crow*, 24; Summerville, *Educating Black Doctors*, 96–97; "Meharry College to Open Endowment Drive," *Tampa Bulletin*, 28 December 1940, clipping, Folder 1253, Box 136, Subseries 1, Series 1, General Education Board Archives, RAC. See also Abraham Flexner to George Eastman, 17 June 1929, Box PER 109, George Eastman's Incoming Personal Letters, George Eastman Legacy Collection, Eastman Museum.

138. See K. Thomas, *Deluxe Jim Crow*, 22–23. See also Fox, "Abraham Flexner's Unpublished Report," 488–89; and Savitt, *Race and Medicine*, 263–64.

139. K. Thomas, *Deluxe Jim Crow*, 25.

140. For more, see Savitt, *Race and Medicine*, 252–66; and Miller and Weiss, "Revisiting Black Medical School Extinctions in the Flexner Era," 226–40. For the medical schools supported by the GEB, see Fosdick, *Adventure in Giving*, 328.

141. K. Thomas, *Deluxe Jim Crow*, 239.

142. Fosdick, *Adventure in Giving*, 174–78, 328.

143. On the gifts, see "Gift Removes Indebtedness for Meharry," *Nashville Banner*, 2 June 1932, clipping, Folder 1253, Box 136, Subseries 1, Series 1, General Education Board Archives, RAC.

144. Abraham Flexner to George Eastman, 17 June 1929.

145. George Eastman to John J. Mullowney, 3 October 1929, George Eastman's Outgoing Personal Letters, vol. 26, George Eastman Legacy Collection, Eastman Museum; John J. Mullowney to W. W. Brierly, 23 April 1930; and G. W. Claridge to W. W. Brierly, 15 April 1930, both in Folder 1234, Box 134, Subseries 1, Series 1, General Education Board Archives, RAC.

146. Hine, "Pursuit of Professional Equality," 174–75, 183–89.

147. Ward, *Black Physicians in the Jim Crow South*, 33. See also Fosdick, *Adventure in Giving*, 328.

148. "Report of the Treasurer of Meharry Medical College in Connection with the Building of the New Plant and the Equipment and Other Costs," 6 November 1931, two pages attached to John J. Mullowney to Trevor Arnett, 6 November

1931, Folder 1235, Box 134; William G. Kaelber to H. J. Thorkelson, 20 September 1928, Folder 1233, Box 133, both in Subseries 1, Series 1, General Education Board Archives, RAC; G. Robinson, "Vanderbilt University School of Medicine," 8–9.

149. "The New Plant Actually Started," *Meharry News* 27, no. 2 (October 1930): 10; H. J. Thorkelson, "Memorandum re Meharry Medical College and Fisk University, Nashville, Tennessee," 1 December 1926, Folder 1231, Box 133, Subseries 1, Series 1, General Education Board Archives, RAC; G. Robinson, "Vanderbilt University School of Medicine," 8.

150. For quotation and Vanderbilt numbers, see G. Robinson, "Vanderbilt University School of Medicine," 11. On Meharry, see "New Plant Actually Started," 10.

151. On the growing emphasis on research between the world wars, see Ludmerer, *Time to Heal*, 49–51.

152. Gamble, *Making a Place for Ourselves*, 125.

153. Ludmerer, *Learning to Heal*, 193, 205–6; P. Starr, *Social Transformation of American Medicine*, 121.

154. Miller and Weiss, "Revisiting Black Medical School Extinctions in the Flexner Era," 223–24.

155. Miller and Weiss, "Revisiting Black Medical School Extinctions in the Flexner Era," 225.

156. Miller and Weiss, "Revisiting Black Medical School Extinctions in the Flexner Era," 225.

157. Abraham Flexner to W. C. McNeill, 13 December 1912, Folder 256, Box 28, Subseries 1, Series 1, General Education Board Archives, RAC (letter also quoted in H. Epps, "Howard University Medical Department in the Flexner Era," 908).

158. Edward A. Balloch, Paul Bartsch, and William C. McNeill to General Education Board, 30 December 1912, Folder 256, Box 28, Subseries 1, Series 1, General Education Board Archives, RAC.

159. H. Epps, "Howard University Medical Department in the Flexner Era," 908.

160. See Ward, *Black Physicians in the Jim Crow South*, 26.

161. "Dedication and Formal Opening of the New Medical School Building," program, Folder "Medical Building," Box 4, Howard University Buildings, Howard University Archives.

162. "Public Health Work Stressed," 1931 newspaper clipping, Folder 1253, Box 136, Subseries 1, Series 1, General Education Board Archives, RAC.

163. "Location and Buildings," *The Meharry: Meharry Medical College with Departments of Medicine, Dentistry, Pharmacy, Nurse Training, and School for Dental Hygienists* (Meharry Medical College catalog) 29, no. 1 (July 1932): 19. For drawings with and without the auditorium, see architectural plans located in the Office of Facilities and Security at Meharry Medical College.

164. John J. Mullowney to George Eastman, 31 August 1929, Box PER 110, George Eastman's Incoming Personal Letters, George Eastman Legacy Collection, Eastman Museum.

165. On the size of Harkness's gift, see John J. Mullowney to W. W. Brierly, 23 April 1930, Folder 1234, Box 134, Subseries 1, Series 1, General Education Board Archives, RAC.

166. "Location and Buildings," 19.

167. John J. Mullowney to Robert A. Lambert, 11 February 1931, Folder 1235, Box 134, Subseries 1, Series 1, General Education Board Archives, RAC. See also Robert A. Lambert to John J. Mullowney, 18 February 1931, Folder 1235, Box 134, Subseries 1, Series 1, General Education Board Archives, RAC. For a description of the curriculum in this subject, see "Preventive Medicine and Public Health," *The Meharry: Meharry Medical College with Departments of Medicine, Dentistry, Pharmacy, Nurse Training, and School for Dental Hygienists* (Meharry Medical College catalog) 29, no. 1 (July 1932): 34.

168. Mullowney, "Meharry," 7.

169. *Souvenir of the Dedication of Meharry's New Educational and Hospital Buildings . . .* (Nashville: Meharry Medical College, 1931), Exchange with the University of Rochester, D.138, Folder 7, Box 8, George Eastman Legacy Collection, Eastman Museum.

170. Ward, *Black Physicians in the Jim Crow South*, 251.

171. On the borrowing of space, see "Memorandum re Vanderbilt University Medical School," 20 March 1935, 6–7 (quote, 7), Folder 1416, Box 153, Subseries 1, Series 1, General Education Board Archives, RAC.

172. On the regional variance in public health, see K. Thomas, *Deluxe Jim Crow*, 10–11.

173. On the grant, see Abraham Flexner to James Kirkland, 29 February 1924, Folder 1410, Box 152, Subseries 1, Series 1, General Education Board Archives, RAC. For Leathers's credentials, see G. Robinson, *Adventures in Medical Education*, 179–80.

174. Leathers, "Vanderbilt University School of Medicine," 82.

175. Abraham Flexner, Memorandum for Mr. Fosdick, 23 September 1924, Folder 1410, Box 152, Subseries 1, Series 1, General Education Board Archives, RAC (emphasis added).

176. Wickliffe Rose to G. Canby Robinson, 31 March 1926, Folder 1421, Box 153, Subseries 1, Series 1, General Education Board Archives, RAC. See also Rothstein, *American Medical Schools*, 154. On the state of preventive medicine and public health at US medical schools in this period, see Weiskotten et al., *Medical Education in the United States*, 207.

177. Nicoll and Williams, "Albany Medical College," 69.

178. "Gifts Improve V.U. Med School."

179. On the relationship between the designs for the medical school–hospitals at Vanderbilt University and the University of Rochester, see G. Robinson, "Vanderbilt University School of Medicine," 8. For Flexner's involvement in bringing Gordon and Kaelber from the University of Rochester to Meharry Medical College, see Rhees to Flexner, 6 November 1926.

180. "Program of the Dedication Exercises of the New Meharry Medical College Buildings . . . ," Folder 1251, Box 136, Subseries 1, Series 1, General Education Board Archives, RAC; John J. Mullowney, "Radio Talk over Station WLAC: Medical and Dental Education as a Factor in Disease Prevention," 3, Folder "Mullowney, John J.—Meharry Medical College—President: Writings, Addresses, Articles, etc. Medical and Dental Education as a Factor in Disease Prevention," Box 1, John J. Mullowney Papers, Meharry Medical College; John J. Mullowney, "Training for Medicine and Dentistry," reprint, *Opportunity: Journal for Negro Life*

(December 1936), n.p., Folder 1251; "Meharry Medical School Dedicated: New Building Constructed at Cost of $2,100,000 Accepted," photocopy of 1931 newspaper clipping, Folder 1253, both in Box 136, Subseries 1, Series 1, General Education Board Archives, RAC.

181. Mullowney, "Training for Medicine and Dentistry," n.p.

182. R. Collins, "Dr William DeMonbreun," 464. On the lack of research at Meharry, see Hine, "Pursuit of Professional Equality," 185.

183. K. Thomas, *Deluxe Jim Crow*, 24–25.

184. On this general trend, see P. Starr, *Social Transformation of American Medicine*, 125–26.

185. Roberts, "President's Annual Address," 25.

186. On the nearly complete exclusion of Black faculty from predominantly white universities and the first Black professors to obtain appointments, see Slater, "First Black Faculty Members at the Nation's Highest Ranked Universities," esp. 99.

187. Hine, "Pursuit of Professional Equality," 173.

188. See Minot, "Further Study of the Unit System of Laboratory Construction," 409.

189. Bunzell, "Chemistry at the Woman's Medical College of Pennsylvania," 5.

190. Martha Tracy, "Report of Woman's Medical College of Pennsylvania to the Alumnae Association, June 13, 1930," in *Transactions of the Fifty-Fifth Annual Meeting of the Alumnae Association of the Woman's Medical College of Pennsylvania* (Philadelphia: Alumnae Association, 1930), 28; Minutes, 13 December 1929, Minutes of the Stated Meeting of the Faculty, Woman's Medical College of Pennsylvania, Drexel.

191. Vida Hunt Francis to Mrs. John Martin, 9 April 1930, Folder untitled, Box 1, ACC 293, Drexel.

192. Martha Tracy, "Report to the Alumnae Association of the Woman's Medical College of Pennsylvania, June 1929," in *Transactions of the Fifty-Fourth Annual Meeting of the Woman's Medical College of Pennsylvania* (Philadelphia: Alumnae Association, 1929), 26; "Editorial," *Bulletin of the Woman's Medical College of Pennsylvania* 79, no. 4 (1929), 2; Minutes, 20 November 1929, Minutes of the November Meeting of the Board of Corporators of the Woman's Medical College of Pennsylvania, Drexel.

193. Charles Coolidge to Charles W. Eliot, 26 July 1904; Charles Coolidge to Charles W. Eliot, 4 August 1904, both in Folder "Shepley, Rutan, and Coolidge, 1903–1906," Box 120, General Correspondence Group 3, Records of the President of Harvard University, Charles W. Eliot, UAI 5.150, Harvard University Archives.

194. On the tension between physicians and architects with regard to hospital design, see Adams, *Medicine by Design*, 104–8.

195. Gifford, *Evolution of a Medical Center*, 50. On Abele, see King, "Discovery of an Architect," 6–21.

196. Gifford, *Evolution of a Medical Center*, 55–65.

197. Stevens, *American Hospital of the Twentieth Century*, 2nd ed., chap. 15; Shepley, "Considerations in Planning a Teaching Hospital," 91–96; Biscoe, "University of Colorado School of Medicine and Hospital at Denver," 319–24.

198. "Designing Procedure of Coolidge, Shepley, Bulfinch and Abbott," 90.

199. Shepley, "Considerations in Planning a Teaching Hospital," 95–96. On the engineers' work at Harvard Medical School, see Coburn, "Mechanical Plant

of the Harvard Medical School," 62–67. On the engineers' work at New York Hospital–Cornell Medical College, see "Structure and Equipment of the New York Hospital," 118–24.

200. "Designing Procedure of Coolidge, Shepley, Bulfinch and Abbott," 88–92 (quote, 88).

201. For both quotes, see Van Poznak, "'Last Smile of Skyscraper Romanticism,'" 14. See also Heskel, *Shepley Bulfinch Richardson and Abbott*, 57–59.

202. On Cassell's life and career, see Lebovich, "Albert Irvin Cassell (1895–1969)."

203. For the planned connection between hospital and medical school, see Herman G. Weiskotten, "The College of Medicine Becomes the Central Unit of the Medical Center," 19 September 1958, 2, Folder "Memoirs," Box 16, Papers of Herman G. Weiskotten, SUNY Upstate.

204. Irma Walker and James T. Wollon, Jr., "George Archer," Baltimore Architecture Foundation, accessed 18 January 2019, http://baltimorearchitecture.org/biographies/george-archer/.

205. Wheatley, *Politics of Philanthropy*, 90–97.

206. On Harkness and Rogers's relationship, see Schiff, "Memorial Quadrangle's Beginnings." On the commissions, see Minutes, 26 May 1921, Minutes of the Joint Administrative Board, Columbia Health Sciences.

207. P. Turner, *Campus*, 177–80.

208. Henry B. Ward to Holabird and Roche, 18 June 1909, Folder "Medical College (Omaha) 1909–1921," Box 2, RG 05/10/04, University of Nebraska.

209. Samuel Avery to C. S. Allen, 24 July 1909, Folder 3, Box 1, RG 05/10/03, University of Nebraska.

210. "The Significance of Harvard's New Buildings," *Bulletin of the University of Nebraska College of Medicine* 1, no. 4 (1906): 185–86; Charles S. Minot to Charles W. Eliot, 26 February 1907, Folder "Medical School 1904–09," Box 103, General Correspondence Group 3, Records of the President of Harvard University, Charles W. Eliot, UAI 5.150, Harvard University Archives; "College Notes," 63. See also C. W. M. Poynter, "History of the Omaha Medical College," 21, Folder 6, Box "C. W. M. Poynter, Dean—University of Nebraska College of Medicine 1930–1946, Miscellaneous Papers," University of Nebraska Medical Center.

211. "Perspective View of the Medical Department of the University of Nebraska," following 440.

212. Young, "College of Medicine of the University of Nebraska," 590.

213. Charles W. Eliot to J. Collins Warren, 28 June 1900, Letterbook 4 (17 January 1898 to 23 March 1903), Box 158, Records of the President of Harvard University, Charles W. Eliot, UAI 5.150, Harvard University Archives.

214. J. Collins Warren to Charles W. Eliot, 10 June 1900; and J. Collins Warren to Charles W. Eliot, 12 June 1900, both in Folder "J. Collins Warren, 1894, 1896–1903," Box 69, General Correspondence Group 2, Records of the President of Harvard University, Charles W. Eliot, UAI 5.150, Harvard University Archives.

215. On the firm, see Forbes, "Shepley, Bulfinch, Richardson and Abbott," 19–31; and Heskel, *Shepley Bulfinch Richardson and Abbott*.

216. Woods, *From Craft to Profession*, 102, 106–10.

217. On designers' anonymity, see Forbes, "Shepley, Bulfinch, Richardson and Abbott," 19.

218. Woods, *From Craft to Profession*, 4, 116–37.

219. Kisacky, *Rise of the Modern Hospital*, 290. See also Adams, *Medicine by Design*, chap. 4.

220. See Heskel, *Shepley Bulfinch Richardson and Abbott*, 37.

221. John D. Rockefeller Jr. to Charles W. Eliot, 4 February 1903, Folder "John D. Rockefeller Jr., 1902–1903," Box 62, General Correspondence Group 2, Records of the President of Harvard University, Charles W. Eliot, UAI 5.150, Harvard University Archives.

222. Heskel, *Shepley Bulfinch Richardson and Abbott*, 31; McLean, "University of Chicago," 7.

223. Bowers, *Western Medicine in a Chinese Palace*, 59; C. A. Coolidge, "Trip to Peking China," undated, File "Peking Union Medical College," Shepley Bulfinch.

224. Abraham Flexner to James H. Kirkland, 7 November 1919.

225. Abraham Flexner to George Eastman, 17 June 1929.

226. Abraham Flexner to James H. Kirkland, 26 January 1920 (quote); Abraham Flexner to James H. Kirkland, 11 October 1920; Abraham Flexner to James H. Kirkland, 1 November 1920, all in Folder 1407, Box 152, Subseries 1, Series 1, General Education Board Archives, RAC.

227. James H. Kirkland to Abraham Flexner, 4 November 1919. On the growing role of the hospital consultant, see Kisacky, *Rise of the Modern Hospital*, 176–77, 290–93. See also Adams, *Medicine by Design*, 102–4.

228. G. Canby Robinson, *Adventures in Medical Education*, 159 (see also 202).

229. Several iterations of the firm published on the topic: Shepley, "New Buildings for the Medical School," 18–22; Coolidge and Shattuck, Smith, and Robinson, "New Plant of the Vanderbilt University Medical School and Hospital," 109–18; Coolidge and Hodgdon and Seem, "Chicago to Have Notable Medical Education and Hospital Buildings," 402–13; Shepley, "Considerations in Planning a Teaching Hospital," 91–96.

Chapter 4. School Buildings and the Marketing of Modern Medical Education

1. Gieryn, "Two Faces on Science," 423. See also Leslie, "Laboratory Architecture," 41.

2. Starr, *Social Transformation of American Medicine*, 13–17, 143.

3. Lupkin, "Manhood Factories," 44 (quote, 40).

4. Kingsley, "Architecture of Nursing," 63, 70, 90. James Hopkins also relates medical school design to the profession's shifting identity. See Hopkins, "(Dis) assembling of Form," 36–39, 48.

5. Frederic S. Lee and Frank H. Pike, "A Letter on the Future Location of the College of Physicians and Surgeons and the University Hospital," 9 April 1913, 18–19, Folder "545 Medical Center Development, 1910–1918," Box 631, Office of the Vice President for Health Sciences Central Records, Columbia Health Sciences.

6. Shepley, "Considerations in Planning a Teaching Hospital," 91.

7. Davison, *Duke University Medical Center*, 29–30.

8. "Report of the Faculty Committee on the Location of the Medical School and Hospitals," Folder 6, Box 18, Records of Charles F. Thwing, 1DB6, Case.

9. Minutes, 3 June 1914, 2, Folder 6, Box 18, Records of Charles F. Thwing, 1DB6, Case.

10. Kisacky, *Rise of the Modern Hospital*, 245, 247.

11. P. Turner, *Campus*, 18.

12. Isadore Rosenfield and Edgar C. Hayhow, "Planning, Building, and Equipping a Hospital," *Modern Hospital* 29, no. 6 (1927): 90, quoted in Kisacky, *Rise of the Modern Hospital*, 246.

13. *Bulletin of the University of Nebraska: Twenty-Second Biennial Report . . .* (Lincoln: University of Nebraska, 1915), 13.

14. Boster and Howell, *Medicine at Michigan*, 13–17, 73, 81–91.

15. Lamb, *Presbyterian Hospital and the Columbia-Presbyterian Medical Center*, 91.

16. Weiskotten et al, *Medical Education in the United States*, 31.

17. G. Robinson, "Vanderbilt University School of Medicine," 8.

18. "Comments on Suggested Plan of Medical Buildings[,] Vanderbilt University, West Campus," Folder 21, Box 98, RG 300, Vanderbilt University.

19. G. Robinson, "Vanderbilt University School of Medicine," 8.

20. "Woman's Medical College of Pennsylvania," Defense of Budget, 1931, Folder untitled, Box 1, ACC 268, Drexel.

21. "Greater Woman's Medical College Finds a Site," 3–4.

22. For an examination of the two neighborhoods, see Peitzman, *New and Untried Course*, 156–57.

23. "Woman's Medical College of Pennsylvania," Defense of Budget, 1931.

24. [Jay Gates?] to S. C. Kingsley, 12 April 1926, Folder 11, Box 9, ACC 42, Drexel. On the racial composition of Woman's Medical College in the 1920s, see Peitzman, *New and Untried Course*, 160–61.

25. [Ellen Culver Potter?] to My dear Fellow Alumna, 10 January 1927, Butler Scrapbook, ACC 123, Drexel.

26. Minutes, 8 March 1929, Minutes of the Stated Meeting of the Faculty [of Woman's Medical College of Pennsylvania], Drexel.

27. Peitzman, *New and Untried Course*, 159.

28. See Bluestone, "From Pasture to Pasteur," chap. 3.

29. Shattuck, "Dramatic Story of the New Harvard Medical School," 1060; Warren, *To Work in the Vineyard of Surgery*, 196, 204–05; A. Lawrence Lowell, "President's Report for 1909–10," in *Reports of the President and the Treasurer of Harvard College, 1909–10* (Cambridge, MA: Harvard University, 1911), 16–17; Bluestone, "From Pasture to Pasteur," 113–16.

30. Shattuck, "Dramatic Story of the New Harvard Medical School," 1060; Bluestone, "From Pasture to Pasteur," 112, 117–24.

31. For more on the Back Bay Fens and the development of the area, see Morgan, *Buildings of Massachusetts*, 181–82.

32. For a fuller discussion of the development of the roadway, see Bluestone, "From Pasture to Pasteur," 126–34.

33. For more on the close relationship between Shepley, Rutan, and Coolidge and the Olmsted office, see Morgan, Cushing, and Reed, *Community by Design*, 72–78, 245–46.

34. Bluestone, "From Pasture to Pasteur," 126–28.

35. C. S. Sargent to J. P. Morgan, 17 November 1905, MHS, quoted in Bluestone, "From Pasture to Pasteur," 129.

36. Nercessian, *Legacy So Enduring*, 9. On the eponym of Oscar C. Tugo Circle, see Gonzalez Castro, "On the Significance of the Circle of Tugo," 28–35.

37. Hine, "Pursuit of Professional Equality," 175.

38. Hine, "Pursuit of Professional Equality," 178–79 (quote, 179).

39. Fosdick, *Adventure in Medical Education*, 180; Hine, "Pursuit of Professional Equality," 186–89.

40. Ward, *Black Physicians in the Jim Crow South*, 33–34.

41. Johnson, *Spirit of a Place Called Meharry*, 55; Summerville, *Educating Black Doctors*, 65–66; Edwin R. Embree to Trevor Arnett, telegram, 5 November 1928; Edwin R. Embree to Trevor Arnett, 15 October 1928; John J. Mullowney to Richard M. Pearce, 24 October 1928; Richard M. Pearce to John J. Mullowney, 25 October 1928 (quote), all in Folder 1233, Box 133, Subseries 1, Series 1, General Education Board Archives, RAC.

42. See Avery, *Philanthropy in Black Higher Education*, app. A, 183–87.

43. Hoffschwelle, "General Education Board (GEB)."

44. J. Smith, "From Andrew Carnegie to John Hope Franklin."

45. Summerville, *Educating Black Doctors*, 97.

46. See, for example, H. J. Thorkelson, "Memorandum re Meharry Medical College, Nashville, Tennessee—July 13 and 14, 1927," Folder 1258, Box 136; and G. Canby Robinson to Abraham Flexner, 3 December 1926, Folder 1231, Box 133, both in Subseries 1, Series 1, General Education Board Archives, RAC.

47. Regarding these sites, see John J. Mullowney to Thomas Nicholson, 29 June 1926, Folder 1231, Box 133; and James H. Kirkland to H. J. Thorkelson, 30 March 1927, Folder 1258, Box 136, both in Subseries 1, Series 1, General Education Board Archives, RAC.

48. G. Canby Robinson to Abraham Flexner, 19 January 1927, Folder 1258, Box 136, Subseries 1, Series 1, General Education Board Archives, RAC. See also John J. Mullowney to Abraham Flexner, 21 January 1927; and G. W. Claridge to John J. Mullowney, 5 February 1927, both in Folder 1258, Box 136; and H. J. Thorkelson, "Memorandum re Meharry Medical College and Fisk University, Nashville, Tennessee," 1 December 1926, Folder 1231, Box 133, all in Subseries 1, Series 1, General Education Board Archives, RAC.

49. James H. Kirkland to H. J. Thorkelson, 14 March 1927, Folder 1258, Box 136, Subseries 1, Series 1, General Education Board Archives, RAC.

50. H. J. Thorkelson, "Memorandum re Meharry Medical College, Nashville, Tennessee—July 13 and 14, 1927."

51. James H. Kirkland to H. J. Thorkelson, 30 March 1927, Folder 1258, Box 136, Subseries 1, Series 1, General Education Board Archives, RAC. For mention of the homeowners' race, see H. J. Thorkelson, "Memorandum re Visit to Meharry Medical College, Nashville, Tennessee August 10 and 11, 1927," Folder 1258, Box 136, Subseries 1, Series 1, General Education Board Archives, RAC.

52. John J. Mullowney to Abraham Flexner, 5 February 1927, excerpted in W. W. Brierley to Raymond B. Fosdick, "Meharry Medical College," interoffice correspondence, 26 May 1938, 5, Folder 1259, Box 136, Subseries 1, Series 1, General Education Board Archives, RAC.

53. H. J. Thorkelson to Trevor Arnett, 20 July 1927, Folder 1258, Box 136, Subseries 1, Series 1, General Education Board Archives, RAC. On the closure of Alameda Avenue, see James H. Kirkland to H. J. Thorkelson, 20 July 1927, Folder 1258, Box 136, Subseries 1, Series 1, General Education Board Archives, RAC.

54. H. J. Thorkelson, "Memorandum re Meharry Medical Property, Nashville, Tennessee," 21 December 1927, Folder 1258, Box 136, Subseries 1, Series 1, General Education Board Archives, RAC.

55. See reprint of earlier communication related to the purchase of the site for Meharry Medical College in W. W. Brierley to Raymond B. Fosdick, "Meharry Medical College," interoffice correspondence, 26 May 1938, 6–8. See also Robert A. Lambert to W. W. Brierley, 6 July 1938, Folder 1259, Box 136, Subseries 1, Series 1, General Education Board Archives, RAC. See also "Warranty Deeds," *Tennessean*, 14 March 1928, 8.

56. William G. Kaelber to John J. Mullowney, 11 May 1929; Charles Nelson to Trevor Arnett, 4 October 1929; Jackson Davis to Charles Nelson, 11 October 1929, all in Folder 1259, Box 136, Subseries 1, Series 1, General Education Board Archives, RAC.

57. John J. Mullowney to Trevor Arnett, 14 May 1929, Folder 1259, Box 136, Subseries 1, Series 1, General Education Board Archives, RAC.

58. H. J. Thorkelson to Trevor Arnett, 20 July 1927.

59. See reprint of earlier communication related to the purchase of the site for Meharry Medical College in W. W. Brierley to Raymond B. Fosdick, "Meharry Medical College," interoffice correspondence, 26 May 1938, 9. See also "To the Members of the Executive Committee," 27 July 1927, Folder 1258, Box 136, Subseries 1, Series 1, General Education Board Archives, RAC.

60. On the officers' doubts about Mullowney, see Hine, "Pursuit of Professional Equality," 183–86.

61. Summerville, *Educating Black Doctors*, 67.

62. Goldstein, "Student Recollections," 78.

63. Ludmerer, *Learning to Heal*, 131, 136–38, 214–17.

64. P. Turner, *Campus*, 167.

65. John B. Pine, "Notes on the Building of a University," *American Architect* 106, no. 2032 (2 December 1914): 333, quoted in P. Turner, *Campus*, 167; and Nieves, *Architecture of Education*, 53.

66. P. Turner, *Campus*, 167.

67. P. Turner, *Campus*, 196, 202.

68. P. Turner, *Campus*, 251.

69. Kisacky, *Rise of the Modern Hospital*, 328.

70. Charles Coolidge to James H. Kirkland, 16 March 1922, Folder 12, Box 100, RG 300, Vanderbilt University.

71. Charles Coolidge to James H. Kirkland, 16 March 1922.

72. James H. Kirkland to Charles Coolidge, 30 January 1922, Folder 12, Box 100, RG 300, Vanderbilt University.

73. Block, *Uses of Gothic*, 148.

74. Winford Smith to Charles Hodgson, 4 May 1920, Folder 1, Box 11, Presidents' Papers, 1889–1925, University of Chicago Archives, quoted in Block, *Uses of Gothic*, 147.

75. Harry Pratt Judson to Martin A. Ryerson, 28 June 1919, Folder 1, Box 11, Presidents' Papers, 1889–1925, University of Chicago Archives, quoted in Block, *Uses of Gothic*, 147.

76. Wallace Heckman to Ernest DeWitt Burton, 14 April 1923, Folder 1, Box 11, Presidents' Papers, 1889–1925, University of Chicago Archives, quoted in Block, *Uses of Gothic*, 148.

77. Block, *Uses of Gothic*, 147–51.

78. Davison, *Duke University Medical Center*, 16.

79. On the associations with permanency and venerability, see P. Turner, *Campus*, 116–17.

80. Welch address quoted in "Dedication of the New Medical School," 246 (also quoted in Nercessian, *Legacy So Enduring*, 10).

81. Adams, "Modernism and Medicine," 58. See also Adams, *Medicine by Design*, 109–29.

82. Adams, "Modernism and Medicine," 48, 56.

83. Warner, "Aesthetic Grounding of Modern Medicine," 18–21, 25, 29–31, 45–46 (quote, 21).

84. James Collins Jr. makes similar points with regard to the Lewis Thomas Laboratory at Princeton. See Collins, "Design Process for the Human Workplace," 406. See also Whipple, *Planning and Construction Period of the School and Hospitals*, 12.

85. Adams, "Art Deco Medicine," 174.

86. "Richard C. Darcy was born . . . ," *Caduceus*, vol. 1 (1929): 153.

87. Charles W. Eliot to J. Collins Warren, 6 June 1906, J. C. Warren Papers, MHS, quoted in Nercessian, *Legacy So Enduring*, 17. Nercessian mistakenly links this letter to the building's dedication, which did not take place until September.

88. J. Collins Warren to Charles W. Eliot, 6 June 1906, Folder "J. Collins Warren, 1903–1908," Box 129, General Correspondence Group 3, Records of the President of Harvard University, Charles W. Eliot, UAI 5.150, Harvard University Archives (also quoted [and erroneously connected to the quadrangle's dedication] in Nercessian, *Legacy So Enduring*, 17).

89. Peitzman, *New and Untried Course*, 42.

90. On women's dormitories, see Yanni, *Living on Campus*, 116.

91. Peitzman, *New and Untried Course*, 159.

92. Speech of Frances Heath quoted in "College Drive Started with Over $250,000," *Roxborough News*, 28 December 1927, clipping, p. 882l, Clippings Scrapbook #14, July 1926–May 1936, ACC 133, Drexel.

93. "College Drive Started with Over $250,000" clipping.

94. Martha Tracy, "Report of Woman's Medical College of Pennsylvania to the Alumnae Association," 13 June 1930, 2, Folder 6, Box 3, ACC 290, Drexel.

95. Nieves, *Architecture of Education*, 98–99 (quote, 99).

96. Weiss, *Robert R. Taylor and Tuskegee*, xviii.

97. Weiss, *Robert R. Taylor and Tuskegee*, xviii.

98. Cobb, "Howard Dedicates Preclinical Medical Science Buildings," 470 (emphasis added).

99. Cordell, *Historical Sketch of the University of Maryland School of Medicine*, 22n2.

100. Abraham Flexner, Memorandum for Mr. Fosdick, 23 September 1924, Folder 1410, Box 152, Subseries 1, Series 1, General Education Board Archives, RAC.

101. "The Breaking of Ground for a Medical Center in the City of New York," Folder "Columbia-Presbyterian Medical Center: Groundbreaking, Jan. 31, 1925," Programs and Invitations, A–O, Columbia Health Sciences. See also Lamb, "Story of the Founding of the Columbia-Presbyterian Medical Center," 760.

102. "Presidential Party Greeted by 4,000 on Campus Visit," *Syracuse Daily Orange*, 30 September 1936, clipping, Folder: "Historical—College of Medicine," Box

13, Papers of Herman G. Weiskotten, SUNY Upstate; "City Praised by Roosevelt for Progress," *Syracuse Herald*, 30 September 1936; "Syracuse Public Invited to Hear Roosevelt Talk at New Medical College," *Syracuse Herald*, 27 September 1936.

103. "Meharry Makes Progress," 3.

104. Mullowney, "Meharry," 8 (original emphasis).

105. "Reception at the New Medical Building," *Schedule of Clinics, Conferences and Entertainments: Fourth Annual Alumni Clinical Week of the University of Nebraska, College of Medicine* ([Omaha?]: [University of Nebraska College of Medicine?], [1913?]), 31, University of Nebraska Medical Center.

106. Davison, *Duke University Medical Center*, 19.

107. "Woman's Medical College Dedicates $1,000,000 Building," *Philadelphia Inquirer*, 25 September 1930, clipping, p. 882aad, Clippings Scrapbook #14, July 1926–May 1936, ACC 133, Drexel.

108. "Educators Praise $1,000,000 College," *Public Ledger*, 25 January 1931, clipping, p. 882aaj, Clippings Scrapbook #14, July 1926–May 1936, ACC 133, Drexel.

109. "Educators Praise $1,000,000 College."

110. Harvard Medical School, "The Harvard Medical School, 1782–1906," *On-View: Digital Collections and Exhibits*, accessed 29 October 2019, https://collections.countway.harvard.edu/onview/items/show/12730. The commemorative volume was Harvard Medical School, *Harvard Medical School, 1782–1906*.

111. See *Souvenir of the Dedication of Meharry's New Educational and Hospital Buildings . . .* (Nashville: Meharry Medical College, 1931), Exchange with the University of Rochester, D.138, Folder 7, Box 8, George Eastman Legacy Collection, Eastman Museum.

112. Davison, *Duke University Medical Center*, 4.

113. Warren, *To Work in the Vineyard of Surgery*, 210–12.

114. Hopkins, "(Dis)assembling of Form," 32.

115. Harold C. Ernst to J. Collins Warren, 9 December 1912, Dormitory Scrap Book, Vanderbilt Hall, vol. 1: 1908–25, Archives DE 3.A119, Countway. See also Burrell, "New Duty of the Medical Profession," 854.

116. Burrell, "New Duty of the Medical Profession," 851–55 (quotes, 855).

117. On scientists' preference for the phrase "animal experimentation," see Ross, "Recruiting 'Friends of Medical Progress,'" 366n4.

118. Burrell, "New Duty of the Medical Profession," 854.

119. Guerrini, *Experimenting with Humans and Animals*, 112–13.

120. Lederer, "Political Animals," 65.

121. Lederer, "Political Animals," 67–68 (quote, 68, originally from George Hoyt Whipple to Cark Nixon, 14 January 1927, Folder 7, Box 2, George Hoyt Whipple Papers, Edward G. Miner Library Archives, University of Rochester School of Medicine and Dentistry, Rochester, New York).

122. On the resurgence of antivivisectionist activity in this decade, see Ross, "Recruiting 'Friends of Medical Progress,'" 367, 376–79.

123. To the Board of Trustees, memorandum, 16 November 1921, 3–4, Folder 12, Box 18, Records of Charles F. Thwing, 1DB6, Case (see also 9–10, 12).

124. On the animal houses, see "Animal House, 1924," Case Western Reserve University Archives, accessed 4 February 2021, https://case.edu/its/archives/Buildings/anihou1924.htm; and "Animal House, 1930," Case Western Reserve University

Archives, accessed 4 February 2021, https://case.edu/its/archives/Buildings/ani hou1930.htm.

125. To the Board of Trustees, memorandum, 16 November 1921, 10.

126. Whipple, "University of Rochester School of Medicine and Dentistry: Animal House," 15–19, (quotes, 18, 19).

127. Lederer, "Political Animals," 68–71.

128. Scholars have noted the practice of housing animals unobtrusively in recent laboratories as well. See, for instance, Kaji-O'Grady and Smith, *LabOratory*, 139, 152–54.

129. Holyoke, *Centennial Trilogy of the University of Nebraska College of Medicine*, 77.

130. Gesell, "Department of Physiology," 50–52 (quotes, 51, 50, respectively). On antivivisectionists' focus on dogs, see Lederer, "Political Animals," 62–68, 71–73.

131. Sappol, *Traffic of Dead Bodies*, 2–6 (quote, 5), 75–76, 171–73, 192–93, 315–19.

132. "Teaching and Opportunities in the Harvard Medical School of To-day," 69.

133. "Teaching and Opportunities in the Harvard Medical School of To-day," 68.

134. On the history of the museum, see Nercessian, *Legacy So Enduring*, 28–29.

135. Mall, "Anatomical Course and Laboratory of the Johns Hopkins University," 88.

136. Sappol, *Traffic of Dead Bodies*, 3–4, 137.

137. Warren, *To Work in the Vineyard of Surgery*, 66–67n7.

138. Cassell, "New Medical Building," 78.

139. Brenner, "Human Body Preservation," 325.

140. C. C. Burlingame, Executive Officer's Notes on Expediting Committee Meeting, 19 October 1923, Joint Administrative Board: Executive Committee, Expediting Committee, Committee for Laundry, Committee on Building and Grounds, March 1923–December 1940, Columbia Health Sciences.

141. On the decrease in body snatching, see Warner, "Witnessing Dissection," 19–20.

142. On dissection and the breech of funerary practices, see Sappol, *Traffic of Dead Bodies*, 3–5.

143. Warner, "Witnessing Dissection," 7 (quote), 11–13, 15–21, 23–26, 61; Warner, "Aesthetic Grounding of Modern Medicine," 4, 10 (quote), 18 (quote). On anatomy instruments and books in dissection imagery, see Hansen, *Picturing Medical Progress from Pasteur to Polio*, 26.

144. "Home of Osteopathy," *Macon (MO) Times*, 18 January 1895, quoted in Walter, *First School of Osteopathic Medicine*, 20.

145. Terry, "Washington University School of Medicine," 1.

146. Joe E. Holoubek, "Memories of My Medical School Years and Internship at the University of Nebraska College of Medicine, 1934–1939," [2001?], n.p., University of Nebraska Medical Center.

147. Cobb, "Howard Department of Anatomy," 424.

148. Bickings-Thornton, "Department of Anatomy," 18.

149. Biscoe, "University of Colorado School of Medicine and Hospital at Denver," 323.

150. Bergengren, "New Harvard Medical School," 57.

151. Hansen, *Picturing Medical Progress from Pasteur to Polio*, 114–15.

152. "New Medical College Ready for Dedication," *Syracuse Herald*, 21 November 1937.

153. "3,000 at Dedication of Medical Centre," *New York Times*, 13 October 1928.

154. On criticism of the Rockefeller foundations, see Ludmerer, *Learning to Heal*, 195–97; and Curti and Nash, *Philanthropy in the Shaping of American Higher Education*, 221–22.

155. Hoffschwelle, *Rosenwald Schools of the American South*, 256.

156. G. Robinson, "Influence of Environment in Medical Education," 11.

157. To the Board of Trustees, memorandum, 16 November 1921, 1.

158. Walter Riker Jr., "Postscript: Wally Remembers," *Cornell Medicine* 3, no. 1 (1998): 54, quoted in Gotto and Moon, *Weill Cornell Medicine*, 63.

159. Joe E. Holoubek to Alice Baker, 28 October 1937, reprinted in A. Holoubek and J. Holoubek, *Courtship of Two Doctors*, 38.

160. Lupkin, *Manhood Factories*, 102–3.

161. C. A. Hamann, "Report of the Dean of the School of Medicine," in *Western Reserve University Bulletin: Reports of the President and Other Officers, 1924–1925* (Cleveland, OH: Western Reserve University, [1925?]), 52.

162. Carl J. Wiggers to Torald Sollmann, 24 April 1925, printed in *Western Reserve University Bulletin: Reports of the President and Other Officers, 1924–1925*, 65.

163. Carl J. Wiggers to Torald Sollmann, 24 April 1925.

164. On the transfer of the medical school, see Luft, *SUNY Upstate Medical University*, 120–21.

165. Hine, "Pursuit of Professional Equality," 174.

166. Summerville, *Educating Black Doctors*, 67, 78–79. For more on Mullowney, see Hine, "Pursuit of Professional Equality," 174–75, 183–86.

167. Edward L. Turner to Robert Lambert, 29 January 1937, Box 134, General Education Board Papers, RAC, quoted in Hine, "Pursuit of Professional Equality," 187.

168. Tucker, *Miss Susie Slagle's*, 31–32.

Chapter 5. Constructing a Profession

1. See especially Horowitz, *Alma Mater*, 172–78; and Leslie, "Laboratory Architecture," 41.

2. For the leaky roof, see "Anatomy," *Pulse* (University of Nebraska College of Medicine student newspaper), 1 October 1913, 16. For the description of smoking on the porch, see Kampmeier, *Recollections*, 32.

3. Sappol, *Traffic of Dead Bodies*, 3 (emphasis added; see also 319).

4. "Anatomy," 16–17.

5. Adams, "Designing the Medical Museum," 179.

6. R. Collins, "Pictures at the North Portico," 22–24.

7. On this tradition, see Warner, "Witnessing Dissection," 129, 143.

8. Rudolph Kampmeier compares these two images in Kampmeier, *Vanderbilt University School of Medicine*, 101. I expand on Kampmeier's analysis.

9. "P&S Alumni Urged to Expand Influence," 14.

10. For Vanderbilt, see G. Canby Robinson to James H. Kirkland, 5 November 1925, Folder 26, Box 100, RG 300, Vanderbilt University. For Woman's Medical College, see Martha Tracy, "Nurses' Commencement, Hospital of the Woman's Medical College, November 26, 1934" (speech transcript), 1, Folder 24, Box 2, ACC 290, Drexel; and Florence H. Hill, "Professional Recognition for Women a Long Struggle—But Successful," 9 March 1935, 8–9, Folder "Misc. Items (incl. Macfarlane research report)," Box 1, ACC 268, Drexel.

11. Johnson, *Spirit of a Place Called Meharry*, 76.

12. Joe Holoubek to Alice Baker, 2 May 1938, reprinted in A. Holoubek and J. Holoubek, *Courtship of Two Doctors*, 112–13.

13. Corner, "Foundation and Earliest Years," 48.

14. *Proceedings of the Semi-Centennial of Vanderbilt University*, 5–7, 11–12.

15. Clarence P. Connell to Dr. Douglas, 12 October 1925; "Visitors to Be Entertained in the Hospital"; "Additions to Printed List"; "Assignments of Space to Guests in the Hospital," all in Folder "Semi-Centennial and Dedication of the Medical School," Box 1c, Dean Robinson's Files, Eskind.

16. "Hub of Medical Universe: Boston Will Radiate Its Hospitality on Thousands of Visiting Physicians This Week," *Boston Daily Globe*, 3 June 1906.

17. *College of Medicine: Syracuse University; Announcement, 1898–1899* (Syracuse, NY: [Syracuse University?], 1898), photographs following p. 34.

18. Davison, *Duke University Medical Center*, 17 (for the list of honorees, see 18).

19. "Woman Physician—A Symbolic Study," 204.

20. Before 1946, the sculpture was in the auditorium. See Marion Fay to Rosalie S. Morton, 14 September 1946, Folder "Slaughter-Morton, R. B.; 1897," Box 11, ACC 266, Drexel.

21. For discussion of African American students and international students at Woman's Medical College, see Peitzman, *New and Untried Course*, 95, 116–20, 160–61.

22. I have found references to three portraits in the boardroom in Tracy, "Nurses' Commencement," 1; and Hill, "Professional Recognition for Women," 8–9.

23. Camilla Graham quoted in Peitzman, *New and Untried Course*, 242 (see also 310n35, 310n37).

24. Peitzman, *New and Untried Course*, 242.

25. Extensive scholarship documents the discrimination against women, Jews, and African Americans; see, for example, Morantz-Sanchez, *Sympathy and Science*; Heynick, *Jews and Medicine*; and Savitt, *Race and Medicine*. On discrimination against Catholics and immigrants, see Rothstein, *American Medical Schools*, 153.

26. For these statistics, see Ward, *Black Physicians in the Jim Crow South*, 52–53. For more recent scholarship on the number of Black women who graduated from Woman's Medical College of Pennsylvania, see Gamble, "'Sisters of a Darker Race,'" 171.

27. Ludmerer, *Time to Heal*, 74–75; Leroy M. S. Miner to C. Sidney Burwell, 28 April 1937, Folder 11:617, Box 15, Series 00267, Harvard Medical School, Office of the Dean, Subject files, 1899–1953, Countway.

28. Warner, "Witnessing Dissection," 58–59.

29. Bonner, *To the Ends of the Earth*, 140–42; Boster and Howell, *Medicine at Michigan*, 29–33 (quote, 33).

30. Hayden, "Urban Landscape History," 120.

31. Sappol, *Traffic of Dead Bodies*, 80–81, 88–89.

32. Davenport, *Not Just Any Medical School*, 9–10.

33. Pauline Stitt oral history, in Morantz, Pomerleau, and Fenichel, *In Her Own Words*, 110 (also quoted in part in Sappol, *Traffic of Dead Bodies*, 90).

34. Ludmerer, *Time to Heal*, 74–75.

35. For a description of the locker and toilet facilities, see Mall, "Anatomical Course and Laboratory of the Johns Hopkins University," 99.

36. On smoking, see Rudy, *Freedom to Smoke*, 14, quoted in Adams, "Place of Manliness," 131n28.

37. Baserga, "Early Years of Coeducation," 181, 184–85.

38. Morantz-Sanchez, *Sympathy and Science*, 244–55 (quote, 254).

39. Ludmerer, *Time to Heal*, 59, 70–72 (quotes, 70, 59). See also Stern and Papadakis, "Developing Physician," 1795–96. Ludmerer hints at the architectural component of the "hidden curriculum" in *Time to Heal*, 74–75.

40. Ludmerer, *Time to Heal*, 72.

41. Allison, *Doctor Mary in Arabia*, 13.

42. Ludmerer, *Time to Heal*, 72.

43. Allison, *Doctor Mary in Arabia*, 19.

44. Ludmerer, *Time to Heal*, 72–73.

45. Joe E. Holoubek, "Memories of My Medical School Years and Internship at the University of Nebraska College of Medicine, 1934–1939," [2001?], n.p., University of Nebraska Medical Center.

46. Ludmerer, *Time to Heal*, 75.

47. Walter B. Cannon to Francis M. Rackemann, 31 January 1927, Dormitory Scrap Book, Vanderbilt Hall, vol. 2: 1925–1928, Archives DE 3.A119, Countway. This two-volume scrapbook, bound in 1933, contains official documents and personal papers related to the Harvard Medical School Dormitory Fund collected by Francis M. Rackemann, Harvard Medical School class of 1912 and general secretary of the Dormitory Fund Committee.

48. On the scarcity of medical school dormitories, see Ludmerer, *Time to Heal*, 72.

49. Rosof, "Quiet Feminism of Dr. Florence Sabin," 9; Worthington, "Osler Interns Remember," 25.

50. "Professional Men Get Dormitory," 19.

51. "Expenses," *77th Annual Announcement of the Woman's Medical College of Pennsylvania, Session of 1926–1927* (Philadelphia: [Woman's Medical College of Pennsylvania?], [1926?]), 21; Minutes, 30 September 1925 and 19 May 1926, Minutes of the Regular Meeting of the Corporation of the Woman's Medical College of Pennsylvania, Drexel; "Memorandum re Brinton Hall and Charter of the Young Women's Christian Association of the Woman's Medical College of Pennsylvania," Folder 15, Box 9, ACC 42, Drexel.

52. Warren, *To Work in the Vineyard of Surgery*, 252.

53. General Secretary [Francis M. Rackemann], "'Vanderbilt Hall,'" 6–9.

54. Samuel W. Lambert, *Memorandum on the Ideal Development of Hospital and Medical School Addressed to the Trustees of Columbia University and the Managers of the Presbyterian Hospital* (New York: [Samuel Lambert?], 1912): 17, Folder "545 Medical Center Development, 1910–1918," Box 631, Office of the Vice President for Health Sciences Central Records, Columbia Health Sciences.

55. Francis M. Rackemann to C. C. Burlingame, 24 February 1927, in Dormitory Scrap Book, Vanderbilt Hall, vol. 2: 1925–1928, Archives DE 3.A119, Countway. See also C. C. Burlingame, telegram to Francis M. Rackemann, 4 March 1927, Dormitory Scrap Book, Vanderbilt Hall, vol. 2: 1925–1928, Archives DE 3.A119, Countway.

56. Flood, *P&S*, 305–6; Edward Harkness to Nicholas Murray Butler, 26 December 1928, Folder "535 Bard Hall, 1928–30," Box 560, Office of the Vice President for Health Sciences Central Records, Columbia Health Sciences.

57. On the friendship between Darrach, Harkness, and Rogers, see Timothy Wagner, "The History of Bard Hall," in the program "An Evening of Celebration: Columbia University Bard Hall, December 4, 1991," in Folder "Bard Hall; Programs, Invitations," Programs and Invitations, A–O, Columbia Health Sciences.

58. "Need for Dormitories as Expressed by the Students," 314; Edsall, "Need for Dormitories at the Medical School," 313. See also Henry A. Christian to J. Collins Warren, 20 March 1913; "To All Harvard Medical School Graduates," 1 May 1924; and Francis M. Rackemann to "All Friends of Medical Education," 1 December 1924, all in Dormitory Scrap Book, Vanderbilt Hall, vol. 1: 1908–1925, Archives DE 3.A119, Countway.

59. For Harold Vanderbilt's gift, see "Harvard Medical School: Jubilee Celebration of the Founding of Vanderbilt Hall," 5–6, Folder 11:612, Box 15, Series 00267, Harvard Medical School, Office of the Dean, Subject files, 1899–1953, Countway.

60. General Secretary [Francis M. Rackemann] to "Editor [of the] New York Times," 29 April 1925, Dormitory Scrap Book, Vanderbilt Hall, vol. 2: 1925–1928, Archives DE 3.A119, Countway.

61. Christian to Warren, 20 March 1913.

62. Ludmerer, *Time to Heal*, 301.

63. "To All Harvard Medical School Graduates," 1 May 1924; Warren, "Social Side of Student Life," 1005; Rackemann to "All Friends of Medical Education," 1 December 1924 (quote).

64. Francis M. Rackemann to "All Graduates and Friends of the Harvard Medical School," 15 September 1923, Dormitory Scrap Book, Vanderbilt Hall, vol. 1: 1908–1925, Archives DE 3.A119, Countway. For the housing and feeding of instructors, see Rackemann to "All Friends of Medical Education," 1 December 1924.

65. Warren, "Social Side of Student Life," 1005–6 (quote, 1006).

66. Rackemann to "All Friends of Medical Education," 1 December 1924.

67. Warren, "Social Side of Student Life," 1005.

68. Nicholas Murray Butler, "Report of the President of Columbia University," in *Annual Report of the President and Treasurer to the Trustees with Accompanying Documents for the Year Ending June 30, 1929* (New York: [Columbia University?], [1930?]), 49.

69. Nicholas Murray Butler to Edward S. Harkness, 27 December 1928, Folder "535 Bard Hall, 1928–30," Box 560, Office of the Vice President for Health Sciences Central Records, Columbia Health Sciences. For discussion of recruitment, see William Darrach to Nicholas Murray Butler, 5 April 1929, Folder "535 Bard Hall, 1928–30," Box 560, Office of the Vice President for Health Sciences Central Records, Columbia Health Sciences.

70. Duke, *Importing Oxbridge*, 1, 7, 39–45; Yanni, *Living on Campus*, 117–18, 121–23. See also P. Turner, *Campus*, 215–16.

71. On Harkness, see Yanni, *Living on Campus*, 145.

72. David Edsall to Harold S. Vanderbilt, 27 April 1929, Folder 11:609, Box 15, Series 00267, Harvard Medical School, Office of the Dean, Subject files, 1899–1953, Countway.

73. Samuel W. Lambert, "The Development of the Medical Center in Columbia University," *Columbia University Quarterly* 18, no. 1 (December 1915): 4, reprint in *P. and S. Vault Pamphlets 79–102*, Columbia Health Sciences. For similar sentiments at Harvard Medical School, see Warren, "Social Side of Student Life," 1004–5.

74. "Harvard Medical School: Vanderbilt Hall; From the Alumni Committee on the Medical Dormitories to the Students of the Harvard Medical School," Dormitory Scrap Book, Vanderbilt Hall, vol. 2: 1925–1928, Archives DE 3.A119, Countway.

75. David L. Edsall to A. Lawrence Lowell, 2 May 1929, Folder 11:609, Box 15, Series 00267, Harvard Medical School, Office of the Dean, Subject files, 1899–1953, Countway; "Vanderbilt Hall" (1930), 13.

76. William Darrach, "Memorandum," 15 October 1930; "Bard Hall," May 1931, both in Folder "535 Bard Hall, 1928–30," Box 560, Office of the Vice President for Health Sciences Central Records, Columbia Health Sciences.

77. Wagner, "History of Bard Hall."

78. Warren, "Social Side of Student Life," 1005.

79. On the undergraduate dormitories, see Yanni, *Living on Campus*, 152.

80. Yanni, *Living on Campus*, 130.

81. Duke, *Importing Oxbridge*, 113, 122 (quote).

82. Rackemann to "All Friends of Medical Education," 1 December 1924; "Harvard Medical School: Vanderbilt Hall; Plans and Price List, 1927–28," Vanderbilt Hall—Plans and Price List, HUB 1866.71, Box 31, Harvard University Archives.

83. Leroy M. S. Miner to C. Sidney Burwell, 28 April 1937.

84. Nercessian, *Against All Odds*, 139 (quote), 275–77.

85. Poindexter, *My World of Reality*, 99–100.

86. Kemeny, *Princeton in the Nation's Service*, 10–11, 163–64, 219 (quote).

87. Photograph of the lounge interior, in Folder 10, Box 154, Subseries 3, Series VII, Historical Photograph Collection, UA #003, Columbia University. Architectural drawings are located in the Avery Architectural and Fine Arts Library at Columbia University.

88. Wellington H. Tinker to Frederick T. Van Beuren Jr., 1 July 1931 (quote), Folder "535 Athletics—Bard Hall," Box 561; "Bard Hall," May 1931, 10, Folder "535 Bard Hall, 1928–30," Box 560, both in Office of the Vice President for Health Sciences Central Records, Columbia Health Sciences.

89. For discussion of fundraising, see Francis M. Rackemann to A. Lawrence Lowell, 23 November 1923, Dormitory Scrap Book, Vanderbilt Hall, vol. 1: 1908–1925, Archives DE 3.A119, Countway.

90. For undergraduate examples, see P. Turner, *Campus*, 227, 240.

91. "Vanderbilt Hall: From the Alumni Committee on the Medical Dormitories," 20.

92. See invitation to "All Harvard Medical Students," 16 November 1927, Folder 12:640, Box 16, Series 00267, Harvard Medical School, Office of the Dean, Subject files, 1899–1953, Countway.

93. Zug, *Squash*, 46–62, 79–81, 86–92 (quote, 59).

94. David L. Edsall to Arthur L. Endicott, 29 April 1931; R. B. Johnson to David L. Edsall, 5 February 1932, both in Folder 11:609, Box 15, Series 00267, Harvard Medical School, Office of the Dean, Subject files, 1899–1953, Countway.

95. E. S. Emery to David Edsall, 7 February 1931; W. B. Cannon to Worth Hale, 20 March 1931, both in Folder 11:616, Box 15, Series 00267, Harvard Medical School, Office of the Dean, Subject files, 1899–1953, Countway.

96. Reginald Fitz to David Edsall, 27 May 1931, Folder 11:615, Box 15, Series

00267, Harvard Medical School, Office of the Dean, Subject files, 1899–1953, Countway.

97. Moore, *Miracle and a Privilege*, 19.

98. Henry A. Christian to C. Sidney Burwell, 12 June 1939, Folder 11:615, Box 15, Series 00267, Harvard Medical School, Office of the Dean, Subject files, 1899–1953, Countway.

99. Edsall to Vanderbilt, 27 April 1929.

100. Edsall, "Additions to the Dormitory," 11–12.

101. Edsall, "Additions to the Dormitory," 13.

102. Darrach to Butler, 5 April 1929.

103. Darrach to Butler, 5 April 1929.

104. William Darrach, "School of Medicine: Report of the Dean for the Academic Year Ending June 30, 1927," in *Annual Report of the President and Treasurer to the Trustees with Accompanying Documents for the Year Ending June 30, 1927* (New York: [Columbia University?], 1928), 78.

105. Willard C. Rappleye to Nicholas Murray Butler, 20 October 1931, Folder "535 Bard Hall 1931," Box 560, Office of the Vice President for Health Sciences Central Records, Columbia Health Sciences.

106. Nicholas Murray Butler to Willard C. Rappleye, 5 December 1931, Folder "535 Bard Hall 1931," Box 560, Office of the Vice President for Health Sciences Central Records, Columbia Health Sciences. For statistics on the composition of the student body, see "P&S Draws Student Body of 400," 8.

107. For dental students' living and financial situations, see Rappleye to Butler, 20 October 1931.

108. Willard C. Rappleye to Nicholas Murray Butler, 20 January 1932, Folder "535 Bard Hall 1932–1934," Box 560, Office of the Vice President for Health Sciences Central Records, Columbia Health Sciences.

109. Yanni, "Coed's Predicament," 26.

110. See plans for Bard Hall at Avery Architectural and Fine Arts Library at Columbia University. See also the photograph of the foyer in Folder 10, Box 154, Historical Photograph Collection, Columbia University.

111. Frederick T. van Beuren Jr. to William Darrach, 18 April 1931, Folder "535 Bard Hall 1931," Box 560, Office of the Vice President for Health Sciences Central Records, Columbia Health Sciences; "Bard Hall Club of the College of Physicians and Surgeons, Columbia University, By-Laws"; "House Rules: Bard Hall Club of the College of Physicians and Surgeons," [1932?], both in Folder "535 Bard Hall 1932–1934," Box 560, Office of the Vice President for Health Sciences Central Records, Columbia Health Sciences.

112. Minutes, 17 December 1928, Columbia University: College of P&S; Minutes of the Meetings of the Committee on Administration, Columbia Health Sciences.

113. Adams, "Place of Manliness," 109–31.

114. Adams, "Place of Manliness," 120.

115. Adams uses the smoking room and heraldic motifs in the Strathcona Building, the building for McGill University's Faculty of Medicine that opened in 1911, to connect that building's design and associations of class and gender to private men's clubs. See Adams, "Designing the Medical Museum," 179.

116. On the differences between staircase and single-entrance designs, see Yanni, "Coed's Predicament," 40–41.

117. For this element of men's clubs, see Adams, "Place of Manliness," 126; for eating and conversing as part of club life, 123.

118. For the club as escape, see Adams, "Place of Manliness," 123.

119. Yanni, "Coed's Predicament," 26 (original emphasis).

120. For use of this moniker, see Alice Baker to Joe E. Holoubek, 10 March 1938, reprinted in A. Holoubek and J. Holoubek, *Courtship of Two Doctors*, 94.

121. For paucity of housing in the area, see Flood, *P&S*, 305.

122. Alice Baker to Joe E. Holoubek, 9 April 1938, reprinted in A. Holoubek and J. Holoubek, *Courtship of Two Doctors*, 107.

123. Alice Baker to Joe E. Holoubek, 9 November 1937, reprinted in A. Holoubek and J. Holoubek, *Courtship of Two Doctors*, 42.

124. Morantz-Sanchez, *Sympathy and Science*, 254.

125. Reverby, *Ordered to Care*, 60–61.

126. For the increasing authority of physicians relative to nurses in the late nineteenth century, see Reverby, *Ordered to Care*, 74–76.

127. Reverby, *Ordered to Care*, 3, 47, 60–64.

128. D'Antonio, *American Nursing*, 24–27, 29–30, 39–41.

129. Reverby, *Ordered to Care*, 3, 47, 63–65.

130. Kisacky, *Rise of the Modern Hospital*, 146.

131. Kingsley, "Architecture of Nursing," 63, 67–75, 90 (quote).

132. Kisacky, *Rise of the Modern Hospital*, 147.

133. Goldenberg, *Nurses of a Different Stripe*, 27–35, 114–15, 135.

134. "Memorandum on the School of Nursing in Vanderbilt University," 2, attached to Waller S. Leathers to Mary Beard, 6 June 1929, Folder 1516, Box 122, Series 200 C, RG 1.1, Rockefeller Foundation Archives, RAC.

135. Goldenberg, *Nurses of a Different Stripe*, 135.

136. Nancy Caroline King Cost quoted in *Vanderbilt School of Nursing*, 31.

137. "Statement of Needs and Program of Development Proposed for Vanderbilt University," 1 May 1939, 4, Folder 1398, Box 151, Subseries 1, Series 1, General Education Board Archives, RAC.

138. For the difference in titles as representative of the work in nursing education, see Reverby, *Ordered to Care*, 63.

139. Goldenberg, *Nurses of a Different Stripe*, 122–23, 135.

140. For fuller discussion of nurses' struggle to professionalize, see Reverby, *Ordered to Care*, especially the introduction and chap. 7.

141. Goldenberg, *Nurses of a Different Stripe*, 127–31. See also "Anna C. Maxwell Hall," *Quarterly Magazine* (student publication of the Presbyterian Hospital School of Nursing) 22, no. 2 (January 1928): 3–10.

142. *School of Nursing[,] The Presbyterian Hospital in the City of New York: Announcement 1928* ([New York?]: [Presbyterian Hospital?], [1928?]), 19.

143. Goldenberg, *Nurses of a Different Stripe*, 129.

144. Quoted in Goldenberg, *Nurses of a Different Stripe*, 131.

145. Kisacky, *Rise of the Modern Hospital*, 273–74.

146. See Kingsley, "Architecture of Nursing," 76–78. Prominent hospital architect Edward F. Stevens makes similar recommendations in Stevens, *American Hospital of the Twentieth Century*, 2nd ed., chap. 16.

147. Adams, *Medicine by Design*, 79–81.

148. This analysis follows Adams's interpretation of similar furnishings and activities in the nurses' residence constructed in the early twentieth century at the Royal Victoria Hospital in Montreal. See Adams, *Medicine by Design*, 79–80.

149. *Announcement of the Presbyterian Hospital School of Nursing, 1935–1936* (New York: [Presbyterian Hospital?], [1935?]), 30.

150. Adams, *Medicine by Design*, 81.

151. Adams, *Medicine by Design*, 71. See also Kingsley, "Architecture of Nursing," 75; and Dodd, "Nurses' Residences," 190.

152. *Stripes: 1936* ([New York?]: Presbyterian Hospital, 1936), 46.

153. For examples of supervision and surveillance at the Royal Victoria Hospital's school for nurses, see Adams, *Medicine by Design*, 83, 86. See also Dodd, "Nurses' Residences," 190–91.

154. Goldenberg, *Nurses of a Different Stripe*, 134 (quote).

155. Goldenberg, *Nurses of a Different Stripe*, 39–42 (quote, 40). See also Dodd, "Nurses' Residences," 201.

156. Goldenberg, *Nurses of a Different Stripe*, 41 (quote).

157. Schneckloth, *University of Nebraska College of Nursing*, 116.

158. Schneckloth, *University of Nebraska College of Nursing*, 115.

159. Goldenberg, *Nurses of a Different Stripe*, 41.

160. Warner, "Witnessing Dissection," 179; Ludmerer, *Time to Heal*, 73.

161. J. Holoubek, "Memories of My Medical School Years."

162. Suzanne Festersen, *Student Handbook*, 1959, quoted in Goldenberg, *Nurses of a Different Stripe*, 39 (see also 40–42).

163. Abbott, *White Linen Nurse*, 59–60 (original emphasis). Reverby quotes this passage as part of her discussion of the public image of student nurses, but does not examine uniforms; see Reverby, *Ordered to Care*, 65.

164. For the different room types in Bard, see William Darrach, "Memorandum," 15 October 1930, Folder "535 Bard Hall, 1928–30," Box 560, Office of the Vice President for Health Sciences Central Records, Columbia Health Sciences.

165. "House Rules," [1932?].

166. On faculty living in the hall, see "Anna C. Maxwell Hall," 6; and Goldenberg, *Nurses of a Different Stripe*, 130.

167. "Anna C. Maxwell Hall," 5. See also the later plans in Joint Administrative Board, Columbia-Presbyterian Medical Center, *Medical Center, New York, N.Y., Units Cooperating . . .* (1928), in CUIMC Publications: CPMC Floor Plans, 1920s, Columbia Health Sciences.

168. "Programme for Medical School Housing," attached to James Gamble Rogers to William Darrach, 20 March 1929, Folder "535 Bard Hall, 1928–30," Box 560, Office of the Vice President for Health Sciences Central Records, Columbia Health Sciences.

169. Frederick T. van Beuren Jr. to John J. Caffey, 17 August 1931, Folder "535 Bard Hall 1931," Box 560, Office of the Vice President for Health Sciences Central Records, Columbia Health Sciences.

170. Similarly, Vanessa Heggie argues that female doctors identified first as physicians and then as women. See Heggie, "Women Doctors and Lady Nurses," 273–74.

171. For a brief description of the nursing students' housing, see *Year Book Graduating Class 1931 Woman's Medical College Hospital of Pennsylvania* ([Philadelphia?]: [Woman's Medical College Hospital of Pennsylvania?], [1931?]), 23.

172. Adams, *Medicine by Design*, 86–88.

173. Kampmeier, *Recollections*, 32.

174. On this program, see Davison, *Duke University Medical Center*, 34, 42.

175. Kampmeier, *Vanderbilt University School of Medicine*, 26.

176. Conkin, *Gone with the Ivy*, 260–61.

177. Cobb, "First Hundred Years of the Howard University College of Medicine," 416; "School of Medicine Including the Medical, Dental, and Pharmaceutical Colleges," *Howard University Bulletin* 7, no. 7 (June 1928): 13.

178. Charles W. Eliot, "President's Report for 1907–08," *Reports of the President and the Treasurer of Harvard College, 1907–08* (Cambridge, MA: Harvard University, 1909), 30.

179. "Dental Entering Class Drawn from 12 Colleges," 11.

180. Minutes, 23 January 1925, 30 January 1925, vol. 1, Minutes of Committee on Plans, Joint Administrative Board, Columbia University and Presbyterian Hospital, Columbia Health Sciences.

181. "Memorandum to the Committee on Administration," included in Minutes, 20 March 1922, vol. 15, Minutes of the Meetings of the Faculty, Columbia University College of Physicians and Surgeons, Columbia Health Sciences.

182. "Dental Entering Class Drawn from 12 Colleges," 11.

183. Caption for photograph of entrance to the College of Physicians and Surgeons, *Columbia Alumni News* 20, no. 4 (19 October 1928): 4.

184. "Better Dental Service for New York," 6, Folder "Dental and Oral Surgery, School of: Fundraising Appeal, c. 1931; Development/Promotional," Development/Promotional Literature, A–N, Columbia Health Sciences.

185. For the budget of each school, see "Budget: Current Receipts and Expenses Estimated for the Year 1926–1927," 18 May 1926, Folder 1231, Box 133, Subseries 1, Series 1, General Education Board Archives, RAC.

Epilogue

1. Leslie, "'Different Kind of Beauty,'" 173.

2. Leslie, "'Different Kind of Beauty,'" 176.

3. L. R. Chandler to C. Sidney Burwell, 20 August 1945, Folder 4:198, Box 6, Series 00267, Harvard Medical School, Office of the Dean, Subject files, 1899–1953, Countway.

4. C. Sidney Burwell to L. R. Chandler, 22 September 1945, Folder 4:198, Box 6, Series 00267, Harvard Medical School, Office of the Dean, Subject files, 1899–1953, Countway (emphasis added).

5. R. Collins, "Pictures at the North Portico," 24.

6. Conversation between Cyril Stewart and the author, 29 August 2006. Stewart was director of facility planning at Vanderbilt University Medical Center from 1990 to 2013. He reviewed my paraphrase of our conversation.

7. Cobb, "Numa P. G. Adams," 48–50.

8. US Department of Education, Office for Civil Rights, "Historically Black Colleges and Universities and Higher Education Desegregation," March 1991, https://www2.ed.gov/about/offices/list/ocr/docs/hq9511.html.

9. "The Medical Schools with the Most Black Students," *Journal of Blacks in Higher Education*, 29 January 2018, https://www.jbhe.com/2018/01/the-medical -schools-with-the-most-black-students/.

10. On historically Black colleges and universities generally, see, for example, "The Challenges Facing HBCU Campuses," *Weekend Edition Saturday*, NPR, 25 May 2019, https://www.npr.org/2019/05/25/726941875/the-challenges-facing -hbcu-campuses.

11. Adam Harris, "Why America Needs Its HBCUs," *The Atlantic*, 16 May 2019, https://www.theatlantic.com/education/archive/2019/05/howard-universitys -president-why-america-needs-hbcus/589582/.

12. "Diversity in Medicine: Facts and Figures 2019," Association of American Medical Colleges, figure 6, accessed 15 January 2020, https://www.aamc.org/ data-reports/workforce/interactive-data/figure-6-percentage-acceptees-us -medical-schools-race/ethnicity-alone-academic-year-2018-2019.

13. Melissa Bailey, "Harvard Medical School Students Decry Lack of Diversity," STAT, 8 February 2016, https://www.statnews.com/2016/02/08/harvard-medical -school-diversity/.

14. Christina Mangurian, Eleni Linos, Urmimala Sarkar, Carolyn Rodriguez, and Reshma Jagsi, "What's Holding Women in Medicine Back from Leadership," *Harvard Business Review*, 19 June 2018, updated 7 November 2018, https://hbr.org /2018/06/whats-holding-women-in-medicine-back-from-leadership.

15. "The Large Racial Gap in Medical School Faculty," *Journal of Blacks in Higher Education*, 5 February 2018, https://www.jbhe.com/2018/02/the-large-racial -gap-in-medical-school-faculty/.

16. White Coats for Black Lives, *Racial Justice Report Card: Full Report with Supplemental Materials*, 2018, 7, https://whitecoats4blacklives.org/wp-content/ uploads/2018/04/WC4BL-Racial-Justice-Report-Card-2018-Full-Report -2.pdf.

17. White Coats for Black Lives, *Racial Justice Report Card*, 2018, 43–44 (see also 13 for the schools' ratings). For more on Holmes (the father of United States Supreme Court justice Oliver Wendell Holmes Jr.), see M. R. F. Buckley, "Winds of Change," *Harvard Gazette*, 23 September 2020, https://news.harvard.edu/ gazette/story/2020/09/harvard-medical-schools-holmes-academic-society -renamed/.

18. White Coats for Black Lives, *Racial Justice Report Card: Full Report with Supplemental Materials*, 2019, 81–82, https://whitecoats4blacklives.org/wp-content/ uploads/2019/08/RJRC-2019-Full-Report-Final-8.28.19.pdf; see also Harvard Medical School Institutional Response from Associate Dean, Chief Communications Officer, 2019, 2–3, https://drive.google.com/drive/folders/15LF76iZ3nI-HaUFN h1GtIC-orJ-UieE0.

19. Buckley, "Winds of Change." See also M. R. F. Buckley, "Portrait of a Pioneer," Harvard Medical School, News and Research, 13 September 2019, https:// hms.harvard.edu/news/portrait-pioneer.

20. Fitzsousa, Anderson, and Reisman, "'This Institution Was Never Meant for Me,'" 2738; Wellbery and Mishori, "Deck the Halls with Diverse Portraits," 528–30. See also Yanni, *Living on Campus*, 225–30.

21. Fitzsousa, Anderson, and Reisman, "'This Institution Was Never Meant for Me,'" 2738.

22. Quoted in Nell Greenfieldboyce, "Academic Science Rethinks All-Too-White 'Dude Walls' of Honor," *Weekend Edition Sunday*, NPR, 25 August 2019,

https://www.npr.org/sections/health-shots/2019/08/25/749886989/academic-science
-rethinks-all-too-white-dude-walls-of-honor.

23. Quoted in Liz Kowalczyk, "In an About-Face, Hospital Will Disperse Portraits of Past White Male Luminaries, Put the Focus on Diversity," *Boston Globe*, 13
June 2018, https://www.bostonglobe.com/metro/2018/06/13/about-face-hospital
-will-disperse-portraits-past-white-male-luminaries-put-focus-diversity/opICgb
psw7QoHFFJQQEZOJ/story.html.

24. Ludmerer, *Time to Heal*, 209–12, 281, 334.

25. Dalen and Ryan, "United States Medical School Expansion," 1241;
Association of American Medical Colleges, "U.S. Medical School Enrollment
Surpasses Expansion Goal," press release, 25 July 2019, https://www.aamc.org/
news-insights/press-releases/us-medical-school-enrollment-surpasses-expansion
-goal; Anemona Hartocollis, "Expecting a Surge in U.S. Medical Schools," *New
York Times*, 14 February 2010, https://www.nytimes.com/2010/02/15/education/
15medschools.html; Whitcomb, "Development of New MD-Granting Medical
Schools in the United States in the 21st Century," 340–43.

26. On the rise of internship and residency training, see Ludmerer, *Let Me
Heal*, 44–46, 123. On the racially discriminatory policies toward Black graduates
seeking internships, see Gamble, "'Sisters of a Darker Race,'" 182.

27. On the shortage of residency positions, see, for example, Lindsay Kalter,
"U.S. Medical School Enrollment Rises 30%," Association of American Medical
Colleges, 25 July 2019, https://www.aamc.org/news-insights/us-medical-school
-enrollment-rises-30.

28. DeZee et al., "Medical Education in the United States of America," 523.
See also Scott P. Kelsey, "The New American Medical School," *Contract*, 5 March
2015, https://www.contractdesign.com/practice/design/the-new-american-medical
-school/.

29. For the Carnegie Foundation report, see Cooke, Irby, and O'Brien,
Educating Physicians.

30. Zinski et al., "Is Lecture Dead?," 326; Kelsey, "New American Medical
School"; discussion following L. Smith, "New Medical Schools in the United
States," 236–37.

31. On the lack of long-term reform, see discussion following L. Smith, "New
Medical Schools in the United States," 236–37.

32. Ludmerer, *Time to Heal*, 307–9, 475n67.

33. Ludmerer, "Internal Challenges to Medical Education," 247.

34. Ludmerer, *Time to Heal*, 308.

35. Brendan Murphy, "Why Some Medical Students Are Cutting Class to Get
Ahead," American Medical Association, 4 February 2019, https://www.ama-assn
.org/residents-students/medical-school-life/why-some-medical-students-are
-cutting-class-get-ahead; Orly Nadell Farber, "Medical Students Are Skipping
Class in Droves—and Making Lectures Increasingly Obsolete," STAT, 14 August
2018, https://www.statnews.com/2018/08/14/medical-students-skipping-class/.

36. Quoted in Farber, "Medical Students Are Skipping Class in Droves."

37. A number of authors have compared the reforms made one hundred years
ago and those needed now. See Ludmerer, *Time to Heal*, 381–83; and Irby, Cooke,
and O'Brien, "Calls for Reform of Medical Education."

38. Quoted in Canan Yetmen, "Collective Learning," *Texas Architect*, January–February 2017, https://magazine.texasarchitects.org/2017/01/09/collective-learning/.

39. Quoted in Sean Price, "Dell's Different Direction," *Texas Medicine* 113, no. 5 (May 2017), last updated 23 August 2018, https://www.texmed.org/Template.aspx?id=44650.

40. Quoted in Price, "Dell's Different Direction."

41. On these ideas at Dell Medical School and elsewhere, see Martha M. Jablow, "New Schools of Thought," Association of American Medical Colleges, 20 March 2018, https://www.aamc.org/news-insights/new-schools-thought; and Kelsey, "New American Medical School."

42. Quoted in Yetmen, "Collective Learning."

43. Yetmen, "Collective Learning."

44. For an overview of the curriculum, see "Leading EDGE Curriculum," Dell Medical School, accessed 17 January 2020, https://dellmed.utexas.edu/education/academics/undergraduate-medical-education/leading-edge-curriculum.

45. "Curriculum," in *The University of Texas at Austin Medical School Catalog, 2018–2019* ([Austin?]: University of Texas at Austin, [2018?]), 28.

46. Quoted in Nupur Shah, "Dr. Sue Cox, Chair of Medical Education at the Dell Medical School at the University of Texas at Austin," Osmosis Blog, 9 June 2016, https://www.osmosis.org/blog/2016/06/09/leaders-in-medical-education-dr-sue-cox-chair-of-medical-education-at-the-dell-medical-school-at-the-university-of-texas-at-austin.

47. Quoted in Yetmen, "Collective Learning."

48. Ludmerer, "Internal Challenges to Medical Education," 242–43 (quote, 242).

49. "Health Discovery Building—Interaction Space," Dell Medical School, accessed 13 May 2017, https://dellmed.utexas.edu/hdb/interaction-space (site discontinued).

50. Quoted in Dell Medical School, *Commitment, Compassion, Leadership, and Care: Education and Training* (brochure), [2019?], 40, collection of the author.

51. "Design in Health: A Radical Problem-Solving Toolbox," Design Institute for Health, Dell Medical School, accessed 17 January 2020, https://dellmed.utexas.edu/units/design-institute-for-health.

52. Whitcomb, "Development of New MD-Granting Medical Schools in the United States in the 21st Century," 342.

53. Dan Zehr, "Officials Launch Nonprofit to Oversee New Medical School's Innovation Zone," *Austin American-Statesman*, 11 March 2016, updated 24 September 2018, https://www.statesman.com/news/20160311/officials-launch-nonprofit-to-oversee-new-medical-schools-innovation-zone.

54. Zehr, "Officials Launch Nonprofit to Oversee New Medical School's Innovation Zone."

55. "Created by Our Community," Dell Medical School, accessed 13 May 2017, https://dellmed.utexas.edu/community-investment (site discontinued).

56. "Building the Health Professions Pipeline," Dell Medical School, accessed 14 January 2020, https://dellmed.utexas.edu/case-studies/building-the-health-pro-

fessions-pipeline; "Health Science Summer Camps: Inspiring Future Leaders," Dell Medical School, accessed 14 January 2020, https://dellmed.utexas.edu/education/academics/programs-for-youth-and-undergrads/health-sciences-summer-camps. See also Mara Gordon, "A Push for Diversity in Medical School Is Slowly Paying Off," *Health Inc.*, NPR, 4 December 2018, https://www.npr.org/sections/health-shots/2018/12/04/673318859/the-push-for-diversity-in-medical-school-is-slowly-paying-off.

BIBLIOGRAPHY

Unpublished archival materials (such as letters, minute books, and memoranda), yearbooks, announcements, annual reports, unsigned reviews, most online publications and blogs, and newspaper articles appear only in the notes but are fully cited there.

Abbott, Andrew. "Library Research Infrastructure for Humanistic and Social Scientific Scholarship in the Twentieth Century." In *Social Knowledge in the Making*, edited by Charles Camic, Neil Gross, and Michèle Lamont, 43–87. Chicago: University of Chicago Press, 2011.

Abbott, Eleanor Hallowell. *The White Linen Nurse*. New York: Century, 1913.

Adams, Annmarie. "Art Deco Medicine." In *The Routledge Companion to Art Deco*, edited by Bridget Elliott and Michael Windover, 160–76. London: Routledge, 2019.

Adams, Annmarie. "Designing the Medical Museum." In *Healing Spaces, Modern Architecture, and the Body*, edited by Sarah Schrank and Didem Ekici, 171–85. London: Routledge, 2017.

Adams, Annmarie. "Designing Penfield: Inside the Montreal Neurological Institute." *Bulletin of the History of Medicine* 93, no. 2 (2019): 207–40.

Adams, Annmarie. *Medicine by Design: The Architect and the Modern Hospital, 1893–1943*. Minneapolis: University of Minnesota Press, 2008.

Adams, Annmarie. "Modernism and Medicine: The Hospitals of Stevens and Lee, 1916–1932." *Journal of the Society of Architectural Historians* 58, no. 1 (1999): 42–61.

Adams, Annmarie. "The Place of Manliness: Architecture, Domesticity, and Men's Clubs." In *Making Men, Making History: Canadian Masculinities across Time and Place*, edited by Peter Gossage and Robert Rutherdale, 109–31. Vancouver: UBC Press, 2018.

Adams, Annmarie. "Rooms of Their Own: The Nurses' Residences at Montreal's Royal Victoria Hospital." In *Restoring Women's History through Historic Preservation*, edited by Gail Lee Dubrow and Jennifer B. Goodman, 131–44. Baltimore: Johns Hopkins University Press, 2003.

Adams, Annmarie, and Thomas Schlich. "Design for Control: Surgery, Science, and Space at the Royal Victoria Hospital, Montreal, 1893–1956." *Medical History* 50, no. 3 (2006): 303–24.

Adolph, Edward F. "Perspectives of the First Faculty." In *To Each His Farthest Star: University of Rochester Medical Center, 1925–1975*, edited by John Romano, Edward C. Atwater, Gilbert B. Forbes, Raymond Gramiak, Milton B. Lederman, Henry L. Lemkau, Lucretia W. McClure, William D. McHugh, Gordon M. Meade, and

William L. Morgan Jr., 55–69. [Rochester, NY?]: University of Rochester Medical Center, 1975.

Allison, Mary Bruins. *Doctor Mary in Arabia: Memoirs by Mary Bruins Allison, M.D.* Edited by Sandra Shaw. Austin: University of Texas Press, 1994.

Avery, Vida L. *Philanthropy in Black Higher Education: A Fateful Hour Creating the Atlanta University System.* New York: Palgrave Macmillan, 2013.

Bailey, Moya. "The Flexner Report: Standardizing Medical Students through Region-, Gender-, and Race-Based Hierarchies." *American Journal of Law and Medicine* 43, no. 2–3 (2017): 209–23.

Baker, Robert B., Harriet A. Washington, Ololade Olakanmi, Todd L. Savitt, Elizabeth A. Jacobs, Eddie Hoover, and Matthew K. Wynia. "Creating a Segregated Medical Profession: African American Physicians and Organized Medicine, 1846–1910." *Journal of the National Medical Association* 101, no. 6 (2009): 501–12.

Barker, Lewellys F., and Charles R. Bardeen. "An Outline of the Course in Normal Histology and Microscopic Anatomy." *Johns Hopkins Hospital Bulletin* 7, no. 62–63 (1896): 100–109.

Barzansky, Barbara. "The Growth and Divergence of the Basic Sciences." In *Beyond Flexner: Medical Education in the Twentieth Century*, edited by Barbara Barzansky and Norman Gevitz, 19–34. New York: Greenwood Press, 1992.

Baserga, Susan J. "The Early Years of Coeducation at the Yale University School of Medicine." *Yale Journal of Biology and Medicine* 53, no. 3 (1980): 181–90.

Beecher, Henry K., and Mark D. Altschule. *Medicine at Harvard: The First Three Hundred Years.* Hanover, NH: University Press of New England, 1977.

Ben-David, Joseph. "The Universities and the Growth of Science in Germany and the United States." *Minerva* 7, no. 1–2 (1968–1969): 1–35.

Bergengren, Ralph. "The New Harvard Medical School: The Most Perfectly Equipped Institution of Its Kind in the World Begins Its Activities with the Opening of the Present College Year." *Indoors and Out* 3, no. 2 (1906): 53–61.

Berliner, Howard S. *A System of Scientific Medicine: Philanthropic Foundations in the Flexner Era.* New York: Tavistock, 1985.

Bethell, John T. *Harvard Observed: An Illustrated History of the University in the Twentieth Century.* Cambridge, MA: Harvard University Press, 1998.

Betsky, Aaron. *James Gamble Rogers and the Architecture of Pragmatism.* New York: Architectural History Foundation; Cambridge, MA: MIT Press, 1994.

Bickings-Thornton, Mary. "The Department of Anatomy." *Bulletin of the Woman's Medical College of Pennsylvania* 82, no. 3 (1931): 16–18.

Billings, John Shaw. "Ideals of Medical Education." *Boston Medical and Surgical Journal* 125, no. 1 (2 July 1891): 1–4.

Billings, John Shaw. "The Plans and Purposes of the Johns Hopkins Hospital: An Address Delivered at the Opening of the Hospital, May 7, 1889." *Medical News* 54, no. 19 (11 May 1889): 505–10.

Billroth, Theodor. *The Medical Sciences in the German Universities: A Study in the History of Civilization.* 1876. New York: Macmillan, 1924.

Biscoe, Maurice B. "The University of Colorado School of Medicine and Hospital at Denver." *Modern Hospital* 20, no. 4 (1923): 319–24.

Blake, John Bapst. "The Laboratories, Hospitals, Libraries and Museums." *Harvard Alumni Bulletin* 17, no. 19 (10 February 1915): 332–35.

Block, Jean F. *The Uses of Gothic: Planning and Building the Campus of the University of Chicago.* Chicago: University of Chicago Library, 1983.

Bluestone, Daniel Michael. "From Pasture to Pasteur: An Architectural and Environ-
    mental History of the 1906 Harvard Medical School." Undergraduate thesis, Harvard
    College, 1975.

Blustein, Bonnie Ellen. *Educating for Health and Prevention: A History of the Department of
    Community and Preventative Medicine of the (Woman's) Medical College of Pennsylvania.*
    Canton, MA: Science History Publications, 1993.

Bonner, Thomas Neville. *American Doctors and German Universities: A Chapter in Interna-
    tional Intellectual Relations, 1870–1914.* Lincoln: University of Nebraska Press, 1963.

Bonner, Thomas Neville. *Becoming a Physician: Medical Education in Britain, France,
    Germany, and the United States, 1750–1945.* Baltimore: Johns Hopkins University Press,
    2000.

Bonner, Thomas Neville. *Iconoclast: Abraham Flexner and a Life in Learning.* Baltimore:
    Johns Hopkins University Press, 2002.

Bonner, Thomas Neville. *To the Ends of the Earth: Women's Search for Education in Medi-
    cine.* Cambridge, MA: Harvard University Press, 1992.

Boster, Dea H., and Joel D. Howell. *Medicine at Michigan: A History of the University of
    Michigan Medical School at the Bicentennial.* Ann Arbor: University of Michigan Press,
    2017.

Bowditch, Henry P. Letter to the editor. *Boston Medical and Surgical Journal* 82 (21 April
    1870): 305–7.

Bowers, John Z. *Western Medicine in a Chinese Palace: Peking Union Medical College,
    1917–1951.* [Philadelphia?]: Josiah Macy Jr. Foundation, 1972.

Brandt, Allan M., and David Charles Sloane. "Of Beds and Benches: Building the
    Modern American Hospital." In *The Architecture of Science*, edited by Peter Galison
    and Emily Thompson, 281–305. Cambridge, MA: MIT Press, 1999.

Brayer, Elizabeth. *George Eastman: A Biography.* Baltimore: Johns Hopkins University
    Press, 1996.

Bremner, Robert H. *American Philanthropy.* 2nd ed. Chicago: University of Chicago
    Press, 1988.

Brenner, Erich. "Human Body Preservation—Old and New Techniques." *Journal of
    Anatomy* 224, no. 3 (2014): 316–44.

Brown, E. Richard. *Rockefeller Medicine Men: Medicine and Capitalism in America.*
    Berkeley: University of California Press, 1979.

Brown, Theodore M. "George Canby Robinson and 'The Patient as a Person.'" In *Greater
    Than the Parts: Holism in Biomedicine, 1920–1950*, edited by Christopher Lawrence and
    George Weisz, 135–60. New York: Oxford University Press, 1998.

"Building the Hospital." *Hopkins Medical News* 10, no. 2 (1986): 12–15.

Bunzell, Herbert H. "Chemistry at the Woman's Medical College of Pennsylvania."
    Bulletin of the Woman's Medical College of Pennsylvania 81, no. 4 (1931): 2–9.

Burns, Sarah. *Painting the Dark Side: Art and the Gothic Imagination in Nineteenth-Century
    America.* Berkeley: University of California Press, 2004.

Burrell, Herbert L. "New Duty of the Medical Profession: The Education of the Public
    in Scientific Medicine." *Boston Medical and Surgical Journal* 158, no. 23 (4 June 1908):
    851–55.

Cameron, John L. "Early Contributions to the Johns Hopkins Hospital by the 'Other'
    Surgeon: John Shaw Billings." *Annals of Surgery* 234, no. 3 (2001): 267–78.

Campbell, Walter E. *Foundations for Excellence: 75 Years of Duke Medicine.* Edited by
    Maura High. Durham: Duke University Medical Center Library, 2006.

Carroll, Katherine L. "Creating the Modern Physician: The Architecture of American Medical Schools in the Era of Medical Education Reform." *Journal of the Society of Architectural Historians* 75, no. 1 (2016): 48–73.

Carroll, Katherine L. "Incorporated Philanthropy: The General Education Board, Abraham Flexner, and the Architecture of American Medical Schools." In *Corporate Patronage of Art and Architecture in the United States: Late Nineteenth Century to the Present*, edited by Monica E. Jovanovich and Melissa Renn, 77–95. New York: Bloomsbury Visual Arts, 2019.

Carroll, Katherine L. "Modernizing the American Medical School, 1893–1940: Architecture, Pedagogy, Professionalization, and Philanthropy." PhD diss., Boston University, 2012.

Cassell, Albert I. "The New Medical Building." *Howard Alumnus* 5, no. 4 (1927): 77–80.

Chernow, Ron. *Titan: The Life of John D. Rockefeller, Sr.* New York: Random House, 1998.

Chesney, Alan M. *The Johns Hopkins Hospital and the Johns Hopkins University School of Medicine: A Chronicle.* 3 vols. Baltimore: Johns Hopkins Press, 1943–1963.

Cobb, W. Montague. "The First Hundred Years of the Howard University College of Medicine." *Journal of the National Medical Association* 59, no. 6 (1967): 408–20.

Cobb, W. Montague. "Howard Dedicates Preclinical Medical Science Buildings." *Journal of the National Medical Association* 50, no. 6 (1958): 468–72.

Cobb, W. Montague. "The Howard Department of Anatomy." *Journal of the National Medical Association* 59, no. 6 (1967): 421–28.

Cobb, W. Montague. "Numa P. G. Adams, M.D., 1884–1940." *Journal of the National Medical Association* 43, no. 1 (1951): 42–54.

Coburn, Frederick W. "The Mechanical Plant of the Harvard Medical School: The Heart and Lungs of an Architectural Group, Incessantly Supplying Hot Water, Fresh Air and Other Necessities to the Building." *Indoors and Out* 3, no. 2 (1906): 62–67.

Coleman, Robert B. *The First Hundred Years of the University of Nebraska College of Medicine.* Omaha: University of Nebraska Medical Center, 1980.

Coleman, William, and Frederic L. Holmes. "Introduction." In *The Investigative Enterprise: Experimental Physiology in Nineteenth-Century Medicine*, edited by William Coleman and Frederic L. Holmes, 1–14. Berkeley: University of California Press, 1988.

"College Notes." *Bulletin of the University of Nebraska College of Medicine* 2, no. 2 (1907): 62–64.

Collins, James, Jr. "The Design Process for the Human Workplace." In *The Architecture of Science*, edited by Peter Galison and Emily Thompson, 399–412. Cambridge, MA: MIT Press, 1999.

Collins, Robert D. *Ahmic Lake Connections: The Founding Leadership of Vanderbilt University.* Nashville, TN: Eveready Press, 2004.

Collins, Robert D. "Dr William DeMonbreun: Description of His Contributions to Our Understanding of Histoplasmosis and Analysis of the Significance of His Work." *Human Pathology* 36, no. 5 (2005): 453–64.

Collins, Robert D. *Ernest William Goodpasture: Scientist, Scholar, Gentleman.* Franklin, TN: Hillsboro Press, 2002.

Collins, Robert D. "Pictures at the North Portico." *Vanderbilt Medicine*, Spring 1994, 22–24.

Collins, William F. "The Sterling Hall of Medicine, Yale University School of Medicine." *Journal of Neurosurgery* 75 (September 1981): 489–90.

Conkin, Paul K. *Gone with the Ivy: A Biography of Vanderbilt University*. With the assistance of Henry Lee Swint and Patricia S. Miletich. Knoxville: University of Tennessee Press, 1985.

Connor, J. T. H. "Bigger Than a Bread Box: Medical Buildings as Museum Artifacts." *Caduceus* 9, no. 2 (1993): 119–30.

Cooke, Molly, David M. Irby, and Bridget C. O'Brien. *Educating Physicians: A Call for Reform of Medical School and Residency*. San Francisco: Jossey-Bass, 2010.

Cooke, Molly, David M. Irby, William Sullivan, and Kenneth M. Ludmerer. "American Medical Education 100 Years after the Flexner Report." *New England Journal of Medicine* 355, no. 13 (28 September 2006): 1339–44.

Coolidge and Hodgdon and Ralph B. Seem. "Chicago to Have Notable Medical Education and Hospital Buildings." *Modern Hospital* 26, no. 5 (1926): 402–13.

Coolidge and Shattuck, Winford H. Smith, and G. Canby Robinson. "The New Plant of the Vanderbilt University Medical School and Hospital." *Modern Hospital* 20, no. 2 (1923): 109–18.

Cordell, Eugene Fauntleroy. *Historical Sketch of the University of Maryland School of Medicine (1807–1890)*. Baltimore: Press of Isaac Friedenwald, 1891.

Corner, George W. "Foundation and Earliest Years." In *To Each His Farthest Star: University of Rochester Medical Center, 1925–1975*, edited by John Romano, Edward C. Atwater, Gilbert B. Forbes, Raymond Gramiak, Milton B. Lederman, Henry L. Lemkau, Lucretia W. McClure, William D. McHugh, Gordon M. Meade, and William L. Morgan Jr., 37–54. [Rochester, NY?]: University of Rochester Medical Center, 1975.

Corner, George W. *A History of the Rockefeller Institute: 1901–1953, Origins and Growth*. New York: Rockefeller Institute Press, 1964.

Corner, George W. "University of Rochester School of Medicine and Dentistry: Department of Anatomy." *Methods and Problems of Medical Education*, 7th ser. (1927): 21–28.

Council on Medical Education and Hospitals (American Medical Association). *A History of the Council on Medical Education and Hospitals of the American Medical Association, 1904–1959*. [Chicago?]: [American Medical Association?], [1960?].

Councilman, W. T. "Ideals and Methods of the New Harvard Medical School." *Harvard Graduates' Magazine* 15, no. 60 (1907): 584–95.

Cox, A. A. "The Johns Hopkins Hospital, Baltimore, Maryland." *American Architect and Building News* 35, no. 837 (9 January 1892): 24–26.

Cullen, Glenn Ernest. "Vanderbilt University School of Medicine: Department of Biochemistry." *Methods and Problems of Medical Education*, 13th ser. (1929): 33–38.

Curti, Merle, and Roderick Nash. *Philanthropy in the Shaping of American Higher Education*. New Brunswick, NJ: Rutgers University Press, 1965.

Cushing, Harvey. "The Binding Influence of a Library on a Subdividing Profession." *Johns Hopkins Hospital Bulletin* 46, no. 1 (1930): 29–42.

Dalen, James E., and Kenneth J. Ryan. "United States Medical School Expansion: Impact on Primary Care." *American Journal of Medicine* 129, no. 12 (2016): 1241–43.

D'Antonio, Patricia. *American Nursing: A History of Knowledge, Authority, and the Meaning of Work*. Baltimore: Johns Hopkins University Press, 2010.

Davenport, Horace W. *Not Just Any Medical School: The Science, Practice, and Teaching of Medicine at the University of Michigan, 1850–1941*. Ann Arbor: University of Michigan Press, 1999.

Davidge Hall: The First 170 Years, 1812–1982. [Baltimore?]: [Medical Alumni Association of the University of Maryland?], [1982?]. http://hdl.handle.net/10713/5366.

Davison, W. C. *The Duke University Medical Center (1892–1960): Reminiscences of W. C. Davison, Dean of the Duke University Medical School, 1927–1960*. [Durham?], [1966?].

"The Dedication of the New Medical School." *Harvard Graduates' Magazine* 15, no. 58 (December 1906): 237–57.

Densmore, Edward D., and Gifford LeClear. "The Mechanical Plant." *Harvard Graduates' Magazine* 14, no. 56 (1906): 626–42.

"Dental Entering Class Drawn from 12 Colleges." *Columbia Alumni News* 20, no. 4 (19 October 1928): 11.

"A Description of the New Building Erected for the Medical School of Harvard University." *Boston Medical and Surgical Journal* 108, no. 15 (12 April 1883): 339–43.

"The Designing Procedure of Coolidge, Shepley, Bulfinch and Abbott, Architects of the New York Hospital–Cornell Medical College Buildings." *Architectural Forum* 58, no. 2 (February 1933): 87–92.

DeZee, Kent J., Anthony R. Artino, D. Michael Elnicki, Paul A. Hemmer, and Steven J. Durning. "Medical Education in the United States of America." *Medical Teacher* 34, no. 7 (2012): 521–25.

Dodd, Dianne. "Nurses' Residences: Using the Built Environment as Evidence." *Nursing History Review* 9 (2001): 185–206.

Donaldson, Mary Louise. *A History of the Vanderbilt University School of Nursing, 1909–1984*. Nashville: Vanderbilt University, 1984.

Duke, Alex. *Importing Oxbridge: English Residential Colleges and American Universities*. New Haven: Yale University Press, 1996.

Dyson, Walter. *Founding the School of Medicine of Howard University, 1868–1873*. Washington, DC: Howard University Press, 1929.

Dyson, Walter. *Howard University: The Capstone of Negro Education; A History, 1867–1940*. Washington, DC: Graduate School, Howard University, 1941.

Edsall, David. "The Additions to the Dormitory." *Bulletin of the Harvard Medical School Alumni Association* 4, no. 1 (1929): 8–13.

Edsall, David. "The Need for Dormitories at the Medical School." *Harvard Alumni Bulletin* 25, no. 11 (7 December 1922): 312–13.

Elenbaas, Robert M., and Dennis B. Worthen. "Transformation of a Profession: An Overview of the 20th Century." *Pharmacy in History* 51, no. 4 (2009): 151–82.

Eliot, Charles. "Exercises in Huntington Hall, Massachusetts Institute of Technology: Remarks of President Eliot." In *The New Century and the New Building of the Harvard Medical School, 1783–1883: Addresses and Exercises at the One Hundredth Anniversary of the Foundation of the Medical School of Harvard University, October 17, 1883*, 36–41. Cambridge, MA: John Wilson and Son and University Press, 1884.

Epps, Anna L. Cherrie, and Patricia Morris Hammock. *An Act of Grace: The Right Side of History*. [Nashville?]: Anna L. Cherrie Epps and Patricia Morris Hammock, 2009.

Epps, Howard R. "The Howard University Medical Department in the Flexner Era: 1910–1929." *Journal of the National Medical Association* 81, no. 8 (1989): 885–86, 888–90, 893–95, 898, 901–2, 904–6, 908, 911.

Ettling, John. *The Germ of Laziness: Rockefeller Philanthropy and Public Health in the New South*. Cambridge, MA: Harvard University Press, 1981.

Fair, Alistair. "'A Laboratory of Heating and Ventilation': The Johns Hopkins Hospital as Experimental Architecture, 1870–90." *Journal of Architecture* 19, no. 3 (2014): 357–81.

Fee, Elizabeth. *Disease and Discovery: A History of the Johns Hopkins School of Hygiene and Public Health, 1916–1939*. Baltimore: Johns Hopkins University Press, 1987.

Fee, Elizabeth, and Barbara Greene. "Science and Social Reform: Women in Public Health." *Journal of Public Health Policy* 10, no. 2 (1989): 161–77.

Fitzgerald, Martha H. "Courtship of Two Doctors: 1930s Letters Spotlight Nebraska Medical Training." *Nebraska History* 92 (Summer 2011): 70–77.

Fitzsousa, Elizabeth, Nientara Anderson, and Anna Reisman. "'This Institution Was Never Meant for Me': The Impact of Institutional Historical Portraiture on Medical Students." *Journal of General Internal Medicine* 34, no. 12 (2019): 2738–39.

Flexner, Abraham. *Abraham Flexner: An Autobiography*. Rev. ed. New York: Simon and Schuster, 1960.

Flexner, Abraham. *Funds and Foundations: Their Policies Past and Present*. With the collaboration of Esther S. Bailey. 1952. N.p.: Arno, 1976.

Flexner, Abraham. *Medical Education: A Comparative Study*. New York: Macmillan, 1925.

Flexner, Abraham. *Medical Education in the United States and Canada: A Report to the Carnegie Foundation for the Advancement of Teaching*. 1910. N.p.: Wm. F. Fell, 1972. http://archive.carnegiefoundation.org/publications/pdfs/elibrary/Carnegie_Flexner_Report.pdf.

Flood, Charles A. *P&S: The College of Physicians and Surgeons, Columbia University*. N.p.: Charles A. Flood, 1989.

Forbes, J. D. "Shepley, Bulfinch, Richardson and Abbott, Architects: An Introduction." *Journal of the Society of Architectural Historians* 17, no. 3 (1958): 19–31.

Forgan, Sophie. "The Architecture of Display: Museums, Universities and Objects in Nineteenth-Century Britain." *History of Science* 32 (June 1994): 139–62.

Forgan, Sophie. "Bricks and Bones: Architecture and Science in Victorian Britain." In *The Architecture of Science*, edited by Peter Galison and Emily Thompson, 181–208. Cambridge, MA: MIT Press, 1999.

Forgan, Sophie. "Building the Museum: Knowledge, Conflict, and the Power of Place." *Isis* 96, no. 4 (2005): 572–85.

Forgan, Sophie. "'But Indifferently Lodged . . .': Perception and Place in Building for Science in Victorian London." In *Making Space for Science: Territorial Themes in the Shaping of Knowledge*, edited by Crosbie Smith and Jon Agar with the assistance of Gerald Schmidt, 195–215. New York: St. Martin's, 1998.

Formicola, Allan J. *The Columbia University College of Dental Medicine, 1916–2016: A Dental School on University Lines*. New York: Columbia University Press, 2016.

Forty, Adrian. "The Modern Hospital in England and France: The Social and Medical Uses of Architecture." In *Buildings and Society: Essays on the Social Development of the Built Environment*, edited by Anthony D. King, 61–93. London: Routledge and Kegan Paul, 1980.

Fosdick, Raymond B. *Adventure in Giving: The Story of the General Education Board, a Foundation Established by John D. Rockefeller*. Based on an unfinished manuscript prepared by the late Henry F. Pringle and Katharine Douglas Pringle. New York: Harper and Row, 1962.

Fosdick, Raymond B. *The Story of the Rockefeller Foundation*. New York: Harper and Brothers, 1952.

Fox, Daniel M. "Abraham Flexner's Unpublished Report: Foundations and Medical Education, 1909–1928." *Bulletin of the History of Medicine* 54, no. 4 (1980): 475–96.

Fye, W. Bruce. "Carl Ludwig and the Leipzig Physiological Institute: 'A Factory of New Knowledge.'" *Circulation* 74, no. 5 (1986): 920–28.

Gallagher, Teresa Catherine. "From Family Helpmeet to Independent Professional:

Women in American Pharmacy, 1870–1940." *Pharmacy in History* 31, no. 2 (1989): 60–77.

Galpin, W. Freeman. *Syracuse University*. Vol. 2, *The Growing Years*. [Syracuse, NY?]: Syracuse University Press, 1960.

Gamble, Vanessa Northington. *Making a Place for Ourselves: The Black Hospital Movement, 1920–1945*. New York: Oxford University Press, 1995.

Gamble, Vanessa Northington. "'Sisters of a Darker Race': African American Graduates of the Woman's Medical College of Pennsylvania, 1867–1925." *Bulletin of the History of Medicine* 95, no. 2 (2021): 169–97.

[General Education Board?]. *The General Education Board: An Account of Its Activities, 1902–1914*. New York: General Education Board, 1915.

General Secretary [Francis M. Rackemann]. "'Vanderbilt Hall,' the Harvard Medical School Dormitory: A History." *Bulletin of the Harvard Medical School Alumni Association* 1, no. 1 (1927): 6–10.

Gesell, Robert. "Department of Physiology: University of Michigan." *Methods and Problems of Medical Education*, 18th ser. (1930): 39–54.

Gevitz, Norman. *The DOs: Osteopathic Medicine in America*. Baltimore: Johns Hopkins University Press, 1982.

Gevitz, Norman. "The Fate of Sectarian Medical Education." In *Beyond Flexner: Medical Education in the Twentieth Century*, edited by Barbara Barzansky and Norman Gevitz, 83–97. New York: Greenwood Press, 1992.

Gevitz, Norman. "From Flexner to Elliott: The Educational Survey Movement and the Health Professions." *Pharmacy in History* 30, no. 3 (1988): 120–28.

Gieryn, Thomas F. "Two Faces on Science: Building Identities for Molecular Biology and Biotechnology." In *The Architecture of Science*, edited by Peter Galison and Emily Thompson, 423–55. Cambridge, MA: MIT Press, 1999.

Gieryn, Thomas F. "What Buildings Do." *Theory and Society* 31, no. 1 (2002): 35–74.

Gifford, James F., Jr. *The Evolution of a Medical Center: A History of Medicine at Duke University to 1941*. Durham: Duke University Press, 1972.

Girsch, Martha. "Corydon La Ford (1813–94) and the Museum of Anatomy." In *Object Lessons and the Formation of Knowledge: The University of Michigan Museums, Libraries, and Collections 1817–2017*, edited by Kerstin Barndt and Carla M. Sinopoli, 107–11. Ann Arbor: University of Michigan Press, 2017.

Goldberg, Barry, and Barbara Shubinski. "Black Education and Rockefeller Philanthropy from the Jim Crow South to the Civil Rights Era." *Re:Source* (blog), Rockefeller Archive Center, 11 September 2020. https://resource.rockarch.org/story/black-education-and-rockefeller-philanthropy-from-the-jim-crow-south-to-the-civil-rights-era/.

Goldberger, Paul. "James Gamble Rogers and the Shaping of Yale in the Twentieth Century." In *Yale in New Haven: Architecture and Urbanism*, by Vincent Scully Jr., Catherine Lynn, Erik Vogt, and Paul Goldberger, 263–91. New Haven: Yale University, 2004.

Goldenberg, Gary. *Nurses of a Different Stripe: A History of the Columbia University School of Nursing, 1892–1992*. New York: Columbia University School of Nursing, 1992.

Goldstein, Jacob D. "Student Recollections, 1925–1929." In *To Each His Farthest Star: University of Rochester Medical Center, 1925–1975*, edited by John Romano, Edward C. Atwater, Gilbert B. Forbes, Raymond Gramiak, Milton B. Lederman, Henry L. Lemkau, Lucretia W. McClure, William D. McHugh, Gordon M. Meade, and William L. Morgan Jr., 70–80. [Rochester, NY?]: University of Rochester Medical Center, 1975.

Gonzalez Castro, Luis Nicolas. "On The Significance of the Circle of Tugo." *Pharos* (Winter 2016): 28–35.

[Gordon and Kaelber?]. *A Monograph of the Work of Gordon and Kaelber Architects*. New York: Architectural Catalog, 1923.

Gotto, Antonio M., and Jennifer Moon. *Weill Cornell Medicine: A History of Cornell's Medical School*. Ithaca, NY: Cornell University Press, 2016.

Gournay, Isabelle. "L'architecture hospitalo-universitaire: Le tournant des années 20." *Journal of Canadian Art History* 13–14, no. 2/1 (1990–1991): 26–43.

Grandison, Kenrick Ian. "Negotiated Space: The Black College Campus as a Cultural Record of Postbellum America." *American Quarterly* 51, no. 3 (1999): 529–79.

Grauer, Neil A. *Leading the Way: A History of Johns Hopkins Medicine*. Baltimore: Johns Hopkins Medicine in association with Johns Hopkins University Press, 2012.

"The Greater Woman's Medical College Finds a Site." *Bulletin of the Woman's Medical College of Pennsylvania* 76, no. 5 (1926): 3–4.

Grubiak, Margaret M. *White Elephants on Campus: The Decline of the University Chapel in America, 1920–1960*. Notre Dame: University of Notre Dame Press, 2014.

Guerrini, Anita. *Experimenting with Humans and Animals: From Galen to Animal Rights*. Baltimore: Johns Hopkins University Press, 2003.

Gyure, Dale Allen. "Creating Friendly School Environments: 'Casual' High Schools, Progressive Education, and Child-Centred Culture in Postwar America." In *Designing Schools: Space, Place, and Pedagogy*, edited by Kate Darian-Smith and Julie Willis, 68–82. New York: Routledge: 2017.

Gyure, Dale Allen. "The Heart of the University: A History of the Library as Architectural Symbol of American Higher Education." *Winterthur Portfolio* 42, no. 2–3 (2008): 107–32.

Hansen, Bert. *Picturing Medical Progress from Pasteur to Polio: A History of Mass Media Images and Popular Attitudes in America*. New Brunswick, NJ: Rutgers University Press, 2009.

Harrington, Thomas Francis. *The Harvard Medical School: A History, Narrative, and Documentary, 1782–1905*. Vol. 3. Edited by James Gregory Mumford. New York: Lewis, 1905.

Harvard Medical School. *The Harvard Medical School, 1782–1906*. Edited by Harold C. Ernst. [Boston?], [1906?].

"The Harvard Medical School Dormitory." *Boston Medical and Surgical Journal* 189, no. 23 (6 December 1923): 961–62.

Harvey, A. McGehee. "G. Canby Robinson: Peripatetic Medical Educator." *Johns Hopkins Medical Journal* 143, no. 3 (1978): 84–103.

Harvey, A. McGehee, Gert H. Brieger, Susan L. Abrams, Jonathan M. Fishbein, and Victor A. McKusick. *A Model of Its Kind*. Vol. 2, *A Pictorial History of Medicine at Johns Hopkins*. Baltimore: Johns Hopkins University Press, 1989.

Harvey, A. McGehee, Gert H. Brieger, Susan L. Abrams, and Victor A. McKusick. *A Model of Its Kind*. Vol. 1, *A Centennial History of Medicine at Johns Hopkins*. Baltimore: Johns Hopkins University Press, 1989.

Hayden, Dolores. "Urban Landscape History: The Sense of Place and the Politics of Space." In *Understanding Ordinary Landscapes*, edited by Paul Groth and Todd W. Bressi, 111–33. New Haven: Yale University Press, 1997.

Heggie, Vanessa. "Women Doctors and Lady Nurses: Class, Education, and the Professional Victorian Woman." *Bulletin of the History of Medicine* 89, no. 2 (2015): 267–92.

Hertzler, Arthur E. *The Horse and Buggy Doctor*. New York: Harper and Brothers, 1938.

Heskel, Julia. *Shepley Bulfinch Richardson and Abbott: Past to Present*. Boston: SBRA, 1999.

Heynick, Frank. *Jews and Medicine: An Epic Saga*. Hoboken, NJ: KTAV, 2002.

H. H. L. "The New Medical Buildings at Yale University." *Scientific Monthly* 40, no. 4 (1935): 388–90.

Hine, Darlene Clark. "The Pursuit of Professional Equality: Meharry Medical College, 1921–1938, a Case Study." In *New Perspectives on Black Educational History*, edited by Vincent P. Franklin and James D. Anderson, 173–92. Boston: G. K. Hall, 1978.

Hoffschwelle, Mary S. "General Education Board (GEB)." In *Tennessee Encyclopedia*. Tennessee Historical Society, last updated 1 March 2018. http://tennesseeencyclopedia.net/entries/general-education-board-geb/.

Hoffschwelle, Mary S. *The Rosenwald Schools of the American South*. Gainesville: University Press of Florida, 2006.

Holoubek, Alice Baker, and Joe Edward Holoubek. *The Courtship of Two Doctors: A 1930s Love Story of Letters, Hope and Healing*. Edited by Martha Holoubek Fitzgerald. Shreveport, LA: Little Dove, 2012.

Holt, Anna C. "The Library of the Harvard Medical School 1847 and 1947." *Harvard Library Bulletin* 2 (Winter 1948): 32–43.

Holyoke, Edward A. *Centennial Trilogy of the University of Nebraska College of Medicine*. Vol. 2, *Golden Anniversary*. Omaha: University of Nebraska Medical Center, 1980.

Hopkins, James. "The (Dis)assembling of Form: Revealing the Ideas Built into Manchester's Medical School." *Journal of the History of Medicine and Allied Sciences* 75, no. 1 (2020): 24–53.

Horowitz, Helen Lefkowitz. *Alma Mater: Design and Experience in the Women's Colleges from Their Nineteenth-Century Beginnings to the 1930s*. 2nd ed. Amherst: University of Massachusetts Press, 1993.

Howell, Joel D. "The Changing Structure of Medical Education: A Historical Perspective." In *Leadership Careers in Medical Education*, edited by Louis Pangaro, 15–29. Philadelphia: ACP Press, 2010.

Howell, Joel D. *Technology in the Hospital: Transforming Patient Care in the Early Twentieth Century*. Baltimore: Johns Hopkins University Press, 1995.

Hudson, Robert P. "Abraham Flexner in Perspective: American Medical Education, 1865–1910." *Bulletin of the History of Medicine* 46, no. 6 (1972): 545–61.

Ingleby, Helen. "The Department of Pathology." *Bulletin of the Woman's Medical College of Pennsylvania* 83, no. 3 (1932): 11–14.

Irby, David M., Molly Cooke, and Bridget C. O'Brien. "Calls for Reform of Medical Education by the Carnegie Foundation for the Advancement of Teaching: 1910 and 2010." *Academic Medicine* 85, no. 2 (2010): 220–27.

Jacobson, Timothy C. *Making Medical Doctors: Science and Medicine at Vanderbilt since Flexner*. Tuscaloosa: University of Alabama Press, 1987.

Jarrett, William H., II. "Raising the Bar: Mary Elizabeth Garrett, M. Carey Thomas, and the Johns Hopkins Medical School." *Baylor University Medical Center Proceedings* 24, no. 1 (2011): 21–26.

Johns, Elizabeth. "*The Gross Clinic*, or *Portrait of Professor Gross*." In *Reading American Art*, edited by Marianne Doezema and Elizabeth Milroy, 232–63. New Haven: Yale University Press, 1998.

Johnson, Charles W., Sr. *The Spirit of a Place Called Meharry: The Strength of Its Past to Shape the Future*. Franklin, TN: Hillsboro Press, 2000.

Jonas, Gerald. *The Circuit Riders: Rockefeller Money and the Rise of Modern Science*. New York: Norton, 1989.

Joyce, H. Horatio. "New York's Harvard House and the Origins of an Alumni Culture in America." In *Experiencing Architecture in the Nineteenth Century: Buildings and Society in the Modern Age*, edited by Edward Gillin and H. Horatio Joyce, 89–100. London: Bloomsbury Visual Arts, 2019.

Kaji-O'Grady, Sandra, and Chris L. Smith. *LabOratory: Speaking of Science and Its Architecture*. Cambridge, MA: MIT Press, 2019.

Kaji-O'Grady, Sandra, Chris L. Smith, and Russell Hughes, eds. *Laboratory Lifestyles: The Construction of Scientific Fictions*. Cambridge, MA: MIT Press, 2018.

Kampmeier, Rudolph H. *Recollections: The Department of Medicine, Vanderbilt University School of Medicine, 1925–1959*. Nashville: Vanderbilt University Press, 1980.

Kampmeier, Rudolph H. *Vanderbilt University School of Medicine: The Story in Pictures from Its Beginning to 1963*. [Nashville?]: Vanderbilt University Medical Center, 1990.

Karsner, Howard T. "Institute of Pathology of Western Reserve University and the University Hospitals of Cleveland." *Methods and Problems of Medical Education*, 20th ser. (1932): 85–114.

Karsner, Howard T. "Western Reserve University School of Medicine: Department of Pathology." *Methods and Problems of Medical Education*, 3rd ser. (1925): 79–89.

Kasses, Carol D., Susan D. Taylor, and C. Lee Jones. "Departmental Libraries: Curse or Blessing?" *Bulletin of the Medical Library Association* 66, no. 2 (1978): 177–84.

Keegan, J. Jay. "The University of Nebraska Hospital at Omaha." *Nebraska State Medical Journal* 12, no. 11 (1927): 406–11.

Keeling, Arlene Wynbeek. *Nursing and the Privilege of Prescription, 1893–2000*. Columbus: Ohio State University Press, 2007.

Keiller, William. "The Teaching of Anatomy: Lecture III—The Dissecting Room; Practical Anatomy and Lectures." *New York Medical Journal*, 3 November 1894, 545–49.

Kemeny, P. C. *Princeton in the Nation's Service: Religious Ideals and Educational Practice, 1868–1928*. New York: Oxford University Press, 1998.

King, William E. "The Discovery of an Architect: Duke University and Julian F. Abele." *Southern Cultures* 15, no. 1 (2009): 6–21.

Kingsley, Karen. "The Architecture of Nursing." In *Images of Nurses: Perspectives from History, Art, and Literature*, edited by Anne Hudson Jones, 63–94. Philadelphia: University of Pennsylvania Press, 1988.

Kisacky, Jeanne. "Restructuring Isolation: Hospital Architecture, Medicine, and Disease Prevention." *Bulletin of the History of Medicine* 79 (2005): 1–49.

Kisacky, Jeanne. *Rise of the Modern Hospital: An Architectural History of Health and Healing, 1870–1940*. Pittsburgh: University of Pittsburgh Press, 2017.

Knowles, Scott G., and Stuart W. Leslie. "'Industrial Versailles': Eero Saarinen's Corporate Campuses for GM, IBM, and AT&T." *Isis* 92, no. 1 (2001): 1–33.

Kremer, Richard L. "Building Institutes for Physiology in Prussia, 1836–1846: Contexts, Interests and Rhetoric." In *The Laboratory Revolution in Medicine*, edited by Andrew Cunningham and Perry Williams, 72–109. Cambridge: Cambridge University Press, 1992.

Kuhlenbeck, Hartwig. "The Department of Anatomy and Histology." *Club Woman's Journal*, February 1937, 14.

Kwolek-Folland, Angel. *Engendering Business: Men and Women in the Corporate Office, 1870–1930*. Baltimore: Johns Hopkins University Press, 1994.

Lagemann, Ellen Condliffe. *Private Power for the Public Good: A History of the Carnegie Foundation for the Advancement of Teaching.* Middletown, CT: Wesleyan University Press, 1983.

Lamb, Albert R. *The Presbyterian Hospital and the Columbia-Presbyterian Medical Center, 1868–1943: A History of a Great Medical Adventure.* New York: Columbia University Press, 1955.

Lamb, Albert R. "The Story of the Founding of the Columbia-Presbyterian Medical Center." *American Journal of Medicine* 15, no. 6 (1953): 754–60.

Langone, John. "The Racial Integration of Harvard Medical School." *Journal of Blacks in Higher Education* 8 (Summer 1995): 66–70.

Lavoie, Catherine C. "Davidge Hall" [Baltimore, Maryland]. In *SAH Archipedia*, edited by Gabrielle Esperdy and Karen Kingsley. Charlottesville: University of Virginia Press, 2012–. Accessed 17 August 2018. http://sah-archipedia.org/buildings/MD-01-510-0021.

Lawrence, Christopher, and George Weisz. "Medical Holism: The Context." In *Greater Than the Parts: Holism in Biomedicine, 1920–1950*, edited by Christopher Lawrence and George Weisz, 1–22. New York: Oxford University Press, 1998.

Leathers, Waller S. "Vanderbilt University School of Medicine: Department of Preventive Medicine and Public Health." *Methods and Problems of Medical Education*, 13th ser. (1929): 73–82.

Lebovich, William. "Albert Irvin Cassell (1895–1969)." In *African American Architects: A Biographical Dictionary 1865–1945*, edited by Dreck Spurlock Wilson, 125–32. New York: Routledge, 2004.

Lederer, Susan E. "Political Animals: The Shaping of Biomedical Research Literature in Twentieth-Century America." *Isis* 83, no. 1 (1992): 61–79.

Lee, Eleanor. *History of the School of Nursing of the Presbyterian Hospital, New York, 1892–1942.* New York: G. P. Putnam's Sons, 1942.

Lemkau, Henry L. "Crossroads: The Story of the Medical Library." In *To Each His Farthest Star: University of Rochester Medical Center, 1925–1975*, edited by John Romano, Edward C. Atwater, Gilbert B. Forbes, Raymond Gramiak, Milton B. Lederman, Henry L. Lemkau, Lucretia W. McClure, William D. McHugh, Gordon M. Meade, and William L. Morgan Jr., 145–61. [Rochester, NY?]: University of Rochester Medical Center, 1975.

Lenoir, Timothy. "Science for the Clinic: Science Policy and the Formation of Carl Ludwig's Institute in Leipzig." In *The Investigative Enterprise: Experimental Physiology in Nineteenth-Century Medicine*, edited by William Coleman and Frederic L. Holmes, 139–78. Berkeley: University of California Press, 1988.

Leroy, Robert. "The Columbia-Presbyterian Medical Center." *Architecture* 55, no. 4 (1927): 185–87.

Leslie, Stuart W. "'A Different Kind of Beauty': Scientific and Architectural Style in I. M. Pei's Mesa Laboratory and Louis Kahn's Salk Institute." *Historical Studies in the Natural Sciences* 38, no. 2 (2008): 173–221.

Leslie, Stuart W. "Laboratory Architecture: Building for an Uncertain Future." *Physics Today* 63, no. 4 (2010): 40–45.

Leslie, Stuart W. "The Strategy of Structure: Architectural and Managerial Style at Alcoa and Owens-Corning." *Enterprise and Society* 12, no. 4 (2011): 863–902.

Lewis, Frederic T. "Charles Sedgwick Minot: An Address. . . ." *Anatomical Record* 10, no. 3 (1916): 133–64.

Long, Diana E. "The Medical World of *The Agnew Clinic*: A World We Have Lost?"
  Prospects: An Annual of American Cultural Studies 11 (1987): 185–98.

Ludmerer, Kenneth M. "The Internal Challenges to Medical Education." *Transactions of
  the American Clinical and Climatological Association* 114 (2003): 241–53.

Ludmerer, Kenneth M. *Learning to Heal: The Development of American Medical Education.*
  New York: Basic Books, 1985.

Ludmerer, Kenneth M. *Let Me Heal: The Opportunity to Preserve Excellence in American
  Medicine.* Oxford: Oxford University Press, 2015.

Ludmerer, Kenneth M. "Reform of Medical Education at Washington University."
  Journal of the History of Medicine and Allied Sciences 35, no. 2 (1980): 149–73.

Ludmerer, Kenneth M. *Time to Heal: American Medical Education from the Turn of the
  Century to the Era of Managed Care.* Oxford: Oxford University Press, 1999.

Ludmerer, Kenneth M. "Washington University and the Creation of the Teaching Hospital." *Journal of the American Medical Association* 226, no. 14 (9 October 1991): 1981–83.

Luft, Eric von der. *SUNY Upstate Medical University: A Pictorial History.* North Syracuse,
  NY: Gegensatz Press, 2005.

Lupkin, Paula. "Manhood Factories: Architecture, Business, and the Evolving Urban
  Role of the YMCA, 1865–1925." In *Men and Women Adrift: The YMCA and the YWCA
  in the City*, edited by Nina Mjagkij and Margaret Spratt, 40–64. New York: New York
  University Press, 1997.

Lupkin, Paula. *Manhood Factories: YMCA Architecture and the Making of Modern Urban
  Culture.* Minneapolis: University of Minnesota Press, 2010.

Lyttle, Hulda M. "A School for Negro Nurses: At the George W. Hubbard Hospital and
  Meharry Medical College Nashville, Tennessee." *American Journal of Nursing* 39, no.
  2 (1939): 133–38.

Mall, Franklin P. "The Anatomical Course and Laboratory of the Johns Hopkins
  University." *Johns Hopkins Hospital Bulletin* 7, no. 62–63 (1896): 85–100.

Mallory, Frank B. "The Medical School." *Harvard Graduates' Magazine* 15, no. 60 (1907): 669–71.

Manning, Kenneth R. "A History of Black Medical Education, 1868–1929." In *African-
  American Medical Pioneers*, by Charles H. Epps Jr., Davis G. Johnson, and Audrey L.
  Vaughan, 8–14. Rockville, MD: Betz, 1994.

Marshall, Clara. *The Woman's Medical College of Pennsylvania: An Historical Outline.*
  Philadelphia: P. Blakiston, Son and Co., 1897.

McBride, David. *Integrating the City of Medicine: Blacks in Philadelphia Health Care,
  1910–1965.* Philadelphia: Temple University Press, 1989.

McClelland, Charles E. *Queen of the Professions: The Rise and Decline of Medical Prestige
  and Power in America.* Lanham, MD: Rowman and Littlefield, 2014.

McClelland, Charles E. *State, Society, and University in Germany, 1700–1914.* Cambridge:
  Cambridge University Press, 1980.

McIsaac, Peter M. "The Rise and the Fall of the University of Michigan's Medical Mu-
  seums." In *Object Lessons and the Formation of Knowledge: The University of Michigan
  Museums, Libraries, and Collections 1817–2017*, edited by Kerstin Barndt and Carla M.
  Sinopoli, 59–70. Ann Arbor: University of Michigan Press, 2017.

McLean, Franklin C. "University of Chicago History and Development of Medicine in
  the Division of Biological Sciences." *Methods and Problems of Medical Education*, 19th
  ser. (1931): 5–18.

McLeary, Erin Hunter. "Science in a Bottle: The Medical Museum in North America,
  1860–1940." PhD diss., University of Pennsylvania, 2001.

Meader, Charles N. "The University of Colorado School of Medicine and Hospital." *Colorado Medicine* 21, no. 10 (1924): 287–303.

Medical College of Pennsylvania. *Pioneer-Pacesetter-Innovator: The Story of the Medical College of Pennsylvania.* New York: Newcomen Society in North American, 1971.

"Meharry Makes Progress." *Meharry News* 27, no. 2 (1930): 3.

Meister, Maureen. "At a Crossroads: Architect Charles Rutan and His Photo Album." *Nineteenth Century* 37, no. 2 (2017): 2–7.

Miller, Lynn E., and Richard M. Weiss. "Revisiting Black Medical School Extinctions in the Flexner Era." *Journal of the History of Medicine and Allied Sciences* 67, no. 2 (2012): 217–43.

Miner, Leroy M. S. "The Dental School." In *The Development of Harvard University since the Inauguration of President Eliot: 1869–1929*, edited by Samuel Eliot Morison, 595–602. Cambridge, MA: Harvard University Press, 1930.

Minot, Charles S. "A Further Study of the Unit System of Laboratory Construction." *Science*, n.s., 13, no. 324 (15 March 1901): 409–15.

Minot, Charles S. "The Unit System of Laboratory Construction." *Philadelphia Medical Journal* 6, no. 9 (1 September 1900): 390–91.

Moore, Francis D. *A Miracle and a Privilege: Recounting a Half Century of Surgical Advance.* Washington, DC: Joseph Henry, 1995.

Moran, Bronte. "The Role of the Medical Departmental Library." *Bulletin of the Medical Library Association* 84, no. 1 (1996): 25–31.

Morantz, Regina Markell, Cynthia Stodola Pomerleau, and Carol Hansen Fenichel, eds. *In Her Own Words: Oral Histories of Women Physicians.* New Haven: Yale University Press, 1982.

Morantz-Sanchez, Regina. *Sympathy and Science: Women Physicians in American Medicine.* 1985. Chapel Hill: University of North Carolina Press, 2000.

Morgan, Keith N., ed. *Buildings of Massachusetts: Metropolitan Boston.* Charlottesville: University of Virginia Press, 2009.

Morgan, Keith N., Elizabeth Hope Cushing, and Roger G. Reed. *Community by Design: The Olmsted Firm and the Development of Brookline, Massachusetts.* Amherst: University of Massachusetts Press, 2013.

Morrison, William, ed. *The Work of Dwight James Baum.* New York: Acanthus, 2008.

Morton-Young, Tommie. *Nashville, Tennessee.* Charleston, SC: Arcadia, 2000.

Mould, Ward L. "Dr. Ward L. Mould Remembers." *Alumni Journal* (SUNY Upstate Medical University), Summer 1986, 12–13.

Mullowney, John J. "Meharry: Her Past, Her Future." *Meharry News* 27, no. 3 (1931): 3–8.

Munby, Alan E. "The Design of Science Buildings." *Journal of the Royal Institute of British Architects* 37 (7 December 1929): 75–84.

Munger, D. "Robert Brookings and the Flexner Report: A Case Study of the Reorganization of Medical Education." *Journal of the History of Medicine and Allied Sciences* 23 (1968): 356–71.

"National Plans of Campaign Are Discussed." *Bulletin of the Woman's Medical College of Pennsylvania* 77, no. 3 (1926): 7–8.

"The Need for Dormitories as Expressed by the Students." *Harvard Alumni Bulletin* 25, no. 11 (7 December 1922): 313–14.

Nercessian, Nora N. *Against All Odds: The Legacy of Students of African Descent at Harvard Medical School before Affirmative Action, 1850–1968.* [Boston?]: Harvard Medical School, 2004.

Nercessian, Nora N. *A Legacy So Enduring: An Account of the Administration Building at Harvard Medical School from Its Foundation to Its Rededication as the Gordon Hall of Medicine*. [Cambridge, MA?]: President and Fellows of Harvard College, 2001.

"The New Harvard Medical School: The Architects' Work." *Harvard Graduates' Magazine* 14, no. 56 (1906): 616–26.

Nicoll, Matthias, Jr., and Huntington Williams. "Albany Medical College: Department of Public Health." *Methods and Problems of Medical Education*, 15th ser. (1929): 69–70.

Nieves, Angel David. *An Architecture of Education: African American Women Design the New South*. Rochester, NY: University of Rochester Press, 2018.

Numbers, Ronald L., and John Harley Warner. "The Maturation of American Medical Science." In *Sickness and Health in America: Readings in the History of Medicine and Public Health*, edited by Judith Walzer Leavitt and Ronald L. Numbers, 130–42. 3rd ed. Madison: University of Wisconsin Press, 1997.

O'Connor, Candace. *Beginning a Great Work: Washington University in St. Louis, 1853–2003*. [St. Louis?]: Washington University in St. Louis, 2003.

Ogata, Amy F. "Building for Learning in Postwar American Elementary Schools." *Journal of the Society of Architectural Historians* 67, no. 4 (2008): 562–91.

Ogata, Amy F. *Designing the Creative Child: Playthings and Places in Midcentury America*. Minneapolis: University of Minnesota Press, 2013.

Ogata, Amy F. "Educational Facilities Laboratories: Debating and Designing the Postwar American Schoolhouse." In *Designing Schools: Space, Place, and Pedagogy*, edited by Kate Darian-Smith and Julie Willis, 55–67. New York: Routledge: 2017.

O'Gorman, James F. *H. H. Richardson and His Office: A Centennial of His Move to Boston, 1874; Selected Drawings*. [Cambridge, MA?]: Department of Printing and Graphic Arts, Harvard College Library, 1974.

O'Neal, William B. *Pictorial History of the University of Virginia*. Charlottesville: University Press of Virginia, 1968.

Ophir, Adi, and Steven Shapin. "The Place of Knowledge: A Methodological Survey." *Science in Context* 4, no. 1 (1991): 3–21.

Osler, William. "On the Library of a Medical School." *Johns Hopkins Hospital Bulletin* 18, no. 193 (1907): 109–11.

"Our Proudest Possessions." *Bulletin of the Woman's Medical College of Pennsylvania* 79, no. 4 (1929): 3–4.

"P&S Alumni Urged to Expand Influence: New Medical Center Offers Opportunity for Wider Activity, Speakers Tell 200 at Dinner." *Columbia Alumni News* 20, no. 4 (19 October 1928): 13–14.

"P&S Draws Student Body of 400 from 82 Colleges." *Columbia Alumni News* 20, no. 4 (19 October 1928): 8.

Parham, Sandra Martin. "Member Spotlight: Why Meharry Medical College Library Is Open during COVID-19." *SEA Currents* (blog), Network of the National Library of Medicine, 9 July 2020. https://news.nnlm.gov/sea/2020/07/09/member-spotlight-why-meharry-medical-college-library-is-open-during-covid-19/.

Pearce, Richard M. "Prefatory Note." *Methods and Problems of Medical Education*, 1st ser. (1924): 3.

Peitzman, Steven J. *A New and Untried Course: Woman's Medical College and Medical College of Pennsylvania, 1850–1998*. New Brunswick, NJ: Rutgers University Press, 2000.

Peitzman, Steven J. "Style and Space: Designing a Medical School Building for Women in the 1870s." *Medical Humanities Review* 13, no. 2 (1999): 28–43.

Peitzman, Steven J. "Why Support a Women's Medical College? Philadelphia's Early Male Medical Pro-Feminists." *Bulletin of the History of Medicine* 77, no. 3 (2003): 576–99.

"Perspective View of the Medical Department of the University of Nebraska, to Be Located at Dewey Avenue and Forty-Second Street." *Western Medical Review* 14, no. 8 (15 August 1909): following 440.

Peterson, Glenn A., Gina Shaw, and Stephen E. Novak. *Seventy-Five Years of Healing on the Heights: Columbia University Medical Center Celebrates the 75th Anniversary of Columbia-Presbyterian Medical Center, 1928–2003.* [New York?]: [Columbia University Medical Center?], [2003?].

Pistor, Moritz. *Anstalten und Einrichtungen des öffentlichen Gesundheitswesens in Preussen: Festschrift zum X. internationalen medizinischen Kongress, Berlin 1890.* Berlin: Julius Springer, 1890.

Pitrof, Larry. *University of Maryland School of Medicine: The First Two Centuries.* Baltimore: Medical Alumni Association of the University of Maryland, 2006.

Poindexter, Hildrus A. *My World of Reality.* Detroit: Balamp, 1973.

Porter, W. T. "Charles Sedgwick Minot, M.D." *Boston Medical and Surgical Journal* 172, no. 13 (1 April 1915): 467–70.

"Present Ideals of the Physical Plant in Medical Education" (discussion). *Journal of the American Medical Association* 80, no. 14 (7 April 1923): 1009–10.

Prior, Lindsay. "The Architecture of the Hospital: A Study of Spatial Organization and Medical Knowledge." *British Journal of Sociology* 39, no. 1 (March 1988): 86–113.

Proceedings of the Semi-Centennial of Vanderbilt University Celebrated during the Four Days, October 15 to October 18, 1925, at Nashville, Tennessee. Nashville: Vanderbilt University, [1925?].

"Professional Men Get Dormitory." *Howard Alumni Journal*, December 1933, 19.

"Progress of the College." *Bulletin of the University of Nebraska College of Medicine* 4, no. 2 (1909): 65–66.

Prutkin, Jordan M. "Abraham Flexner and the Development of the Yale School of Medicine." *Yale Journal of Biology and Medicine* 72, no. 4 (1999): 269–79.

Pusey, William Allen. "The Importance of Being Historically Minded." *Journal of the American Medical Association* 89, no. 25 (17 December 1927): 2079–82.

Rappleye, W. C. "Survey of Medical Education." *Journal of the American Medical Association* 88, no. 11 (12 March 1927): 843–44.

Reinarz, Jonathan. "The Age of Museum Medicine: The Rise and Fall of the Medical Museum at Birmingham's School of Medicine." *Social History of Medicine* 18, no. 3 (2005): 419–37.

Reverby, Susan. *Ordered to Care: The Dilemma of American Nursing, 1850–1945.* Cambridge: Cambridge University Press, 1987.

Robert, Alfred L. "The Libraries at P. and S." *Columbia Alumni News* 4, no. 15 (20 December 1912): 214–16.

Roberts, Carl Glennis. "President's Annual Address." *Journal of the National Medical Association* 20, no. 1 (1928): 23–32.

Robinson, Clare. "Architecture in Support of Citizenry: Vernon DeMars and the Berkeley Student Union." *Journal of Architectural Education* 70, no. 2 (2016): 236–46.

Robinson, Clare. "Student Union: The Architecture and Social Design of Postwar Campus Community Centers in California." PhD diss., University of California, Berkeley, 2012.

Robinson, G. Canby. *Adventures in Medical Education: A Personal Narrative of the Great Advance of American Medicine.* Cambridge, MA: Harvard University Press, 1957.

Robinson, G. Canby. "The Influence of Environment in Medical Education." *Southern Medical Journal* 18, no. 1 (1925): 9–12.

Robinson, G. Canby. "The Principles of Planning: The New York Hospital–Cornell Medical College Buildings." *Architectural Forum* 58, no. 2 (February 1933): 85–86.

Robinson, G. Canby. "The Relation of Medical Education to the Medical Plant." *Journal of the American Medical Association* 81, no. 4 (28 July 1923): 321–23.

Robinson, G. Canby. "Vanderbilt University School of Medicine: History and General Description." *Methods and Problems of Medical Education*, 13th ser. (1929): 1–14.

Robinson, Harry G., III, and Hazel Ruth Edwards. *The Long Walk: The Placemaking Legacy of Howard University*. Washington, DC: Moorland-Spingarn Research Center, Howard University, 1996.

Roman, Charles Victor. *Meharry Medical College: A History*. Nashville: Sunday School Publication Board of the National Baptist Convention, 1934.

Rose, S. Brandt. "The Department of Bacteriology and Immunology." *Bulletin of the Woman's Medical College of Pennsylvania* 83, no. 3 (1932): 15–17.

Rosenberg, Charles E. *The Care of Strangers: The Rise of America's Hospital System*. New York: Basic Books, 1987.

Rosof, Patricia J. F. "The Quiet Feminism of Dr. Florence Sabin: Helping Women Achieve in Science and Medicine." *Gender Forum*, no. 24 (2009): 1–10. genderforum.org/apparatus-xy-issue-24-2009.

Ross, Karen D. "Recruiting 'Friends of Medical Progress': Evolving Tactics in the Defense of Animal Experimentation, 1910s and 1920s." *Journal of the History of Medicine and Allied Sciences* 70, no. 3 (2015): 365–93.

Rothstein, William G. *American Medical Schools and the Practice of Medicine: A History*. New York: Oxford University Press, 1987.

Rudy, Jarrett. *Freedom to Smoke: Tobacco Consumption and Identity*. Montreal and Kingston: McGill-Queen's University Press, 2005.

Sander, Kathleen Waters. *Mary Elizabeth Garrett: Society and Philanthropy in the Gilded Age*. Baltimore: Johns Hopkins University Press, 2008.

Sappol, Michael. *A Traffic of Dead Bodies: Anatomy and Embodied Social Identity in Nineteenth-Century America*. Princeton: Princeton University Press, 2002.

Savitt, Todd L. *Race and Medicine in Nineteenth- and Early-Twentieth-Century America*. Kent, OH: Kent State University Press, 2007.

Schiff, Judith. "The Memorial Quadrangle's Beginnings." *Yale Alumni Magazine*, September–October 2017. https://yalealumnimagazine.com/articles/4540-the-memorial -quadrangles-beginnings.

Schlich, Thomas. "Surgery, Science and Modernity: Operating Rooms and Laboratories as Spaces of Control." *History of Science* 45, no. 3 (2007): 231–56.

Schlich, Thomas, and Audrey Hasegawa. "Order and Cleanliness: The Gendered Role of Operating Room Nurses in the United States (1870s–1930s)." *Social History of Medicine* 31, no. 1 (1 February 2018): 106–21.

Schneckloth, Nancy W. *The University of Nebraska College of Nursing, 1917–1987*. Omaha: University of Nebraska Medical Center, 1987.

Setran, David P. *The College "Y": Student Religion in the Era of Secularization*. New York: Palgrave Macmillan, 2007.

Shattuck, Frederick C. "The Dramatic Story of the New Harvard Medical School." *Boston Medical and Surgical Journal* 193, no. 23 (3 December 1925): 1058–61.

Shattuck, Frederick C., and J. Lewis Bremer. "The Medical School: 1869–1929." In *The

Development of Harvard University since the Inauguration of President Eliot: 1869–1929, edited by Samuel Eliot Morison, 555–94. Cambridge, MA: Harvard University Press, 1930.

Shepley, George. "New Buildings for the Medical School." *Quarterly of the Harvard Medical Alumni Association*, no. 1 (July 1901): 18–22.

Shepley, Henry R. "Considerations in Planning a Teaching Hospital." *Modern Hospital Year Book*, 6th ed. (1926): 91–96.

Shepley, Rutan, and Coolidge. "The New Harvard Medical School Buildings, Boston, Mass." *American Architect* 92, no. 1669 (21 December 1907): 203–6.

Shikes, Robert H., and Henry N. Claman. *The University of Colorado School of Medicine: A Centennial History, 1883–1983*. Denver: University of Colorado School of Medicine, 1983.

"The Significance of Harvard's New Buildings." *Bulletin of the University of Nebraska College of Medicine* 1, no. 4 (1906): 185–86.

Slater, Robert Bruce. "The First Black Faculty Members at the Nation's Highest-Ranked Universities." *Journal of Blacks in Higher Education*, no. 22 (Winter 1998–1999): 97–106.

Sloane, David Charles, and Beverlie Conant Sloane. *Medicine Moves to the Mall*. Baltimore: Johns Hopkins University Press, 2003.

Smith, Jessica Carney. "From Andrew Carnegie to John Hope Franklin: Library Development at Fisk University." *Tennessee Libraries* 59, no. 4 (2009). https://www.tnla.org/page/290/TL-v59n4-Fisk-University-Library-.htm.

Smith, Lawrence. "New Medical Schools in the United States: Forces of Change Past and Present." *Transactions of the American Clinical and Climatological Association* 120 (2009): 227–38.

Smith, Margaret Supplee. "*The Agnew Clinic*: 'Not Cheerful for Ladies to Look At.'" *Prospects: An Annual of American Cultural Studies* 11 (1987): 161–83.

Sokoloff, Leon. "The Rise and Decline of the Jewish Quota in Medical School Admissions." *Bulletin of the New York Academy of Medicine* 68, no. 4 (1992): 497–518.

Sollmann, Torald. "Departmental Libraries of the School of Medicine of Western Reserve University." *Methods and Problems of Medical Education*, 10th ser. (1928): 177–83.

Souers, Clark, and Christopher G. Parnall. "The New Medical Unit at the University of Iowa." *Modern Hospital* 33, no. 4 (1929): 73–78.

Spock, Benjamin, and Mary Morgan. *Spock on Spock: A Memoir of Growing Up with the Century*. New York: Pantheon Books, 1989.

Starr, Paul. *The Social Transformation of American Medicine*. Updated ed. New York: Basic Books, 2017.

Starr, Sarah Logan Wister. "To the Alumnae of the Woman's Medical College of Pennsylvania." *Special Bulletin of the Woman's Medical College of Pennsylvania* 73, no. 5 (1923): 1–9.

Stefanacci, Michal A., M. Sandra Wood, and Laura D. Huff. "Departmental Libraries: Why Do They Exist?" *Bulletin of the Medical Library Association* 65, no. 4 (1977): 433–37.

Stern, David T., and Maxine Papadakis. "The Developing Physician—Becoming a Professional." *New England Journal of Medicine* 355, no. 17 (26 October 2006): 1794–99.

Stevens, Edward F. *The American Hospital of the Twentieth Century: A Treatise on the Development of Medical Institutions, Both in Europe and in America, since the Beginning of the Present Century*. New York: Architectural Record, 1918.

Stevens, Edward F. *The American Hospital of the Twentieth Century: A Treatise on the*

Development of Medical Institutions, Both in Europe and in America, since the Beginning of the Present Century. Rev. ed. New York: Architectural Record, 1921.

Stevens, Edward F. *The American Hospital of the Twentieth Century: A Treatise on the Development of Medical Institutions, Both in Europe and in America, since the Beginning of the Present Century.* 2nd ed. New York: F. W. Dodge, 1928.

Strickland, Thomas. "Passive and Active: Public Space at the McMaster Health Sciences Centre, 1972." In *Healing Spaces, Modern Architecture, and the Body*, edited by Sarah Schrank and Didem Ekici, 203–23. London: Routledge, 2017.

"The Structure and Equipment of the New York Hospital." *Architectural Forum* 58, no. 2 (1933): 118–24.

Summerville, James. *Educating Black Doctors: A History of Meharry Medical College.* University: University of Alabama Press, 1983.

"Teaching and Opportunities in the Harvard Medical School of To-day." *Bulletin [of the] Harvard Medical Alumni Association*, n.s., no. 6 (July 1908): 3–70.

Terry, Robert J. "Washington University School of Medicine: Departments of Anatomy, Neuroanatomy, and Histology." *Methods and Problems of Medical Education*, 5th ser. (1926): 1–25.

Thomas, George E., and David B. Brownlee. *Building America's First University: An Historical and Architectural Guide to the University of Pennsylvania.* Philadelphia: University of Pennsylvania Press, 2000.

Thomas, Karen Kruse. *Deluxe Jim Crow: Civil Rights and American Health Policy, 1935–1954.* Athens: University of Georgia Press, 2011.

Thompson, John D., and Grace Goldin. *The Hospital: A Social and Architectural History.* New Haven: Yale University Press, 1975.

Tilton, Edward L. "William H. Welch Medical Library." *Johns Hopkins Hospital Bulletin* 46 (January 1930): 10–21.

"Triennial Dinner." *Quarterly of the Harvard Medical Alumni Association*, no. 10 (October 1903): 604–27.

Tuchman, Arleen M. "From the Lecture to the Laboratory: The Institutionalization of Scientific Medicine at the University of Heidelberg." In *The Investigative Enterprise: Experimental Physiology in Nineteenth-Century Medicine*, edited by William Coleman and Frederic L. Holmes, 65–99. Berkeley: University of California Press, 1988.

Tucker, Augusta. *Miss Susie Slagle's.* 1939. Baltimore: Johns Hopkins University Press, 1987.

Turner, Paul Venable. *Campus: An American Planning Tradition.* Rev. ed. New York: Architectural History Foundation; Cambridge, MA: MIT Press, 1990.

Turner, Thomas B. *Heritage of Excellence. The Johns Hopkins Medical Institutions, 1914–1947.* Baltimore: Johns Hopkins University Press, 1974.

Tyler, Albert F., ed., and Ella F. Auerbach, comp. *History of Medicine in Nebraska.* A reprint of the 1928 edition augmented by Bernice M. Hetzner. Omaha: University of Nebraska Medical Center, 1977.

"Vanderbilt Hall." *Bulletin of the Harvard Medical School Alumni Association* 5, no. 1 (1930): 13.

"Vanderbilt Hall: From the Alumni Committee on the Medical Dormitories [sic] to the Students of the Harvard Medical School." *Bulletin of the Harvard Medical School Alumni Association* 1, no. 1 (1927): 20–21.

The Vanderbilt School of Nursing: Celebrating One Hundred Years, 1908–2008. Nashville: Turner, 2008.

Van Poznak, Alan. "'The Last Smile of Skyscraper Romanticism.'" *Cornell University Medical College Alumni Quarterly* 45, no. 3–4 (1982): 14–16.

Van Slyck, Abigail A. *Free to All: Carnegie Libraries and American Culture, 1890–1920.* Chicago: University of Chicago Press, 1995.

Van Slyck, Abigail A. *A Manufactured Wilderness: Summer Camps and the Shaping of American Youth, 1890–1960.* Minneapolis: University of Minnesota Press, 2006.

Van Slyck, Abigail A. "'The Utmost Amount of Effectiv [*sic*] Accommodation': Andrew Carnegie and the Reform of the American Library." *Journal of the Society of Architectural Historians* 50, no. 4 (1991): 359–83.

Verderber, Stephen, and David J. Fine. *Healthcare Architecture in an Era of Radical Transformation.* New Haven: Yale University Press, 2000.

Wailoo, Keith. "Sovereignty and Science: Revisiting the Role of Science in the Construction and Erosion of Medical Dominance." *Journal of Health Politics, Policy and Law* 29, no. 4–5 (2004): 643–59.

Waite, Frederick Clayton. *Western Reserve University Centennial History of the School of Medicine.* Cleveland, OH: Western Reserve University Press, 1946.

Walker, Matthew. "Architecture, Anatomy, and the New Science in Early Modern London: Robert Hooke's College of Physicians." *Journal of the Society of Architectural Historians* 72, no. 4 (2013): 475–502.

Walsh, Mary Roth. *"Doctors Wanted: No Women Need Apply"; Sexual Barriers in the Medical Profession, 1835–1975.* New Haven: Yale University Press, 1977.

Walter, Georgia Warner. *The First School of Osteopathic Medicine: A Chronicle.* Kirksville: Thomas Jefferson University Press at Northeast Missouri State University, 1992.

Ward, Thomas J., Jr. *Black Physicians in the Jim Crow South.* Fayetteville: University of Arkansas Press, 2003.

Warner, John Harley. "The Aesthetic Grounding of Modern Medicine." *Bulletin of the History of Medicine* 88, no. 1 (2014): 1–47.

Warner, John Harley. "The Art of Medicine in an Age of Science: Reductionism, Holism, and the Doctor-Patient Relationship in the United States, 1890–1960." *Senri Ethnological Reports* 120 (2014): 55–91.

Warner, John Harley. "Grand Narrative and Its Discontents: Medical History and the Social Transformation of American Medicine." *Journal of Health Politics, Policy and Law* 29, nos. 4–5 (2004): 757–80.

Warner, John Harley. "Witnessing Dissection: Photography, Medicine, and American Culture." In *Dissection: Photographs of a Rite of Passage in American Medicine, 1880–1930,* by John Harley Warner and James M. Edmonson, 7–192. New York: Blast, 2009.

Warren, J. Collins. "The Social Side of Student Life." *Harvard Alumni Bulletin* 25, no. 34 (31 May 1923): 1004–6.

Warren, J. Collins. *To Work in the Vineyard of Surgery: The Reminiscences of J. Collins Warren (1842–1927).* Edited by Edward D. Churchill. Cambridge, MA: Harvard University Press, 1958.

Washington University School of Medicine. *The Dedication of the New Buildings of Washington University Medical School.* [St. Louis, MO?], [1915?].

Watson, Wilbur H. *Against the Odds: Blacks in the Profession of Medicine in the United States.* New Brunswick, NJ: Transaction, 1999.

Weed, Lewis H. "The William H. Welch Medical Library." *Johns Hopkins Hospital Bulletin* 46 (1930): 3–9.

Weindling, Paul. "Scientific Elites and Laboratory Organisation in *Fin de Siècle* Paris and Berlin: The Pasteur Institute and Robert Koch's Institute for Infectious Diseases Compared." In *The Laboratory Revolution in Medicine*, edited by Andrew Cunningham and Perry Williams, 170–88. Cambridge: Cambridge University Press, 1992.

Weiskotten, Herman G. "A History of Syracuse University College of Medicine." In *Onondaga County Medical Society, 1906–1956: Sesquicentennial*, 40–56. [Syracuse, NY?]: [Onondaga County Medical Society?], 1956.

Weiskotten, Herman G., Alphonse M. Schwitalla, William D. Cutter, and Hamilton H. Anderson. *Medical Education in the United States: 1934–1939*. Chicago: American Medical Association, 1940.

Weiss, Ellen. *Robert R. Taylor and Tuskegee: An African American Architect Designs for Booker T. Washington*. Montgomery, AL: NewSouth Books, 2012.

Weiss, Ellen. "Tuskegee: Landscape in Black and White." *Winterthur Portfolio* 36, no. 1 (2001): 19–37.

Wellbery, Caroline, and Ranit Mishori. "Deck the Halls with Diverse Portraits." *Journal of the American Medical Association* 320, no. 6 (14 August 2018): 528–30.

Wheatley, Steven C. *The Politics of Philanthropy: Abraham Flexner and Medical Education*. Madison: University of Wisconsin Press, 1989.

Whipple, George Hoyt. "Autobiographical Sketch." *Perspectives in Biology and Medicine* 2, no. 3 (1959): 253–89.

Whipple, George Hoyt. *Planning and Construction Period of the School and Hospitals, 1921–1925*. Rochester, NY: University of Rochester, 1957.

Whipple, George Hoyt. "University of Rochester School of Medicine and Dentistry: Animal House." *Methods and Problems of Medical Education*, 7th ser. (1927): 15–19.

Whipple, George Hoyt. "University of Rochester School of Medicine and Dentistry: School and Hospital Plans." *Methods and Problems of Medical Education*, 7th ser. (1927): 1–14.

Whitcomb, Michael E. "The Development of New MD-Granting Medical Schools in the United States in the 21st Century." *Academic Medicine* 95, no. 3 (2020): 340–43.

Wiebe, Robert H. *The Search for Order, 1877–1920*. New York: Hill and Wang, 1967.

Wiggers, Carl J. "Western Reserve University School of Medicine: Department of Physiology." *Methods and Problems of Medical Education*, 3rd ser. (1925): 47–61.

Wilcox, Marrion. "New York's Great Medical Center." *Architectural Record* 58, no. 2 (1925): 101–15.

"The Woman Physician—A Symbolic Study." *Woman's Medical Journal* 26, no. 8 (1916): 204.

Woods, Mary N. *From Craft to Profession: The Practice of Architecture in Nineteenth-Century America*. Berkeley: University of California Press, 1999.

Worthen, Dennis B. "Early Pharmacy Education at the University of Illinois." *Pharmacy in History* 48, no. 2 (2006): 55–68.

Worthington, Janet Farrar. "Osler Interns Remember." *Hopkins Medical News* 11, no. 3 (1988): 24–27.

Wright, Kenneth W. *Foundations Well and Truly Laid: A History Leading to the Formation of the State University of New York Health Science Center at Syracuse*. [Syracuse, NY?]: Alumni Association of the SUNY Health Science Center at Syracuse, 1994.

Yanni, Carla. *The Architecture of Madness: Insane Asylums in the United States*. Minneapolis: University of Minnesota Press, 2007.

Yanni, Carla. "The Coed's Predicament: The Martha Cook Building at the University of

Michigan." *Buildings and Landscapes: Journal of the Vernacular Architecture Forum* 24, no. 1 (2017): 26–45.

Yanni, Carla. "History and Sociology of Science: Interrogating the Spaces of Knowledge." *Journal of the Society of Architectural Historians* 64, no. 4 (2005): 423–25.

Yanni, Carla. "Housing Lunatics and Students: Nineteenth-Century Asylums and Dormitories." *Change over Time* 6, no. 2 (2016): 154–72.

Yanni, Carla. "The Linear Plan for Insane Asylums in the United States before 1866." *Journal of the Society of Architectural Historians* 62, no. 1 (2003): 24–49.

Yanni, Carla. *Living on Campus: An Architectural History of the American Dormitory.* Minneapolis: University of Minnesota Press, 2019.

Yanni, Carla. *Nature's Museums: Victorian Science and the Architecture of Display.* Baltimore: Johns Hopkins University Press, 1999.

Young, Blaine A. "The College of Medicine of the University of Nebraska." *Western Medical Review* 18, no. 11 (1913): 590–91.

Zinski, Ann, Kristina T. C. Panizzi Woodley Blackwell, F. Mike Belue, and William S. Brooks. "Is Lecture Dead? A Preliminary Study of Medical Students' Evaluation of Teaching Methods in the Preclinical Curriculum." *Journal of Medical Education* 8 (22 September 2017): 326–33.

Zug, James. *Squash: A History of the Game.* New York: Scribner, 2003.

Zunz, Olivier. *Philanthropy in America: A History.* Princeton: Princeton University Press, 2012.

FIGURE SOURCES
AND CREDITS

Introduction

I.1. Harvard Medical School.

I.2. Philadelphia Museum of Art: Gift of the Alumni Association to Jefferson Medical College in 1878 and purchased by the Pennsylvania Academy of the Fine Arts and the Philadelphia Museum of Art in 2007 with the generous support of more than 3,600 donors, 2007, 2007–1-1.

I.3. Item 1994.42.007. Courtesy of the Maryland Historical Society.

I.4. Courtesy of Medical Alumni Association of the University of Maryland, Inc.

I.5. Image 97.242, Series 00097, Record Group M-CL02, Harvard Medical Library in the Francis A. Countway Library of Medicine.

I.6. Image 96.078, Series 00096, Record Group M-CL02, Harvard Medical Library in the Francis A. Countway Library of Medicine.

Chapter 1

1.1. Image 96.172, Series 00096, Record Group M-CL02, Harvard Medical Library in the Francis A. Countway Library of Medicine.

1.2. [Marvin Willard?] Wiles, photographer. Photograph 12, Folder 2, Box 1, Historical Photographs 1800s Collection, Meharry Medical College Library and Archives.

1.3. Marie Kucera Holoubek, photographer. Courtesy of Martha Holoubek Fitzgerald.

1.4. Item 233748, Buildings Photograph Collection, The Alan Mason Chesney Medical Archives of The Johns Hopkins Medical Institutions.

1.5. Item 184857, Buildings Photograph Collection, The Alan Mason Chesney Medical Archives of The Johns Hopkins Medical Institutions.

1.6. Item 184854, Buildings Photograph Collection, The Alan Mason Chesney Medical Archives of The Johns Hopkins Medical Institutions.

1.7. Map image courtesy of The Johns Hopkins Hospital, © 2020.

1.8. Moritz Pistor, *Anstalten und Einrichtungen des öffentlichen Gesundheitswesens in Preussen: Festschrift zum X. internationalen medizinischen Kongress, Berlin 1890* (Berlin: Julius Springer, 1890), 325.

1.9. Drawing by Aya Abdallah, based on plan published in Helen Ingleby, "The Department of Pathology," *Bulletin of the Woman's Medical College of Pennsylvania* 83, no. 3 (1932): 12, Legacy Center, Drexel University College of Medicine.

1.10. Franklin P. Mall, "The Anatomical Course and Laboratory of the Johns Hopkins University," *Johns Hopkins Hospital Bulletin* 7, no. 62–63 (1896): following 96.

1.11. Franklin P. Mall, "The Anatomical Course and Laboratory of the Johns Hopkins University," *Johns Hopkins Hospital Bulletin* 7, no. 62–63 (1896): 88.

1.12. Item 113618, People at Work Photograph Collection, The Alan Mason Chesney Medical Archives of The Johns Hopkins Medical Institutions.

1.13. Franklin P. Mall, "The Anatomical Course and Laboratory of the Johns Hopkins University," *Johns Hopkins Hospital Bulletin* 7, no. 62–63 (1896): 89.

1.14. Franklin P. Mall, "The Anatomical Course and Laboratory of the Johns Hopkins University," *Johns Hopkins Hospital Bulletin* 7, no. 62–63 (1896): 92.

1.15. Franklin P. Mall, "The Anatomical Course and Laboratory of the Johns Hopkins University," *Johns Hopkins Hospital Bulletin* 7, no. 62–63 (1896): following 94.

1.16. Elmer Chickering, photographer. Image 97.488, Series 00097, Record Group M-CL02, Harvard Medical Library in the Francis A. Countway Library of Medicine.

1.17. "Harvard University Medical School, Original Medical School Buildings, Boston, MA, #0148, 1906" files. Courtesy of the Archives of Shepley Bulfinch Richardson and Abbott, Boston, Massachusetts.

1.18. Henry P. Bowditch, letter to the editor (with plan), *Boston Medical and Surgical Journal* 82 (21 April 1870): 306.

1.19. "A Description of the New Building Erected for the Medical School of Harvard University," *Boston Medical and Surgical Journal* 108, no. 15 (12 April 1883): 341.

1.20. Thomas S. Kirkbride, *On the Construction, Organization, and General Arrangements of Hospitals for the Insane*, 2nd ed. (Philadelphia: J. B. Lippincott, 1880), 155.

1.21. Bond Brothers, photographer. Photograph P-2885, Box 1979, Legacy Center, Drexel University College of Medicine.

1.22. Albert I. Cassell, "The New Medical Building," *Howard Alumnus* 5, no. 4 (1927): 79. Courtesy of Moorland-Spingarn Research Center, Howard University.

1.23. T. Wingate Todd, "Western Reserve University School of Medicine: Laboratory of Anatomy," *Methods and Problems of Medical Education*, 3rd ser. (1925): 92.

1.24. William F. Whitney, *The Warren Anatomical Museum of the Harvard Medical School and the Arrangement of Its Collection* (n.p., 1911), frontispiece.

1.25. VC170269, Becker Medical Library, Washington University School of Medicine.

1.26. Charles S. Minot, "A Further Study of the Unit System of Laboratory Construction," *Science*, n.s., 13, no. 324 (15 March 1901): 415.

1.27. Charles S. Minot, "A Further Study of the Unit System of Laboratory Construction," *Science*, n.s., 13, no. 324 (15 March 1901): 412.

1.28. Carl J. Wiggers, "Western Reserve University School of Medicine: Department of Physiology," *Methods and Problems of Medical Education*, 3rd ser. (1925): 52.

Chapter 2

2.1. Isaac U. Doust, photographer. McBride Street Campus Folder #3, Box 32, Subject Files, Syracuse University College of Medicine Collection. Courtesy of the Archives and Special Collections at the SUNY Upstate Health Sciences Library.

2.2. Plan reproduced in J. Howard Ferguson, "A Chronological Calendar of Events of the College of Medicine at Syracuse, 1872–1968, with Some Later Additions." Courtesy of the Archives and Special Collections at the SUNY Upstate Health Sciences Library.

2.3. Folder "B+G/Medicine, College of/Exterior—3rd building," Box 27836, RG 50, Syracuse University Photograph Collection, University Archives, Special Collections Research Center, Syracuse University Libraries.

2.4. *The Syracuse University College of Medicine, Exercises of Dedication, November 14–22, 1937* [Syracuse, 1937?], following 28. Item 2015.0263. Courtesy of the Archives and Special Collections at the SUNY Upstate Health Sciences Library.

2.5. Item 2015.0264. Courtesy of the Archives and Special Collections at the SUNY Upstate Health Sciences Library.

2.6. Unsigned sketch attached to G. Canby Robinson to James H. Kirkland, 11 May 1920, Folder 21, Box 100, RG 300, Vanderbilt University Special Collections and University Archives.

2.7. Drawing by Aya Abdallah, based on Vanderbilt Training Hospital, General Plan #4, revised 8 July 1920, Coolidge and Shattuck, architects, located in Folder "Blueprints: V.U. Hospital and Medical School," Box 1b, Dean Robinson's Files, History of Medicine Collections, Eskind Biomedical Library, Vanderbilt University.

2.8. Robert J. Terry, "Washington University School of Medicine: Departments of Anatomy, Neuroanatomy, and Histology," *Methods and Problems of Medical Education*, 5th ser. (1926): 2.

2.9. Sketch attached to Winford Smith to Charles Coolidge, 7 January 1921, Folder 12, Box 100, RG 300, Vanderbilt University Special Collections and University Archives.

2.10. Folder 2, G. Canby Robinson Biographical File, History of Medicine Collections, Eskind Biomedical Library, Vanderbilt University. Courtesy of George Canby Robinson II.

2.11. "Vanderbilt University, Medical School, Nurses Home and Power House, Nashville, TN, #028, 1926" files. Courtesy of the Archives of Shepley Bulfinch Richardson and Abbott, Boston, Massachusetts.

2.12. G. Canby Robinson, "Vanderbilt University School of Medicine: History and General Description," *Methods and Problems of Medical Education*, 13th ser. (1929): 4.

2.13. G. Canby Robinson, "Vanderbilt University School of Medicine: History and General Description," *Methods and Problems of Medical Education*, 13th ser. (1929): 5.

2.14. G. Canby Robinson, "Vanderbilt University School of Medicine: History and General Description," *Methods and Problems of Medical Education*, 13th ser. (1929): 3.

2.15. Box 2, William Smith Ely Collection. Courtesy of Edward G. Miner Library, University of Rochester Medical Center.

2.16. Item 90743, Buildings Photograph Collection, The Alan Mason Chesney Medical Archives of The Johns Hopkins Medical Institutions.

2.17. G. Canby Robinson, "Vanderbilt University School of Medicine: History and General Description," *Methods and Problems of Medical Education*, 13th ser. (1929): 9.

2.18. Folder 1, Series 5 Faculty-House Staff, Photographic Archive. Courtesy of History of Medicine Collections, Eskind Biomedical Library, Vanderbilt University.

2.19. *Bulletin of the Woman's Medical College of Pennsylvania* 65, no. 4 (1914): 4, Legacy Center, Drexel University College of Medicine.

2.20. Maurice B. Biscoe, "The University of Colorado School of Medicine and Hospital at Denver," *Modern Hospital* 20, no. 4 (1923): 320.

2.21. Joint Administrative Board, Columbia-Presbyterian Medical Center, *Medical Center, New York, N.Y., Units Cooperating . . .* (1928) in CUIMC Publications: CPMC Floor Plans, 1920s, Archives and Special Collections, Columbia University Health Sciences Library, New York, New York.

2.22. Fairchild Aerial Surveys Inc., photographer. Image C-000070, Archives and Special Collections, Columbia University Health Sciences Library, New York, New York.

2.23. *Bulletin of the Woman's Medical College of Pennsylvania* 83, no. 3 (1932): 2, Legacy Center, Drexel University College of Medicine.

Chapter 3

3.1. Aaron Levin, photographer. The Alan Mason Chesney Medical Archives of The Johns Hopkins Medical Institutions.

3.2. Davis and Sanford, photographers. Box P38, Subseries Prints, Series 1003 (FA447), John D. Rockefeller Family Photographs. Courtesy of Rockefeller Archive Center.

3.3. VC410, Becker Medical Library, Washington University School of Medicine.

3.4. Photograph P-2916, WMCP Photograph Collection, Legacy Center, Drexel University College of Medicine.

3.5. Drawing by Aya Abdallah, based on plan published in Herbert H. Bunzell, "Chemistry at the Woman's Medical College of Pennsylvania," *Bulletin of the Woman's Medical College of Pennsylvania* 81, no. 4 (1931): 6.

3.6. *Scalpel: 1911* ([1911?]), 119, Legacy Center, Drexel University College of Medicine.

3.7. Drawing by Aya Abdallah, based on plan located in Woman's Medical College of Pennsylvania Architectural Plans for Henry Avenue property and building, 1929, Collection ID nonacc-2021-carroll, Legacy Center, Drexel University College of Medicine.

3.8. Albert I. Cassell, "The New Medical Building," *Howard Alumnus* 5, no. 4 (1927): 76. Courtesy of Moorland-Spingarn Research Center, Howard University.

3.9. [Marvin Willard?] Wiles, photographer. "Meharry Medical School for Negroes, Nashville, Tenn." Card. Published by Southern Latex Company, Nashville, Tennessee. "Tichnor Quality Views," Reg. U.S. Pat. Off. Made Only by Tichnor Bros., Inc., Boston, Massachusetts, 1930. *Digital Commonwealth*, accessed 16 July 2020, https://ark.digitalcommonwealth.org/ark:/50959/bz60d183x. Holding institution Boston Public Library, Arts Department.

3.10. Albert I. Cassell, "The New Medical Building," *Howard Alumnus* 5, no. 4 (1927): 80. Courtesy of Moorland-Spingarn Research Center, Howard University.

3.11. Walter Eugene Garrey and Charles Edwin King, "Vanderbilt University School of Medicine: Department of Physiology," *Methods and Problems of Medical Education*, 13th ser. (1929): 40.

3.12. *Souvenir of the Dedication of Meharry's New Educational and Hospital Buildings . . .* (Nashville: Meharry Medical College, 1931). Exchange with the University of Rochester, Folder 7, Box 8, D.138, George Eastman Legacy Collection. Courtesy of the George Eastman Museum. Copyright Meharry Medical College Library and Archives.

3.13. *Souvenir of the Dedication of Meharry's New Educational and Hospital Buildings . . .* (Nashville: Meharry Medical College, 1931). Exchange with the University of Rochester, Folder 7, Box 8, D.138, George Eastman Legacy Collection. Courtesy of the George Eastman Museum. Copyright Meharry Medical College Library and Archives.

3.14. *Souvenir of the Dedication of Meharry's New Educational and Hospital Buildings . . .* (Nashville: Meharry Medical College, 1931). Exchange with the University of Rochester, Folder 7, Box 8, D.138, George Eastman Legacy Collection. Courtesy of the George Eastman Museum. Copyright Meharry Medical College Library and Archives.

3.15. *Souvenir of the Dedication of Meharry's New Educational and Hospital Buildings . . .* (Nashville: Meharry Medical College, 1931). Exchange with the University of Rochester, Folder 7, Box 8, D.138, George Eastman Legacy Collection. Courtesy of the George Eastman Museum. Copyright Meharry Medical College Library and Archives.

3.16. Waller S. Leathers, "Vanderbilt University School of Medicine: Department of Preventive Medicine and Public Health," *Methods and Problems of Medical Education*, 13th ser. (1929): 74.

3.17. Box 96, University Archives Photograph Collection, David M. Rubenstein Rare Book and Manuscript Library, Duke University.

3.18. Courtesy of the Archives of Shepley Bulfinch Richardson and Abbott, Boston, Massachusetts.

3.19. Aerial Explorations, Inc., photographer. Courtesy of the Archives of Shepley Bulfinch Richardson and Abbott, Boston, Massachusetts.

3.20. "Exhibit B," Folder 164, Box 20, RG 01/01/01, Board of Regents Papers, Archives and Special Collections, University of Nebraska–Lincoln Libraries.

3.21. "Perspective View of the Medical Department of the University of Nebraska, to be located at Dewey Avenue and Forty-Second Street," *Western Medical Review* 14, no. 8 (15 August 1909): following 440.

3.22. Courtesy of the Archives of Shepley Bulfinch Richardson and Abbott, Boston, Massachusetts.

3.23. Photograph located by Maureen Meister. Courtesy of Christopher Hussey.

3.24. Courtesy of the Archives of Shepley Bulfinch Richardson and Abbott, Boston, Massachusetts.

3.25. The Rockefeller University.

Chapter 4

4.1. Vanderbilt Map ca. 1923 Subject File. Courtesy of History of Medicine Collections, Eskind Biomedical Library, Vanderbilt University.

4.2. [Woman's Medical College of Pennsylvania?], *Natural Guardians of the Race* (Philadelphia: Woman's Medical College of Pennsylvania and Holmes Press, 1926), 23. Butler Scrapbook, ACC 123, Legacy Center, Drexel University College of Medicine.

4.3. McLean, photographer. Image 97.115, Series 00097, Record Group M-CL02, Harvard Medical Library in the Francis A. Countway Library of Medicine.

4.4. Elmer Chickering, photographer. Image 97.767, Series 00097, Record Group M-CL02, Harvard Medical Library in the Francis A. Countway Library of Medicine.

4.5. Attached to William G. Kaelber to Trevor Arnett, 23 May 1929, Folder 1259, Box 136, Subseries 1, Series 1, General Education Board Archives. Courtesy of Rockefeller Archive Center.

4.6. Anne Rayner, photographer. Courtesy of Vanderbilt University.

4.7. Samuel Kravitt, photographer. Samuel Kravitt Photographs and Other Materials (MS 1923). Manuscripts and Archives, Yale University Library.

4.8. *Caduceus* 1 (1929): n.p. Courtesy of the McGoogan Health Sciences Library, Special Collections and Archives, University of Nebraska Medical Center.

4.9. Elmer Chickering, photographer. *Boston Medical and Surgical Journal* 155, no. 13 (27 September 1906): n.p.

4.10. Folder "Buildings and Grounds–College of Medicine–Cornerstone–Third Building," Box 27836, RG 50, Syracuse University Photograph Collection, University Archives, Special Collections Research Center, Syracuse University Libraries.

4.11. Kingsley W. Given, photographer. Image 00033, Case Western Reserve University Archives.

4.12. Robert Gesell, "Department of Physiology: University of Michigan," *Methods and Problems of Medical Education*, 18th ser. (1930): 53.

4.13. Edward P. Beckwith, photographer. Accession number P-00049. Courtesy of the Medical Center Archives of New York–Presbyterian/Weill Cornell Medicine.

4.14. Samuel H. Gottscho, photographer. Folder "B+G/Medicine, College of/Interior–3rd building," Box 27836, RG 50, Syracuse University Photograph Collection, University Archives, Special Collections Research Center, Syracuse University Libraries.

4.15. Local Record Number: YSM_anatomy_lab_003, Medical Historical Library, Harvey Cushing/John Hay Whitney Medical Library, Yale University.

4.16. Horton R. Casparis, "Vanderbilt University School of Medicine: Department of Pediatrics," *Methods and Problems of Medical Education*, 13th ser. (1929): 93.

Chapter 5

5.1. White Studio, New York, photographer. Folder 1925–1926, Series 6 Students, Photographic Archive, History of Medicine Collections, Eskind Biomedical Library, Vanderbilt University.

5.2. Folder 1928–1929, Series 6 Students, Photographic Archive. Courtesy of History of Medicine Collections, Eskind Biomedical Library, Vanderbilt University.

5.3. Scurlock Studio Records, Archives Center, National Museum of American History, Smithsonian Institution.

5.4. Folder 2, Box 155, Historical Photograph Collection, University Archives, Rare Book and Manuscript Library, Columbia University Libraries.

5.5. Item Number p2572, Woman's Medical College of Pennsylvania Photograph Collection, Legacy Center, Drexel University College of Medicine.

5.6. J. Jefferson Gibson, photographer. Item Number BL002025, University of Michigan Bentley Historical Library.

5.7. Albert I. Cassell, "The New Medical Building," *Howard Alumnus* 5, no. 4 (1927): 78. Courtesy of Moorland-Spingarn Research Center, Howard University.

5.8. Arthur Haskell, photographer. Image 97.306, Series 00097, Record Group M-CL02, Harvard Medical Library in the Francis A. Countway Library of Medicine.

5.9. A. Tennyson Beals, photographer. Image P-001571. Courtesy of Archives and Special Collections, Columbia University Health Sciences Library, New York, New York.

5.10. *Aesculapiad* [yearbook] (1931), 56, Harvard Medical Library in the Francis A. Countway Library of Medicine.

5.11. Image 97.725, Series 00097, Record Group M-CL02, Harvard Medical Library in the Francis A. Countway Library of Medicine.

5.12. Arthur Haskell, photographer. Image 97.301, Series 00097, Record Group M-CL02, Harvard Medical Library in the Francis A. Countway Library of Medicine.

5.13. Arthur Haskell, photographer. Image 97.733, Series 00097, Record Group M-CL02, Harvard Medical Library in the Francis A. Countway Library of Medicine.

5.14. Sigurd Fischer, photographer. "Harvard University, Medical School, Vanderbilt Hall Dormitory, Boston, MA, #011, 1927" files. Courtesy of the Archives of Shepley Bulfinch Richardson and Abbott, Boston, Massachusetts.

5.15. Courtesy of Martha Holoubek Fitzgerald.

5.16. Courtesy of the College of Nursing, University of Nebraska Medical Center, Omaha, Nebraska.

5.17. Alfred E. Peyser Company, photographer. Image P-006437. Archives and Special Collections, Columbia University Health Sciences Library, New York, New York.

5.18. Image P-004921. Courtesy of Archives and Special Collections, Columbia University Health Sciences Library, New York, New York.

5.19. Image P-007621. Courtesy of Archives and Special Collections, Columbia University Health Sciences Library, New York, New York.

5.20. *Announcement of the Presbyterian Hospital School of Nursing, 1935–1936* (New York: [Presbyterian Hospital?], [1935?]), 30. Courtesy of Archives and Special Collections, Columbia University Health Sciences Library, New York, New York.

5.21. Photograph Collection, University of Nebraska Medical Center College of Nursing History Museum (location of photo currently unknown). Image scanned from Nancy W. Schneckloth, *The University of Nebraska College of Nursing, 1917–1987* (Omaha: University of Nebraska Medical Center, 1987), 114. Courtesy of the College of Nursing, University of Nebraska Medical Center, Omaha, Nebraska.

5.22. Photograph Collection, University of Nebraska Medical Center College of Nursing History Museum (location of photo currently unknown). Image scanned from Nancy W. Schneckloth, *The University of Nebraska College of Nursing, 1917–1987* (Omaha: University of Nebraska Medical Center, 1987), 114. Courtesy of the College of Nursing, University of Nebraska Medical Center, Omaha, Nebraska.

5.23. *Scalpel: 1911* ([1911?]), 42, Legacy Center, Drexel University College of Medicine.

5.24. John E. Hood Studios, photographer. Folder 3, Series 5 Faculty-House Staff, Photographic Archive. Courtesy of History of Medicine Collections, Eskind Biomedical Library, Vanderbilt University.

5.25. Sigurd Fischer, photographer. Folder 10, Box 154, Historical Photograph Collection, University Archives, Rare Book and Manuscript Library, Columbia University Libraries.

5.26. Image 115.003, Series 00115, Record Group M-CL02, Harvard Medical Library in the Francis A. Countway Library of Medicine.

5.27. Item Identifier #1563. Courtesy of Moorland-Spingarn Research Center, Howard University.

5.28. Image 00097.096, Series 00097b, Record Group M-CL02, Harvard Medical Library in the Francis A. Countway Library of Medicine.

5.29. Folder 2, Box 155, Historical Photograph Collection, University Archives, Rare Book and Manuscript Library, Columbia University Libraries.

5.30. Meharry Medical College, Nashville, Tennessee.

5.31. Meharry Medical College, Nashville, Tennessee.

5.32. *The Meharry: Meharry Medical College with Departments of Medicine, Dentistry, Pharmacy, and Nurse-Training, Also School for Dental Hygienists* [Meharry Medical College catalog] (July 1931), 66, Meharry Medical College Library and Archives.

Epilogue

E.1. Photograph by author.

E.2. Lucius Patenaude, photographer. Meharry Medical College.

E.3. H874, Harvard University Portrait Collection, Harvard Medical School. Image used with permission of the artist, Stephen E. Coit. All rights reserved.

E.4. Courtesy of Brigham and Women's Hospital.

E.5. Courtesy of the Dell Medical School at The University of Texas at Austin.

E.6. Photograph by author.

E.7. Photograph by author.

E.8. Photograph by author.

INDEX

Abbott, Andrew, 108, 109

Adams, Annmarie, 5, 6, 63, 221, 225, 256, 288; and student housing, 299, 308

Adams, Numa P. G., 320, 321, 322

admissions, 336; quotas, 263, 269; standards, 7, 13, 27, 78

Adolph, Edward F., 79, 115, 118

Afolabi, Titilayo, 326–27

African Americans, 158, 170–71, 183, 185, 186; and Black institutions, 165, 174–75, 214, 217, 248; at Harvard Medical School, 280–81, 324–25; as medical students, 185, 263, 272, 280, 324; neighborhood community of, 217, 251–52; and racial discrimination, 208–10, 251–52, 263–64, 280. *See also* Black colleges; Black graduates; Black physicians; Black students; *and individual names*

Agnew, D. Hayes, 9, 10

Albany Medical College, 114, 157, 183

Allison, Mary Bruins, 169, 271

alumni, 255, 258, 259, 276, 296, 298, 302; Columbia-Presbyterian Medical Center, 258; Harvard Medical School, 79, 272, 276; Meharry Medical College, 259–60, 322; New York Hospital–Cornell Medical College, 249; Presbyterian Hospital School of Nursing, 298, 301, 302, 304; University of Michigan, 266; University of Nebraska, 260; Woman's Medical College of Pennsylvania, 258, 262, 263, 319; Yale University School of Medicine, 325. *See also individual names*

American Medical Association (AMA), 82, 104, 226, 227, 235; Council on Medical Education, 80–82, 86, 120, 139, 161–63, 172; reports, 79–80, 106, 107, 111, 134, 206

amphitheaters, 9, 11, 12, 20–21, 26, 120, 124; Louis Bornstein Family Amphitheater, 326, 327; McCosh Memorial Amphitheater, 125; at Presbyterian Hospital School of Nursing, 296

anatomy, 7, 12, 20, 45, 46, 60, 133, 239–47; departments, 38, 41, 61, 65, 245; facilities, 20, 43, 255; at Dell, 333; at Harvard Medical School, 14, 25, 56, 57; at Johns Hopkins Medical School, 28, 35, 42; at Nebraska, 255–56, 163; at Syracuse University College of Medicine, 88; at the University of Michigan, 22; at Vanderbilt University, 92, 99, 296; at Washington University School of Medicine, 65. *See also* dissection; gross anatomy

animal experimentation, 3, 59, 93, 204, 234–39, 246–47

antivivisectionists, 234, 235, 237, 239

Archer, George, 29, 38, 39, 40, 44, 47, 191

architects, 190–91, 193, 197–98; Julian Abele, 186; Josh Coleman, 334; Frank Furness and George E. Hewitt, 120; Addison Hutton,